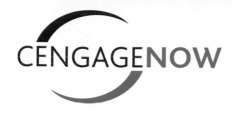

Just What You Need to Know and Do NOW!

CengageNOW is an online teaching and learning resource that provides you more control in less time and delivers better student outcomes—NOW!

What instructors are saying...

> The evidence I have from my students is that this (CengageNOW Personalized Study) is terrific value added.
>
> —**Kevin Smith**, University of Nebraska–Lincoln

> What I like most about CengageNOW is the simplicity of using it...
>
> —**Mina Yavari**, Hancock College

CENGAGENOW IS AN ONLINE TEACHING AND LEARNING RESOURCE.

CengageNOW offers all of your teaching and learning resources in one intuitive program organized around the essential activities you perform for class - lecturing, creating assignments, grading, quizzing, and tracking student progress and performance. CengageNOW's intuitive "tabbed" design allows you to navigate to all key functions with a single click and a unique homepage tell you just what needs to be done and when. CengageNOW, in most cases, provides students access to an integrated eBook, interactive tutorials, videos, animations, games, and other multimedia tools to help them get the most out of your course.

CENGAGENOW PROVIDES MORE CONTROL IN LESS TIME

CengageNOW's flexible assignment and grade book options provides you more control while saving you valuable time in planning and managing your course assignments. With CengageNOW, you can automatically grade all assignments, weigh grades, choose points or percentages and set the number of attempts and due dates per problem to best suit your overall course plan.

CENGAGENOW DELIVERS BETTER STUDENT OUTCOMES

CengageNOW Personalized Study; a diagnostic tool (featuring a chapter specific Pre-test, Study Plan, and Post-test) empowers students to master concepts, prepare for exams, and be more involved in class. It's easy to assign and if you want, results will automatically post to your grade book. Results to Personalize Study provide immediate and ongoing feedback regarding what students are mastering and why they're not - to both you and the student. In most cases, Personalized Study links to an integrated eBook so students can easily review topics.

academic.cengage.com/now

CengageNOW MAKES IT EASIER TO DO WHAT YOU ALREADY DO.

Designed by instructors for instructors, CengageNOW mirrors your natural workflow and provides time-saving, performance-enhancing tools for you and your students—all in one program!

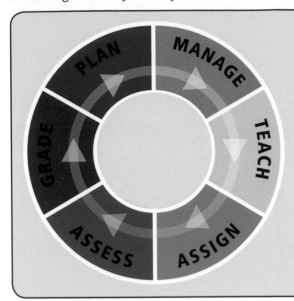

YOU CAN USE CENGAGENOW TO...

▶ **Plan** your curriculum;
▶ **Manage** your course and communicate with students;
▶ **Teach** with more freedom;
▶ **Assign** practice or homework to reinforce key concepts;
▶ **Assess** student performance outcomes;
▶ **Grade** with efficiency and control to get the results you want.

STUDENTS CAN USE CENGAGENOW TO...

▶ **Manage** their time;
▶ **Prepare** for class;
▶ **Practice & Reinforce** key concepts learned in class;
▶ **Study** for exams more effectively;
▶ **Get the Grade** they want.

The flexibility of CengageNOW allows you to use a single aspect of the program, or for maximum power and effectiveness, to use all of the teaching and learning resources to create and customize your own material to match your course objectives.

CENGAGENOW SEAMLESSLY INTEGRATES WITH POPULAR COURSE MANAGEMENT PROGRAMS

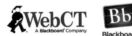

CengageNOW on Blackboard, WebCT, and eCollege provides students with seamless single sign-on access to CengageNOW through the school's course management system (CMS). After entering a simple access code just once at the beginning of the term, students get seamless access to both their CMS and CengageNOW textbook specific assignments and activities, with results flowing to your Blackboard, WebCT, or eCollege gradebook. Rich content, seamless integration with CengageNOW functionality, and only one gradebook to manage.

INTERESTED IN GIVING CENGAGENOW A TEST DRIVE IN YOUR CLASS?

Contact your Cengage Learning sales representative for more information about the **CengageNOW Class Test Program**.

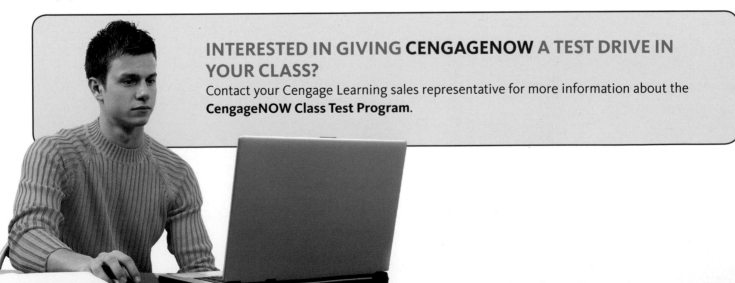

academic.cengage.com/now

Principles and Labs for Fitness and Wellness

FIRST CANADIAN EDITION

Werner W.K. Hoeger Boise State University

Sharon A. Hoeger Fitness & Wellness, Inc.

Marius Locke University of Toronto

Lara Lauzon University of Victoria

NELSON / EDUCATION

NELSON / EDUCATION

Principles and Labs for Fitness and Wellness, First Canadian Edition
by Werner W.K. Hoeger, Sharon A. Hoeger, Marius Locke, and Lara Lauzon

Associate Vice President, Editorial Director:
Evelyn Veitch

Editor-in-Chief, Higher Education:
Anne Williams

Executive Editor:
Paul Fam

Marketing Manager:
Sean Chamberland

Developmental Editor:
My Editor Inc.

Photo Researcher and Permissions Coordinator:
Terri Rothman

Content Production Manager:
Susan Wong

Production Service:
Pre-Press PMG

Copy Editor:
Wendy Thomas

Proofreader:
Janice Austin

Indexer:
Jessica McCurdy Crooks

Manufacturing Coordinator:
Ferial Suleman

Design Director:
Ken Phipps

Managing Designer:
Katherine Strain

Interior Design:
Norman Baugher

Cover Design:
Johanna Liburd

Cover Image:
Dennis O'Clair/Photographer's Choice/Getty Images

Compositor:
Pre-Press PMG

Printer:
RR Donnelley

Library and Archives Canada Cataloguing in Publication Data

Principles and labs for fitness and wellness / Werner W.K. Hoeger ... [et al.]. —1st Canadian ed.

ISBN-13 978-0-17-610404-7

1. Physical fitness—Textbooks.
2. Health—Textbooks.   I. Hoeger, Werner W.K.

RA781.P75 2009 613.7 C2008-905628-0

ISBN-13: 978-0-17-610404-7
ISBN-10: 0-17-610404-6

brief contents

contents

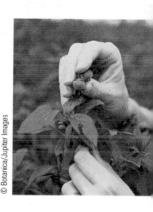
© Botanica/Jupiter Images

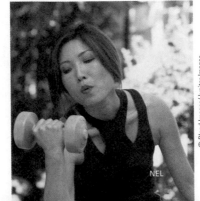

© Blend Images/Jupiter Images

© Digital Vision/Getty Images

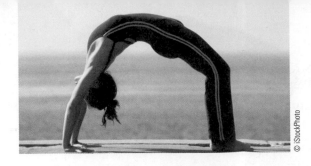
© iStockPhoto

preface

The current Canadian way of life does not provide the human body with sufficient physical activity to maintain adequate health and improve quality of life.

Many present lifestyle patterns are such a serious threat to our health that they actually increase the deterioration rate of the human body and often lead to premature morbidity and mortality.

People who lead an active and healthy lifestyle live longer and enjoy a better quality of life. Many Canadians, however, do not reap the benefit because they are either led astray by a multi-billion-dollar "quick fix," fad industry or simply do not know how to develop their own lifestyle program.

There is ample evidence that lack of physical activity is detrimental to good health. As a result, sound fitness programs have become even more important. Both Health Canada and the Canadian Society for Exercise Physiology (CSEP) have provided leadership on a national and international level with regard to developing recommended physical activity guidelines for adults, children and youths, and older adults. Current health literature suggests that regular physical activity can reduce the risk for a variety of chronic health conditions, premature mortality, and diseases. Health Canada has also identified physical fitness as one of the top health priorities, along with increased consumption of fruits and vegetables and smoking cessation. These fundamental health factors are thoroughly addressed in this textbook.

Principles and Labs for Fitness and Wellness, First Canadian Edition, serves as a guide to implement a complete lifetime fitness and wellness program. It points out the need to go beyond the basic components of fitness to achieve total well-being. In addition to a thorough discussion on physical fitness, including all health- and skill-related components, extensive and up-to-date information is provided on behaviour modification, nutrition, weight management, cardiovascular and cancer risk reduction as well as exercise and aging. Furthermore, the information will provide the necessary tools and guidelines for lifetime exercise and a wellness way of life.

As you work through the various chapters and laboratories, you will be able to develop and regularly update your own lifetime program to improve fitness components and personal wellness. The emphasis throughout the book is on teaching and how to take control of personal health and lifestyle habits so that you can make a constant and deliberate effort to stay healthy and achieve your highest potential for well-being.

A Quick Tour of Features

Turning active learning into active living, *Principles and Labs for Fitness and Wellness,* First Canadian Edition, guides students through the development of an attainable and enjoyable fitness and wellness program.

Behaviour modification continues to be an integrated theme throughout this text. The authors cover the topic early (Chapter 2) and then relate it to other topics throughout the book.

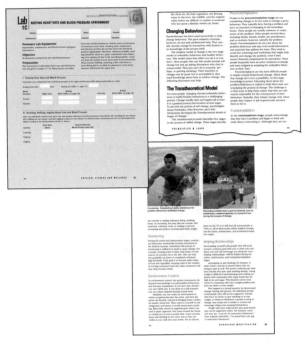

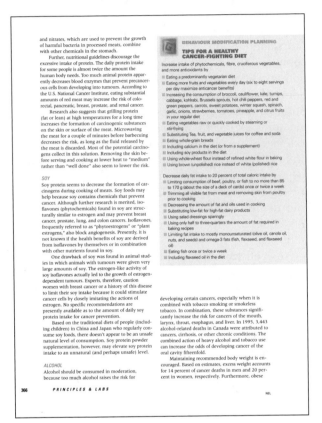

There are also "Behaviour Modification Planning" icons integrated in the text and in the labs, where appropriate. Students are taught how behaviour modification affects everything from nutrition to addictive behaviours. Covering behaviour modification early also enables students to understand the process of change as they eliminate unhealthy habits and adopt new healthy behaviours.

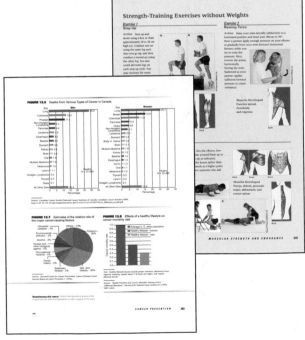

With over 150 pieces of art that make this text truly engaging, the book gives students the motivation and techniques they need to apply their learning experiences and knowledge received from their fitness and wellness course.

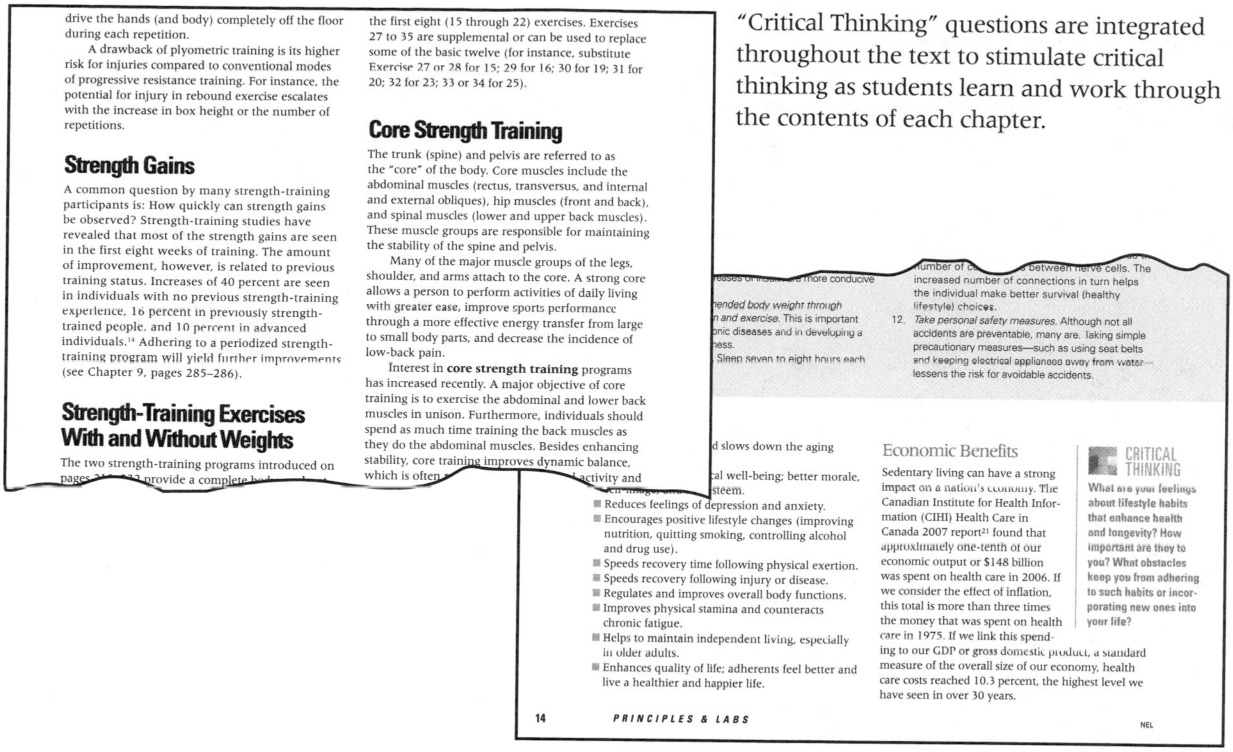

drive the hands (and body) completely off the floor during each repetition.

A drawback of plyometric training is its higher risk for injuries compared to conventional modes of progressive resistance training. For instance, the potential for injury in rebound exercise escalates with the increase in box height or the number of repetitions.

Strength Gains

A common question by many strength-training participants is: How quickly can strength gains be observed? Strength-training studies have revealed that most of the strength gains are seen in the first eight weeks of training. The amount of improvement, however, is related to previous training status. Increases of 40 percent are seen in individuals with no previous strength-training experience, 16 percent in previously strength-trained people, and 10 percent in advanced individuals.[14] Adhering to a periodized strength-training program will yield further improvements (see Chapter 9, pages 285–286).

Strength-Training Exercises With and Without Weights

The two strength-training programs introduced on pages ... provide a complete ...

the first eight (15 through 22) exercises. Exercises 27 to 35 are supplemental or can be used to replace some of the basic twelve (for instance, substitute Exercise 27 or 28 for 15; 29 for 16; 30 for 19; 31 for 20; 32 for 23; 33 or 34 for 25).

Core Strength Training

The trunk (spine) and pelvis are referred to as the "core" of the body. Core muscles include the abdominal muscles (rectus, transversus, and internal and external obliques), hip muscles (front and back), and spinal muscles (lower and upper back muscles). These muscle groups are responsible for maintaining the stability of the spine and pelvis.

Many of the major muscle groups of the legs, shoulder, and arms attach to the core. A strong core allows a person to perform activities of daily living with greater ease, improve sports performance through a more effective energy transfer from large to small body parts, and decrease the incidence of low-back pain.

Interest in **core strength training** programs has increased recently. A major objective of core training is to exercise the abdominal and lower back muscles in unison. Furthermore, individuals should spend as much time training the back muscles as they do the abdominal muscles. Besides enhancing stability, core training improves dynamic balance, which is often ... activity and

...number of c... between nerve cells. The increased number of connections in turn helps the individual make better survival (healthy lifestyle) choices.

12. *Take personal safety measures.* Although not all accidents are preventable, many are. Taking simple precautionary measures—such as using seat belts and keeping electrical appliances away from water—lessens the risk for avoidable accidents.

...d slows down the aging

...al well-being; better morale, ...steem.

- Reduces feelings of depression and anxiety.
- Encourages positive lifestyle changes (improving nutrition, quitting smoking, controlling alcohol and drug use).
- Speeds recovery time following physical exertion.
- Speeds recovery following injury or disease.
- Regulates and improves overall body functions.
- Improves physical stamina and counteracts chronic fatigue.
- Helps to maintain independent living, especially in older adults.
- Enhances quality of life; adherents feel better and live a healthier and happier life.

Economic Benefits

Sedentary living can have a strong impact on a nation's economy. The Canadian Institute for Health Information (CIHI) Health Care in Canada 2007 report[21] found that approximately one-tenth of our economic output or $148 billion was spent on health care in 2006. If we consider the effect of inflation, this total is more than three times the money that was spent on health care in 1975. If we link this spending to our GDP or gross domestic product, a standard measure of the overall size of our economy, health care costs reached 10.3 percent, the highest level we have seen in over 30 years.

CRITICAL THINKING

What are your feelings about lifestyle habits that enhance health and longevity? How important are they to you? What obstacles keep you from adhering to such habits or incorporating new ones into your life?

14 PRINCIPLES & LABS NEL

"Critical Thinking" questions are integrated throughout the text to stimulate critical thinking as students learn and work through the contents of each chapter.

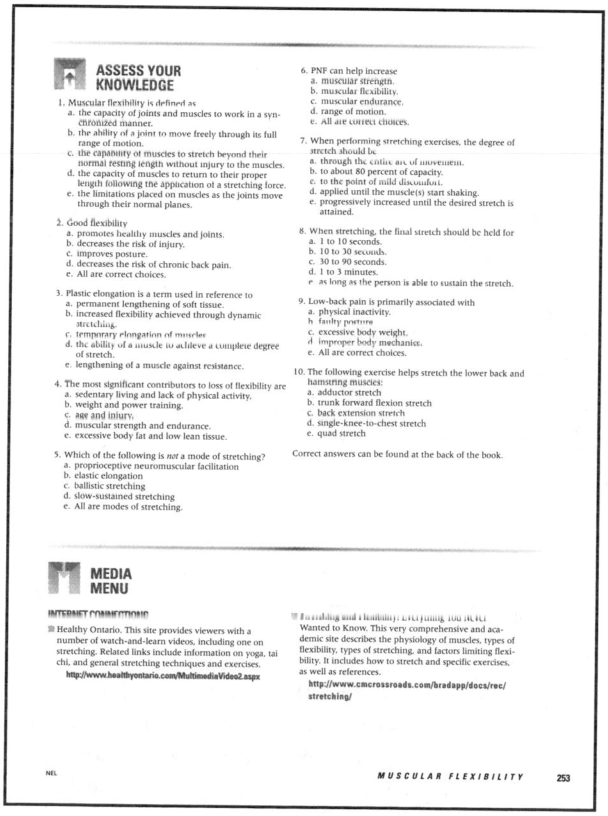

ASSESS YOUR KNOWLEDGE

1. Muscular flexibility is defined as
   a. the capacity of joints and muscles to work in a synchronized manner.
   b. the ability of a joint to move freely through its full range of motion.
   c. the capability of muscles to stretch beyond their normal resting length without injury to the muscles.
   d. the capacity of muscles to return to their proper length following the application of a stretching force.
   e. the limitations placed on muscles as the joints move through their normal planes.
2. Good flexibility
   a. promotes healthy muscles and joints.
   b. decreases the risk of injury.
   c. improves posture.
   d. decreases the risk of chronic back pain.
   e. All are correct choices.
3. Plastic elongation is a term used in reference to
   a. permanent lengthening of soft tissue.
   b. increased flexibility achieved through dynamic stretching.
   c. temporary elongation of muscles.
   d. the ability of a muscle to achieve a complete degree of stretch.
   e. lengthening of a muscle against resistance.
4. The most significant contributors to loss of flexibility are
   a. sedentary living and lack of physical activity.
   b. weight and power training.
   c. age and injury.
   d. muscular strength and endurance.
   e. excessive body fat and low lean tissue.
5. Which of the following is *not* a mode of stretching?
   a. proprioceptive neuromuscular facilitation
   b. elastic elongation
   c. ballistic stretching
   d. slow-sustained stretching
   e. All are modes of stretching.
6. PNF can help increase
   a. muscular strength.
   b. muscular flexibility.
   c. muscular endurance.
   d. range of motion.
   e. All are correct choices.
7. When performing stretching exercises, the degree of stretch should be
   a. through the entire arc of movement.
   b. to about 80 percent of capacity.
   c. to the point of mild discomfort.
   d. applied until the muscle(s) start shaking.
   e. progressively increased until the desired stretch is attained.
8. When stretching, the final stretch should be held for
   a. 1 to 10 seconds.
   b. 10 to 30 seconds.
   c. 30 to 90 seconds.
   d. 1 to 3 minutes.
   e. as long as the person is able to sustain the stretch.
9. Low-back pain is primarily associated with
   a. physical inactivity.
   b. faulty posture.
   c. excessive body weight.
   d. improper body mechanics.
   e. All are correct choices.
10. The following exercise helps stretch the lower back and hamstring muscles:
    a. adductor stretch
    b. trunk forward flexion stretch
    c. back extension stretch
    d. single-knee-to-chest stretch
    e. quad stretch

Correct answers can be found at the back of the book.

MEDIA MENU

INTERNET CONNECTIONS

- Healthy Ontario. This site provides viewers with a number of watch-and-learn videos, including one on stretching. Related links include information on yoga, tai chi, and general stretching techniques and exercises.
  http://www.healthyontario.com/MultimediaVideo2.aspx
- Stretching and Flexibility: Everything You Never Wanted to Know. This very comprehensive and academic site describes the physiology of muscles, types of flexibility, types of stretching, and factors limiting flexibility. It includes how to stretch and specific exercises, as well as references.
  http://www.cmcrossroads.com/bradapp/docs/rec/stretching/

NEL MUSCULAR FLEXIBILITY 253

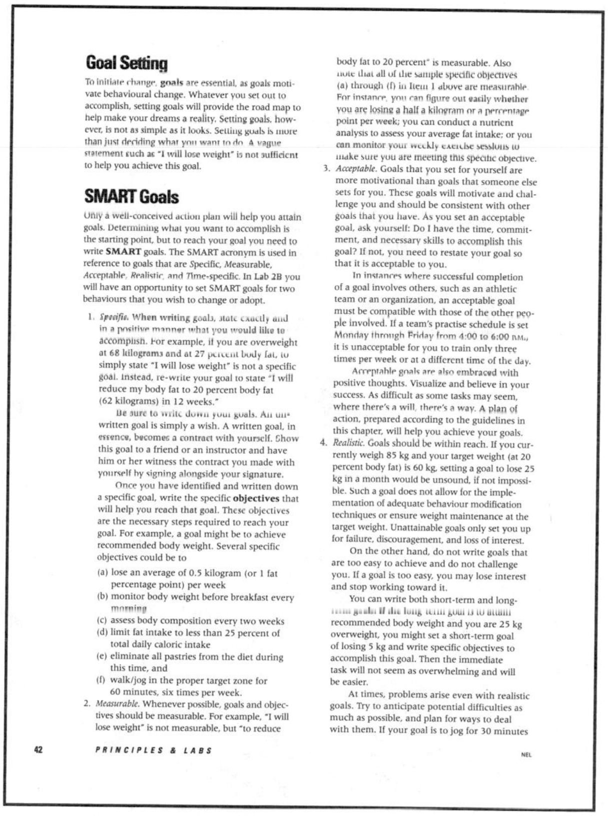

Goal Setting

To initiate change, **goals** are essential, as goals motivate behavioural change. Whatever you set out to accomplish, setting goals will provide the road map to help make your dreams a reality. Setting goals, however, is not as simple as it looks. Setting goals is more than just deciding what you want to do. A vague statement such as "I will lose weight" is not sufficient to help you achieve this goal.

SMART Goals

Only a well-conceived action plan will help you attain goals. Determining what you want to accomplish is the starting point, but to reach your goal you need to write **SMART** goals. The SMART acronym is used in reference to goals that are *S*pecific, *M*easurable, *A*cceptable, *R*ealistic, and *T*ime-specific. In Lab 2B you will have an opportunity to set SMART goals for two behaviours that you wish to change or adopt.

1. *Specific.* When writing goals, state exactly and in a positive manner what you would like to accomplish. For example, if you are overweight at 68 kilograms and at 27 percent body fat, to simply state "I will lose weight" is not a specific goal. Instead, re-write your goal to state "I will reduce my body fat to 20 percent body fat (62 kilograms) in 12 weeks."

   Be sure to write down your goals. An unwritten goal is simply a wish. A written goal, in essence, becomes a contract with yourself. Show this goal to a friend or an instructor and have him or her witness the contract you made with yourself by signing alongside your signature.

   Once you have identified and written down a specific goal, write the specific **objectives** that will help you reach that goal. These objectives are the necessary steps required to reach your goal. For example, a goal might be to achieve recommended body weight. Several specific objectives could be to

   (a) lose an average of 0.5 kilogram (or 1 fat percentage point) per week
   (b) monitor body weight before breakfast every morning
   (c) assess body composition every two weeks
   (d) limit fat intake to less than 25 percent of total daily caloric intake
   (e) eliminate all pastries from the diet during this time, and
   (f) walk/jog in the proper target zone for 60 minutes, six times per week.
2. *Measurable.* Whenever possible, goals and objectives should be measurable. For example, "I will lose weight" is not measurable, but "to reduce body fat to 20 percent" is measurable. Also note that all of the sample specific objectives (a) through (f) in Item 1 above are measurable. For instance, you can figure out easily whether you are losing a half a kilogram or a percentage point per week; you can conduct a nutrient analysis to assess your average fat intake; or you can monitor your weekly exercise sessions to make sure you are meeting this specific objective.
3. *Acceptable.* Goals that you set for yourself are more motivational than goals that someone else sets for you. These goals will motivate and challenge you and should be consistent with other goals that you have. As you set an acceptable goal, ask yourself: Do I have the time, commitment, and necessary skills to accomplish this goal? If not, you need to restate your goal so that it is acceptable to you.

   In instances where successful completion of a goal involves others, such as an athletic team or an organization, an acceptable goal must be compatible with those of the other people involved. If a team's practise schedule is set Monday through Friday from 4:00 to 6:00 P.M., it is unacceptable for you to train only three times per week or at a different time of the day.

   Acceptable goals are also embraced with positive thoughts. Visualize and believe in your success. As difficult as some tasks may seem, where there's a will, there's a way. A plan of action, prepared according to the guidelines in this chapter, will help you achieve your goals.
4. *Realistic.* Goals should be within reach. If you currently weigh 85 kg and your target weight (at 20 percent body fat) is 60 kg, setting a goal to lose 25 kg in a month would be unsound, if not impossible. Such a goal does not allow for the implementation of adequate behaviour modification techniques or ensure weight maintenance at the target weight. Unattainable goals only set you up for failure, discouragement, and loss of interest.

   On the other hand, do not write goals that are too easy to achieve and do not challenge you. If a goal is too easy, you may lose interest and stop working toward it.

   You can write both short-term and long-term goals. If the long-term goal is to attain recommended body weight and you are 25 kg overweight, you might set a short-term goal of losing 5 kg and write specific objectives to accomplish this goal. Then the immediate task will not seem as overwhelming and will be easier.

   At times, problems arise even with realistic goals. Try to anticipate potential difficulties as much as possible, and plan for ways to deal with them. If your goal is to jog for 30 minutes

42 PRINCIPLES & LABS NEL

"Assess Your Knowledge" reviews questions at the end of each chapter and includes 10 multiple-choice questions, which focuses students on the core concepts discussed in the chapter while allowing them to evaluate what they have learned. Answers can be found at the end of the text. The same questions are also included within the CengageNOW site.

Updated end-of-chapter "Internet Connections" boxes provide a list of current websites that contain interactive activities and assessments for extended learning opportunities.

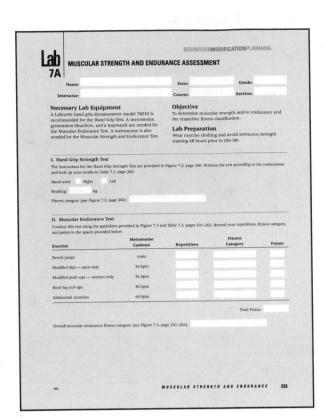

Perforated laboratory worksheets found at the end of each chapter allow readers to analyze and understand the concepts that they have learned and move to the next state of behavioural modification.

In the final lab, "Life Expectancy and Physiological Age Prediction Questionnaire," the authors summarize the fitness and wellness concepts presented throughout the book and give students an opportunity to reassess themselves and estimate their "real" physiological age based on current lifestyle habits.

The emphasis in the First Canadian Edition is on teaching individuals how to take control of their personal health and lifestyle habits so they can make a constant and deliberate effort to stay healthy and realize their highest potentials for well-being.

New in the Canadian Edition

The First Canadian Edition of *Principles and Labs for Fitness and Wellness* has been revised and updated to include new information reported in literature and professional health, physical education, and sports medicine meetings. The most significant changes in this new edition are as follows:

■ Chapter 1 provides a general overview on various aspects of health, fitness, and wellness as they relate to the Canadian population. Wherever possible, the latest data on the Canadian population for topics such as deaths from the major diseases have been provided. As you will see, physical inactivity plays a major role.

■ Chapter 2 discusses the issues relating to the behavioural choices that may lead one to participate or not to participate in physical activity. Topics such as barriers to physical activity and the transtheoretical model are discussed in relation to Canadian examples.

■ In 2007, a new Canada Food Guide was released. This guide is included in Chapter 3. Current information regarding how nutrition can influence the health and wellness of Canadians is also included, complete with examples of the nutritional content of numerous fast-food outlets.

■ Body composition is always of interest to athletes and fitness buffs. Chapter 4 explains the methods of evaluating body composition with metric tables and measurements.

■ In Chapter 5, Weight Management, trends of the obesity epidemic are explained and graphically illustrated. Canadian data on eating disorders and methods of achieving a normal body weight are discussed.

■ In Chapter 6, methods of evaluating cardiorespiratory endurance are provided and discussed. The caloric costs of various seasonal physical activities are also provided.

■ Skeletal muscle is a vital component to one's health and fitness. In Chapter 7, information about muscular strength and endurance is provided as are various exercise routines and methods of influencing the size and composition of skeletal muscle. A variety of tests are included to allow the reader to evaluate his or her own muscular strength and endurance.

■ No text on fitness would be complete without a chapter on muscular flexibility. In Chapter 8, the various factors that influence flexibility as well as its importance are discussed. Many stretches are illustrated and several easy-to-conduct tests are supplied to help the reader evaluate his or her own flexibility.

■ Chapter 9, Skill Fitness and Fitness Programming, brings many aspects of the book together to help the reader understand the importance of fitness as it relates to certain sports. It also provides the reader with information on how to best set up and optimize a complete individual fitness program.

■ Stress management is becoming increasingly important, and Chapter 10 provides information on how various aspects of stress may influence health. A variety of methods to evaluate one's level of stress are provided.

■ Chapter 11 deals with preventing cardiovascular disease (CVD) and clearly outlines the need for Canadians to pay close attention to the numerous health risks associated with this disease. While Canadians have made progress in this area, there is still much to be learned about the benefits of regular physical activity and the prevention of CVD.

■ Research suggests that cancer may soon become the major killer of Canadians and thus understanding the most recent trends and how to provide protection against certain forms of cancer is a national concern. Chapter 12 provides the latest data on our struggle to control this disease.

■ In the final chapter (13), Lifetime Fitness and Wellness, various aspects of the textbook are brought together to allow one to create a picture of how to live a high quality of life. The role of age in various fitness and wellness components is discussed, and methods of prediction of one's long-term health is shared.

Ancillaries

■ **CENGAGENOW.** This dynamic CengageNOW online learning tool is assessment-driven and student-centred to provide students with a personalized learning plan. Results from a diagnostic pretest generate a customized learning path for each individual student. Instant Access Card ISBN 0-17-647457-9.

■ **INSTRUCTOR'S RESOURCE CD.** Managing classroom resources is now easier for instructors. The Canadian Edition Instructor's Resource CD contains all key instructor supplements:

■ **INSTRUCTOR'S MANUAL.** The Instructor's Manual helps instructors plan and coordinate their lectures by offering detailed outlines of each chapter with specific PowerPoint references. A lab list accompanies Instructor's Activities for each chapter. These activities offer instructors ideas for incorporating the material into classroom activities and discussions.

■ **COMPUTERIZED TEST BANK.** Create and deliver custom tests and study guides (both print and online) in minutes with this easy-to-use assessment and tutorial system. ExamView offers the Quick Test Wizard, which guides instructors through the process of creating tests while allowing them to see the test they are creating on the screen exactly as it will print or display online.

■ **TEST BANK.** A full test bank is extracted from the computerized test bank program in Microsoft Word format for instructors to have easy access to the database of questions.

■ **POWERPOINT LECTURE SLIDES.** This lecture presentation tool features more than 100 PowerPoint slides for classroom teaching and reviewing of individual chapters. Order the Instructor's Resource CD from your local sales representative. ISBN 0-17-610517-4.

■ **FITNESS AND WELLNESS WEBSITE** (www.fitness.nelson.com). When instructors adopt *Principles and Labs for Fitness and Wellness*, First Canadian Edition, their students have access to an array of learning resources not found elsewhere. Resources include self-quizzes, web links, suggested online readings, and more!

■ **INFOTRAC® COLLEGE EDITION.** This extensive online library gives instructors and students access to the latest news and research articles online—updated daily and spanning 20 years. Conveniently accessible from a personal computer or the library, InfoTrac College Edition opens the door to the full extent of articles from hundreds of scholarly and popular journals and publications.

other outstanding supplements

■ **WADSWORTH VIDEO LIBRARY FOR FITNESS, WELLNESS, AND PERSONAL HEALTH.** This comprehensive library of U.S. videos includes such topics as weight control and fitness, AIDS, sexual communication, and peer pressure. Available to qualified adopters. Please consult your local sales representative for details.

■ **TRIGGER VIDEO SERIES.** Exclusive to Cengage and Nelson Education Ltd., these U.S. videos are designed to promote classroom discussion on a variety of important topics related to physical fitness and stress. Each 60-minute video contains five 8-to-10-minute clips, followed by questions for discussion and material appropriate to the chapters in the text. Available to qualified adopters. Please consult your local sales representative for details.

■ **PERSONAL DAILY LOG.** The Personal Daily Log contains study and exercise tips, a goal-setting worksheet, a cardio-respiratory exercise record form, a strength training record form, a daily nutrient diary, and helpful U.S. Internet links. ISBN 0-534-58966-4.

■ **BEHAVIOR CHANGE WORKBOOK.** This book includes a brief discussion of the current theories behind making positive lifestyle changes, along with exercises to help students affect those changes in their daily lives. ISBN 0-495-01145-2.

■ **WELLNESS WORKSHEETS.** These detachable self-assessment and wellness worksheets are handy, are easy to use, and make a terrific bundle item. ISBN 0-534-57788-1.

■ **HEALTH AND WELLNESS RESOURCE CENTRE** (www.gale.cengage.com/health). Gale's Health and Wellness Resource Centre is a new, comprehensive website that provides easy-to-find answers to health questions.

■ **WALK4LIFE ELITE MODEL PEDOMETER.** This pedometer tracks steps, elapsed time, distance, and calories burned. Whether used as a class activity or simply to encourage students to track their steps and walk toward better fitness, this is a valuable item for everyone. ISBN 0-495-0315-3.

Acknowledgments

Many individuals unselfishly contributed to the creation of the original text and the revision of the First Canadian Edition of *Principles and Labs for Fitness and Wellness*. In particular we wish to express our most sincere gratitude to

■ teachers, students, researchers, coaches, and friends who have shared their expertise, time, talents, and energy with us.

■ colleagues throughout Canada and the United States who evaluated this and previous editions of *Principles and Labs for Fitness and Wellness*. The feedback and input of the following instructors especially enhanced the preparation of this First Canadian Edition:

Adele Thompson, *College of the Rockies*
Ralph Hofmann, *Durham College*
Tracy Gedies, *Fanshawe College*
Leigh Goldie, *Grande Prairie Regional College*
Bertil Johansson, *Lethbridge Community College*
Enrique Garcia Bengoechea, *McGill University*
Heather Ray, *Mount Royal College*
Peggy Gallant, *St. Francis Xavier University*
Anna Morrison, *Sault College*
Deanna Schick, *Trinity Western University*
Gordon Bell, *University of Alberta*

To the staff at Nelson Education Ltd., we are grateful for your diligence, kindness, and enthusiasm for this project. Special thanks to Cara Yarzab and Kevin Smulan, Executive Editors, who brought us together for this project; to Paul Fam, Executive Editor, for overseeing the project to completion; and to developmental editors Katherine Goodes and Jennifer Oliver at My Editor Inc. for their patience and guidance in assessing the needs of the Canadian market. Our gratitude to photo researcher and permissions editor, Terri Rothman. Finally, we thank content production manager, Susan Wong; copyeditor, Wendy Thomas; and Pre-Press PMG for their hard work in polishing this text. We feel privileged to have worked with each of you.

Marius Locke
Lara Lauzon
Toronto and Vancouver
August 2008

brief author biographies

ERNER W.K. HOEGER is the most successful Fitness and Wellness college textbook author. Dr. Hoeger is a Full Professor and Director of the Human Performance Laboratory at Boise State University. He completed his undergraduate and Master's degrees in physical education at the age of 20 and at the age of 24 received his doctorate degree with an emphasis in exercise physiology. Dr. Werner Hoeger is a fellow of the American College of Sports Medicine. In 2002, he was recognized as the Honored Alumnus from the College of Health and Human Performance at Brigham Young University. He is also the recipient of the first (2004) Presidential Award for Research and Scholarship in the College of Education at Boise State University.

Dr. Hoeger uses his knowledge and personal experiences to write engaging, informative books that thoroughly address today's fitness and wellness issues in a format accessible to students. He has written several textbooks for Thomson/Wadsworth, including *Lifetime Physical Fitness and Wellness*, eighth edition; *Fitness and Wellness*, sixth edition, *Principles and Labs for Physical Fitness*, fifth edition; *Wellness: Guidelines for a Healthy Lifestyle*, fourth edition; and *Water Aerobics for Fitness and Wellness*, third edition (with Terry-Ann Spitzer Gibson).

He was the first author to write a college fitness textbook that incorporated the "wellness" concept. In 1986, with the release of the first edition of *Lifetime Physical Fitness and Wellness*, he introduced the principle that to truly improve fitness, health, and quality of life and achieve wellness, a person needed to go beyond the basic health-related components of physical fitness. His work was so well received that almost every fitness author immediately followed his lead in the field.

As an innovator in the field, Dr. Hoeger has developed many fitness and wellness assessment tools, including fitness tests such as the modified sit-and-reach, total body rotation, shoulder rotation, muscular endurance, and muscular strength and endurance, and "soda pop" coordination tests. Proving that he "practises what he preaches," at 48, he was the oldest male competitor in the 2002 Winter Olympics in Salt Lake City, Utah. He raced in the sport of luge along with his 17-year-old son, Christopher. This was the first time in Winter Olympics history that father and son competed in the same event.

SHARON A. HOEGER Sharon A. Hoeger is vice-president of Fitness & Wellness, Inc. of Boise, Idaho. Sharon received her degree in computer science from Brigham Young University. She is the author of the software that accompanies all of the Hoegers' fitness and wellness textbooks. Her innovations in this area since the publication of the first edition of *Lifetime Physical Fitness & Wellness* set the standard for fitness and wellness computer software used in this market today.

Sharon is a coauthor in five of the seven fitness and wellness titles. Husband and wife have been jogging and strength training together for over 28 years. They are the proud parents of five children, all of whom are involved in sports and lifetime fitness activities. Their motto: "Families that exercise together, stay together."

MARIUS LOCKE Marius Locke is an Associate Professor in the Faculty of Physical Education and Health at the University of Toronto. He completed undergraduate degrees in both physical education and biology at the University of Western Ontario. During this time he was a varsity football player. After obtaining his Ph.D. in Kinesiology (UWO), he spent three years as a post-doctoral fellow at the Deborah Research Institute in Browns Mills, New Jersey, where he studied cellular responses of the heart during exercise. Since arriving at the University of Toronto in 1996, he has continued to study the cellular stress responses of striated muscle. In 1999 he received a New Investigator Award from the American College of Sports Medicine. He currently teaches first-year physical education students about the biophysical aspects of physical activity and health, and fourth-year students about the cellular and physiological responses to exercise. In addition to his teaching and research, he has coached numerous sports, including baseball, soccer, hockey, and football at various levels. He currently lives in Toronto with his wife and four children.

LARA LAUZON Lara Lauzon is an Assistant Professor in the Faculty of Exercise Science, Physical and Health Education at the University of Victoria. Her teaching and research focus is human wellness and potential and active health. She has worked for non-profit, municipal, provincial, and private health and fitness agencies. Professor Lauzon co-produced and hosted a long-running internationally syndicated health and fitness show called *Body Moves*. She has won many awards, including a Faculty of Education Teaching Excellence Award, a Graduate Student Award for Teaching Excellence, the Victoria "Y" Women of Distinction Award for the fitness and health category, the B.C. Promotion Plus Leadership Award for promotion of girls and women in fitness and sport, a B.C. Paraplegic Association Award for the production of two fitness videos for persons with disabilities, and a Community Wellness Award. She has written numerous fitness and health columns for newspapers and magazines and has published a number of fitness and health journal articles. Lara has co-authored a textbook titled *An Invitation to Health*, First Canadian Edition, along with Diane Hales, and is also a popular keynote speaker and workshop presenter.

Chapter 1

Physical Fitness and Wellness

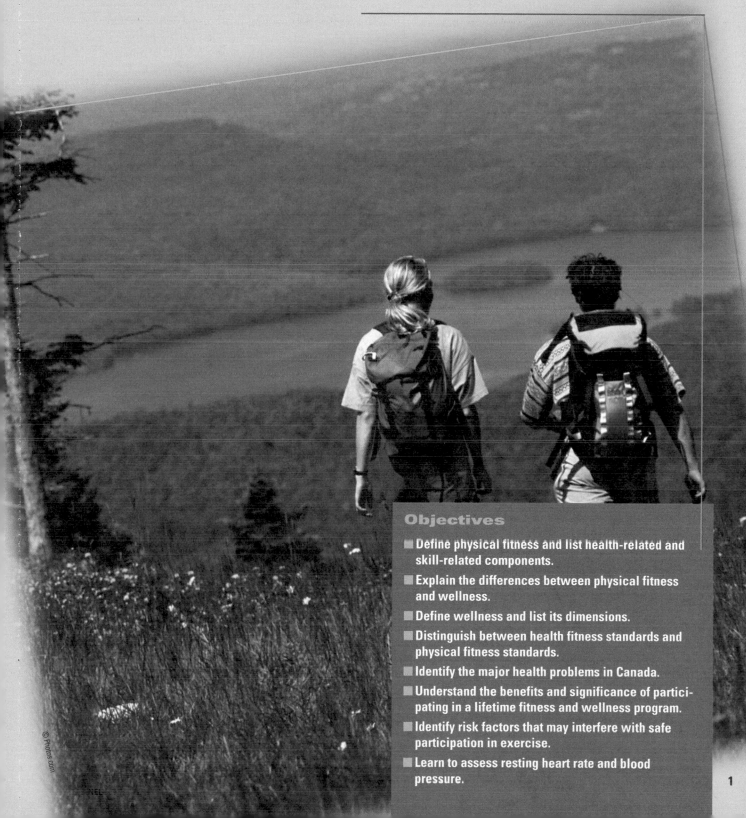

Objectives

- Define physical fitness and list health-related and skill-related components.
- Explain the differences between physical fitness and wellness.
- Define wellness and list its dimensions.
- Distinguish between health fitness standards and physical fitness standards.
- Identify the major health problems in Canada.
- Understand the benefits and significance of participating in a lifetime fitness and wellness program.
- Identify risk factors that may interfere with safe participation in exercise.
- Learn to assess resting heart rate and blood pressure.

Widespread interest in **health** and preventive medicine over the last three decades has led to an increase in the number of people participating in organized fitness and wellness programs. From an initial fitness fad in the early 1970s, physical activity and wellness programs became a trend that now is very much a part of the North American way of life. The growing number of participants is attributed primarily to scientific evidence linking regular physical activity and positive lifestyle habits to better health, longevity, quality of life, and total well-being. In Canada, we have seen the percentage of population that can be considered at least moderately active increase significantly between 1994–95 and 2004–05. See Figure 1.1.

Research findings in the last few years have shown that physical inactivity and a negative lifestyle seriously threaten health and hasten the deterioration rate of the human body. Physically active people live longer than their inactive counterparts, even if activity begins later in life.

However, despite the evidence suggesting health benefits can be derived from physical activity,

research from the 2004/2005 Canadian Community Health Survey shows that only 49 percent of Canadians aged 20 and older are at least moderately active during their leisure time. Of that 49 percent, only 24 percent are classified as active.[1]

The human organism needs movement and activity to grow, develop, and maintain health. Advances in modern technology, however, have almost completely eliminated the necessity for physical exertion in daily life. Physical activity is no longer a natural part of our existence. We live in an automated society, where most of the activities that used to require strenuous exertion can be accomplished by machines with the simple pull of a handle or push of a button. This epidemic of physical inactivity is a great threat to Canadian public health and has been termed **Sedentary Death Syndrome**, or **SeDS**.[2]

At the beginning of the 20th century, **life expectancy** for a child born in Canada was about 50 years. The most common health problems in the Western world were infectious diseases, such as tuberculosis, diphtheria, influenza, kidney disease, polio, and other illnesses of infancy. Progress in the medical field largely eliminated these diseases. Then, as more North American people started to enjoy the "good life" (sedentary living and overuse of alcohol, fatty foods, excessive sweets, tobacco, drugs), we saw an increase in deaths resulting from **chronic diseases** such as hypertension, coronary heart disease, atherosclerosis, strokes, diabetes, cancer, emphysema, and cirrhosis of the liver (see Table 1.1).

As the incidence of chronic diseases climbed, we recognized that prevention is the best medicine. Consequently, a fitness and wellness movement developed gradually in the 1980s. People began to realize that good health is mostly self-controlled and

FIGURE 1.1 Physical activity trends of adults, 1994–95 to 2004–05

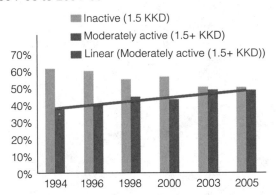

Physical activity trends of adults, 1994–95 to 2004–05

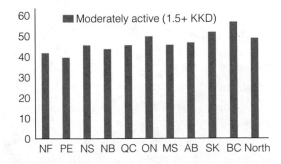

Source: Christine Cameron, Rebecca Wolfe, and Cora Craig. *Physical Activity and Sport: Encouraging Children to Be Active.* Canadian Fitness and Lifestyle Research Institute, 2005 Physical Activity and Sport Monitor (June 05, 2007). Available online from: http://www.cflri.ca/eng/statistics/surveys/documents/PAM2005.pdf (p. 7). Used with permission of the Canadian Fitness and Lifestyle Research Institute. www.cflri.ca

TABLE 1.1 Major Causes of Death in Canada for 2004

	Males	Females	Total
Cardiovascular Diseases	35,800	36,500	72,300
Cancer	35,200	31,800	67,000
Heart Disease	27,100	24,900	52,000
Respiratory (lung) Diseases	5,300	4,700	10,000
Accidents	5,400	3,600	9,000
Influenza and Pneumonia	2,600	3,200	5,800
Suicide	2,700	900	3,600
Kidney Diseases	1,800	1,700	3,500
Liver Diseases	1,500	800	2,300

Adapted from Statistics Canada publication *Mortality, Summary List of Causes,* 2004, Catalogue 84F0209XIE, pp. 20–21, http://www.statcan.ca/english/freepub/84F0209XIE/84F0209XIE2004000.pdf

TABLE 1.2   Life Expectancy and Healthy Life Expectancy for Selected Countries

Country	Life expectancy at birth, in years (year data obtained)		Healthy life expectancy at birth, in years (year data obtained)	
	Males	Females	Males	Females
Australia	79.0 (2005)	84.0 (2005)	71.0 (2002)	74.0 (2002)
Canada	78.0 (2005)	83.0 (2005)	70.0 (2002)	74.0 (2002)
China	71.0 (2005)	74.0 (2005)	63.0 (2002)	65.0 (2002)
Japan	79.0 (2005)	86.0 (2005)	72.0 (2002)	78.0 (2002)
New Zealand	77.0 (2005)	82.0 (2005)	69.0 (2002)	72.0 (2002)
Switzerland	79.0 (2005)	84.0 (2005)	71.0 (2002)	75.0 (2002)
United States	75.0 (2005)	80.0 (2005)	67.0 (2002)	71.0 (2002)

Source: World Health Organization. Healthy life expectancy (HALE) at birth (years). Selected Countries. Retrieved January 3, 2008. Used with permission © World Health Organization (WHO), 2008.

that the leading causes of illness and premature death in North America could be prevented by adhering to positive lifestyle habits. Whereas we all desire to live a long life, wellness programs focus on enhancing the overall quality of life—for as long as we live.

Life Expectancy Versus Healthy Life Expectancy

According to Statistics Canada, the average life expectancy in Canada is about 79.9 years.[3] In a break with tradition, the World Health Organization also began calculating **healthy life expectancy** (HLE, sometimes called HALE—Healthy Adjusted Life Expectancy) in the year 2000. HLE is obtained by subtracting the years of ill health from total life expectancy. Canada ranked 11th in this report, with an HLE of 72 years; Japan was first with an HLE of 75 years[4] (see Table 1.2). It was a major surprise that Canada was not ranked among the top countries, given its status as a developed country with one of the best medical care systems in the world. The rating indicates that Canadians die earlier and spend more time disabled than people in most other advanced countries. The WHO report points to several factors that may account for this unexpected finding:

1. The extremely poor health of some groups, such as First Nations and the inner-city poor. Their health status is more characteristic of poor developing nations than a rich industrialized country.
2. The HIV epidemic, which causes more deaths and disabilities in North America than in other areas.

3. The high incidence of tobacco use.
4. The high incidence of coronary heart disease.

Leading Health Problems in Canada

When heart disease is grouped with cerebrovascular disease and diseases of the arteries and other blood vessels, it is termed cardiovascular disease (CVD). In 1979, the leading cause of death in Canada was cardiovascular disease—47 percent of all deaths. Fortunately, this rate has declined over the years. Data collected by Statistics Canada indicate that by 2004 the percentage of deaths due to CVD was down to 32 percent.[5] However, the economic costs are great: over $18 billion a year goes to health care costs for cardiovascular disease.[6]

In Canada, degenerative diseases of the cardiovascular system such as coronary artery disease (CAD) contribute greatly to premature deaths. An examination of the main risk factors for CAD shows that in the late 1990s almost 30 percent of

Health   A state of complete well-being, and not just the absence of disease or infirmity.

Sedentary Death Syndrome (SeDS)   A term used to describe deaths that are attributed to a lack of regular physical activity.

Life expectancy   Number of years a person is expected to live based on the person's birth year.

Chronic diseases   Illnesses that develop and last a long time.

Healthy Life Expectancy (HLE)   Number of years a person is expected to live in good health; this number is obtained by subtracting ill-health years from overall life expectancy.

Canadians smoked, 20 percent had elevated blood pressure, 26 percent had high blood cholesterol, and over 60 percent were inactive. And, as previously mentioned, physical inactivity or Sedentary Death Syndrome represents many "hypokinetic" (hypo = diminished, kinetic = movement) diseases that currently threaten the Canadian public. In 1999, about $2.1 billion in health care costs in Canada were attributable to physical inactivity. This represented 2.5 percent of the total direct health care costs for that year. More importantly, it was reported that 33 percent of deaths from CAD, colon cancer and type 2 diabetes could have been prevented if physical inactivity was eliminated.[7]

The percentage of deaths due to cancer, Canada's second main cause of death, increased from 23 percent in 1979 to 30 percent in 2004. Researchers suggest that deaths due to cancer may soon surpass those caused by cardiovascular disease. Combined, these diseases caused about 6 out of every 10 deaths in 2004 (see Figure 1.2).

Lung, breast, prostate, and colorectal cancers are the most predominant cancers. Other conditions that are responsible for death of Canadians include chronic obstructive pulmonary disease, unintentional injuries, followed by pneumonia and influenza and diabetes. These disease all have strong lifestyle components.[8]

Lifestyle as a Health Problem

As the incidence of chronic diseases rose, it became clear that prevention was—and remains—the best medicine. Some research does suggest that a certain percentage of disease can be directly attributed to lifestyle.[9] While it is difficult to say with absolute certainty exactly what percentage that might be, self-care most certainly does make a difference.

Because of the unhealthy lifestyles that many young adults lead, their bodies may be middle-aged or older! Healthy choices made today influence health for decades. Many physical education programs do not emphasize the skills necessary for youths to maintain a high level of fitness and health throughout life. The intent of this book is to provide those skills and help to prepare you for a lifetime of physical fitness and wellness. A healthy lifestyle is self-controlled, and you can learn how to be responsible for your own health and fitness. Other factors include the environment you live in, access to health care, and your genetic make-up (see Figure 1.3).

There are also other things to consider that have come to be defined as the Social Determinants of Health. These include income inequality, job security, working conditions, housing and food security, education, care in early life, and social exclusion of certain individuals or groups.[10] An in-depth discussion of these determinants is better suited for a health textbook, but students who plan to work in the area of health promotion might want to access a Public Health Agency of Canada article titled *The Social Determinants of Health: An Overview of the Implications for Policy and the Role of the Health Sector*, to become more knowledgeable about health determinants. This article is available at http://www.phac-aspc.gc.ca/ph-sp/phdd/overview_implications/01_overview.html.

FIGURE 1.2 Share of deaths due to cardiovascular diseases, cancer, and both causes, Canada, 1979–2004

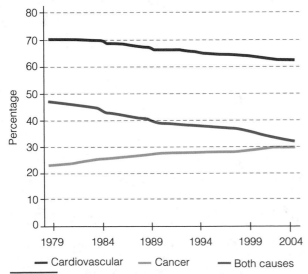

Source: Adapted from Statistics Canada publication *Mortality, Summary List of Causes*, 2004, Catalogue 84F0209XWE, Chart 3 http://www.statcan.ca/english/freepub/84F0209XIE/2004000/ct003_en.htm

FIGURE 1.3 Approximate contributions of factors that affect health and well-being

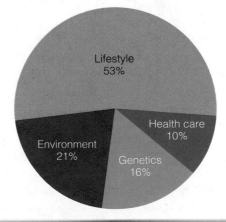

Physical Activity and Exercise Defined

Abundant scientific research over the last three decades has established a distinction between physical activity and exercise. **Physical activity** is bodily movement produced by skeletal muscles. It requires energy expenditure and produces progressive health benefits. Physical activity typically requires only a low to moderate intensity of effort. Examples of physical activity are walking to and from work, taking the stairs instead of elevators and escalators, gardening, doing household chores, dancing, and washing the car by hand. Physical inactivity, on the other hand, implies a level of activity that is lower than that required to maintain good health.

Exercise is a type of physical activity that requires planned, structured, and repetitive bodily movement to improve or maintain one or more components of physical fitness. Examples of exercise are walking, running, cycling, aerobics, swimming, and strength training. Exercise is usually viewed as an activity that requires a high-intensity effort.

Increasing Physical Activity in Canada—Coalition for Active Living

The Coalition for Active Living (CAL) is made up of over one hundred different organizations across Canada that form a national action group. This group is dedicated to creating a country-wide co-ordinated system that will ensure all Canadians have access to venues where they can engage in regular physical activity.[11] Members of the coalition believe that physical activity plays an important role in good health and that supportive and well-equipped environments encourage us to be physically active.

"A Business Plan to Increase Physical Activity in Canada"[12] is a document also developed by the coalition and complements the federal, provincial, and territorial sport and health strategies that are already in place. The aim of the plan is to increase the proportion of Canadians who participate in regular physical activity by 20 percent by 2015.

Research suggests that physical *inactivity* in Canada costs the country $5.3 billion. The cost of obesity in health care expenditures alone is approximately $4.3 billion. Medical experts tell us that chronic disease resulting from obesity is a serious health and economic issue that threatens our health care system. Regular physical activity is an important investment that can help us prevent chronic disease, lower health care costs, and improve our quality of life.

The strategic directions of this plan include the following:

- Physical Activity Goals—education, improving community environments, and reducing differences in physical activity levels related to ability, culture, race, gender, age, income, education, or geography.
- System Goals—a coordinated effort between federal departments of health, sport, and transportation, provincial and territorial governments and departments, municipal governments, regional businesses, voluntary sector organizations, school boards, recreation centres, and private sector companies.
- Strategic Priorities and Actions—the development of healthy public policy, community physical environments, and supportive social environments.
- Federal Government Investment—a recommendation to increase the current health care funding for physical activity of $300 to $475 million annually to an investment of $100 million annually—which would save $3 billion a year in health care costs.

Wellness

Most people recognize that participating in fitness programs improves their quality of life. At the end of the 20th century, however, we came to realize that physical fitness alone was not always sufficient to lower the risk for disease and ensure better health. For example, individuals who run 5 km a day, lift weights regularly, participate in stretching

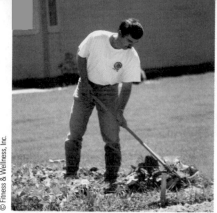

Exercise and an active lifestyle increases health, quality of life, and longevity.

CRITICAL THINKING

Do you consciously incorporate physical activity into your daily lifestyle? Can you provide examples? Do you think you get sufficient daily physical activity to maintain good health?

Physical activity Bodily movement produced by skeletal muscles; requires expenditure of energy and produces progressive health benefits.

Exercise A type of physical activity that requires planned, structured, and repetitive bodily movement with the intent of improving or maintaining one or more components of physical fitness.

exercises, and watch their body weight might be easily classified as having good or excellent fitness. Offsetting these good habits, however, might be **risk factors**, including high blood pressure, smoking, excessive stress, drinking excessive alcohol, and eating too many fatty foods. These factors place people at risk for cardiovascular disease and other chronic diseases of which they may not be aware.

Even though most people are aware of their unhealthy behaviours, they seem satisfied with life as long as they are free from symptoms of disease or illness. They do not contemplate change until they suffer a major health problem. Present lifestyle habits, however, dictate the health and well-being of tomorrow.

Good health is no longer viewed as simply the absence of illness. The notion of good health has evolved notably in the last few years and continues to change as scientists learn more about lifestyle factors that bring on illness and affect wellness. Furthermore, once the idea took hold that fitness by itself would not always decrease the risk for disease and ensure better health, the **wellness** concept developed. Wellness living requires implementing positive programs to change behaviour to improve health and quality of life, prolong life, and achieve total well-being.

The Seven Dimensions of Wellness

Wellness has seven dimensions: physical, emotional, mental, social, environmental, occupational, and other (see Figure 1.4). These dimensions are interrelated: One frequently affects the others. For example, a person who is emotionally down often has no desire to exercise, study, socialize with friends, attend church, and may be more susceptible to illness and disease.

The seven dimensions of wellness show how the concept clearly goes beyond the absence of disease. Wellness incorporates factors such as adequate fitness, proper nutrition, stress management, disease prevention, not smoking or abusing drugs, personal safety, regular physical examinations, health education, and environmental support.

For a wellness way of life, not only must individuals be physically fit and manifest no signs of disease, but they must also be free of risk factors for disease (such as hypertension, hyperlipidemia, cigarette smoking, negative stress, faulty nutrition, careless sex). The relationship between adequate fitness and wellness is illustrated in the continuum in Figure 1.5. Even though an individual tested in a fitness centre may demonstrate adequate or even excellent fitness, indulgence in unhealthy lifestyle behaviours will still increase the risk for chronic diseases and diminish the person's well-being.

Physical Wellness

Physical wellness is the dimension most commonly associated with being healthy. It entails confidence and optimism about one's ability to protect one's physical health and take care of health problems.

Physically well individuals are active, exercise regularly, eat a well-balanced diet, maintain recommended body weight, get sufficient sleep, practise safe sex, minimize exposure to environmental contaminants, avoid harmful drugs (including tobacco and excessive alcohol), and seek medical care and exams as needed. Physically well people also exhibit good cardiorespiratory endurance, adequate muscular strength and flexibility, proper body composition, and the ability to carry out ordinary and unusual demands of daily life safely and effectively. These concepts are discussed in subsequent chapters.

Emotional Wellness

Emotional wellness involves the ability to understand one's own feelings, accept one's limitations, and achieve emotional stability. Furthermore, it implies the ability to express emotions appropriately, adjust to change, cope with stress in a healthy way, and enjoy life despite its occasional disappointments and frustrations.

Emotional wellness brings with it a certain stability, an ability to look both success and failure squarely in the face and to keep moving along a predetermined course. When success is evident, the emotionally well person radiates the expected joy and confidence. When failure seems evident, the emotionally well person responds by making the

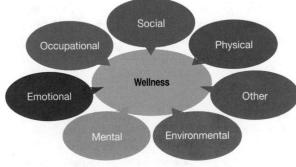

FIGURE 1.4 Dimensions of wellness

FIGURE 1.5 Wellness continuum

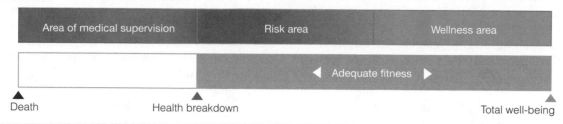

best of circumstances and moving beyond the failure. Wellness enables one to move ahead with optimism and energy instead of spending time and talent worrying about failure. You learn from it, identify ways to avoid it in the future, and then go on with the business at hand.

And emotional wellness involves happiness—an emotional anchor that gives meaning and joy to life. Happiness is a long-term state of mind that permeates the various facets of life and influences our outlook. Although there is no simple recipe for creating happiness, researchers agree that happy people are usually participants in some category of a supportive family unit where they feel loved themselves. Healthy, happy people enjoy friends, work hard at something fulfilling, get plenty of exercise, and enjoy play and leisure time. They know how to laugh, and they laugh often. They give of themselves freely to others and seem to have found deep meaning in life.

An attitude of true happiness signals freedom from the tension and depression that many people endure. Emotionally well people are obviously subject to the same kinds of depression and unhappiness that occasionally plague us all, but the difference lies in their ability to bounce back. Emotionally well people take minor setbacks in stride and have the ability to enjoy life despite it all. They don't waste energy or time recounting the situation, wondering how they could have changed it, or dwelling on the past.

Mental Wellness

Mental wellness, also referred to as intellectual wellness, implies that the mentally well person can apply the things he or she has learned, create opportunities to learn more, and engage the mind in lively interaction with the outside world. When you are mentally well, you are not intimidated by facts and figures with which you are unfamiliar but instead embrace the chance to learn something new. Your confidence and enthusiasm enable you to

approach any learning situation with eagerness that leads to success.

Mental wellness brings with it vision and promise. More than anything else, mentally well people are open-minded and accepting of others. Instead of being threatened by people who are different from themselves, they show respect and curiosity without feeling they have to conform. They are faithful to their own ideas and philosophies and allow others the same privilege. Their self-confidence guarantees that they can take their place among others in the world without having to give up part of themselves and without requiring others to do the same.

Social Wellness

Social wellness, with its accompanying positive self-image, endows a person with the ease and confidence to be outgoing, friendly, and affectionate toward others. Social wellness involves not only a concern for oneself but also an interest in humanity and the environment as a whole.

One of the hallmarks of social wellness is the ability to relate to others and to reach out to other people both within the family and outside it. Similar to emotional wellness, it involves being comfortable with one's emotions and thus helps the socially

Risk factors Lifestyle and genetic variables that may lead to disease.

Wellness The constant and deliberate effort to stay healthy and achieve the highest potential for well-being. It encompasses seven dimensions—physical, emotional, mental, social, environmental, occupational, and other—and integrates them all into a quality life.

Physical wellness Good physical fitness and confidence in one's personal ability to take care of health problems.

Emotional wellness The ability to understand one's own feelings, accept limitations, and achieve emotional stability.

Mental wellness A state in which one's mind is engaged in lively interaction with the surrounding world; also called intellectual wellness.

Social wellness The ability to relate well to others, both within and outside the family unit.

well person understand and accept the emotions of others. One's own balance and sense of self enable extending respect and tolerance to others. Healthy people are honest and loyal. This dimension of wellness leads to the ability to maintain close relationships with other people.

Environmental Wellness

Environmental wellness refers to the effect that our surroundings have on our well-being. Our planet is a delicate **ecosystem**, and its health depends on the continuous recycling of its elements. Unfortunately, the man-made toxicity of the environment has a direct effect on personal wellness.

To enjoy health, we require clean air, pure water, quality food, adequate shelter, satisfactory work conditions, personal safety, and healthy relationships. Health is negatively affected when we live in a polluted, toxic, unkind, and unsafe environment. To enjoy environmental wellness, it is our personal responsibility not only to educate and protect ourselves against environmental hazards but also to protect the environment so that we, our children, and future generations can enjoy a safe and clean environment.

Occupational Wellness

Occupational wellness is not tied to high salary, prestigious position, or extravagant working conditions. Any job can bring occupational wellness if it provides rewards that are important to the individual. Salary might be the most important factor to one person, whereas another might place a much greater value on creativity. People who are occupationally well have their own "ideal" job, which allows them to thrive.

People who are occupationally well face demands on the job, but they also have some say over demands that are placed on them. Any job has routine demands, but occupational wellness means that routine demands are mixed with new, unpredictable challenges that keep a job exciting. Occupationally well people are able to maximize their skills, and they have the opportunity to broaden their existing skills or gain new ones. Their occupation offers opportunities for advancement and recognition for achievement. Occupational wellness encourages collaboration and interaction among co-workers, which fosters a sense of teamwork and support.

Other Wellness

Other wellness includes aspects of wellness that do not fall within the other six dimensions of wellness. For example, some people believe that spiritual

wellness provides a unifying power that integrates other aspects of wellness. Basic characteristics of spiritual people include a sense of meaning and direction in life and a relationship to a higher being. This leads to personal freedom and encompasses prayer, faith, love, closeness to others, peace, joy, fulfillment, and altruism. Although not everyone claims affiliation with a certain religion or denomination, based on an Ipsos-Reid survey, 78 percent of the Canadian population believes in God or a universal spirit functioning as God.

Several studies have reported positive relationships among spiritual well-being, emotional well-being, and satisfactions with life.[13] Although the ways by which religious or spiritual affiliation enhances wellness are difficult to determine, possible benefits include the promotion of healthy lifestyle behaviours, social support, assistance in times of crisis and need, and counselling to overcome weaknesses. Spiritual beliefs also seem to help people overcome crises and aid them in developing better coping techniques to deal with future trauma.[14]

ALTRUISM

Altruism, a key attribute of spiritual people, seems to enhance health and longevity. Studies indicate that people who perform regular volunteer work live longer. Doing good for others is good for oneself, especially for the immune system. Research has found that health benefits of altruism are so powerful that even watching films of altruistic endeavours enhances the formation of an immune-system chemical that helps fight disease.

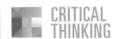

CRITICAL THINKING

Now that you understand the seven dimensions of wellness, rank them in order of importance to you and explain your rationale in doing so.

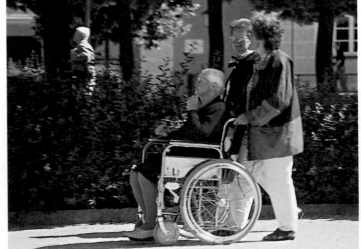

Altruism enhances health and well-being.

Wellness requires a balance among all of its seven dimensions. There can be a relationship between other dimensions (spirituality) and wellness, which therefore can make it meaningful in our quest for a better quality of life. As with the other parameters listed above, optimum wellness requires development of the spiritual dimension to its fullest potential.

Wellness, Fitness, and Longevity

During the second half of the 20th century, scientists began to realize the importance of good fitness and improved lifestyle in the fight against chronic diseases, particularly those of the cardiovascular system. The first major study in this area was conducted among 16,936 Harvard University alumni, linking physical activity habits and mortality rates. The results showed that as the amount of physical activity increased, the risk of cardiovascular deaths decreased. The largest decrease in cardiovascular deaths was observed among alumni who used more than 2,000 calories per week through physical activity.[15] Figure 1.6 graphically illustrates the study results.

A landmark study subsequently conducted at the Cooper Institute in Dallas, Texas, upheld the findings of the Harvard alumni study.[16] Based on data from 13,344 people followed over an average of eight years, the study revealed a graded and consistent inverse relationship between physical activity levels and mortality, regardless of age and other risk factors. As illustrated in Figure 1.7, the higher the level of physical activity, the longer the lifespan. The death rate during the eight-year study from all causes for the least-fit men was 3.4 times higher than that of the most-fit men. For the least-fit women, the death rate was 4.6 times higher than that of most-fit women.

The same study also reported a greatly reduced rate of premature death, even at the moderate fitness levels that most adults can achieve easily. Greater protection is attained by combining higher fitness levels with reduction in other risk factors such as hypertension, high serum cholesterol, cigarette smoking, and excessive body fat.

A five-year follow-up study on fitness and mortality found a substantial (44 percent) reduction in mortality risk when people abandoned a **sedentary** lifestyle and become moderately fit.[17] The lowest death rate was found in people who were fit at the start of the study and remained fit; the highest death rate was found in men who were unfit at the beginning of the study and remained unfit.

In another major research study, a healthy lifestyle was shown to contribute to some of the lowest mortality rates ever reported in the litera-

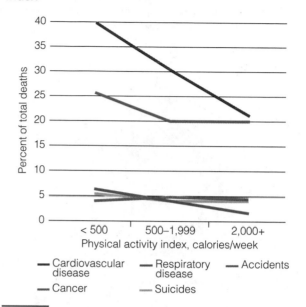

FIGURE 1.6 U.S. death rates by physical activity index

Note: The graph represents cause-specific death rates per 10,000 person-years of observation among 16,936 Harvard alumni, 1962–1978, by physical activity index; adjusted for differences in age, cigarette smoking, and hypertension.

Source: R. S. Paffenbarger, R. T. Hyde, A. L. Wing, and C. H. Steinmetz, "A Natural History of Athleticism and Cardiovascular Health," *Journal of the American Medical Association* 252 (1984): 491–495. Used by permission Copyright © (1984), American Medical Association. All rights reserved.

ture.[18] The investigators in this study looked at three general health habits among the participants: regular physical activity, sufficient sleep, and lifetime abstinence from smoking. In addition, study participants abstained from alcohol, drugs, and all forms of tobacco.

Compared with the general population, this group of more than 10,000 people had much lower cancer, cardiovascular, and overall death rates. Men in the study had one-third the death rate from cancer, one-seventh the death rate from cardiovascular

Environmental wellness The capability to live in a clean and safe environment that is not detrimental to health.

Ecosystem A community of organisms interacting with each other in an environment.

Occupational wellness The ability to perform one's job skillfully and effectively under conditions that provide personal and team satisfaction and adequately reward each individual.

Other wellness Aspects of wellness that do not fall within the other six dimensions; for some people, other wellness may include spirituality.

Altruism True concern for the welfare of others.

Sedentary A lifestyle characterized by relative inactivity and a lot of sitting.

FIGURE 1.7 Death rates by physical fitness groups

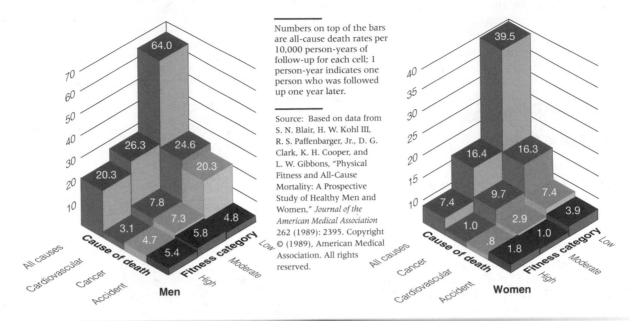

Numbers on top of the bars are all-cause death rates per 10,000 person-years of follow-up for each cell; 1 person-year indicates one person who was followed up one year later.

disease, and one-fifth the rate of overall mortality. Women had about half the rate of cancer and overall mortality and one-third the death rate from cardiovascular disease. Life expectancies for 25-year-olds who adhered to the three health habits were 85 and 86 years, respectively.

Current studies also support these historical studies. Both Kesteloot[19] and Gasser[20] found that physical activity can help prevent cardiovascular disease and also assist in the treatment of various diseases. The lessons learned from these studies clearly indicate that fitness improves wellness, quality of life, and longevity. **Vigorous activity** is preferable to the extent of one's capabilities because it is more clearly associated with longer life.

Types of Physical Fitness

As the fitness concept grew at the end of the last century, it became clear that several specific components contribute to an individual's overall level of fitness. **Physical fitness** can be classified into health-related and motor skill-related fitness.

The four **health-related fitness** components are (see Figure 1.8):

1. cardiorespiratory (aerobic) endurance
2. muscular strength and endurance
3. muscular flexibility
4. body composition

The **skill-related fitness** components consist of (see Figure 1.9):

1. agility
2. balance
3. coordination
4. reaction time
5. speed
6. power

These skill-related fitness components are related primarily to athletic success and may not be as crucial as the health-related components to better health.

With regard to preventive medicine, the main emphasis of fitness programs should be on the health-related components. Nevertheless, total fitness is achieved by taking part in specific programs to improve both health-related and skill-related components.

Fitness Standards: Health Versus Physical Fitness

The assessments of fitness components are presented in Chapters 4, 6, 7, 8, and 9. A meaningful debate regarding age- and gender-related fitness standards, however, has resulted in two standards: health fitness (also referred to as criterion-referenced fitness) and physical fitness.

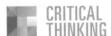

CRITICAL THINKING

What role do the four health-related components of physical fitness play in your life? Can you rank them in order of importance to you and explain the rationale you used?

FIGURE 1.8 Health-related components of physical fitness

Cardiorespiratory endurance

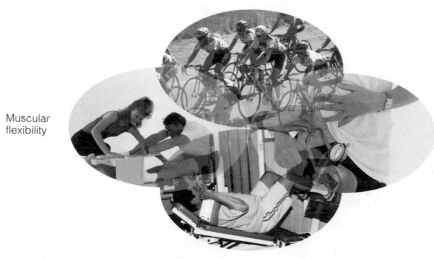

Muscular
flexibility

Body
composition

Muscular strength and endurance

Photos © Fitness & Wellness, Inc.

FIGURE 1.9 Motor skill-related components of physical fitness

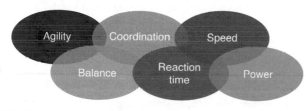

Agility   Coordination   Speed

Balance   Reaction time   Power

glucose tolerance, and improved cholesterol levels) can be notable despite little or no weight loss or improvement in aerobic capacity. **Metabolic fitness** can be attained through an active lifestyle and moderate physical activity.

Vigorous activity Any exercise that requires a MET level equal to or greater than 6 METs (21 mL/kg/min); 1 MET is the energy expenditure at rest, 3.5 mL/kg/min, whereas METs are defined as multiples of the resting metabolic rate (examples of activities that require a 6-MET level are aerobics, walking uphill at 5.6 km/h, cycling at 16 to 19.3 km/h, playing doubles in tennis, and vigorous strength training).

Physical fitness The ability to meet the ordinary as well as the unusual demands of daily life safely and effectively without being overly fatigued and still have energy left for leisure and recreational activities.

Health-related fitness Fitness programs that are prescribed to improve the individual's overall health; components are cardio-respiratory endurance, muscular strength and endurance, muscular flexibility, and body composition.

Skill-related fitness Fitness components important for success in activities and athletic events requiring high skill levels; encompasses agility, balance, coordination, power, reaction time, and speed.

Health fitness standards The lowest fitness requirements for maintaining good health, decreasing the risk for chronic diseases, and lowering the incidence of muscular-skeletal injuries; also referred to as criterion-referenced standards.

Metabolic profile A measurement to assess risk for diabetes and cardiovascular disease through plasma insulin, glucose, lipid, and lipoprotein levels.

Metabolic fitness Denotes improvements in the metabolic profile through a moderate-intensity exercise program in spite of little or no improvement in physical fitness standards.

Health Fitness Standards

The **health fitness standards** proposed here are based on data linking minimum fitness values to disease prevention and health. Attaining the health fitness standard requires only moderate physical activity. For example, a 3 km walk in less than 30 minutes, five or six times per week, seems to be sufficient to achieve the health-fitness standard for cardiorespiratory endurance.

As illustrated in Figure 1.11, significant health benefits can be reaped with such a program, although improvements in fitness, expressed in terms of oxygen uptake or VO₂max (explained on page 12 and in Chapter 6) are not as notable. Nevertheless, health improvements are quite striking, and only slightly greater benefits are obtained with a more intense exercise program. These benefits include reduction in blood lipids, lower blood pressure, weight loss, stress release, decreased risk for diabetes, and lower risk for disease and premature mortality.

More specifically, improvements in the **metabolic profile** (measured by insulin sensitivity,

FIGURE 1.10 Canada's Physical Activity Guide for Healthy Living

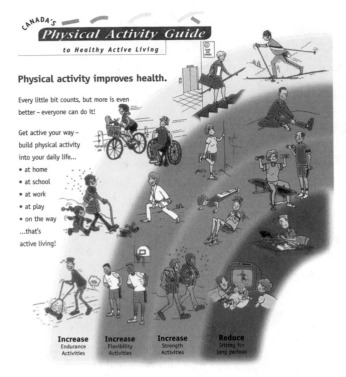

Source: *Canada's Physical Activity Guide to Healthy Active Living* (1998), http://www.phac-aspc.gc.ca/pau-uap/fitness/pdf/handbook_e.pdf, Health Canada. Reproduced with the permission of the Minister of Public Works and Government Services Canada, 2008.

An assessment of health-related fitness uses **cardiorespiratory endurance**, measured by the maximal amount of oxygen the body is able to utilize per minute of physical activity (maximal oxygen uptake, or VO_2max), essentially, a measure of how efficiently the heart, lungs, and muscles can operate during aerobic exercise (see Chapter 6). VO_2max is commonly expressed in millilitres (mL) of oxygen (volume of oxygen) per kilogram (kg) of body weight per minute (mL/kg/min). Individual

values can range from about 10 mL/kg/min in cardiac patients to more than 80 mL/kg/min in world-class runners, cyclists, and cross-country skiers.

Research data from the study presented in Figure 1.6 reported that achieving VO_2max values of 35 and 32.5 mL/kg/min for men and women, respectively, may be sufficient to lower the risk for all-cause mortality significantly. Although greater improvements in fitness yield a slightly lower risk for premature death, the largest drop is seen between the least fit and the moderately fit. Therefore, the 35 and 32.5 mL/kg/min values could be selected as the health fitness standards.

Physical Fitness Standards

Physical fitness standards are set higher than the health fitness standards and require a more intense exercise program. Physically fit people of all ages have the freedom to enjoy most of life's daily and recreational activities to their fullest potential. Current health fitness standards may not be enough to achieve these objectives.

Sound physical fitness gives the individual a measure of independence throughout life that many people in Canada no longer enjoy. Most adults should be able to carry out activities similar to those they conducted in their youth, though not with the same intensity. These standards do not require being a championship athlete, but activities such as climbing several flights of stairs, playing hockey or basketball, mountain biking, playing soccer with children or grandchildren, walking several kilometres around a lake or hiking do require more than the current "average fitness" level in Canada. For example, a person who has attained a high *physical fitness standard* would theoretically be able to exercise at a higher percentage of their maximum heart rate for a longer duration than an average person who had attained a *health fitness standard*. In addition, this individual might also be able to play a team sport, such as basketball or hockey, and demonstrate a consistent level of performance throughout the game with little, if any, signs of fatigue.

Your own objectives will determine the fitness program you use. If the main objective of your fitness program is to lower the risk of disease, attaining the health fitness standards may be enough to ensure better health. If, however, you want to participate in vigorous fitness activities, achieving a high physical fitness standard is recommended. This book gives both health fitness standards and physical fitness standards for each fitness test so you can personalize your approach.

FIGURE 1.11 Health and fitness benefits based on type of lifestyle and physical activity program

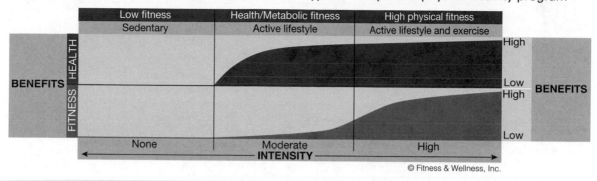

© Fitness & Wellness, Inc.

Benefits of a Comprehensive Wellness Program

An inspiring story illustrating what fitness can do for a person's health and well-being is that of David from Toronto, Ontario. At age 25, David was a very fit 75 kg, 173 cm man, who cycled 10 to 15 hours per week. At age 26, David started his own business and over the years 10-hour days and 3-minute local fast-food meals resulted in a weight gain of 50 kg. By age 46, he weighed 125 kg. Apart from his increased weight, his overall health was good. However, when he eventually developed a sleeping disorder, his doctor told him he could either sleep using a special mask for the rest of his life or lose some weight. David started a balanced diet, following the servings recommended by Canada's Food Guide. He started a walking regimen until he hit 106 kg and became fit enough to start running lightly. He joined a gym where he discovered spinning and would do this three or four times a week as well as undertaking a weight training program. Over a nine-month period, he lost 38 kg of fat and gained some muscle along the way. He now has significantly more energy, sleeps better, takes three-hour bike rides on the weekend, and has taken up boxing.

Health Benefits

Most people exercise because it improves their personal appearance and makes them feel good about themselves. Although many benefits accrue from participating in a regular fitness and wellness program and active people generally live longer, the greatest benefit of all is that physically fit individuals enjoy a better quality of life. These people live life to its fullest, with fewer health problems than inactive individuals (who may also indulge in other negative lifestyle behaviours). Although it would be difficult to compile an all-inclusive list, participating in a fitness and wellness program:

- Improves and strengthens the cardiorespiratory system.
- Maintains better muscle tone, muscular strength, and endurance.
- Improves muscular flexibility.
- Enhances athletic performance.
- Helps to maintain recommended body weight.
- Helps to preserve lean body tissue.
- Increases resting metabolic rate.
- Improves the body's ability to use fat during physical activity.
- Improves posture and physical appearance.
- Improves functioning of the immune system.
- Lowers the risk for chronic diseases and illness (such as cardiovascular diseases and cancer).
- Decreases the mortality rate from chronic diseases.
- Thins the blood so it doesn't clot as readily (thereby decreasing the risk for coronary heart disease and strokes).
- Helps the body to manage cholesterol levels more effectively.
- Prevents or delays the development of high blood pressure and lowers blood pressure in people with hypertension.
- Helps to prevent and control diabetes.
- Helps to achieve peak bone mass in young adults and maintain bone mass later in life, thereby decreasing the risk for osteoporosis.
- Helps people sleep better.
- Helps to prevent chronic back pain.
- Relieves tension and helps in coping with life stresses.
- Raises levels of energy and job productivity.

Cardiorespiratory endurance The ability of the lungs, heart, and blood vessels to deliver adequate amounts of oxygen to the cells to meet the demands of prolonged physical activity.

Physical fitness standards A fitness level that allows a person to sustain moderate-to-vigorous physical activity without undue fatigue and the ability to closely maintain this level throughout life.

Research indicates that adhering to the following 12 lifestyle habits will significantly improve health and extend life.

1. *Participate in a lifetime physical activity program.* Exercise regularly at least three times per week and try to accumulate a minimum of 60 minutes of moderate-intensity physical activity each day of your life. The 60 minutes should include 20 to 30 minutes of aerobic exercise at least three times per week, along with strengthening and stretching exercises two to three times per week.

2. *Do not smoke cigarettes.* Cigarette smoking is the largest preventable cause of illness and premature death in Canada. If we include all related deaths, smoking is responsible for more than 47,000 unnecessary deaths each year.

3. *Eat right.* Eat a good breakfast and two additional well-balanced meals every day. Avoid eating too many calories and foods with a lot of sugar, fat, and salt. Increase your daily consumption of fruits, vegetables, and whole-grain products.

4. *Avoid snacking.* Some researchers recommend refraining from frequent between-meal snacks. Every time a person eats, insulin is released to remove sugar from the blood. Such frequent spikes in insulin may contribute to the development of heart disease. Less frequent increases of insulin are more conducive to good health.

5. *Maintain recommended body weight through adequate nutrition and exercise.* This is important in preventing chronic diseases and in developing a higher level of fitness.

6. *Get enough rest.* Sleep seven to eight hours each night.

7. *Lower your stress levels.* Reduce your vulnerability to stress and practise stress management techniques as needed.

8. *Be wary of alcohol.* Drink alcohol moderately or not at all. Alcohol abuse leads to mental, emotional, physical, and social problems.

9. *Surround yourself with healthy friendships.* Unhealthy friendships contribute to destructive behaviours and low self-esteem. Associating with people who strive to maintain good fitness and health reinforces a positive outlook in life and encourages positive behaviours. Constructive social interactions enhance well-being. Researchers have also found that mortality rates are much higher among people who are socially isolated. People who aren't socially integrated are more likely to "give up when seriously ill"—which accelerates dying.

10. *Be informed about the environment.* Seek clean air, clean water, and a clean environment. Be aware of pollutants and occupational hazards: asbestos fibres, nickel dust, chromate, uranium dust, and so on. Take precautions when using pesticides and insecticides.

11. *Increase education.* Data indicate that people who are more educated live longer. The idea is that as education and hence learning increases, so do the number of connections between nerve cells. The increased number of connections in turn helps the individual make better survival (healthy lifestyle) choices.

12. *Take personal safety measures.* Although not all accidents are preventable, many are. Taking simple precautionary measures—such as using seat belts and keeping electrical appliances away from water—lessens the risk for avoidable accidents.

- Extends longevity and slows down the aging process.
- Promotes psychological well-being; better morale, self-image, and self-esteem.
- Reduces feelings of depression and anxiety.
- Encourages positive lifestyle changes (improving nutrition, quitting smoking, controlling alcohol and drug use).
- Speeds recovery time following physical exertion.
- Speeds recovery following injury or disease.
- Regulates and improves overall body functions.
- Improves physical stamina and counteracts chronic fatigue.
- Helps to maintain independent living, especially in older adults.
- Enhances quality of life; adherents feel better and live a healthier and happier life.

Economic Benefits

Sedentary living can have a strong impact on a nation's economy. The Canadian Institute for Health Information (CIHI) Health Care in Canada 2007 report[21] found that approximately one-tenth of our economic output or $148 billion was spent on health care in 2006. If we consider the effect of inflation, this total is more than three times the money that was spent on health care in 1975. If we link this spending to our GDP or gross domestic product, a standard measure of the overall size of our economy, health care costs reached 10.3 percent, the highest level we have seen in over 30 years.

CRITICAL THINKING

What are your feelings about lifestyle habits that enhance health and longevity? How important are they to you? What obstacles keep you from adhering to such habits or incorporating new ones into your life?

FIGURE 1.12 Total health expenditures in Canada, 1977–2000

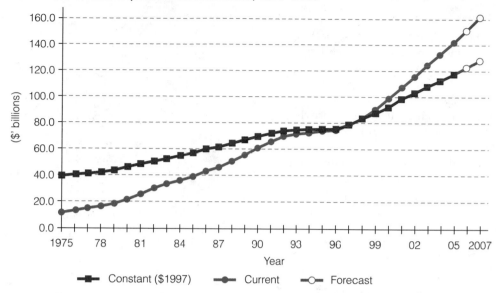

Source: Canadian Institute for Health Information, National Health Expenditure Trends, 1975–2007. Ottawa: CIHI, 2007 (p. 3). http://secure.cihi.ca/ cihiweb/products/NHET_1975_2007_e.pdf. © 2007 Canadian Institute for Health Information. Used with permission.

FIGURE 1.13 Total health expenditure per capita 2005 and outlook for 2006–2007

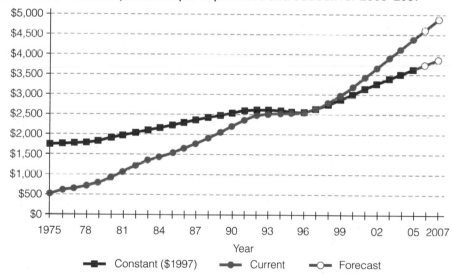

Source: Canadian Institute for Health Information, National Health Expenditure Trends, 1975–2007. Ottawa: CIHI, 2007 (p. 5). http://secure.cihi.ca/ cihiweb/products/NHET_1975_2007_e.pdf. © 2007 Canadian Institute for Health Information. Used with permission.

In 2006, health care costs were approximately $4,548 per person, varying from province and territory due to the cost of providing health services in different parts of Canada. Health care spending is lower in Canada than in the United States and Switzerland, but more than Denmark and the United Kingdom.

It has been suggested that one of the reasons for the increased costs is our overemphasis on state-of-the-art cures instead of prevention programs. The saying that "a gram of prevention is worth a kilogram of cure" still remains true. Our emphasis should be on primary and secondary modes of disease prevention.

The Wellness Challenge of the Future

Because a better and healthier life is something every person should strive for, our biggest challenge is to teach people how to take control of their personal health habits and adhere to a positive lifestyle. A wealth of information on the benefits of fitness and wellness programs indicates that improving the quality and possible length of our lives is a matter of personal choice.

Even though people believe a positive lifestyle has a great impact on health and longevity, most do not reap the benefits because they don't know how to implement a safe and effective fitness and wellness program. Others are exercising incorrectly and, therefore, are not reaping the full benefits of their program. How, then, can we meet the health challenges of the future? That is the focus of this book—to provide the tools necessary to enable you to write, implement, and regularly update your personal lifetime fitness and wellness program.

Wellness Education: Using this Book

Most people go to university or college to learn how to make a living, but a fitness and wellness course will teach you how to *live*—how to truly live life to its fullest potential. Some people seem to think that success is measured by how much money they make. Making a good living will not help you unless you live a wellness lifestyle that will allow you to enjoy what you earn.

Although everyone would like to enjoy good health and wellness, most people don't know how to reach this objective. Lifestyle is the most important factor affecting personal well-being. Granted, some people live long because of genetic factors, but quality of life during middle age and the "golden years" is more often related to wise choices initiated during youth and continued throughout life. In a few short years, lack of wellness can lead to a loss of vitality and gusto for life, as well as premature morbidity and mortality.

A Personalized Approach

Because fitness and wellness needs vary significantly from one individual to another, all exercise and wellness prescriptions must be personalized to obtain best results. The Wellness Lifestyle Questionnaire in Lab 1A will provide an initial rating of your current efforts to stay healthy and well. Subsequent chapters of this book and their respective laboratory experiences

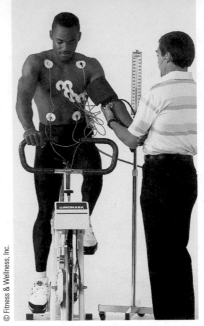

© Fitness & Wellness, Inc.

An exercise tolerance test (stress test) with 12-lead electrocardiographic monitoring may be required of some individuals prior to initiating an exercise program.

present the components of a wellness lifestyle and set forth the necessary guidelines that will allow you to develop a personal lifetime program that will improve your fitness and promote your own preventive health care and personal wellness.

The laboratory experiences have been prepared on tear-out sheets so they can be turned in to class instructors. As you study this book and complete the worksheets, you will learn to do the following:

- Implement motivational and behaviour modification techniques that will help you adhere to a lifetime fitness and wellness program.
- Determine whether medical clearance is needed for your safe participation in exercise.
- Conduct nutritional analyses and follow the recommendations for adequate nutrition.
- Write sound diet and weight-control programs.
- Assess the health-related components of fitness (cardiorespiratory endurance, muscular strength and endurance, muscular flexibility, and body composition).
- Write exercise prescriptions for cardiorespiratory endurance, muscular strength and endurance, and muscular flexibility.
- Assess the skill-related components of fitness (agility, balance, coordination, power, reaction time, and speed).
- Understand the relationship between fitness and aging.
- Determine your levels of tension and stress, lessen your vulnerability to stress, and implement a stress management program, if necessary.
- Determine your potential risk for cardiovascular disease and implement a risk-reduction program.
- Follow a cancer risk-reduction program.
- Implement a smoking cessation program, if applicable.

- Avoid chemical dependency and know where to find assistance, if needed.
- Learn the health consequences of sexually transmitted diseases, including HIV/AIDS, and guidelines for preventing STDs.
- Write objectives to improve your fitness and wellness and learn how to chart a wellness program for the future.
- Differentiate myths and facts of exercise and health-related concepts.

Exercise Safety

Even though testing and participation in exercise are relatively safe for most apparently healthy individuals under age 45, the reaction of the cardiovascular system to higher levels of physical activity cannot be totally predicted.[22] Consequently, a small but real risk exists for exercise-induced abnormalities in people with a history of cardiovascular problems and those who are at higher risk for disease. These include abnormal blood pressure, irregular heart rhythm, fainting, and, in rare instances, a heart attack or cardiac arrest.

Before you start to engage in an exercise program or participate in any exercise testing, you should fill out the questionnaire in Lab 1B. If your answer to any of the questions is yes, you should see a physician before participating in a fitness program. Exercise testing and participation is not wise under some of the conditions listed in Lab 1B and may require a medical evaluation, including a stress electrocardiogram (ECG) test. If you have any questions regarding your current health status, consult your doctor before initiating, continuing, or increasing your level of physical activity.

Resting Heart Rate and Blood Pressure Assessment

In Lab 1C you will learn how to determine your heart rate and blood pressure. Heart rate can be obtained by counting your pulse either on the wrist over the radial artery or over the carotid artery in the neck (see Chapter 6, page 167).

You may count your pulse for 30 seconds and multiply by 2 or take it for a full minute. The heart rate usually is at its lowest point (resting heart rate) late in the evening after you have been sitting quietly for about half an hour watching a relaxing TV show or reading in bed, or early in the morning just before you get out of bed.

Unless you have a pathological condition, a lower resting heart rate indicates a stronger heart. To adapt to cardiorespiratory or aerobic exercise, blood volume increases, the heart enlarges, and the muscle gets stronger. A stronger heart can pump more blood with fewer strokes.

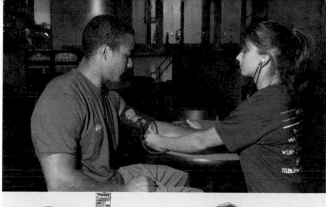
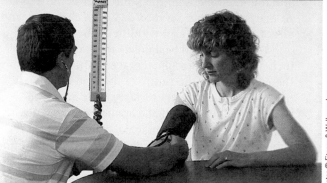

Photos © Fitness & Wellness, Inc.

A mercury gravity manometer can be used to measure blood pressure.

TABLE 1.3 Resting Heart Rate Ratings

Heart Rate (beats/minute)	Rating
≤59	Excellent
60–69	Good
70–79	Average
80–89	Fair
≥90	Poor

Resting heart rate ratings are given in Table 1.3. Although resting heart rate decreases with training, the extent of **bradycardia** depends not only on the amount of training but also on genetic factors. Although most highly trained athletes have a resting heart rate around 40 beats per minute, occasionally, one of these athletes has a resting heart rate in the 60s or 70s even during peak training months of the season. For most individuals, however, the resting heart rate decreases as the level of cardiorespiratory endurance increases.

In recent years, heart rate monitors have become easily accessible and affordable. These devices detect the electrical activity of the heart and relay the information to a wristwatch-like monitor. They are excellent ways of tracking heart rates during training and can be purchased at most stores that sell sporting goods.[23]

Bradycardia Slower heart rate than normal.

Blood pressure is assessed using a **sphygmomanometer** and a stethoscope. Use a cuff of the appropriate size to get accurate readings. Size is determined by the width of the inflatable bladder, which should be about 40 percent of the circumference of the midpoint of the arm.

Blood pressure usually is measured while the person is in the sitting position, with the forearm and the manometer at the same level as the heart. At first, the pressure is recorded from each arm, and after that from the arm with the highest reading.

The cuff should be applied approximately an inch above the antecubital space (natural crease of the elbow), with the centre of the bladder directly over the medial (inner) surface of the arm. The stethoscope head should be applied firmly, but with little pressure, over the brachial artery in the antecubital space. The arm should be flexed slightly and placed on a flat surface.

To determine how high the cuff should be inflated, the person recording the blood pressure monitors the subject's radial pulse with one hand, and with the other hand inflates the manometer's bladder to about 30 to 40 mm Hg above the point at which the feeling of the pulse in the wrist disappears. Next, the pressure is released, followed by a wait of about one minute, and then the bladder is inflated to the predetermined level to take the blood pressure reading. The cuff should not be overinflated, as this may cause blood vessel spasm, resulting in higher blood pressure readings. The pressure should be released at a rate of 2 to 4 mm Hg per second.

As the pressure is released, **systolic blood pressure** is recorded as the point where the sound of the pulse becomes audible. The **diastolic blood pressure** is the point where the sound disappears. The recordings should be expressed as systolic over diastolic pressure—for example, 124/80.

If you take more than one reading, be sure the bladder is completely deflated between readings and allow at least a full minute before making the next recording. The person measuring the pressure also should note whether the pressure was recorded from the left or the right arm. Resting blood pressure ratings are given in Table 1.4.

In some cases the pulse sounds become less intense (point of muffling sounds) but still can be heard at a lower pressure (50 or 40 mm Hg) or even all the way down to zero. In this situation the diastolic pressure is recorded at the point of a clear, definite change in the loudness of the sound (also referred to as fourth phase), and at complete disappearance of the sound (fifth phase) (for example, 120/78/60 or 120/82/0).

To establish the real values for resting blood pressure, have different people take readings at different times of the day. A single reading may not be an accurate value because of the various factors that can affect blood pressure.

Sphygmomanometer Inflatable bladder contained within a cuff and a mercury gravity manometer (or aneroid manometer) from which the pressure is read.

Systolic blood pressure Pressure exerted by blood against walls of arteries during forceful contraction (systole) of the heart.

Diastolic blood pressure Pressure exerted by the blood against the walls of the arteries during the relaxation phase (diastole) of the heart.

TABLE 1.4 Blood Pressure Guidelines (expressed in mm Hg)

Rating	Systolic	Diastolic
Normal	≤120	≤80
Prehypertension	120–139	80–89
Hypertension	≥140	≥90

Source: National Heart, Lung and Blood Institute, April 2008

ASSESS YOUR KNOWLEDGE

1. Bodily movement produced by skeletal muscles is called
   a. physical activity.
   b. kinesiology.
   c. exercise.
   d. aerobic exercise.
   e. muscle strength.

2. Most people in Canada
   a. get adequate physical activity on a regular basis.
   b. meet health-related fitness standards.
   c. regularly participate in skill-related activities.
   d. Choices a, b, and c are correct.
   e. do not get sufficient physical activity to maintain good health.

3. The constant and deliberate effort to stay healthy and achieve the highest potential for well-being is defined as
   a. health.
   b. physical fitness.
   c. wellness.
   d. health-related fitness.
   e. metabolic fitness.

4. The ability to understand your own feelings and accept your limitations is known as
   a. mental wellness.
   b. social wellness.
   c. intellectual wellness.
   d. spiritual wellness.
   e. emotional wellness.

5. Research on the effects of fitness on mortality indicates that the largest drop in premature mortality is seen between
   a. the average and excellent fitness groups.
   b. the least fit and moderately fit groups.
   c. the good and high fitness groups.
   d. the moderately fit and good fitness groups.
   e. the drop is similar between all fitness groups.

6. Which of the following is *not* a component of health-related fitness?
   a. cardiorespiratory endurance
   b. body composition
   c. agility
   d. muscular strength and endurance
   e. muscular flexibility

7. Metabolic fitness can be achieved
   a. with an active lifestyle and moderate physical activity.
   b. through a high-intensity speed-training program.
   c. through an increased basal metabolic rate.
   d. with anaerobic training.
   e. through an increase in lean body mass.

8. The leading cause of death in Canada is
   a. cancer.
   b. accidents.
   c. CLRD.
   d. diseases of the cardiovascular system.
   e. drug-related deaths.

9. During the last few decades, health care costs in Canada
   a. have decreased.
   b. have stayed about the same.
   c. have continued to increase.
   d. have increased in some years and decreased in others.
   e. are unknown.

10. What is the greatest benefit of being physically fit?
    a. absence of disease
    b. a higher quality of life
    c. improved sports performance
    d. better personal appearance
    e. maintenance of ideal body weight

Correct answers can be found at the back of the book.

MEDIA MENU

INTERNET CONNECTIONS

■ Health Canada. This comprehensive government website supplies detailed data on the health of Canadians.

   http://www.hc-sc.gc.ca

■ Canadian Society for Exercise Physiology (CSEP). CSEP is a voluntary organization composed of professionals interested and involved in the scientific study of exercise physiology, exercise biochemistry, fitness, and health. The website offers the most up-to-date information regarding fitness and exercise for Canadians.

   http://www.csep.ca

■ The Canadian Health Network (CHN). CHN is a national, bilingual, health promotion designed to help Canadians find information on how to stay healthy and prevent disease. The network of health information providers includes the public Health Agency of Canada,

Health Canada, and national and provincial/territorial non-profit organizations, as well as universities, hospitals, libraries, and community organizations.

   http://www.canadian-health-network.ca

■ The Canadian Institute for Health Information (CIHI). CIHI is an independent, not-for-profit organization that provides essential data and analysis on Canada's health system and the health of Canadians. The institute's data and reports focus on health care services, health spending, health human resources, and population health.

   http://secure.cihi.ca/

■ LifeMD.com. This informative site provides essential fundamental health information to assist Canadians evaluate the vast amounts of medical news that becomes available every day around the world.

   http://www.lifemd.com/index.php

Notes

1. Christine Cameron, Rebecca Wolfe, and Cora Craig. *Physical Activity and Sport: Encouraging Children to Be Active*. Canadian Fitness and Lifestyle Research Institute, 2005 Physical Activity and Sport Monitor (June 5, 2007). Retrieved December 15, 2007, from http://www.cflri.ca/eng/archives.php.

2. Frank Booth, et al. "Physiologists Claim 'ScDS' Is Second Greatest Threat to U.S. Public Health," *Medical Letter on CDC & FDA*, June 24, 2001.

3. Statistics Canada. "Deaths 2003," The Daily, Wednesday, December 21, 2005. Retrieved December 18, 2007, from http://www.statcan.ca/Daily/English/051221/d051221b.htm.

4. World Health Organization, Core *Health Indicators.* http://www.who.int/whosis/database/core. 2006.

5. Statistics Canada. "Mortality, Summary, List of Causes 2004," *The Daily,* Friday, April 27, 2007. Retrieved December 20, 2007, from http://statcan.ca/Daily/English/070427/d070427b.htm.

6. Public Health Agency of Canada. *Economic Burden of Illness in Canada, 1998.* Released 2002.

7. P. T. Katzmarzyk, N. Gledhill, and R. J. Shephard, "The Economic Burden of Physical Inactivity in Canada," *Canadian Medical Association Journal* 28: 1435–440.

8. Statistics Canada, "Mortality, Summary, List of Causes 2004." Retrieved December 15, 2007, from http://statcan.ca/Daily/English/070427/d070427b.htm.

9. T.A. Murphy and D. Murphy, *The Wellness for Life Workbook* (San Diego: Fitness Publications, 1987).

10. S. E. Johannsson and J. Sundquist, "Change in Lifestyle Factors and Their Influence on Health Status and All-cause Mortality," *International Journal of Epidemiology* 28, 1073–080.

11. Coalition for Active Living, "About CAL." Retrieved December 12, 2007, from http://www.activeliving.ca/English/index.cfm?fa=About.Main.

12. Coalition for Active Living, "Investing in Prevention: A Business Plan to Increase Physical Activity in Canada," September 2006. Retrieved December 18, 2007, from http://www.activeliving.ca/pdf/PABusinessplanfinal.pdf.

13. H.G. Koenig, "The Healing Power of Faith," *Bottom Line/Health* 18 (May 2004): 3–4; "The Spiritual Side of Recovery," *Harvard Mental Health Letter* 24: 6; R. D. Fallot "Spirituality and Religion in Recovery: Some Current Issues, *Psychiatric Rehabilitation Journal* 30: 261–70.

14. K. Mystakidou, E. Tsilika, E. Parpa, M. Symrnoioti, and L. Viahos, "Assessing Spirituality and Religiousness in Advanced Cancer Patients," *American Journal and Palliative Medicine* 23: 457–63.

15. R. S. Paffenbarger, Jr., R. T. Hyde, A. L. Wing, and C. H. Steinmetz, "A Natural History of Athleticism and Cardiovascular Health," *Journal of the American Medical Association* 252: 491–95.

16. S. N. Blair, H. W. Kohl III, R. S. Paffenbarger, Jr., D. G. Clark, K. H. Cooper, and L.W. Gibbons, "Physical Fitness and All-Cause Mortality: A Prospective Study of Healthy Men and Women," *Journal of the American Medical Association* 262: 2395–401.

17. S. N. Blair, H. W. Kohl III, C. E. Barlow, R. S. Paffenbarger, Jr., L. W. Gibbons, and C.A. Macera, "Changes in Physical Fitness and All-Cause Mortality: A Prospective Study of Healthy and Unhealthy Men," *Journal of the American Medical Association* 273: 1193–198.

18. J. E. Enstrom, "Health Practices and Cancer Mortality Among Active California Mormons," *Journal of the National Cancer Institute* 81: 1807–814.

19. H. E. Kesteloot, "All Cause and Cardiovascular Mortality Worldwide: Lessons from Geopathology," *Journal of Cardiology* 37: 1–14.

20. G. A. Gaesser, "Exercise for Prevention and Treatment of Cardiovascular Disease, Type 2 Diabetes, and Metabolic Syndrome," *Current Diabetes Reports* 7: 14–19.

21. Canadian Institute for Health Information, *Health Care in Canada* 2007 (Ottawa: CIHI, 2007). Retrieved January 10, 2007, from http://secure.cihi.ca/cihiweb/products/hcic2007_e.pdf.

22. American College of Sports Medicine, *Guidelines for Exercise Testing and Prescription* (Baltimore: Williams and Wilkins, 2000).

23. D. Terbizan, B. Dolezal, and C. Albano, "Validity of Seven Commercially Available Heart Rate Monitors," *Measurement in Physical Education & Exercise Science.* 6: 243–47.

Suggested Readings

American College of Sports Medicine. ACSM Fit Society Page. http://acsm.org/health+fitness/fit_society.htm.

Blair, S. N., et al. "Influences of Cardiorespiratory Fitness and Other Precursors on Cardiovascular Disease and All-cause Mortality in Men and Women." *Journal of the American Medical Association* 276 (1996): 205–210.

Booth, F. W., and B. S. Tseng. "America Needs to Exercise for Health." *Medicine and Science in Sports and Exercise* 27 (1995): 462–465.

Hales, D., and L. Lauzon. *An Invitation to Health,* First Canadian ed. Toronto: Thomson Nelson, Canada Ltd. ,2007.

Hoeger, W. W. K., L. W. Turner, and B. Q. Hafen. *Wellness: Guidelines for a Healthy Lifestyle.* Belmont, CA: Wadsworth/Thomson Learning, 2002.

Katzmarzyk, P. T., C. L. Craig, and L. Gauvin. "Adiposity, Physical Fitness and Incident Diabetes: The Physical Activity Longitudinal Study." *Diabetologia* 50 (2007): 538–544.

Mason, C. Brien et al. "Musculoskeletal Fitness and Weight Gain in Canada." *Medicine Science in Sports Exercise* 39 (2007): 38–43.

National Academy of Sciences, Institute of Medicine. *Dietary Reference Intakes for Energy, Carbohydrates, Fiber, Fat, Protein and Amino Acids (Macronutrients).* Washington, DC: National Academy Press, 2002.

Nieman, D. C. *The Exercise-Health Connection.* Champaign, IL: Human Kinetics, 1998.

Pate, R., et al. "Physical Activity and Public Health: A Recommendation from the Centers for Disease Control and Prevention and the American College of Sports Medicine." *Journal of the American Medical Association* 273 (1995): 402–407.

Public Health Agency of Canada. "*Canada's Physical Activity Guide for Healthy Living.*" http://www.phac-aspc.gc.ca/pau-uap/fitness/pdf/handbook_e.pdf.

Lab 1C

RESTING HEART RATE AND BLOOD PRESSURE ASSESSMENT

Name: _____   Date: _____   Grade: _____

Instructor: _____   Course: _____   Section: _____

Necessary Lab Equipment

Stopwatches, stethoscopes, and blood pressure sphygmo-manometers.

Objective

To determine resting heart rate and blood pressure.

Preparation

The instructions to determine heart rate and blood pressure are given on pages 17–18. Many factors can affect heart rate and blood pressure. Factors such as excitement, nervousness, stress, food, smoking, pain, temperature, and physical exertion all can alter heart rate and blood pressure significantly. Therefore, whenever possible, readings should be taken in a quiet, comfortable room following a few minutes of rest in the recording position. Avoid any form of exercise several hours prior to the assessment. Wear exercise clothing, including a shirt with short or loose-fitting sleeves to allow for placement of the blood pressure cuff around the upper arm.

I. Resting Heart Rate and Blood Pressure

Determine your resting heart rate and blood pressure in the right and left arms while sitting comfortably in a chair.

Resting Heart Rate: _____ bpm   Rating (see Table 1.3, page 17): _____

Blood Pressure:	Right Arm	Rating (from Table 1.4, page 18)	Left Arm	Rating (from Table 1.4, page 18)
Systolic				
Diastolic				

II. Standing, Walking, Jogging Heart Rate, and Blood Pressure

Have one individual measure your heart rate and another individual your blood pressure immediately after standing for one minute, after walking for one minute, and after jogging in place for one minute. For blood pressure assessment use the arm that showed the highest reading in the sitting position (in Part I, above).

Activity	Heart Rate (bpm)	Systolic/Diastolic Blood Pressure (mm Hg)
Standing		/
Walking		/
Jogging		/

III. Effects of Aerobic Activity on Resting Heart Rate

Using your actual resting heart rate (RHR) from Part I of this lab, compute the total number of times your heart beats each day and each year:

A. Beats per day = _____ (RHR bpm) × 60 (min per hour) × 24 (hours per day) = _____ beats per day

B. Beats per year = _____ (heart rate in beats per day, use item A) × 365 = _____ beats per year

If your RHR dropped 20 bpm through an aerobic exercise program, determine the number of beats that your heart would save each year at that lower RHR:

C. Beats per day = _____ (RHR, use your current RHR) − 20 × 60 × 24 = _____ beats per day

D. Beats per year = _____ (heart rate in beats per day, use item C) × 365 = _____ beats per year

E. Number of beats saved per year (B − D) = _____ − _____ = _____ beats saved per year

Assuming that you will reach the average Canadian life expectancy of 82 years for women or 77 for men, determine the additional number of "heart rate life years" available to you if your RHR was 20 bpm lower:

F. Years of life ahead = _____ (use 82 for women and 77 for men) − _____ (current age) = _____ years

G. Number of beats saved = _____ (use item E) × _____ (use item F) = _____ beats saved

H. Number of heart rate life years based on the lower RHR = _____ (use item G) ÷ _____ (use item D) = _____ years

IV. Mean Blood Pressure Computation

During a normal resting contraction/relaxation cycle of the heart, the heart spends more time in the relaxation (diastolic) phase than in the contraction (systolic) phase. Accordingly, mean blood pressure (MBP) cannot be computed by taking an average of the systolic (SBP) and diastolic (DBP) blood pressures. The following equations are, therefore, used to determine MBP:

MBP = DBP + ⅓ PP   Where PP = pulse pressure or the difference between the systolic and diastolic pressures.

A. Compute your MBP using your own blood pressure results:

PP = _____ (systolic) − _____ (diastolic) = _____ mm Hg

MBP = _____ (DBP) + $\dfrac{\text{(PP)}}{3}$ = _____ mm Hg

B. Determine the MBP for a person with a BP of 130/80 and a second person with a BP of 120/90.

130/80	120/90

Which subject has the lower MBP? _____

V. What I Learned

Draw conclusions based on your observed resting and activity heart rates and blood pressures. Discuss the importance of a lower resting heart rate to your health and comment on the effects of a higher systolic versus diastolic blood pressure on the mean arterial blood pressure.

_____

_____

_____

_____

_____

_____

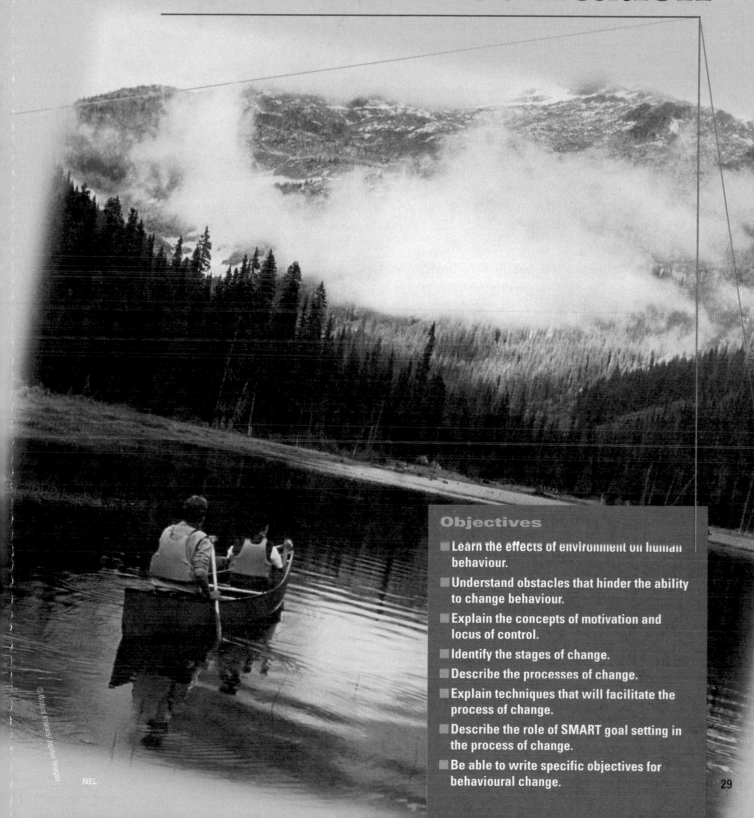

Chapter 2

Behaviour Modification

Objectives

- Learn the effects of environment on human behaviour.
- Understand obstacles that hinder the ability to change behaviour.
- Explain the concepts of motivation and locus of control.
- Identify the stages of change.
- Describe the processes of change.
- Explain techniques that will facilitate the process of change.
- Describe the role of SMART goal setting in the process of change.
- Be able to write specific objectives for behavioural change.

Research studies during the last three decades have convincingly documented the benefits of physical activity and healthy lifestyles. Two-thirds of Canadians strongly agree that a healthy lifestyle contributes to long-term benefits and the majority of Canadians fully intend to be active in the next six months.[1] However, 70 percent of new and returning exercisers are at risk for early dropout.[2] And, although the scientific evidence continues to mount each day and the data are impressive, most people still do not adhere to a healthy lifestyle program.

Let's look at an all-too-common occurrence on university and college campuses. Most students understand that they should be exercising and they contemplate enrolling in a fitness course. The motivating factor might be enhanced physical appearance, health benefits, or simply fulfillment of a college requirement. They sign up for the course, participate for a few months, finish the course—and stop exercising! A wide array of excuses are offered: too busy, no one to exercise with, already have the grade, inconvenient open-gym hours, or job conflicts. A few months later they realize once again that exercise is vital and repeat the cycle (see Figure 2.1).

The information in this book will be of little value to you if you are unable to abandon negative habits and adopt and maintain new, healthy behaviours. Before looking at physical fitness and wellness guidelines, you will need to take a critical look at your behaviours and lifestyle—and most likely make some permanent changes to promote your overall health and wellness.

The science of behavioural therapy has established that most of the behaviours we adopt are a product of our environment—the forces of social influences we encounter and the thought processes we go through. This environment includes family, friends, peers, homes, schools, workplaces, television, radio, and movies, as well as our communities, country, and culture in general.

Unfortunately, when it comes to fitness and wellness, we live in a "toxic environment." From a young age, we are transported by parents, relatives, and friends who drive us nearly any place we need to go. We also watch them drive short distances to run errands. We see them take escalators and elevators and ride moving sidewalks at malls and airports. We notice that they use remote controls, pagers, and cell phones. We observe as they stop at fast-food restaurants and pick up super-sized, calorie-dense, high-fat meals. They watch television and surf the Net for hours at a time. Some smoke, some drink heavily, and some have hard-drug addictions. Others engage in risky behaviours by not wearing seat belts, drinking and driving, and having unprotected sex. All of these unhealthy habits can be passed along, unquestioned, to the next generation.

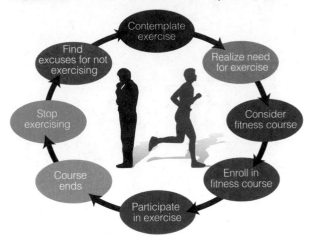

FIGURE 2.1 Exercise/exercise dropout cycle

Even modern-day architecture reinforces unhealthy behaviours, and elevators and escalators are often of the finest workmanship and located in convenient places. Many of our newest, showiest shopping centres and convention centres don't provide accessible stairwells, so people are all but forced to ride escalators. If they want to walk up the escalator, they can't because the people in front of them obstruct the way. Entrances to buildings provide electric sensors and automatic door openers. Without a second thought, people walk through automatic doors instead of taking the time to push a door open.

Walking, jogging, and bicycle trails are too sparse in our cities, further discouraging physical activity. Places for safe exercise are hard to find in many metropolitan areas, motivating many people to remain indoors during leisure hours for fear of endangering their personal safety and well-being.

Food portions in restaurants have substantially increased in size. Patrons consume huge amounts of food, almost as if this were the last meal they will ever have. They drink entire pitchers of soft drinks or beer instead of the traditional 250 mL size. Most restaurants are colourful, well-lit, and nicely decorated to enhance comfort and appetite and increase the length of stay to entice more eating.

All of these examples influence our thought process and hinder our ability to be physically active and adopt healthy behaviours. From childhood through young adulthood, we observe, we learn, we emulate, and gradually, without realizing it, we incorporate many of these unhealthy behaviours into our personal lifestyle.

Let's look at weight gain. Most people do not start life with a weight problem. By age 20, a man may weigh 70 kg. A few years later, the weight starts to

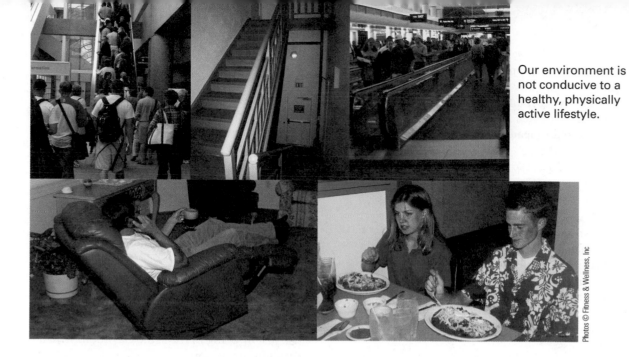

Our environment is not conducive to a healthy, physically active lifestyle.

climb and may reach 75 kg. He now adapts and accepts 75 kg as his weight. He may go on a diet but not make the necessary lifestyle changes. Gradually his weight climbs to 80, 85, 90 kg. Although he may not like it and would like to weigh less, once again he adapts and accepts 90 kg as his stable weight.

The time comes, usually around middle age, when most people want to make changes in their lives but find this difficult to accomplish, illustrating the adage that "old habits die hard." Acquiring positive behaviours that will lead to better health and well-being is a long-lasting process and requires continual effort. Understanding why so many people are unsuccessful at changing their behaviours and are unable to live a healthy lifestyle may increase your readiness and motivation for change. Next we will examine barriers to change, what motivates people to change, the various stages of change, the process of change, techniques for change, and actions required to make permanent changes in behaviour.

Barriers to Change

In spite of the best intentions, people make unhealthy choices daily. The most common reasons are:

1. **Procrastination.** People seem to think that tomorrow, next week, or after the holiday is the best time to start change.

    Tip to initiate change. Ask yourself: Why wait until tomorrow when you can start changing today? Lack of motivation is a key factor in procrastination (motivation is discussed on page 33).

2. **Preconditioned cultural beliefs.** If we accept the principle that we are a product of our environment, our cultural beliefs and our physical surroundings pose significant barriers to change.

    Tip to initiate change. Find a like-minded partner. In the pre-Columbian era, people thought the world was flat. Few dared to sail long distances for fear that they would fall off the edge. If your health and fitness are at stake, preconditioned cultural beliefs shouldn't keep you from making changes. Finding people who are willing to "sail" with you will help overcome this barrier.

3. **Gratification.** People prefer instant gratification to long-term benefits. Therefore, they will overeat (instant pleasure) instead of using self-restraint to eat moderately to prevent weight gain (long-term satisfaction). We like tanning (instant gratification) and avoid paying much attention to skin cancer (long-term consequence).

    Tip to initiate change. Think ahead and ask yourself the following questions: How did you feel the last time you engaged in this behaviour? How did it affect you? Did you really feel good about yourself or about the results? In retrospect, was it worth it?

4. **Risk complacency.** Consequences of unhealthy behaviours often don't manifest themselves until years later. People tell themselves, "If I get heart disease, I'll deal with it then. For now, let me eat, drink, and be merry."

    Tip to initiate change. Ask yourself these questions: How long do you want to live? How do you want to live the rest of your life and what type of health do you want to have? What do you want to be able to do when you are 60, 70, or 80 years old?

5. **Complexity.** People think the world is too complicated, with too much to think about. If you are living the typical lifestyle, you may feel overwhelmed by everything that seems to be required to lead a healthy lifestyle, for example:

- Getting exercise
- Decreasing saturated fat intake
- Eating high-fibre meals and cutting total calories
- Controlling use of substances
- Managing stress
- Wearing seat belts
- Practising safe sex
- Getting annual physicals, including blood tests, Pap smears, and so on
- Fostering spiritual, social, and emotional wellness

   Tip to initiate change. Take it one step at a time. Work on only one or two behaviours at a time so the task won't seem insurmountable.

6. **Indifference and helplessness.** A defeatist thought process often takes over, and we may believe that the way we live won't really affect our health, that we have no control over our health, or that our destiny is all in our genes (also see discussion of locus of control, page 33).

   Tip to initiate change. In Canada, about two-thirds of all deaths are due to cardiovascular disease (heart disease and stroke), cancer, chronic obstructive lung disease (bronchitis and emphysema), and diabetes. It is very unfortunate as these deaths are largely preventable.[3] Realize that only you can take control over your personal health and lifestyle habits and affect the quality of your life. Implementing many of the behavioural modification strategies and programs outlined in this book will get you started on a wellness way of life.

7. **Rationalization.** Even though people are not practising healthy behaviours, they often tell themselves that they do get sufficient exercise, that their diet is fine, that they have good solid relationships, or that they really don't smoke/drink/get high enough to affect their health.

   Tip to initiate change. Learn to recognize when you're glossing over or minimizing a problem. You'll need to face the fact that you have a problem before you can really commit to change. Your health and your life are at stake. Monitoring lifestyle habits through daily logs and then analyzing the results can help you make necessary changes in self-defeating behaviours.

8. **Illusions of invincibility.** At times people believe that unhealthy behaviours will not harm them. Young adults often have the attitude that "I can smoke now, and in a few years I'll quit before it causes any damage." Unfortunately, nicotine is one of the most addictive drugs known to us, so quitting smoking is not an easy task. Health problems may arise before you quit, and the risk of lung cancer lingers for years after you quit. Another example is drinking and driving. The feeling of "I'm in control" or "I can handle it" while under the influence is a deadly combination.

   Others perceive low risk when engaging in negative behaviours with people they like (for example, sex with someone you've recently met and feel attracted to) but perceive themselves at risk just by being in the same classroom with an HIV-infected person.

   Tip to initiate change. No one is immune to sickness, disease, and tragedy. The younger you are when you implement a healthy lifestyle, the better are your odds for a long and healthy life. Thus, initiating change right now will help you enjoy the best possible quality of life for as long as you live.

When health and appearance begin to deteriorate—usually around middle age—people seek out health care professionals in search of a "magic pill" to reverse and cure the many ills accumulated during years of abuse and overindulgence. The sooner we implement a healthy lifestyle program, the greater will be the health benefits and quality of life that lie ahead.

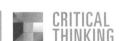

CRITICAL THINKING

What barriers to exercise do you encounter most frequently? How about barriers that keep you from managing your daily caloric intake?

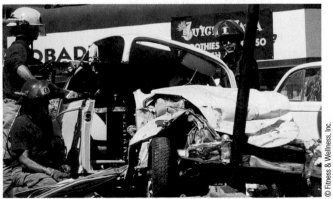

Feelings of invincibility are a strong barrier to change that can bring about life-threatening consequences.

Motivation and Locus of Control

The explanation given for why some people succeed and others do not is often **motivation**. Although motivation comes from within, external factors trigger the inner desire to accomplish a given task. These external factors, then, control behaviour.

When studying motivation, understanding **locus of control** is helpful. People who believe they have control over events in their lives are said to have an *internal locus of control*. People with an *external locus of control* believe that what happens to them is a result of chance or the environment and is unrelated to their behaviour. People with an internal locus of control generally are healthier and have an easier time initiating and adhering to a wellness program than those who perceive that they have no control and think of themselves as powerless and vulnerable. The latter people also are at greater risk for illness. When illness does strike a person, establishing a sense of control is vital to recovery.

Few people have either a completely external or a completely internal locus of control. They fall somewhere along a continuum. The more external one's locus of control is, the greater is the challenge to change and adhere to exercise and other healthy lifestyle behaviours. Fortunately, people can develop a more internal locus of control. Understanding that most events in life are not determined genetically or environmentally helps people pursue goals and gain control over their lives. Three impediments, however, can keep people from taking action: lack of competence, confidence, and motivation.[4]

1. *Problems of competence.* Lacking the skills to get a given task done leads to reduced competence. If your friends play hockey or basketball regularly but you don't know how to play, you might be inclined not to participate. The solution to this problem of competence is to master the skills you need to participate. Most people are not born with all-inclusive natural abilities, including playing sports.

   Another alternative is to select an activity in which you are skilled. It may be aerobics. Don't be afraid to try new activities. Similarly, if your body weight is a problem, you could learn to cook healthy, low-calorie meals. Try different recipes until you find foods that you like.

2. *Problems of confidence.* Problems with confidence arise when you have the skill but don't believe you can get it done. Fear and feelings of inadequacy often interfere with ability to perform the task. You shouldn't talk yourself out of something until you have given it a fair try. If the skills are there, the sky is the limit. Initially, try to visualize yourself doing the task and getting it done. Repeat this several times, then actually try it. You will surprise yourself.

   Sometimes, lack of confidence arises when the task seems insurmountable. In these situations, dividing a goal into smaller, more realistic objectives helps to accomplish the task. You might know how to swim but may need to train for several weeks to swim a continuous distance. Set up your training program so you swim a little farther each day until you are able to swim the entire desired distance. If you don't meet your objective on a given day, try it again, reevaluate, cut back a little, and, most important, don't give up.

3. *Problems of motivation.* With problems of motivation, both the competence and the confidence are there, but individuals are unwilling to change because the reasons to change are not important to them. For example, people begin contemplating a smoking cessation program only when the reasons for quitting outweigh the reasons for smoking. The primary causes of unwillingness to change are lack of knowledge and lack of goals. Knowledge often determines goals, and goals determine motivation. How badly you want something dictates how hard you'll work at it.

An interesting study by Kilpatrick et al. (2005) on college student's motivation for physical activity found that when participants engaged in a sport activity, they reported intrinsic motives such as enjoyment and challenge. When participating in an exercise program, they reported more extrinsic factors such as appearance and weight management. The authors suggest that participation in sport activities might be more desirable to students wanting to adhere to suggested physical activity recommendations.[5]

There are numerous other theories that attempt to explain why some individuals are motivated to adhere to exercise programs and others are not, such as the Theory of Planned Behaviour[6] and the Self-Determination Theory.[7] However, it may also be that some people are just unaware of the magnitude of the benefits of a wellness program. When it comes to a healthy lifestyle, however, you may not get a second chance. A stroke, a heart attack, or cancer can have irreparable or fatal consequences. Greater understanding of what leads to disease may be all you need to initiate change.

Motivation The desire and will to do something.

Locus of control A concept examining the extent to which a person believes he or she can influence the external environment.

BEHAVIOUR MODIFICATION

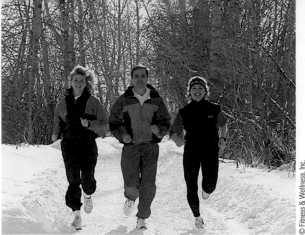
The higher quality of life experienced by people who are physically fit is hard to explain to someone who has never achieved good fitness.

Also, feeling physically fit is difficult to explain unless you have experienced it yourself. Feelings of fitness, self-esteem, confidence, health, and better quality of life cannot be conveyed to someone who is constrained by sedentary living. In a way, wellness is like reaching the top of a mountain. The quiet, the clean air, the lush vegetation, the flowing water in the river, the wildlife, and the majestic valley below are difficult to explain to someone who has spent a lifetime within city limits.

Changing Behaviour

Psychotherapy has been used successfully to help change behaviour. The great majority of people, however, do not seek professional help. They usually attempt change by themselves with limited or no knowledge of the process itself.

The simplest model of change is the two-stage model of unhealthy behaviour and healthy behaviour. This model states that either you do it or you don't. Most people who use this model attempt self-change but end up asking themselves why they're unsuccessful: They just can't do it (exercise, perhaps, or quitting smoking). Their intention to change may be good, but to accomplish it, they need knowledge about how to achieve change. The following discussion may help.

The Transtheoretical Model

For most people, changing chronic/unhealthy behaviours to stable/healthy behaviours is a challenging process. Change usually does not happen all at once. It is a gradual process that involves several stages. To aid with the process of self-change, psychologists James Prochaska, John Norcross, and Carlo DiClemente developed the Transtheoretical Model of Stages of Change.[8]

The transtheoretical model identifies five stages in the process of willful change. These stages describe underlying processes that people go through to change most problem behaviours and adopt healthy behaviours, and understanding the five stages will help you use this process. A sixth stage (termination/adoption) has subsequently been added to this model. Most frequently, the model is used to change health-related behaviours such as physical inactivity, smoking, poor nutrition, weight problems, stress, and alcohol abuse.

The six stages of change are precontemplation, contemplation, preparation, action, maintenance, and termination/adoption (see Figure 2.2). After years of study, researchers indicate that applying specific behavioural-change processes during each stage of the model increases the success rate for change (specific processes for each stage are shown in Table 2.1, page 37). Understanding each stage of this model will help you determine where you are in relation to your personal healthy-lifestyle behaviours. It will also help you identify processes to make successful changes.

Precontemplation

People in the **precontemplation stage** are not considering change or do not want to change a given behaviour. They typically deny having a problem and have no intention of changing in the immediate future. These people are usually unaware or under-aware of the problem. Other people around them, including family, friends, health care practitioners, and co-workers, however, identify the problem clearly. Precontemplators do not care about the problem behaviour and may even avoid information and materials that address the issue. They tend to avoid free screenings and workshops that might help identify and change the problem, even if they receive financial compensation for attendance. These people frequently have an active resistance to change and seem resigned to accepting the unhealthy behaviour as their "fate."

Precontemplators are the most difficult people to inspire toward behavioural change. Many think that change isn't even a possibility. At this stage, knowledge is power. Educating them about the problem behaviour is critical to help them start contemplating the process of change. The challenge is to find ways to help them realize that they are ultimately responsible for the consequences of their behaviour. Typically, they initiate change only when people they respect or job requirements pressure them to do so.

Contemplation

In the **contemplation stage**, people acknowledge that they have a problem and begin to think seriously about overcoming it. Although they are not

FIGURE 2.2 Stages of change model

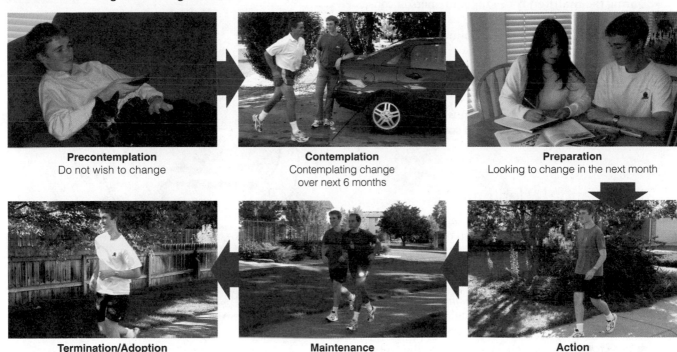

Precontemplation
Do not wish to change

Contemplation
Contemplating change
over next 6 months

Preparation
Looking to change in the next month

Termination/Adoption
Change has been maintained
for more than 5 years

Maintenance
Maintaining change for 5 years

Action
Implementing change for 6 months

quite ready for change, they are weighing the pros and cons of changing. Even though people may remain in this stage for years, in their minds they are planning to take some action within the next six months. Education and peer support remain valuable during this stage.

Preparation

In the **preparation stage**, people are seriously considering change and planning to change a behaviour within the next month. They are taking initial steps for change and may even try the new behaviour for a short while, such as stopping smoking for a day or exercising a few times during the month. During this stage, people define a general goal for behavioural change (for example, to quit smoking by the last day of the month) and write specific objectives to accomplish this goal (see the section on "Goal Setting" later in this chapter). Continued peer and environmental support are helpful during the preparation stage.

Action

This stage requires the greatest commitment of time and energy on the part of the individual.

Here people are actively doing things to change or modify the problem behaviour or to adopt a new health behaviour. The **action stage** requires that the person follow the specific guidelines set forth for that behaviour. For example, a person has actually stopped smoking completely, is exercising aerobically three times per week according to exercise prescription guidelines, or is maintaining a healthy diet. Relapse is common during this stage, and the individual may regress to previous stages. Once people maintain the action stage for six consecutive months, they move into the maintenance stage.

Precontemplation stage Stage of change in the transtheoretical model in which people are unwilling to change behaviour.

Contemplation stage Stage of change in the transtheoretical model in which people are considering changing behaviour within the next six months.

Preparation stage Stage of change in the transtheoretical model in which people are getting ready to make a change within the next month.

Action stage Stage of change in the transtheoretical model in which people are actively changing a negative behaviour or adopting a new, healthy behaviour.

Maintenance

During the **maintenance stage**, the person continues the new behaviour for up to five years. The maintenance phase requires continued adherence to the specific guidelines that govern the behaviour (such as complete smoking cessation, exercising aerobically three times per week, practising proper stress management techniques). At this time, the person works to reinforce the gains made through the various stages of change and strives to prevent lapses and relapse.

Termination/Adoption

Once a behaviour has been maintained for more than five years, a person is said to be in the **termination** or **adoption stage** and exits from the cycle of change without fear of relapse. In the case of negative behaviours that are terminated, the stage of change is referred to as *termination*. If a positive behaviour has been successfully adopted for over five years, this stage is designated as *adoption*. Some researchers have also labelled this stage the "transformed" stage of change because the word literally means "to have changed."[9]

Many experts believe that, once an individual enters the termination/adoption stage, former addictions, problems, or lack of compliance with healthy behaviours no longer present an obstacle in the quest for wellness. The change has now become part of one's lifestyle. This phase is the ultimate goal for all people searching for a healthier lifestyle.

For addictive behaviours such as alcoholism and hard drug use, however, many health care practitioners believe that the individual never enters the termination stage. Chemical dependency is so strong that most former alcoholics and hard-drug users must make a lifetime effort to prevent relapse. Similarly, some behavioural scientists suggest that the adoption stage might not be applicable to health behaviours such as exercise and weight control, because the likelihood of relapse is always high.[10]

Use the guidelines provided in Lab 2A to determine where you stand in respect to behaviours you want to change or new ones you wish to adopt. As you follow the guidelines, you will realize that you might be at different stages for different behaviours. For instance, you might be in the preparation stage for aerobic exercise and smoking cessation, in the action stage for strength training, but only in the contemplation stage for a healthy diet. Realizing where you are with respect to different behaviours will help you design a better action plan for a healthy lifestyle.

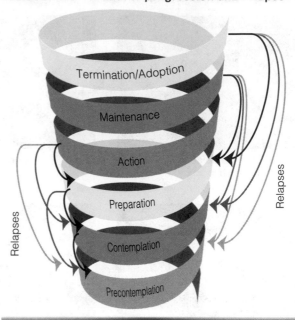

FIGURE 2.3 Model of progression and relapse

Relapse

After the precontemplation stage, **relapse** may occur at any level of the model. Even individuals in the maintenance and termination/adoption stages may regress to any of the first three stages of the model (see Figure 2.3). Relapse, however, does not mean failure. Failure comes only to those who give up and don't use prior experiences as a building block for future success. The chances of moving back up to a higher stage of the model are far better for someone who has previously made it into one of those stages.

The Process of Change

Using the same plan for every individual who wishes to change a behaviour will not work. With exercise, for instance, we provide different prescriptions to people of varying fitness levels (see Chapter 6). The same prescription would not provide optimal results for a person who has been inactive for 20 years, compared to one who already walks regularly three times each week. This principle also holds true for people who are attempting to change behaviours.

Timing is also important in the process of willful change. People respond more effectively to selected **processes of change** according to the stage of change they have reached at any given time.[11] Thus, applying appropriate processes at each stage of change enhances the likelihood of changing behaviour permanently. The following description of 14 of

TABLE 2.1 Applicable Processes of Change During Each Stage of Change

Precontemplation	Contemplation	Preparation	Action	Maintenance	Termination/Adoption
Consciousness-raising	Consciousness-raising	Consciousness-raising			
Social liberation	Social liberation	Social liberation	Social liberation		
	Self-analysis	Self-analysis			
	Emotional arousal	Emotional arousal			
	Positive outlook	Positive outlook	Positive outlook		
		Commitment	Commitment	Commitment	Commitment
		Behaviour analysis	Behaviour analysis		
		Goal setting	Goal setting	Goal setting	
		Self-reevaluation	Self-reevaluation	Self-reevaluation	
			Countering	Countering	
			Monitoring	Monitoring	Monitoring
			Environment control	Environment control	Environment control
			Helping relationships	Helping relationships	Helping relationships
			Rewards	Rewards	Rewards

Source: Adapted from J. O. Prochaska, J. C. Norcross, and C. C. DiClemente, *Changing for Good* (New York: William Morrow, 1994); and W. W. K. Hoeger and S. A. Hoeger, *Fitness & Wellness* (Belmont, CA: Wadsworth/Thomson Learning, 2002).

the most common processes of change will help you develop a personal plan for change. The respective stages of change where each process works best are summarized in Table 2.1.

Consciousness-Raising

The first step in a **behaviour modification** program is consciousness-raising. This process involves obtaining information about the problem so you can make a better decision about the problem behaviour. For example, the problem could be physical inactivity. Learning about the benefits of exercise or the difference in benefits between physical activity and exercise (see Chapter 1) can help you decide the type of fitness program (health or high fitness) that you want to pursue. It is also possible that you don't even know that a certain behaviour is a problem, such as unawareness of saturated and total fat content in many fast-food items. Consciousness-raising may continue from the precontemplation stage through the preparation stage.

Social Liberation

Social liberation stresses external alternatives that make you aware of problem behaviours and contemplate change. Examples of social liberation include pedestrian-only traffic areas, non-smoking areas, health-oriented cafeterias and restaurants,

advocacy groups, civic organizations, policy interventions, and self-help groups. Social liberation often provides opportunities to get involved, stir up emotions, and enhance self-esteem—helping you gain confidence in your ability to change.

Self-Analysis

The next process in modifying behaviour is a decisive desire to do so, called self-analysis. If you have no interest in changing a behaviour, you won't do it. You will remain a precontemplator or a contemplator. A person who has no intention of quitting smoking will not quit, regardless of what anyone may say or how strong the evidence in favour of quitting may be. In your self-analysis, you may want to prepare a list of reasons for continuing or discontinuing the

Maintenance stage Stage of change in the transtheoretical model in which people maintain behavioural change for up to five years.

Termination/adoption stage Stage of change in the transtheoretical model in which people have eliminated an undesirable behaviour or maintained a positive behaviour for more than five years.

Relapse (v.) To slip or fall back into unhealthy behaviour(s); or (n.) failure to maintain healthy behaviours.

Processes of change Actions that help you achieve change in behaviour.

Behavioural modification The process of permanently changing negative behaviours to positive behaviours that will lead to better health and well-being.

behaviour. When the reasons for changing outweigh the reasons for not changing, you are ready for the next stage—either the contemplation stage or the preparation stage.

Emotional Arousal

In emotional arousal, a person experiences and expresses feelings about the problem and its solutions. Also referred to as "dramatic release," this process often involves deep emotional experiences. Watching a loved one die from lung cancer caused by cigarette smoking may be all that is needed to make a person quit smoking. As other examples, emotional arousal might be prompted by a dramatization of the consequences of drug use and abuse, a film about a person undergoing open-heart surgery, or a book illustrating damage to body systems as a result of unhealthy behaviours.

Positive Outlook

Having a positive outlook means taking an optimistic approach from the beginning and believing in yourself. Following the guidelines in this chapter will help you design a plan so you can work toward change and remain enthusiastic about your progress. Also, you may become motivated by looking at the outcome—how much healthier you will be, how much better you will look, or how far you will be able to jog.

Commitment

Upon making a decision to change, you accept the responsibility to change and believe in your ability to do so. During the commitment process, you engage in preparation and may draw up a specific plan of action. Write down your goals and, preferably, share them with others. In essence, you are signing a behavioural contract for change. You will be more likely to adhere to your program if others know you are committed to change.

Behaviour Analysis

Now you determine the frequency, circumstances, and consequences of the behaviour to be altered or implemented, called behaviour analysis. If the desired outcome is to consume less saturated fat, you first must find out what foods in your diet are high in saturated fat, when you eat them, and when you don't eat them—all part of the preparation stage. Knowing when you don't eat them points to circumstances under which you exert control of your diet and will help as you set goals.

BEHAVIOUR MODIFICATION PLANNING

STEPS FOR SUCCESSFUL BEHAVIOUR MODIFICATION

1. Acknowledge that there is a problem.
2. Describe the behaviour to change (increase physical activity, stop overeating, quit smoking).
3. List advantages and disadvantages of changing the specified behaviour.
4. Decide positively that you will change.
5. Identify your stage of change.
6. Set a realistic goal (SMART goal), completion date, and sign a behavioural contract.
7. Define your behavioural change plan: List processes of change, techniques of change, and objectives that will help you reach your goal.
8. Implement the behavioural change plan.
9. Monitor your progress toward the desired goal.
10. Periodically evaluate and reassess your goal.
11. Reward yourself when you achieve your goal.
12. Maintain the successful change for good.

Goals

Goals motivate change in behaviour. The stronger the goal or desire, the more motivated you'll be either to change unwanted behaviours or to implement new, healthy behaviours. The discussion on goal setting (pages 42–43) will help you write goals and prepare an action plan to achieve those goals. This will aid with behaviour modification.

Self-Reevaluation

During the process of self-evaluation, individuals analyze their feelings about a problem behaviour. The pros and cons or advantages and disadvantages of a certain behaviour can be reevaluated at this time. For example, you may decide that strength training will help you tone up and boost your metabolism, but implementing this change will require you to stop watching an hour of TV three times per week. If you presently have a weight problem and are unable to lift certain objects around the house, you may feel good about weight loss and enhanced physical capacity as a result of a strength-training program. You might also visualize what it would be like if you were successful at changing.

Countering

The process whereby you substitute healthy behaviours for a problem behaviour, known as countering, is critical in changing behaviours as part of the action and maintenance stages. You need to replace unhealthy behaviours with new, healthy ones. You can

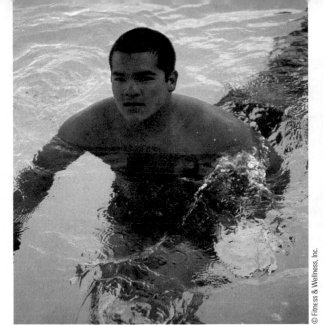

Countering: Substituting healthy behaviours for problem behaviours facilitates change.

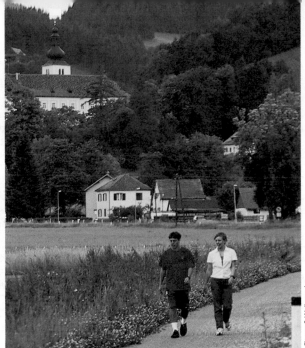

Rewarding oneself when a goal is achieved, such as scheduling a weekend getaway, is a powerful tool during the process of change.

use exercise to combat sedentary living, smoking, stress, or overeating. You may also use exercise, diet, yardwork, volunteer work, or reading to prevent overeating and achieve recommended body weight.

Monitoring

During the action and maintenance stages, continuous behaviour monitoring increases awareness of the desired outcome. Sometimes this process of monitoring is sufficient in itself to cause change. For example, keeping track of daily food intake reveals sources of excessive fat in the diet. This can help you gradually cut down or completely eliminate high-fat foods. If the goal is to increase daily intake of fruit and vegetables, keeping track of the number of servings consumed each day raises awareness and may help increase intake.

Environment Control

In environment control, the person restructures the physical surroundings to avoid problem behaviours and decrease temptations. If you don't buy alcohol, you can't drink any. If you shop on a full stomach, you can reduce impulse-buying of junk food.

Similarly, you can create an environment in which exceptions become the norm, and then the norm can flourish. Instead of bringing home cookies for snacks, bring fruit. Place notes to yourself on the refrigerator and pantry to avoid unnecessary snacking. Place baby carrots or sugarless gum where you used to place cigarettes. Post notes around the house to remind you of your exercise time. Leave exercise shoes and clothing by the entry way so they are visible as you walk into your home. Put an electric

timer on the TV so it will shut off automatically at 7:00 P.M. All of these tactics will be helpful throughout the action, maintenance, and termination/adoption stages.

Helping Relationships

Surrounding yourself with people who will work toward a common goal with you or those who care about you and will encourage you along the way—helping relationships—will be helpful during the action, maintenance, and termination/adoption stages.

Attempting to quit smoking, for instance, is easier when a person is around others who are trying to quit as well. The person could also get help from friends who have quit smoking already. Losing weight is difficult if meal planning and cooking are shared with roommates who enjoy foods that are high in fat and sugar. This situation can be even worse if a roommate also has a weight problem and does not desire to lose weight.

Peer support is a strong incentive for behavioural change. During this process, the individual should avoid people who will not be supportive. Friends who have no desire to quit smoking or to lose weight, or whatever behaviour a person is trying to change, may tempt one to smoke or overeat and encourage relapse into unwanted behaviours.

People who have achieved the same goal already may not be supportive either. For instance, someone may say, "I can do 10 consecutive kilometres." Your response should be, "I'm proud that I can jog 5 consecutive kilometres."

TABLE 2.2 Sample Techniques for Use With Processes of Change

Process	Techniques
Consciousness-Raising	Become aware that there is a problem, read educational materials about the problem behaviour or about people who have overcome this same problem, find out about the benefits of changing the behaviour, watch an instructional program on television, visit a therapist, talk and listen to others, ask questions, take a class.
Social Liberation	Seek out advocacy groups (Overeaters Anonymous, Alcoholics Anonymous), join a health club, buy a bike, join a neighbourhood walking group, work in nonsmoking areas.
Self-Analysis	Become aware that there is a problem, question yourself on the problem behaviour, express your feelings about it, analyze your values, list advantages and disadvantages of continuing (smoking) or not implementing a behaviour (exercise), take a fitness test, do a nutrient analysis.
Emotional Arousal	Practise mental imagery of yourself going through the process of change, visualize yourself overcoming the problem behaviour, do some role-playing in overcoming the behaviour or practising a new one, watch dramatizations (a movie) of the consequences or benefits of your actions, visit an auto salvage yard or a drug rehabilitation centre.
Positive Outlook	Believe in yourself, know that you are capable, know that you are special, draw from previous personal successes.
Commitment	Just do it, set New Year's resolutions, sign a behavioural contract, set start and completion dates, tell others about your goals, work on your action plan.
Behaviour Analysis	Prepare logs of circumstances that trigger or prevent a given behaviour and look for patterns that prompt the behaviour or cause you to relapse.
Goal Setting	Write goals and objectives; design a specific action plan.
Self-Reevaluation	Determine accomplishments and evaluate progress, rewrite goals and objectives, list pros and cons, weigh sacrifices (can't eat out with others) versus benefits (weight loss), visualize continued change, think before you act, learn from mistakes, and prepare new action plans accordingly.
Countering	Seek out alternatives: Stay busy, walk (don't drive), read a book (instead of snacking), attend alcohol-free socials, carry your own groceries, mow your yard, dance (don't eat), go to a movie (instead of smoking), practise stress management.
Monitoring	Use exercise logs (days exercised, sets and resistance used in strength training), keep journals, conduct nutrient analyses, count grams of fat, count number of consecutive days without smoking, list days and type of relaxation technique(s) used.
Environment Control	Rearrange your home (no TVs, ashtrays, large-sized cups), get rid of unhealthy items (cigarettes, junk food, alcohol), then avoid unhealthy places (bars, happy hour), avoid relationships that encourage problem behaviours, use reminders to control problem behaviours (post notes indicating "don't snack after dinner" or "lift weights at 8:00 PM"). Frequent healthy environments (a clean park, a health club, restaurants with low-fat/low-calorie/nutrient-dense menus, friends with goals similar to yours).
Helping Relationships	Associate with people who have and want to overcome the same problem, form or join self-help groups, join community programs specifically designed to deal with your problem (eating disorders, substance abuse control, smoking cessation).
Rewards	Go to a movie, buy a new outfit or shoes, buy a new bike, go on a weekend get-away, reassess your fitness level, use positive self-talk ("good job," "that felt good," "I did it," "I knew I'd make it," "I'm good at this").

Rewards

People tend to repeat behaviours that are rewarded and disregard those that are not rewarded or are punished. Rewarding oneself or being rewarded by others is a powerful tool during the process of change in all stages. If you have successfully cut down your caloric intake during the week, reward yourself by going to a show or buying a new pair of shoes. Do not reinforce yourself with destructive behaviours such as eating a high-fat/calorie-dense dinner. If you fail to change a desired behaviour (or to implement a new one), you may want to put off buying those new shoes you had planned for that week. When a positive behaviour becomes habitual,

give yourself an even better reward. Treat yourself to a weekend away from home or buy a new bicycle.

Techniques of Change

Not to be confused with the processes of change, you can apply any number of **techniques of change** within each process to help you through that specific process (see Table 2.2). For example, following dinner, people with a weight problem often can't resist continuous snacking during the rest of the evening until it is time to retire for the night. In the process of countering, for example, you can use various techniques to avoid unnecessary snacking. Examples include going for a walk, flossing

FIGURE 2.4 Stage of change identification and behaviour modification outline

Please indicate which response most accurately describes your current [_____] behaviour (in the blank space identify the behaviour: smoking, physical activity, stress, nutrition, weight control). Next, select the statement below (select only one) that best represents your current behaviour pattern. To select the most appropriate statement, fill in the blank for one of the first three statements if your current behaviour is a problem behaviour. (For example, you may say, "I currently smoke and I do *not* intend to change in the foreseeable future," or "I currently *do not exercise* but I am contemplating changing in the next six months.") If you have already started to make changes, fill in the blank in one of the last three statements. (In this case, you may say: "I currently *eat a low-fat diet* but I have only done so within the last six months," or "I currently *practise adequate stress management techniques* and I have done so for over six months.") As you can see, you may use this form to identify your stage of change for any type of health-related behaviour.

1. I currently [_____], and I do not intend to change in the foreseeable future.

2. I currently [_____], but I am contemplating changing in the next six months.

3. I currently [_____] regularly, but I intend to change in the next month.

4. I currently [_____], but I have done so only within the last six months.

5. I currently [_____], and I have done so for more than six months.

6. I currently [_____], and I have done so for more than five years.

and brushing your teeth right after dinner, going for a drive, playing the piano, going to a show, or going to bed earlier.

As you develop a behaviour modification plan, you need to identify specific techniques that may work for you within each process of change. A list of techniques for each process is provided in Table 2.2. This is only a sample list; dozens of other techniques may be used as well. For example, Behaviour Modification and Adherence to a Weight Management Program is found on page 143, A Lifetime Commitment to Fitness is presented on page 180, and stress management techniques are provided in Chapter 10. Some of the techniques can also be used with more than one process, visualization, for example, is helpful in emotional arousal and self-reevaluation.

Now that you are familiar with the stages of change in the process of behaviour modification, use Figure 2.4 and Lab 2A to identify two problem behaviours in your life. In this lab you will be asked to determine your stage of change for two behaviours according to six standard statements. Based on your

TABLE 2.3 Stage of Change Classification

Selected Statement (see Figure 2.4 and Lab 2A)	Classification
1	Precontemplation
2	Contemplation
3	Preparation
4	Action
5	Maintenance
6	Termination/Adoption

selection, determine the stage of change classification according to the ratings provided in Table 2.3. Next, develop a behaviour modification plan according to the processes and techniques for change that you have learned in this chapter. It will also be important to remember the results of a study by Marcus and Lewis[17] that individuals have differences across the stages of change. Individualized exercise plans appear to support adherence to the varying stages you will find yourself moving through. (Similar exercises to identify stages of change for other fitness and wellness behaviours are provided in labs for subsequent chapters.)

CRITICAL THINKING

Your friend John is a 20-year-old student who is not physically active. Exercise has never been a part of his life, and it has not been a priority in his family. He has decided to start a jogging and strength-training course in two weeks. Can you identify his current stage of change and list processes and techniques of change that will help him maintain a regular exercise behaviour?

Techniques of change Methods or procedures used during each process of change.

Goals The ultimate aims toward which effort is directed.

Goal Setting

To initiate change, **goals** are essential, as goals motivate behavioural change. Whatever you set out to accomplish, setting goals will provide the road map to help make your dreams a reality. Setting goals, however, is not as simple as it looks. Setting goals is more than just deciding what you want to do. A vague statement such as "I will lose weight" is not sufficient to help you achieve this goal.

SMART Goals

Only a well-conceived action plan will help you attain goals. Determining what you want to accomplish is the starting point, but to reach your goal you need to write **SMART** goals. The SMART acronym is used in reference to goals that are *S*pecific, *M*easurable, *A*cceptable, *R*ealistic, and *T*ime-specific. In Lab 2B you will have an opportunity to set SMART goals for two behaviours that you wish to change or adopt.

1. *Specific.* When writing goals, state exactly and in a positive manner what you would like to accomplish. For example, if you are overweight at 68 kilograms and at 27 percent body fat, to simply state "I will lose weight" is not a specific goal. Instead, re-write your goal to state "I will reduce my body fat to 20 percent body fat (62 kilograms) in 12 weeks."

   Be sure to write down your goals. An unwritten goal is simply a wish. A written goal, in essence, becomes a contract with yourself. Show this goal to a friend or an instructor and have him or her witness the contract you made with yourself by signing alongside your signature.

   Once you have identified and written down a specific goal, write the specific **objectives** that will help you reach that goal. These objectives are the necessary steps required to reach your goal. For example, a goal might be to achieve recommended body weight. Several specific objectives could be to

   (a) lose an average of 0.5 kilogram (or 1 fat percentage point) per week
   (b) monitor body weight before breakfast every morning
   (c) assess body composition every two weeks
   (d) limit fat intake to less than 25 percent of total daily caloric intake
   (e) eliminate all pastries from the diet during this time, and
   (f) walk/jog in the proper target zone for 60 minutes, six times per week.

2. *Measurable.* Whenever possible, goals and objectives should be measurable. For example, "I will lose weight" is not measurable, but "to reduce body fat to 20 percent" is measurable. Also note that all of the sample specific objectives (a) through (f) in Item 1 above are measurable. For instance, you can figure out easily whether you are losing a half a kilogram or a percentage point per week; you can conduct a nutrient analysis to assess your average fat intake; or you can monitor your weekly exercise sessions to make sure you are meeting this specific objective.

3. *Acceptable.* Goals that you set for yourself are more motivational than goals that someone else sets for you. These goals will motivate and challenge you and should be consistent with other goals that you have. As you set an acceptable goal, ask yourself: Do I have the time, commitment, and necessary skills to accomplish this goal? If not, you need to restate your goal so that it is acceptable to you.

   In instances where successful completion of a goal involves others, such as an athletic team or an organization, an acceptable goal must be compatible with those of the other people involved. If a team's practise schedule is set Monday through Friday from 4:00 to 6:00 P.M., it is unacceptable for you to train only three times per week or at a different time of the day.

   Acceptable goals are also embraced with positive thoughts. Visualize and believe in your success. As difficult as some tasks may seem, where there's a will, there's a way. A plan of action, prepared according to the guidelines in this chapter, will help you achieve your goals.

4. *Realistic.* Goals should be within reach. If you currently weigh 85 kg and your target weight (at 20 percent body fat) is 60 kg, setting a goal to lose 25 kg in a month would be unsound, if not impossible. Such a goal does not allow for the implementation of adequate behaviour modification techniques or ensure weight maintenance at the target weight. Unattainable goals only set you up for failure, discouragement, and loss of interest.

   On the other hand, do not write goals that are too easy to achieve and do not challenge you. If a goal is too easy, you may lose interest and stop working toward it.

   You can write both short-term and long-term goals. If the long-term goal is to attain recommended body weight and you are 25 kg overweight, you might set a short-term goal of losing 5 kg and write specific objectives to accomplish this goal. Then the immediate task will not seem as overwhelming and will be easier.

   At times, problems arise even with realistic goals. Try to anticipate potential difficulties as much as possible, and plan for ways to deal with them. If your goal is to jog for 30 minutes on six consecutive days, what are the alternatives if the weather turns bad? Possible solutions are to jog in the rain, find an indoor track, jog at a different time of day when the weather is better, or participate in a different aerobic activity such as stationary cycling, swimming, or step aerobics.

Monitoring your progress as you move toward a goal also reinforces behaviour. Keeping an exercise log or doing a body composition assessment periodically enables you to determine your progress at any given time.

5. *Time-specific.* A goal always should have a specific date set for completion. The above example to reach 20 percent body fat in 12 weeks is time-specific. The chosen date should be realistic but not too distant in the future. Allow yourself enough time to achieve the goal, but not too much time, as this could affect your performance. With a deadline, a task is much easier to work toward.

Goal Evaluation

In addition to the SMART guidelines provided above, you should conduct periodic evaluations of your goals. Reevaluations are vital for success. You may find that after you have fully committed and put all your effort into a goal, that goal may be unreachable. If so, reassess the goal.

Recognize that you will face obstacles, and you will not always meet your goals. Use your setbacks and learn from them. Rewrite your goal and create a plan that will help you get around self-defeating behaviours in the future. Once you achieve a goal, set a new one to improve upon or maintain what you have achieved. Goals keep you motivated.

SMART An acronym used in reference to *S*pecific, *M*easurable, *A*ttainable, *R*ealistic, and *T*ime-specific goals.

Objectives Steps required to reach a goal.

 ## ASSESS YOUR KNOWLEDGE

1. Most of the behaviours that people adopt in life are
   a. a product of their environment.
   b. learned early in childhood.
   c. learned from parents.
   d. genetically determined.
   e. the result of peer pressure.

2. Instant gratification is
   a. a barrier to change.
   b. a factor that motivates change.
   c. one of the six stages of change.
   d. the end result of successful change.
   e. a technique in the process of change.

3. The desire and will to do something is referred to as
   a. invincibility.
   b. confidence.
   c. competence.
   d. external locus of control.
   e. motivation.

4. People who believe they have control over events in their lives
   a. tend to rationalize their negative actions.
   b. exhibit problems of competence.
   c. often feel helpless over illness and disease.
   d. have an internal locus of control.
   e. often engage in risky lifestyle behaviours.

5. A person who is unwilling to change a negative behaviour because the reasons for change are not important enough is said to have problems of
   a. competence.
   b. conduct.
   c. motivation.
   d. confidence.
   e. risk complacency.

6. Which of the following is a stage of change in the Transtheoretical Model?
   a. recognition
   b. motivation
   c. relapse
   d. preparation
   e. goal setting

7. A precontemplator is a person who
   a. has no desire to change a behaviour.
   b. is looking to make a change in the next six months.
   c. is preparing for change in the next 30 days.
   d. willingly adopts healthy behaviours.
   e. is talking to a therapist to overcome a problem behaviour.

8. An individual who is trying to stop smoking and has not smoked for three months is in the
   a. maintenance stage.
   b. action stage.
   c. termination stage.
   d. adoption stage.
   e. evaluation stage.

9. The process of change where an individual obtains information to make a better decision about a problem behaviour is known as
   a. behaviour analysis.
   b. self-reevaluation.
   c. commitment.
   d. positive outlook.
   e. consciousness-raising.

10. A goal is effective when it is
    a. specific.
    b. measurable.
    c. time-specific.
    d. realistic.
    e. all of the above.

Correct answers can be found at the back of the book.

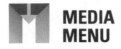

MEDIA MENU

INTERNET CONNECTIONS

■ Canadian Fitness and Lifestyle Research Institute (CFLRI) conducts research, monitors trends, and makes recommendations to increase levels of physical activity and improve the health of all Canadians.

www.cflri.ca

■ The Canadian Health Network (CHN) is a national, bilingual health promotion program with a mission of promoting healthy choices. The CHN's goal is to help Canadians find the information on how to stay healthy and prevent disease. Included as providers are Health Canada, the Public Health Agency of Canada, and many other organizations.

http://www.canadian-health-network.ca

■ Transtheoretical Model—Cancer Prevention Research Centre. This site describes the transtheoretical model, including descriptions of effective interventions to promote health behaviour change, focusing on the individual's decision-making strategies.

http://www.uri.edu/research/cprc/TTM/ detailedoverview.htm

■ Behaviour Change Theories. This very comprehensive site, by the Department of Health Promotion at California Polytechnic University at Pomona, describes all of the theories of behavioural change, including Learning Theories, Transtheoretical Model, Health Belief Model, Relapse Prevention Model, Reasoned Action and Planned Behaviour, Social Learning/Social Cognitive Theory, and Social Support.

http://www.csupomona.edu/~jvgrizzell/best_ practices/bctheory.html

■ How to Fit Exercise into Your Daily Routine. This site describes how you can incorporate simple exercises into your daily schedule—whether you're at home, at work, or spending time away with the family. Make time to exercise!

http://www.cdc.gov/nccdphp/dnpa/phys_act.htm

Notes

1. Advisory Committee on Population Health, "Advancing Integrated Prevention Strategies in Canada: An Approach to Reducing the Burden of Chronic Diseases," Discussion Paper, June 10, 2002.

2. J. Annesi, "Using Emotions to Empower Members for Long-Term Exercise Success," *Fitness Management* 17: 54–58.

3. A. A. Conti, C. Macchi, R. Molino Lova, A. Conti, and G. Gensini, "Relationship Between Physical Activity and Cardiovascular Disease: Selected Historical Highlights," *Journal of Sports Medicine & Physical Fitness* 47: 84–90.

4. G. S. Howard, D. W. Nance, and P. Myers, *Adaptive Counseling and Therapy* (San Francisco: Jossey-Bass, 1987).

5. M. Kilpatrick, E. Herbert, and J. Bartholomew, "College Students' Motivation for Physical Activity: Differentiating Men's and Women's Motives for Sport Participation and Exercise," *Journal of College Health* 54 (2005): 87–94.

6. I. Ajzen, "Perceived Behavioral Control, Self-Efficacy, Locus of Control, and the Theory of Planned Behavior," *Journal of Applied Social Psychology* 32 (2002): 665–83.

7. R. M. Ryan, "Motivation for Physical Activity Research on Persistence, Performance, and Enjoyment in Sport, Exercise, and Everyday Life from a Self-Determination Theory Viewpoint," *Journal of Sport & Exercise Psychology Supplement* 29 (2007): 3–10.

8. J. O. Prochaska, J. C. Norcross, and C. C. DiClemente, *Changing for Good* (New York: William Morrow, 1994.)

9. B. J. Cardinal, "Extended Stage Model of Physical Activity Behavior," *Journal of Human Movement Studies* 37 (1999): 37–54.

10. Cardinal, "Extended Stage Model of Physical Activity Behavior," 37–54.

11. B. H. Marcus, et al., "Evaluation of Motivationally Tailored vs. Standard Self-Help Physical Activity Interventions at the Workplace," *American Journal of Health Promotion* 12 (1998): 246–53.

12. B. Marcus and B. Lewis, "Physical Activity and the Stages of Motivational Readiness for Change Model," *President's Council on Physical Fitness and Sports Research Digest* Series 4. No. 1. March 2003.

Suggested Readings

Blair, S. N., et al. *Active Living Every Day*. Champaign, IL: Human Kinetics, 2001.

Bouchard, C., et al. *Physical Activity, Fitness, and Health*. Champaign, IL: Human Kinetics, 1994.

Brehm, B. *Successful Fitness Motivation Strategies*. Champaign, IL: Human Kinetics, 2004.

Carron, A. V., H. A. Hausenblas, and P. A. Estabrooks. *The Psychology of Physical Activity*. New York: McGraw Hill, 2003.

Dishman, R. *Advances in Exercise Adherence*. Champaign, IL: Human Kinetics, 1994.

Faulkner, G., and A. H. Taylor. *Exercise, Health and Mental Health: Emerging Relationships*. London: Routledge, 2005.

Leith, L. M. *Motivation to Diet and Exercise. Encyclopedia of Applied Psychology* (pp. 456–67). Exeter, UK: Elsevier Publishers, Inc., 2004.

Lox, C., K. A. Martin Ginis, and S. Petruzello. *The Psychology of Exercise: Integrating Theory and Practice* (2nd edition). Scottsdale, AZ: Holcomb Hathaway, 2006.

Marcus, B., and L. Forsyth. *Motivating People To Be Physically Active*. Champaign, IL: Human Kinetics, 2003.

Prochaska, J. O., J. C. Norcross, and C. C. DiClemente. *Changing for Good*. New York: William Morrow, 1994.

Samuelson, M. "Stages of Change: From Theory to Practice." *The Art of Health Promotion* 2 (1998): 1–7.

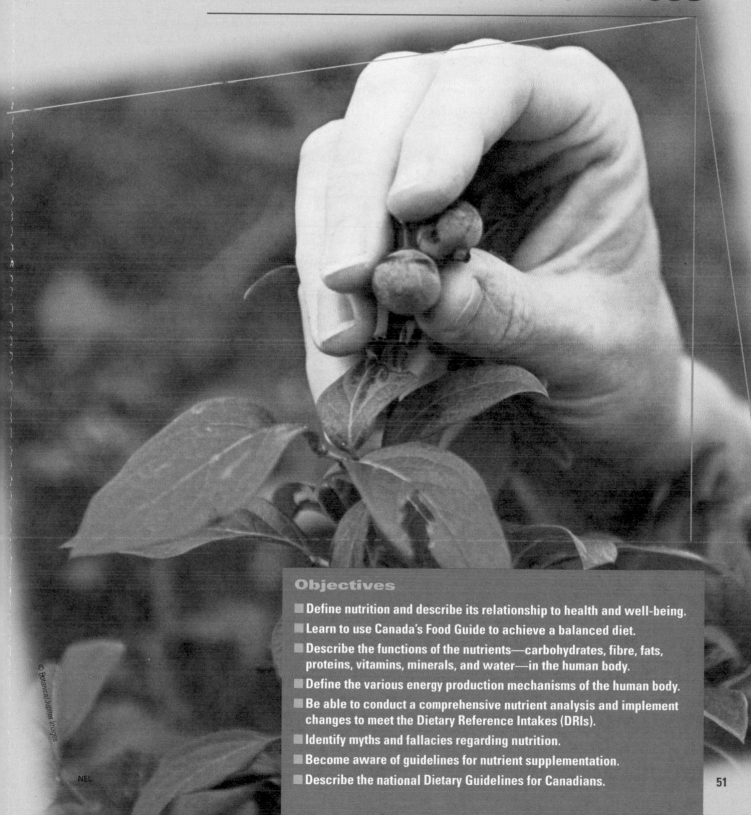

Chapter 3

Nutrition for Wellness

Objectives

- Define nutrition and describe its relationship to health and well-being.
- Learn to use Canada's Food Guide to achieve a balanced diet.
- Describe the functions of the nutrients—carbohydrates, fibre, fats, proteins, vitamins, minerals, and water—in the human body.
- Define the various energy production mechanisms of the human body.
- Be able to conduct a comprehensive nutrient analysis and implement changes to meet the Dietary Reference Intakes (DRIs).
- Identify myths and fallacies regarding nutrition.
- Become aware of guidelines for nutrient supplementation.
- Describe the national Dietary Guidelines for Canadians.

© Botanica/Jupiter Images

Scientific evidence has long linked good **nutrition** to overall health and well-being. Proper nutrition means that a person's diet supplies all the essential nutrients needed to carry out normal tissue growth, repair, and maintenance. The diet should also provide enough **substrates** to produce the energy necessary for work, physical activity, and relaxation. These **nutrients** should be obtained from a wide variety of sources. Figure 3.1 shows Canada's Food Guide with the recommended number of servings from each food group for proper nutrition.

Too much or too little of any nutrient can precipitate serious health problems. The typical North American diet is too high in calories, sugar, fat, saturated fat, and sodium, and not high enough in fibre—factors that undermine good health. Food availability is not the problem. The problem is overconsumption.

Diet and nutrition often play a crucial role in the development and progression of chronic diseases. A diet high in saturated fat and cholesterol increases the risk for atherosclerosis and coronary heart disease. In sodium-sensitive individuals, high salt intake has been linked to high blood pressure. Some researchers believe that 30 to 50 percent of all cancers are diet-related. Obesity, diabetes, and osteoporosis also have been associated with faulty nutrition.

To lower the risk for chronic disease, an effective wellness program must incorporate the nutritional recommendations for Canadians, as follows:

- Provide energy consistent with the maintenance of body weight within the recommended range.
- Include essential nutrients in amounts specified in the Recommended Nutrient Intakes.
- Include no more than 30 percent of energy as fat and no more than 10 percent as saturated fat.
- Provide at least half of energy as carbohydrates from a variety of sources.
- Reduce the amount of sodium.

FIGURE 3.1 Canada's Food Guide

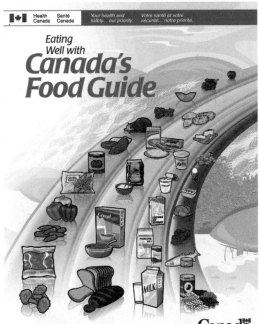

	Children			Teens		Adults			
Age in Years	2-3	4-8	9-13	14-18		19-50		51+	
Sex	Girls and Boys			Females	Males	Females	Males	Females	Males
Vegetables and Fruit	4	5	6	7	8	7-8	8-10	7	7
Grain Products	3	4	6	6	7	6-7	8	6	7
Milk and Alternatives	2	2	3-4	3-4	3-4	2	2	3	3
Meat and Alternatives	1	1	1-2	2	3	2	3	2	3

Recommended Number of *Food Guide Servings* per Day

The chart above shows how many Food Guide Servings you need from each of the four food groups every day.

Having the amount and type of food recommended and following the tips in *Canada's Food Guide* will help:

- Meet your needs for vitamins, minerals and other nutrients.
- Reduce your risk of obesity, type 2 diabetes, heart disease, certain types of cancer and osteoporosis.
- Contribute to your overall health and vitality.

A Closer Examination of Canada's Food Guide

Canada's Food Guide promotes a pattern of eating that will meet nutrient needs, promote health, and minimize the risk of nutrition-related chronic disease. Because the amount of food required every day will depend on a person's age, body size, activity level, sex, pregnancy, or breast-feeding status, the Food Guide provides a range of servings for each food group. Most individuals will select the middle servings, but other groups can choose according to their needs. For example, male teenagers can select the higher number and young children can select the lower number of servings.

Source: *Eating Well with Canada's Food Guide* (2007), http://www.hc-sc.gc.ca/fn-an/food-guide-aliment/index_e.html, Health Canada. Reproduced with the permission of the Minister of Public Works and Government Services Canada, 2008.

- Include no more than 5 percent of total energy as alcohol, or two drinks daily, whichever is less.
- Contain no more caffeine than the equivalent of four cups of regular coffee per day.

In addition, it is recommended that individuals get their drinking water from community water supplies, which must be fluoridated to a minimum level of 1 mg/L.

These guidelines will be discussed throughout this chapter and in later chapters of this book.

Nutrients

The essential nutrients the human body requires are carbohydrates, fat, protein, vitamins, minerals, and water. The first three are called *fuel nutrients* because they are the only substances the body uses to supply the energy (commonly measured in calories) needed for work and normal body functions. The three others—vitamins, minerals, and water—are regulatory nutrients. They have no caloric value, but still are necessary for a person to function normally and maintain good health. Many nutritionists add to this list a seventh nutrient: fibre. This nutrient has received a great deal of attention recently. Recommended amounts seem to provide protection against several diseases, including cardiovascular disease and some cancers.

Carbohydrates, fats, proteins, and water are termed *macronutrients* because we need them in proportionately large amounts daily. Vitamins and minerals are required in only small amounts—grams, milligrams, and micrograms—and nutritionists refer to them as *micronutrients*.

Depending on the amount of nutrients and calories they contain, foods can be classified by their **nutrient density**. Foods that contain few or a moderate number of calories but are packed with nutrients are said to have high nutrient density. Foods that have a lot of calories but few nutrients are of low nutrient density and are commonly called "junk food."

A **calorie** is the unit of measure indicating the energy value of food to the person who consumes it. It is also used to express the amount of energy a person expends in physical activity. Technically, a kilocalorie (kcal) is the amount of heat necessary to raise the temperature of 1 kg of water 1 degree Celsius. Thus, a calorie is the amount of heat necessary to raise the temperature of 1 g of water 1 degree Celsius. Confusion often arises as the public often (and incorrectly) uses the term "calorie" in place of the term "kcal." As we have shown, they are not the same since 1,000 Calories is equal to one kcal. To avoid confusion, the use of a capital "C" in calorie (Calorie) is often used to denote the use of kcals.

For example, if the caloric value of a food is 100 Calories (that is, 100 kcal) the energy in this food would raise the temperature of 100 kg of water 1 degree Celsius. Similarly, walking 1.6 km would burn about 100 Calories (again, 100 kcal).

Carbohydrates

Carbohydrates constitute the major source of calories the body uses to provide energy for work, maintain cells, and generate heat. They also help regulate fat and metabolize protein. Each gram of carbohydrates provides the human body with 4 Calories. The major sources of carbohydrates are breads, cereals, fruits, vegetables, and milk and other dairy products. Carbohydrates are classified into simple carbohydrates and complex carbohydrates (Figure 3.2).

SIMPLE CARBOHYDRATES
Often called "sugars," **simple carbohydrates** have little nutritive value. Examples are candy, soda, and cakes. Simple carbohydrates are divided into monosaccharides and disaccharides. These carbohydrates—whose names end with "-ose"—often take the place of more nutritive foods in the diet.

Monosaccharides The simplest sugars are **monosaccharides**. The three most common monosaccharides are glucose, fructose, and galactose.

1. *Glucose* is a natural sugar found in food and also is produced in the body from other simple and complex carbohydrates. It is used as a source of energy, or it may be stored in the muscles and liver in the form of glycogen (a long chain of glucose molecules hooked together). Excess glucose in the blood is converted to fat and stored in **adipose tissue**.

Nutrition Science that studies the relationship of foods to optimal health and performance.

Substrates Substances acted upon by an enzyme (examples: carbohydrates, fats).

Nutrients Substances found in food that provide energy, regulate metabolism, and help with growth and repair of body tissues.

Nutrient density A measure of the amount of nutrients and calories in various foods.

Calorie The amount of heat necessary to raise the temperature of 1 gram of water 1 degree Celsius; used to measure the energy value of food and cost (energy expenditure) of physical activity.

Carbohydrates A classification of dietary nutrient containing carbon, hydrogen, and oxygen; the major source of energy for the human body.

Simple carbohydrates Formed by simple or double sugar units with little nutritive value; divided into monosaccharides and disaccharides.

Monosaccharides The simplest carbohydrates (sugars), formed by five- or six-carbon skeletons. The three most common monosaccharides are glucose, fructose, and galactose.

FIGURE 3.2 Major types of carbohydrates

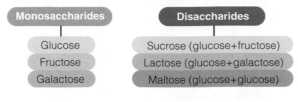

Simple carbohydrates

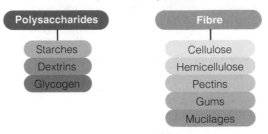

Monosaccharides
- Glucose
- Fructose
- Galactose

Disaccharides
- Sucrose (glucose+fructose)
- Lactose (glucose+galactose)
- Maltose (glucose+glucose)

Complex carbohydrates

Polysaccharides
- Starches
- Dextrins
- Glycogen

Fibre
- Cellulose
- Hemicellulose
- Pectins
- Gums
- Mucilages

2. *Fructose*, or fruit sugar, occurs naturally in fruits and honey and is converted to glucose in the body.
3. *Galactose* is produced from milk sugar in the mammary glands of lactating animals and is converted to glucose in the body.

Disaccharides   The three major **disaccharides** are:

1. *Sucrose* or table sugar (glucose + fructose).
2. *Lactose* (glucose + galactose).
3. *Maltose* (glucose + glucose).

These disaccharides are broken down in the body, and the resulting simple sugars (monosaccharides) are used as indicated above.

COMPLEX CARBOHYDRATES

Complex carbohydrates are also called *polysaccharides*. Anywhere from about ten to thousands of monosaccharide molecules can unite to form a single polysaccharide. Examples of complex carbohydrates are starches, dextrins, and glycogen.

1. *Starch*, the storage form of glucose in plants, is needed to promote their earliest growth. Starch is commonly found in grains, seeds, corn, nuts, roots, potatoes, and legumes. In a healthful diet, grains, the richest source of starch, should supply most of the energy. Once eaten, starch is converted to glucose for the body's own energy use.
2. *Dextrins* are formed from the breakdown of large starch molecules exposed to dry heat, such as in baking bread or producing cold cereals. These complex carbohydrates of plant origin provide many valuable nutrients and can be an excellent source of fibre.

3. **Glycogen** is the animal polysaccharide synthesized from glucose and is found only in tiny amounts in meats. In essence, we manufacture it; we don't consume it. Glycogen constitutes the body's reservoir of glucose. Thousands of glucose molecules are linked, to be stored as glycogen in the liver and muscle. When a surge of energy is needed, enzymes in the muscle and the liver break down glycogen and thereby make glucose readily available for energy transformation. (This process is discussed under "Nutrition for Athletes," starting on page 79.)

FIBRE

Fibre is a form of complex carbohydrate. A high-fibre diet gives a person a feeling of fullness without adding too many calories to the diet. **Dietary fibre** is present mainly in plant leaves, skins, roots, and seeds. Processing and refining foods removes almost all of their natural fibre. In our diet, the main sources of fibre are whole-grain cereals and breads, fruits, vegetables, and legumes.

Fibre is important in the diet because it decreases the risk for cardiovascular disease and cancer. Increased fibre intake also may lower the risk for coronary heart disease, because saturated fats often take the place of fibre in the diet, increasing the absorption and formation of cholesterol. Other health disorders that have been tied to low intake of fibre are constipation, diverticulitis, hemorrhoids, gallbladder disease, and obesity.

Over the past decade, nutrition surveys in Canada have revealed that many Canadians are not meeting the Adequate Intake (AI) recommendations. One example is data collected for the New Brunswick Nutrition survey, where only 1 percent of adult males and females under 50 years of age were meeting the recommendation. And although 15 percent of men 50 years and older were achieving the recommended Adequate Intake for fibre, only about 5 percent of women this age were.[1]

A person can increase fibre intake by eating more fruits, vegetables, legumes, whole grains, and whole-grain cereals. Research provides evidence that increasing fibre intake to 30 g per day leads to a significant reduction in heart attacks, cancer of the colon, breast cancer, diabetes, and diverticulitis. Table 3.1 provides the fibre content of selected foods. A practical guideline to obtain your fibre intake is to eat at least five daily servings of fruits and vegetables and three servings of whole-grain foods (whole-grain bread, cereal, and rice).

Fibre is typically classified according to solubility in water. *Soluble fibre* dissolves in water and forms a gel-like substance that encloses food particles. This property allows soluble fibre to bind and excrete fats from the body. This type of fibre has been shown to

BEHAVIOUR MODIFICATION PLANNING

TIPS TO INCREASE FIBRE IN YOUR DIET

- Eat more vegetables, either raw or steamed.
- Eat salads daily that include a wide variety of vegetables.
- Eat more fruit, including the skin.
- Choose whole-wheat and whole-grain products.
- Choose breakfast cereals with more than 3 g of fibre per serving.
- Sprinkle a spoonful or two of unprocessed bran or 100 percent bran cereal on your favourite breakfast cereal.
- Add high-fibre cereals to casseroles and desserts.
- Add beans to soups, salads, and stews.
- Add vegetables to sandwiches: sprouts, green and red pepper strips, diced carrots, sliced cucumbers, red cabbage, onions.
- Add vegetables to spaghetti: broccoli, cauliflower, sliced carrots, mushrooms.
- Experiment with unfamiliar fruits and vegetables—collards, kale, broccoflower, asparagus, papaya, mango, kiwi, starfruit.
- Blend fruit juice with small pieces of fruit and crushed ice.
- When increasing fibre in your diet, drink plenty of fluids.

lower blood cholesterol and blood sugar levels. Soluble fibre is found primarily in oats, fruits, barley, legumes, and psyllium (an ancient Indian grain added to some breakfast cereals).

Insoluble fibre is not easily dissolved in water, and the body cannot digest it. This type of fibre is important because it binds water, causing a softer and bulkier stool that increases **peristalsis**, the involuntary muscle contractions of intestinal walls that force the stool through the intestines and enable quicker excretion of food residues. Speeding the passage of food residues through the intestines seems to lower the risk for colon cancer, mainly because it reduces the amount of time that cancer-causing agents are in contact with the intestinal wall. Insoluble fibre is also thought to bind with carcinogens (cancer-producing substances), and more water in the stool may dilute the cancer-causing agents, lessening their potency.

Adipose tissue Fat cells in the body.

Disaccharides Simple carbohydrates formed by two monosaccharide units linked together, one of which is glucose. The major disaccharides are sucrose, lactose, and maltose.

Complex carbohydrates Carbohydrates formed by three or more simple sugar molecules linked together; also referred to as polysaccharides.

Glycogen Form in which glucose is stored in the body.

Dietary fibre A complex carbohydrate in plant foods that is not digested but is essential to the digestion process.

Peristalsis Involuntary muscle contractions of intestinal walls that facilitate excretion of wastes.

TABLE 3.1 Dietary Fibre Content of Selected Foods

Food	Portion	Fibre amount (grams)
10 g or more of fibre per serving		
Soybean kernels, roasted	175 mL or ¾ cup	22.5
All bran cereals	30 g or ½ cup or ⅓ cup (Bran Buds)	10–14*
Black beans, cooked or canned baked beans	175 mL or ¾ cup	10–11
6–9.9 g of fibre per serving		
Kidney and baked beans, cooked	175 mL or ¾ cup	~ 8
Lentils, cooked	175 mL or ¾ cup	6.2
4–5.9 g of fibre per serving		
Green peas, cooked	125 mL or ½ cup	5.6
Garbanzo beans (chickpeas), cooked	175 mL or ¾ cup	5.5
Pear, with skin	1 medium	5.0
Bran flakes	30 g or 1 cup	4–5*
Post Raisin Bran, Post Spoon Size Shredded Wheat, Quaker Oat Bran	30 g ~ ½ cup	4.2–4.5*
Split peas, cooked	175 mL or ¾ cup	4.2
Almonds, roasted	60 mL or ¼ cup	4.1
Blackberry or raspberry	125 mL or ½ cup	~ 4
Red River cereal, prepared	175 mL or ¾ cup	4.0
2–3.9 g of fibre per serving		
Mango	1 fruit	3.8
Sunflower seeds kernels, dried	60 mL or ¼ cup	3.8
Potato, with or without skin	1 medium	3.4–3.8
Post Shreddies or Kellogg's Raisin Bran	125 mL or ½ cup	3.4
Brussels sprouts	4 sprouts	3.0
Peanuts, dry, roasted	60 mL or ¼ cup	3.0
Stewed rhubarb, mixed vegetables or parsnips, cooked	125 mL or ½ cup	2.5–2.8
Kiwifruit	1 large	2.7
Cooked Quaker Oat Bran or oatmeal (large oats)	175 mL or ¾ cup	2.2–2.7
Apple with skin	1 medium	2.6
Peanut butter, chunk type	30 mL or 2 tbsp.	2.6
Whole-wheat bread, commercial	35 g or 1 slice	2.4
Whole-wheat spaghetti	125 mL or ½ cup	2.4
Corn, carrot, or broccoli, cooked	125 mL or ½ cup	2–2.3
Pear, canned halves	125 mL or ½ cup	2.1
Banana	1 medium	2.0
Brown rice, medium grain or pearl barley, cooked	125 mL or ½ cup	2.0
Dates, dried	3 dates	2.0
Flax seeds, ground	15 mL or 1 tbsp.	2.0
Snap beans (green, yellow, Italian), raw	125 mL or ½ cup	2.0

*Check the label
Fibre in Foods, BC HealthFile #68h, September 2007.
www.bchealthguide.org/healthfiles/hfile68h.stm#E46E3 Retrieved April, 2008.
Copyright © 2007, Province of British Columbia. Used with permission.

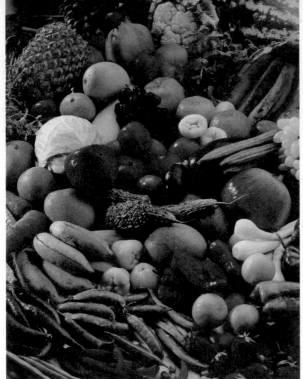

High-fibre foods are essential in a healthy diet.

Sources of insoluble fibre include wheat, cereals, vegetables, and skins of fruits.

The most common types of fibre are:

1. *Cellulose*, water-soluble fibre found in plant cell walls.
2. *Hemicellulose*, water-soluble fibre found in cereal fibres.
3. *Pectins*, water-insoluble fibre found in vegetables and fruits.
4. *Gums and mucilages*, water-insoluble fibre also found in small amounts in foods of plant origin.

Surprisingly, excessive fibre intake can be detrimental to health. It can produce loss of calcium, phosphorus, and iron, not to mention gastrointestinal discomfort. If your fibre intake is below the recommended amount, increase your intake gradually over several weeks to avoid gastrointestinal disturbances. While increasing fibre intake, be sure to drink more water to avoid constipation and even dehydration.

Fats

The human body uses **fats** as a source of energy. Fat is the most concentrated energy source. Each gram of fat supplies 9 Calories to the body (in contrast to 4 for carbohydrates). Fats are a part of the human cell structure. Deposits of fat cells are used as stored energy and as an insulator to preserve body heat. They absorb shock, supply essential fatty acids, and carry the fat-soluble vitamins A, D, E, and K. Fats can be classified into three main groups: simple, compound, and derived (see Figure 3.3). The most familiar sources of fat are whole milk and other dairy products, meats, and meat alternatives such as eggs and nuts.

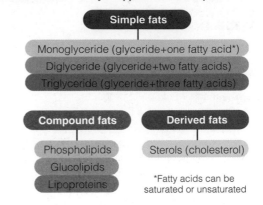

FIGURE 3.3 Major types of fats (lipids)

Simple fats
- Monoglyceride (glyceride+one fatty acid*)
- Diglyceride (glyceride+two fatty acids)
- Triglyceride (glyceride+three fatty acids)

Compound fats
- Phospholipids
- Glucolipids
- Lipoproteins

Derived fats
- Sterols (cholesterol)

*Fatty acids can be saturated or unsaturated

SIMPLE FATS

A simple fat consists of a glyceride molecule linked to one, two, or three units of fatty acids. Depending on the number of fatty acids attached, simple fats are divided into *monoglycerides* (one fatty acid), *diglycerides* (two fatty acids), and *triglycerides* (three fatty acids). More than 90 percent of the weight of fat in foods and more than 95 percent of the stored fat in the human body are in the form of triglycerides.

The length of the carbon atom chain and the amount of hydrogen saturation (that is, the number of hydrogen molecules attached to the carbon chain) in fatty acids varies. Based on the extent of saturation, fatty acids are said to be saturated or unsaturated. Unsaturated fatty acids are classified further into monounsaturated and polyunsaturated. Saturated fatty acids are mainly of animal origin; unsaturated fats are found mostly in plant products.

Saturated Fats   In saturated fatty acids (often called "saturated fats"), the carbon atoms are fully saturated with hydrogen atoms; only single bonds link the carbon atoms on the chain (see Figure 3.4). Foods high in saturated fatty acids are meats, animal fat, lard, whole milk, cream, butter, cheese, ice cream, hydrogenated oils (hydrogenation makes oils saturated), coconut oil, and palm oils. Saturated fats typically do not melt at room temperature. Coconut and palm oils are exceptions. In general, saturated fats raise the blood cholesterol level.

Unsaturated Fats   In unsaturated fatty acids (often called "unsaturated fats"), double bonds form between unsaturated carbons. In monounsaturated fatty acids (MUFA), only one double bond is found along the chain. Examples of monounsaturated fatty acids are olive, canola, rapeseed, peanut, and sesame oils. Polyunsaturated fatty acids (PUFA) contain two or more double bonds between unsaturated carbon

FIGURE 3.4 Chemical structure of saturated and unsaturated fats

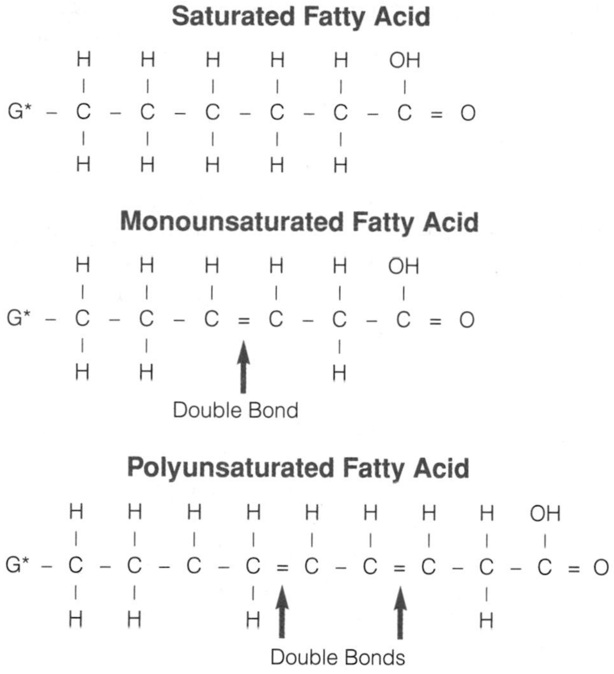

Saturated Fatty Acid

```
      H     H     H     H     H    OH
      |     |     |     |     |     |
G* -  C  -  C  -  C  -  C  -  C  -  C  =  O
      |     |     |     |     |
      H     H     H     H     H
```

Monounsaturated Fatty Acid

```
      H     H     H     H     H    OH
      |     |     |     |     |     |
G* -  C  -  C  -  C  =  C  -  C  -  C  =  O
      |     |                 |
      H     H                 H
                    ↑
               Double Bond
```

Polyunsaturated Fatty Acid

```
      H     H     H     H     H     H     H     H    OH
      |     |     |     |     |     |     |     |     |
G* -  C  -  C  -  C  -  C  =  C  -  C  =  C  -  C  -  C  =  O
      |     |           |                       |
      H     H           H                       H
                        ↑           ↑
                      Double Bonds
```

*Glyceride component

atoms along the chain. Corn, cottonseed, safflower, walnut, sunflower, and soybean oils are high in polyunsaturated fatty acids. Unsaturated fats usually are liquid at room temperature. Shorter fatty acid chains also tend to be liquid at room temperature.

Polyunsaturated and monounsaturated fats tend to lower blood cholesterol. When unsaturated fats replace saturated fats in the diet, the former tend to stimulate the liver to clear cholesterol from the blood.

Other Fatty Acids Hydrogen is often added to monounsaturated and polyunsaturated fats to increase shelf life and to solidify them so they are more spreadable. During this process, called "partial hydrogenation," the position of hydrogen atoms may be changed along the carbon chain, transforming the fat into a **trans fatty acid**.

Margarine and spreads, crackers, cookies, dairy products, meats, and fast foods often contain trans fatty acids. Trans fatty acids are not essential and provide no known health benefit. In fact, health-conscious people minimize their intake of these types of fats, because diets high in trans fatty acids elevate cholesterol. Paying attention to food labels is important, because the words "partially hydrogenated" and "trans fatty acids" indicate that the product carries a health risk just as high as that of saturated fat. Starting in December 2005, Health Canada required that food labels list trans fatty acids so consumers can make healthier choices.

A type of polyunsaturated fatty acids that has gained attention in recent years are the **omega-3 fatty acids** (specifically alpha-linolenic acid), which are heart-healthy. Fish—especially fresh or frozen mackerel, herring, tuna, salmon, and lake trout—and flaxseed contain omega-3 fatty acids. Canned fish also contains omega-3 fatty acids, but the amount may vary considerably and the oil is often drained, a practice that can remove some of the omega-3 fatty acids. Fish stored in water may retain more of its omega-3 content.[2] These fatty acids are also found, but to a lesser extent, in milk, canola oil, walnuts, soybeans, and wheat germ.

One of the simplest ways to increase omega-3 fatty acids is to consume flaxseed, which is also high in fibre and plant chemicals known as *lignans*. The oil in flaxseed is high in alpha-linolenic acid and has been shown to reduce abnormal heart rhythms and prevent blood clots.[3]

Studies are being conducted to investigate the potential cancer-fighting ability of lignans. In one report, the addition of 45 to 55 g of ground flaxseeds to the diet seemed to lead to a decrease in the onset of tumours, preventing their formation, and even led to a shrinkage of tumours.[4]

Amounts of flaxseed in the diet higher than recommended, however, is not recommended. High doses actually may be detrimental to health. Pregnant and lactating women, especially, should not consume large amounts of flaxseed.

Other essential unsaturated fatty acids are the **omega-6** group, in particular linoleic acid. Our diets are typically high in omega-6-rich oils, found in corn, sunflower, and most oils in processed foods. We usually consume 10 to 20 times more omega-6 than omega-3. Excessive omega-6 fatty acids amplify inflammatory processes that can damage organs in the body.

For adults consuming a 2,000 kcal diet, the Adequate Intake (AI) of linoleic acid is 4.44 g/day. However, care must be taken not to overconsume linoleic acid as the excess will be converted into detrimental by-products.

Fats A classification of nutrients containing carbon, hydrogen, some oxygen, and sometimes other chemical elements.

Trans fatty acid Solidified fat formed by adding hydrogen to monounsaturated and polyunsaturated fats to increase shelf life.

Omega-3 fatty acids Polyunsaturated fatty acids found primarily in cold-water seafood, flaxseed, and flaxseed oil; thought to lower blood cholesterol and triglycerides.

Omega-6 fatty acids Polyunsaturated fatty acids found primarily in corn and sunflower oils and most oils in processed foods.

COMPOUND FATS

Compound fats are a combination of simple fats and other chemicals. Examples are:

1. *Phospholipids*: similar to triglycerides, except that choline (or another compound) and phosphoric acid take the place of one of the fatty acid units.
2. *Glucolipids:* a combination of carbohydrates, fatty acids, and nitrogen.
3. *Lipoproteins:* water-soluble aggregates of protein and triglycerides, phospholipids, or cholesterol.

Lipoproteins (a combination of lipids and proteins) are especially important because they transport fats in the blood. The major forms of lipoproteins are high-density (HDL), low-density (LDL), and very-low-density (VLDL) lipoproteins. Lipoproteins play a large role in developing or in preventing heart disease. High HDL levels have been associated with lower risk for coronary heart disease, whereas high LDL levels have been linked to increased risk for this disease. HDL is more than 50 percent protein and contains little cholesterol; LDL is approximately 25 percent protein and nearly 50 percent cholesterol. VLDL contains about 50 percent triglycerides, only about 10 percent protein, and 20 percent cholesterol.

DERIVED FATS

Derived fats combine simple and compound fats. **Sterols** are an example. Although sterols contain no fatty acids, they are considered lipids because they do not dissolve in water. The most often mentioned sterol is cholesterol, which is found in many foods or can be manufactured in the body—primarily from saturated fats.

Proteins

Proteins are the main substances the body uses to build and repair tissues such as muscles, blood, internal organs, skin, hair, nails, and bones. They form a part of hormone, antibody, and **enzyme** molecules. Enzymes play a key role in all of the body's processes. Because all enzymes are formed by proteins, this nutrient is necessary for normal functioning. Proteins also help maintain the normal balance of body fluids.

Proteins can be used as a source of energy, too, but only if sufficient carbohydrates are not available. Each gram of protein yields 4 Calories of energy (the same as carbohydrates). The main sources of protein are meats and alternatives, and milk and other dairy products. Excess proteins may be converted to glucose or fat, or even excreted in the urine.

The human body uses 20 **amino acids** to form different types of protein. Amino acids contain nitrogen, carbon, hydrogen, and oxygen. Of the 20 amino acids, 9 are called "essential amino acids" because the body cannot produce them. The other 11, termed "nonessential amino acids," can be manufactured in the body if food proteins in the diet provide enough nitrogen (see Table 3.2). For the body to function normally, all amino acids shown in the table must be present in the diet.

Proteins that contain all the essential amino acids, known as "complete" or "higher-quality" protein, are usually of animal origin. If one or more of the essential amino acids is missing, the proteins are termed "incomplete" or "lower-quality" protein. Individuals have to take in enough protein to ensure nitrogen for adequate production of amino acids and also to get enough high-quality protein to obtain the essential amino acids.

Protein deficiency is not a problem in the typical Canadian diet. Two glasses of skim milk combined with about 113 g of poultry or fish meet the daily protein requirement. Too much animal protein, on the other hand, can cause serious health problems. Some people eat twice as much protein as they need. Protein foods from animal sources are often high in fat, saturated fat, and cholesterol, which can lead to cardiovascular disease and cancer. Too much animal protein also decreases blood enzymes that prevent precancerous cells from developing into tumours.

As mentioned earlier, a well-balanced diet contains a variety of foods from all the basic food groups, including a wise selection of foods from animal sources (see also "Balancing the Diet," pages 59–62). Based on current nutrition data, meat (poultry and fish included) should be replaced by grains, legumes, vegetables, and fruits as main courses. Meats should be used more for flavouring than for volume. Daily consumption of beef, poultry, or fish should be limited to 85 g (about the size of a deck of cards) to 170 g.

TABLE 3.2 Amino Acids

Essential Amino Acids*	Nonessential Amino Acids
Histidine	Alanine
Isoleucine	Arginine
Leucine	Asparagine
Lysine	Aspartic acid
Methionine	Cysteine
Phenylalanine	Glutamic acid
Threonine	Glutamine
Tryptophan	Glycine
Valine	Proline
	Serine
	Tyrosine

* Must be provided in the diet, because the body cannot manufacture them.

Vitamins

Vitamins are necessary for normal bodily metabolism, growth, and development. Vitamins are classified into two types based on their solubility: fat-soluble (A, D, E, and K) and water-soluble (B complex and C). The body does not manufacture most vitamins, so they can be obtained only through a well-balanced diet. To decrease loss of vitamins during cooking, natural foods should be microwaved or steamed rather than boiled in water that is thrown out later.

A few exceptions, such as vitamins A, D, and K, are formed in the body. Vitamin A is produced from beta-carotene, found mainly in yellow foods such as carrots, pumpkin, and sweet potatoes. Vitamin D is created when ultraviolet light from the sun transforms 7-dehydrocholesterol, a compound in human skin. Vitamin K is created in the body by intestinal bacteria. The major functions of vitamins are outlined in Table 3.3.

Vitamins C, E, and beta-carotene also function as antioxidants, which are thought to play a key role in preventing chronic diseases. The specific function of these antioxidant nutrients and of the mineral selenium (also an antioxidant) are discussed under "Antioxidants" (page 73) and "Folate," (page 76).

Minerals

Approximately 25 **minerals** have important roles in body functioning. Minerals are inorganic substances contained in all cells, especially those in hard parts of the body (bones, nails, teeth). Minerals are crucial to maintaining water balance and the acid–base balance. They are essential components of respiratory pigments, enzymes, and enzyme systems, and they regulate muscular and nervous tissue impulses, blood clotting, and normal heart rhythm.

The four minerals mentioned most often are calcium, iron, sodium, and selenium. Calcium deficiency may result in osteoporosis, and low iron intake can induce iron deficiency anemia (both are discussed under "Special Nutrient Needs of Women," pages 82–83). High sodium intake may contribute to high blood pressure. Selenium seems to be important in preventing certain types of cancer. Specific functions of some of the most important minerals are given in Table 3.4.

Water

The most important nutrient is **water**, as it is involved in almost every vital body process: in digesting and absorbing food, in energy production, in the circulatory process, in body heat regulation, in removing waste products, in building and rebuilding cells, and in transporting other nutrients. Approximately 60 percent of total body weight is water (see Figure 3.5).

Water is contained in almost all foods, but primarily in liquid foods, fruits, and vegetables. Although for decades the recommendation was to consume at least 2 L of water per day, a panel of scientists of the Institute of Medicine of the National Academy of Sciences indicated in 2004 that people are getting enough water from the liquids (milk, juices, sodas, coffee) and the moisture content of solid foods. Most Canadians remain well-hydrated simply by using thirst as their guide. Caffeine-containing drinks are also acceptable as a water source because data indicate that people who regularly consume such beverages do not have a greater 24-hour urine output than those who don't.

An exception of not waiting for the thirst signal to replenish water loss is when an individual exercises in the heat or does so for an extended time (see Chapter 9, page 279). Water lost under these conditions must be replenished regularly. If you wait for the thirst signal, you may have lost too much water already. At 2 percent of body weight lost, a person is dehydrated. At 5 percent, one may become dizzy and disoriented, have trouble with cognitive skills and heart function, and even lose consciousness.

Balancing the Diet

One of the fundamental ways to enjoy good health and live life to its fullest is through a well-balanced diet. Several guidelines have been published to help you accomplish this. As illustrated in Table 3.5, the 2002 recommended guidelines by the National Academy of Sciences (NAS) state that daily caloric

Lipoproteins Lipids covered by proteins, they transport fats in the blood; types are LDL, HDL, and VLDL.

Sterols Derived fats, of which cholesterol is the best-known example.

Proteins A classification of nutrients consisting of complex organic compounds containing nitrogen and formed by combinations of amino acids; the main substances used in the body to build and repair tissues.

Enzymes Catalysts that facilitate chemical reactions in the body.

Amino acids Chemical compounds that contain nitrogen, carbon, hydrogen, and oxygen; the basic building blocks the body uses to build different types of protein.

Vitamins Organic nutrients essential for normal metabolism, growth, and development of the body.

Minerals Inorganic nutrients essential for normal body functions; found in the body and in food.

Water The most important classification of essential body nutrients, involved in almost every vital body process.

TABLE 3.3   Major Functions of Vitamins

Nutrient	Good Sources	Major Functions	Deficiency Symptoms
Vitamin A	Milk, cheese, eggs, liver, yellow and dark green fruits and vegetables	Required for healthy bones, teeth, skin, gums, and hair; maintenance of inner mucous membranes, thus increasing resistance to infection; adequate vision in dim light.	Night blindness; decreased growth; decreased resistance to infection; rough, dry skin
Vitamin D	Fortified milk, cod liver oil, salmon, tuna, egg yolk	Necessary for bones and teeth; needed for calcium and phosphorus absorption.	Rickets (bone softening), fractures, muscle spasms
Vitamin E	Vegetable oils, yellow and green leafy vegetables, margarine, wheat germ, whole-grain breads and cereals	Related to oxidation and normal muscle and red blood cell chemistry.	Leg cramps, red blood cell breakdown
Vitamin K	Green leafy vegetables, cauliflower, cabbage, eggs, peas, potatoes	Essential for normal blood clotting.	Hemorrhaging
Vitamin B_1 (Thiamin)	Whole-grain or enriched bread, lean meats and poultry, fish, liver, pork, poultry, organ meats, legumes, nuts, dried yeast	Assists in proper use of carbohydrates, normal functioning of nervous system, maintenance of good appetite.	Loss of appetite, nausea, confusion, cardiac abnormalities, muscle spasms
Vitamin B_2 (Riboflavin)	Eggs, milk, leafy green vegetables, whole grains, lean meats, dried beans and peas	Contributes to energy release from carbohydrates, fats, and proteins; needed for normal growth and development, good vision, and healthy skin.	Cracking of the corners of the mouth, inflammation of the skin, impaired vision
Vitamin B_6 (Pyridoxine)	Vegetables, meats, whole grain cereals, soybeans, peanuts, potatoes	Necessary for protein and fatty acids metabolism and for normal red blood cell formation.	Depression, irritability, muscle spasms, nausea
Vitamin B_{12}	Meat, poultry, fish, liver, organ meats, eggs, shellfish, milk, cheese	Required for normal growth, red blood cell formation, nervous system and digestive tract functioning.	Impaired balance, weakness, drop in red blood cell count
Niacin	Liver and organ meats, meat, fish, poultry, whole grains, enriched breads, nuts, green leafy vegetables, and dried beans and peas	Contributes to energy release from carbohydrates, fats, and proteins; normal growth and development; and formation of hormones and nerve-regulating substances.	Confusion, depression, weakness, weight loss
Biotin	Liver, kidney, eggs, yeast, legumes, milk, nuts, dark green vegetables	Essential for carbohydrate metabolism and fatty acid synthesis.	Inflamed skin, muscle pain, depression, weight loss
Folic Acid	Leafy green vegetables, organ meats, whole grains and cereals, dried beans	Needed for cell growth and reproduction and for red blood cell formation.	Decreased resistance to infection
Pantothenic Acid	All natural foods, especially liver, kidney, eggs, nuts, yeast, milk, dried peas and beans, green leafy vegetables	Related to carbohydrate and fat metabolism.	Depression, low blood sugar, leg cramps, nausea, headaches
Vitamin C (Ascorbic acid)	Fruits, vegetables	Helps protect against infection; required for formation of collagenous tissue, normal blood vessels, teeth, and bones.	Slow-healing wounds, loose teeth, hemorrhaging, rough scaly skin, irritability

intake should be distributed so that 45 to 65 percent of the total calories come from carbohydrates (mostly complex carbohydrates and less than 25 percent from sugar), 20 to 35 percent from fat, and 10 to 35 percent from protein.[5] These new ranges offer greater flexibility in planning diets according to individual health and physical activity needs.

In addition to the macronutrients, the diet must include all of the essential vitamins, minerals, and water. The source of fat calories is also critical. The Heart and Stroke Foundation of Canada suggests Canadians limit their consumption of fat to 30 percent of energy intake and limit saturated fat to 10 percent of energy intake. The Canadian Dietetic Association has similar recommendations but also suggests polyunsaturated fats be 10 percent of energy of the recommended fat intake.[6] Rating a particular diet accurately is difficult without a complete nutrient analysis. You have an opportunity to perform this analysis in Lab 3A.

The 2002 NAS guidelines are in sharp contrast to those of major national health organizations, which recommend 50 to 60 percent of total calories from carbohydrates, less than 30 percent from fat, and about 15 percent from protein. These percentages are within the ranges recommended by the

TABLE 3.4 Major Functions of Minerals

Nutrient	Good Sources	Major Functions	Deficiency Symptoms
Calcium	Milk, yogurt, cheese, green leafy vegetables, dried beans, sardines, salmon	Required for strong teeth and bone formation; maintenance of good muscle tone, heartbeat, and nerve function.	Bone pain and fractures, periodontal disease, muscle cramps
Copper	Seafood, meats, beans, nuts, whole grains	Helps with iron absorption and hemoglobin formation; required to synthesize the enzyme cytochrome oxidase.	Anemia (although deficiency is rare in humans)
Iron	Organ meats, lean meats, seafoods, eggs, dried peas and beans, nuts, whole and enriched grains, green leafy vegetables	Major component of hemoglobin; aids in energy utilization.	Nutritional anemia, overall weakness
Phosphorus	Meats, fish, milk, eggs, dried beans and peas, whole grains, processed foods	Required for bone and teeth formation and for energy release regulation.	Bone pain and fracture, weight loss, weakness
Zinc	Milk, meat, seafood, whole grains, nuts, eggs, dried beans	Essential component of hormones, insulin, and enzymes; used in normal growth and development.	Loss of appetite, slow-healing wounds, skin problems
Magnesium	Green leafy vegetables, whole grains, nuts, soybeans, seafood, legumes	Needed for bone growth and maintenance, carbohydrate and protein utilization, nerve function, temperature regulation.	Irregular heartbeat, weakness, muscle spasms, sleeplessness
Sodium	Table salt, processed foods, meat	Needed for body fluid regulation, transmission of nerve impulses, heart action.	Rarely seen
Potassium	Legumes, whole grains, bananas, orange juice, dried fruits, potatoes	Required for heart action, bone formation and maintenance, regulation of energy release, acid-base regulation.	Irregular heartbeat, nausea, weakness
Selenium	Seafood, meat, whole grains	Component of enzymes; functions in close association with vitamin E.	Muscle pain, possible heart muscle deterioration, possible hair and nail loss

FIGURE 3.5 Approximate proportions of nutrients in the human body

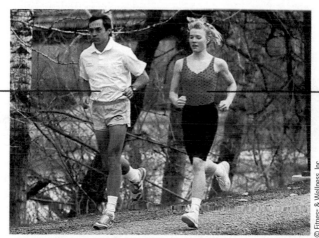

1% Carbohydrates
6% Minerals
16% Protein
17% Fat
61% Water

1% Carbohydrates
5% Minerals
12% Protein
27% Fat
56% Water

© Fitness & Wellness, Inc.

Higher percentage of fat tissue in women is normal and needed for reproduction.

NAS. The most drastic difference appears in the NAS allowed range of fat intake, up to 35 percent of total calories. This higher percentage was included to accommodate individuals with metabolic syndrome (see Chapter 11, page 347) who have an abnormal insulin response to carbohydrates and may need additional fat in the diet.

The NAS recommendations will be effective only if people consistently replace saturated and trans fatty acids with unsaturated fatty acids. The latter will require dramatic changes in the typical "unhealthy" North American diet, which is generally high in red meats, whole dairy products, and fast foods—all of which are high in saturated and/or trans fatty acids.

CALORIC AND FAT CONTENT OF SELECTED FAST FOOD ITEMS

Item	Calories	Total Fat (grams)	Saturated Fat (grams)	Percent Fat Calories
Arby's Regular Roast Beef	320	14	5	120
Arby's Super Roast Beef	400	19	6	170
Arby's Chicken Fillet Sandwich, Grilled	390	17	2.5	150
Arby's Market Fresh® Santa Fe Salad w/Grilled Chicken (no dressing)	240	8	4	80
Subway® Veggie Delite™, 6-inch	230	3	1	30
Subway® Turkey Breast, 6-inch	280	4.5	1.5	40
Subway® Sweet Onion Chicken Teryaki, 6-inch	370	5.0	1.5	45
Subway® Steak & Cheese	400	12	5	110
Subway® Cold Cut Trio, 6-inch Double	660	39	14	390
Subway® Tuna, 6-inch	530	30	7	270
Subway® Oven Roasted Chicken Breast Salad, no dressing	130	2.5	0.5	25
Tim Hortons BLT	450	18	5	36
Tim Hortons Chicken Salad	380	9	1.5	21
Tim Hortons Ham and Swiss	440	12	5	25
Tim Hortons Turkey Bacon Club	440	8	2.5	16
Tim Hortons Breakfast Sandwich Bacon, Egg, Cheese	410	23	4	54
Tim Hortons Iced Cappuccino, with cream, small	250	11	6	40

* Note: Check restaurant websites for the latest nutritional information.

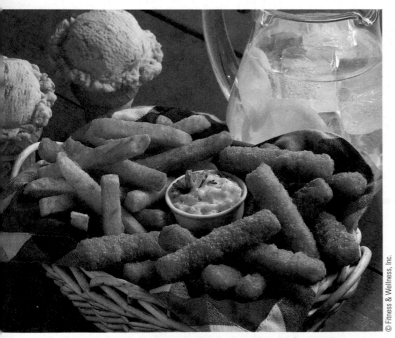

The typical North American diet is too high in fat intake.

TABLE 3.5 The Canadian Diet: Current and Recommended Carbohydrate, Fat, and Protein Intake Expressed as a Percentage of Total Calories

	Current %	Recommended %*
Carbohydrates:	50%	45–65%
Simple	26%	Less than 25%
Complex	24%	20–40%
Fat:	34%	20–35%**
Monounsaturated:	11%	Up to 20%
Polyunsaturated:	10%	Up to 10%
Saturated:	13%	Less than 7%
Protein:	16%	10–35%

* 2002 recommended guidelines by the National Academy of Sciences.

** Less than 30% recommended by most health organizations. A higher amount may be indicated for people with metabolic syndrome.

Diets in most developed countries have changed significantly since the turn of the 20th century. Today, people eat more calories and fat, fewer carbohydrates, and about the same amount of protein. People also weigh more than they did in 1900, an indication that they are eating more calories and are not as physically active as their ancestors were.

Diets also were much healthier at the turn of the 20th century. In North America, at the beginning of the 20th century, carbohydrates accounted for 57 percent of the total daily caloric intake, 67 percent of which were complex carbohydrates. Today, carbohydrate intake has decreased to 50 percent and complex carbohydrates account for only 24 percent of this intake. The proportion of fat has risen from 32 percent to 34 percent, but a higher proportion is in the form of saturated and trans fatty acids.

Nutrition Standards

Nutritionists use a variety of nutrient standards. The most widely known nutrient standard is the RDA, or Recommended Dietary Allowances. This, however, is not the only standard. Among others are the Dietary Reference Intakes and the Daily Values on food labels. Each standard has a different purpose and utilization in dietary planning and assessment.

Dietary Reference Intakes

To help people meet dietary guidelines, the National Academy of Sciences developed a set of dietary nutrient intakes for healthy people in Canada and the United States, the **Dietary Reference Intakes (DRIs)**. The DRIs are based on a review of the most current research on nutrient needs of healthy people. The DRI reports are written by the Food and

Nutrition Board of the Institute of Medicine in cooperation with scientists from Canada.

The general term DRIs includes four types of reference values for planning and assessing diets and for establishing adequate amounts and maximum safe nutrient intakes in the diet: Estimated Average Requirement (EAR), Recommended Dietary Allowance (RDA), Adequate Intakes (AI), and Tolerable Upper Intake Levels (UL). The type of reference value used for a given nutrient and a specific age/gender group is determined according to available scientific information and the intended use of the dietary standard.

EAR

The **Estimated Average Requirement (EAR)** is the amount of a nutrient that is estimated to meet the nutrient requirement of half the healthy people in specific age and gender groups. At this nutrient intake level, 50 percent of the people do not have their nutritional requirements met. If, for example, we look at 300 healthy women at age 26, the EAR would meet the nutritional requirement for only half of these women.

RDA

The **Recommended Dietary Allowance (RDA)** is the daily amount of a nutrient considered adequate to meet the known nutrient needs of nearly all healthy people. Because the committee must decide what level of intake to recommend for everybody, the RDA is set well above the EAR and covers about 98 percent of the population. Stated another way, the RDA recommendation for any nutrient is well above almost everyone's actual requirement. The RDA could be considered a goal for adequate intake. The process for determining the RDA depends on being able to set an EAR, because RDAs are statistically determined from the EAR values. If an EAR cannot be set, no RDA can be established.

AI

When data are insufficient or inadequate to set an EAR, an **Adequate Intakes (AI)** value is determined instead of the RDA. The AI value is derived from approximations of observed nutrient intakes by a group or groups of healthy people. The AI value for children and adults is expected to meet or exceed the nutritional requirements of a corresponding healthy population.

Nutrients for daily DRIs have been set are presented in Table 3.6.

UL

The **Upper Intake Level (UL)** establishes the highest level of nutrient intake that seems to be safe for most healthy people, beyond which exists an increased risk of adverse effects. As intakes increase above the UL, so does the risk of adverse effects. In general terms, the optimum nutrient range for healthy eating is between the RDA and the UL. The established ULs are presented in Table 3.7.

Daily Values

The **Daily Values (DVs)** are reference values for nutrients and food components for use on food labels. The DVs include fat, saturated fat, and carbohydrates (as a percent of total calories); cholesterol, sodium, and potassium (in milligrams); and fibre and protein (in grams). The DVs for total fat, saturated fat, and carbohydrate are expressed as percentages for a 2,000-calorie diet and may therefore require adjustments depending on an individual's daily **Estimated Energy Requirement (EER)** in calories. For example, on a 2,000-calorie diet (EER), recommended carbohydrate intake is about 300 g (about 60 percent of EER), and fat is 65 g (about 30 percent of EER) (see Figure 3.6). The vitamin, mineral, and protein DVs were adapted from the RDAs. The DVs are also not as specific for age and gender groups as are the DRIs. Both the DRIs and the DVs apply only to healthy adults. They are not intended for people who are ill and may require additional nutrients.

Figure 3.6 shows the food label with Recommended Daily Values.

Dietary Reference Intakes (DRIs) A general term that describes four types of nutrient standards that establish adequate amounts and maximum safe nutrient intakes in the diet. These standards are Estimated Average Requirements (EAR), Recommended Dietary Allowances (RDA), Adequate Intakes (AI), and Tolerable Upper Intake Levels (UL).

Estimated Average Requirements (EAR) The amount of a nutrient that meets the dietary needs in half the people.

Recommended Dietary Allowances (RDA) The daily amount of a nutrient (statistically determined from the EARs) considered adequate to meet the known nutrient needs of almost 98 percent of all healthy people.

Adequate Intakes (AI) The recommended amount of a nutrient intake when sufficient evidence is not available to calculate the EAR and subsequent RDA.

Upper Intake Level (UL) The highest level of nutrient intake that appears safe for most healthy people, beyond which exists an increased risk of adverse effects.

Daily Values (DVs) Reference values for nutrients and food components used in food labels.

Estimated Energy Requirement (EER) The average dietary energy (caloric) intake that is predicted to maintain energy balance in a healthy adult of defined age, gender, weight, height, and level of physical activity, consistent with good health.

TABLE 3.6 Dietary Reference Intakes (DRIs): Recommended Dietary Allowances (RDA) and Adequate Intakes (AI) for Selected Nutrients

	Recommended Dietary Allowances (RDA)													Adequate Intakes (AI)					
	Thiamin (mg)	Riboflavin (mg)	Niacin (mg NE)	Vitamin B$_6$ (mg)	Folate (mcg DFE)	Vitamin B$_{12}$ (mcg)	Phosphorus (mg)	Magnesium (mg)	Vitamin A (mg RAE)	Vitamin C (mg)	Vitamin E (mg)	Selenium (mcg)	Iron (mcg)	Calcium (mg)	Vitamin D (mcg)	Fluoride (mg)	Pantothenic acid (mg)	Biotin (mcg)	Choline (mg)
Males																			
14–18	1.2	1.3	16	1.3	400	2.4	1,250	410	900	75	15	55	11	1,300	5	3	5	25	550
19–30	1.2	1.3	16	1.3	400	2.4	700	400	900	90	15	55	8	1,000	5	4	5	30	550
31–50	1.2	1.3	16	1.3	400	2.4	700	420	900	90	15	55	8	1,000	5	4	5	30	550
51–70	1.2	1.3	16	1.7	400	2.4	700	420	900	90	15	55	8	1,200	10	4	5	30	550
>70	1.2	1.3	16	1.7	400	2.4	700	420	900	90	15	55	8	1,200	15	4	5	30	550
Females																			
14–18	1.0	1.0	14	1.2	400	2.4	1,250	360	700	65	15	55	15	1,300	5	3	5	25	400
19–30	1.1	1.1	14	1.3	400	2.4	700	310	700	75	15	55	18	1,000	5	3	5	30	425
31–50	1.1	1.1	14	1.3	400	2.4	700	320	700	75	15	55	18	1,000	5	3	5	30	425
51–70	1.1	1.1	14	1.5	400	2.4	700	320	700	75	15	55	8	1,200	10	3	5	30	425
>70	1.1	1.1	14	1.5	400	2.4	700	320	700	75	15	55	8	1,200	15	3	5	30	425
Pregnant																			
14–18	1.4	1.4	18	1.9	600	2.6	1,250	400	750	80	15	60	27	1,300	5	3	6	30	450
19–30	1.4	1.4	18	1.9	600	2.6	700	350	770	85	15	60	27	1,000	5	3	6	30	450
31–50	1.4	1.4	18	1.9	600	2.6	700	360	770	85	15	60	27	1,000	5	3	6	30	450
Lactating																			
14–18	1.4	1.6	17	2.0	500	2.8	1,250	360	1,200	115	19	70	10	1,300	5	3	7	35	550
19–30	1.4	1.6	17	2.0	500	2.8	700	310	1,300	120	19	70	9	1,000	5	3	7	35	550
31–50	1.4	1.6	17	2.0	500	2.8	700	320	1,300	120	19	70	9	1,000	5	3	7	35	550

* Values for these nutrients do not change with pregnancy or lactation. Use the value listed for women of comparable age.

Source: Adapted with permission from *Dietary Reference Intakes: Essential Guide*, 2006, by the National Academy of Sciences. Courtesy of the National Academies Press, Washington, DC.

TABLE 3.7 Tolerable Upper Intake Levels (UL) of Selected Nutrients for Adults (19–70 years)

Nutrient	UL per Day
Calcium	2.5 gr
Phosphorus	4.0 gr*
Magnesium	350 mg
Vitamin D	50 mcg
Fluoride	10 mg
Niacin	35 mg
Iron	45 mg
Vitamin B$_6$	100 mg
Folate	1,000 mcg
Choline	3.5 gr
Vitamin A	3,000 mcg
Vitamin C	2,000 mg
Vitamin E	1,000 mg
Selenium	400 mcg

* 3.5 gr per day for pregnant women.

Nutrient Analysis

The first step in evaluating your diet is to conduct a nutrient analysis. This can be quite educational, because most people do not realize how harmful and non-nutritious many common foods are. The analysis covers calories, carbohydrates, fats, cholesterol, and sodium, as well as eight crucial nutrients: protein, calcium, iron, vitamin A, thiamin, riboflavin, niacin, and vitamin C. If the diet has enough of these eight nutrients, the foods consumed in natural form to provide these nutrients typically contain all the other nutrients the human body needs.

To do your own nutrient analysis, go to Lab 3A, where you will need to access the web-based Nutrition tool EATracker from Dietitians of Canada (http://www.eatracker.ca). When you are in

FIGURE 3.6 Food label with Recommended Daily Values

1 Nutrition Facts Table

The Nutrition Facts table can help you make healthy food choices and assist you in reducing your risk of chronic diseases such as cancer, diabetes, heart disease and stroke. It includes Calories and 13 nutrients: Fat, Saturated fat, Trans fat, Cholesterol, Sodium, Carbohydrate, Fibre, Sugars, Protein, Vitamin A, Vitamin C and Calcium and Iron. You will find that some foods, such as fresh fruits and vegetables, raw meat and poultry, bakery items, coffee, tea and alcoholic beverages are exempt from the nutrition labelling requirements.

2 Specific Amount of Food

When you read the Nutrition Facts, look first at the specific amount of food that is listed on the table. Then compare this amount to how much food you actually eat. You might notice that the specific amount is described by phrases such as a slice, or a specific number of such as one egg or two cookies, or by some familiar household units such as a mL, a cup, a tablespoon or a unit of food such as ¼ of a pizza. The phrase will be followed by the metric measure of the serving such as grams or mLs.

3 % of Daily Value

The % of Daily Value is used to determine whether the food you choose has a lot or a little of a nutrient in a specific amount of food. These values are based on standards that have been established for health outcomes, healthy growth and development and a reduced risk of nutrition-related chronic disease. They apply to most people. This value is especially useful when you are comparing two food products.

4 Calories and Core Nutrients

Individual caloric needs vary and depend on your age, body size, gender, activity level and whether or not you are pregnant or breastfeeding. It is also important to remember that if you eat more than the amount of food specified in the Nutrition Facts Table you will consume more Calories than what is listed so you will need to calculate what your intake actually is.

5 Nutrition Claims

The Government has specific rules in place that determine whether or not a nutrition claim can be made on a label or advertisement. You should be aware that manufacturers can choose whether or not to put on a nutrition claim on their product if it meets the criteria set out by the government rules for these claims. For example Low Fat means that the food contains no more than 3 grams of fat in the amount of food specified in the Nutrition Facts table. Other examples of nutrition claims include source of fibre (at least 2 grams), cholesterol-free (less than 2 mg and also low in saturated and trans fat), sodium-free (less than 5 mg), reduced in calories (at least 25% less energy than the food it is being compared to, or light (foods reduced in fat or energy or used to describe sensory characteristics such as light tasting or light coloured).

6 List of Ingredients

The list of ingredients is mandatory for all food product packages. They are listed in descending order by weight. The ingredients present in the greatest amount in a product are listed first. This list helps you identify sources of certain nutrients in the food.

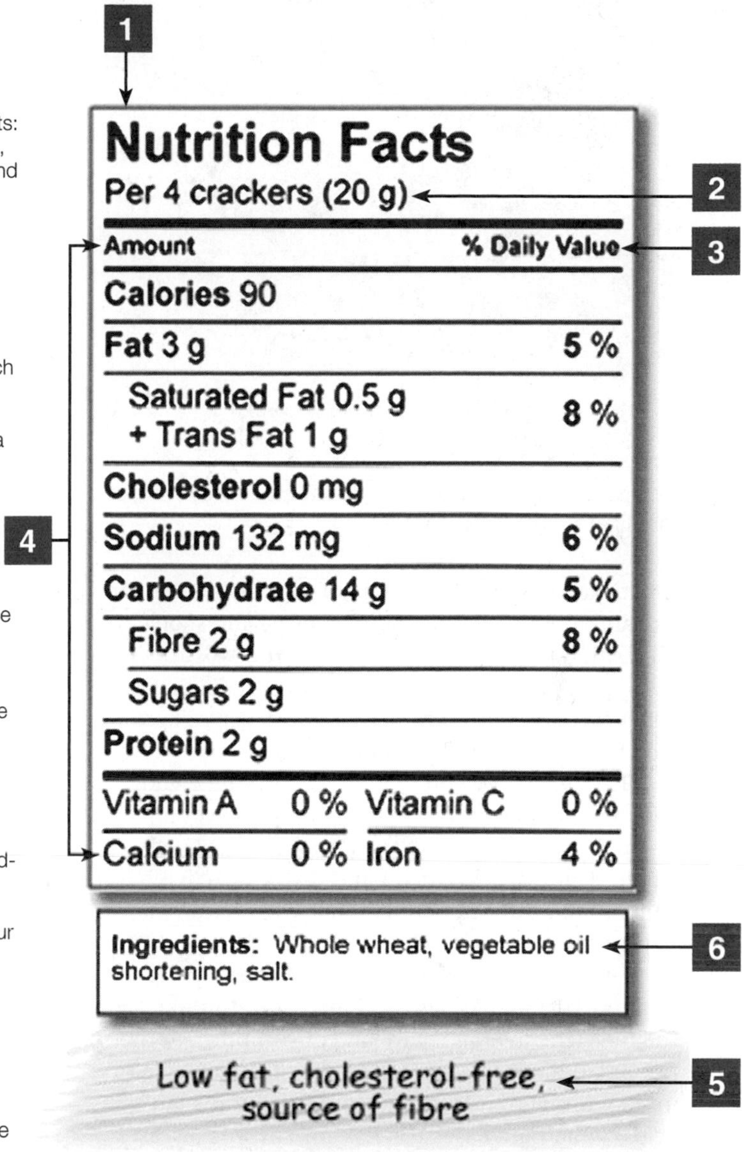

Nutrition Facts
Per 4 crackers (20 g)

Amount	% Daily Value
Calories 90	
Fat 3 g	5 %
Saturated Fat 0.5 g + Trans Fat 1 g	8 %
Cholesterol 0 mg	
Sodium 132 mg	6 %
Carbohydrate 14 g	5 %
Fibre 2 g	8 %
Sugars 2 g	
Protein 2 g	

Vitamin A	0 %	Vitamin C	0 %
Calcium	0 %	Iron	4 %

Ingredients: Whole wheat, vegetable oil shortening, salt.

Low fat, cholesterol-free, source of fibre

Health Canada, Food and Nutrition, *Interactive Nutrition Label: Get the Facts*, 2006. © Reproduced with the permission of the Minister of Public Works and Government Services Canada, 2008. http:// www.hc-sc.gc.ca/fn-an/label-etiquet/nutrition/cons/ inl_main-eng.php

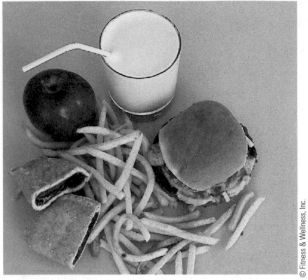

An apple a day will not keep the doctor away if most meals are high in fat content.

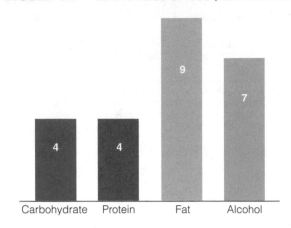

FIGURE 3.7 Caloric value of food (fuel nutrients)

© Fitness & Wellness, Inc.

EATracker, you will be prompted to select a calendar day and to list all the foods, beverages, and supplements that you consumed that day. You will also be asked to enter the physical activities you did on that day. Based on this information, EATracker will provide feedback about your food and activity choices.

This will allow you to track and evaluate your daily food intake and physical activity choices for seven days, and compare them to Canada's Food Guide (Figure 3.1, page 52) and Physical Activity Guide (online at http://www.phac-aspc.gc.ca/pau-uap/paguide/index.html).

Some of the most revealing information learned in a nutrient analysis is the source of fat intake in the diet. The average daily fat consumption in the Canadian diet is about 30 percent of the total caloric intake, much of it from saturated and trans fatty acids, which increases the risk for chronic diseases such as cardiovascular disease, cancer, diabetes, and obesity. Although fat provides a smaller percentage of our total daily caloric intake as compared to three decades ago (40 percent), the decrease in the percentage is simply because we now eat more calories than 30 years ago.

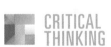
As illustrated in Figure 3.7, 1 gram of carbohydrates or of protein supplies the body with 4 Calories, and fat provides 9 Calories per gram consumed (alcohol yields 7 Calories per gram). Therefore, looking at only the total grams consumed for each type of food can be misleading.

For example, a person who eats 160 g of carbohydrates, 100 g of fat, and 70 g of protein has a total intake of 330 g of food. This indicates that 30 percent of the total grams of food is in the form of fat (100 g of fat ÷ 330 g of total food = .30; .30 × 100 = 30 percent)—and, in reality, almost half of that diet is in the form of fat calories.

In the sample diet, 640 Calories are derived from carbohydrates (160 g × 4 Calories per g), 280 Calories from protein (70 g × 4 Calories per g), and 900 Calories from fat (100 g × 9 Calories per g), for a total of 1,820 Calories. If 900 Calories are derived from fat, almost half of the total caloric intake is in the form of fat (900 ÷ 1,820 × 100 = 49.5 percent).

Each gram of fat provides 9 Calories—more than twice the calories of a gram of carbohydrates or protein. When figuring out the percent fat calories of individual foods, you can multiply the Total Fat grams by 9 and then divide by the total calories in that particular food (per serving). Then you multiply that number by 100 to get the percentage. This simple guideline can help you decrease the fat in your diet.

The fat content of selected foods, given in grams and as a percent of total calories, is presented in Figure 3.9. The percentage of fat is further subdivided into saturated, monounsaturated, polyunsaturated, and other fatty acids.

Beware of products labelled "97 percent fat-free." These products use weight, and not percent of total calories, as a measure of fat. Many of these foods still are in the range of 30 percent fat calories.

Achieving a Balanced Diet

Anyone who has completed a nutrient analysis and has given careful attention to Tables 3.3 (vitamins) and 3.4 (minerals) will probably realize that a well-balanced diet entails eating a variety of foods and

FIGURE 3.8 Canadian Nutrition Facts Table

The nutrient information is based on a specified amount of food. Compare this to the amount you eat.

This number is the amount of the nutrient in the specified quantity of food

The Nutrition Facts table will include this list of Calories and 13 nutrients

The % Daily Value gives a context to the amount of the nutrient in the specified amount of food. The Daily Value are based on recommendations for healthy eating.

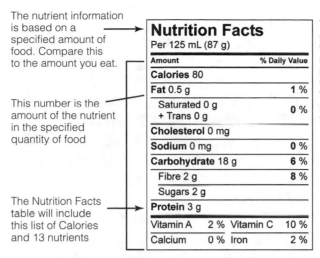

Nutrition Facts	
Per 125 mL (87 g)	
Amount	**% Daily Value**
Calories 80	
Fat 0.5 g	1 %
Saturated 0 g + Trans 0 g	0 %
Cholesterol 0 mg	
Sodium 0 mg	0 %
Carbohydrate 18 g	6 %
Fibre 2 g	8 %
Sugars 2 g	
Protein 3 g	
Vitamin A 2 % Vitamin C 10 %	
Calcium 0 % Iron 2 %	

Source: Health Canada, 2003 © Reproduced with the permission of the Minister of Public Works and Government Services Canada, 2008.

reducing daily intake of fats and sweets. Canada's Food Guide in Figure 3.1 (page 52) contains four major food groups. The recommended daily servings for adults are as follows:

	Gender	19–50 years	51+
1. Vegetables	Females	7–8	7
and Fruits	Males	8–10	7
2. Grain Products	Females	6–7	6
	Males	8	7
3. Milk and	Females	2	3
Alternatives	Males	2	3
4. Meat and	Females	2	2
Alternatives	Males	3	3

The four food groups provide the nutritional base for a healthy diet. Health Canada recommends eating at least one dark green and one orange vegetable a day. Suggestions include broccoli, romaine lettuce and spinach, carrots, sweet potatoes, and winter squash.

In addition to providing nutrients crucial to health, fruits and vegetables are the sole source of **phytochemicals** ("phyto" comes from the Greek word for plant). These compounds, recently discovered by scientists, show promising results in the fight against cancer and heart disease. More than 4,000 phytochemicals have been identified. The main function of phytochemicals in plants is to protect them from sunlight.

In humans, phytochemicals seem to have a powerful ability to block the formation of cancerous tumours. Their actions are so diverse that, at almost every stage of cancer, phytochemicals have the ability to block, disrupt, slow down, or even reverse the process. With regard to heart disease, they may reduce inflammation, inhibit blood clots, or prevent the oxidation of LDL cholesterol.

Grains such as barley, brown rice, oats, and wild rice, whole-grain breads, and whole-wheat pasta are also good choices because they are a good source of complex carbohydrates, which are rich in vitamins, minerals, and other nutrients. It is wise to choose grain products that are lower in fat, sugar, or salt.

Lower fat dairy products are also recommended. Try skim milk or 1 or 2 percent milk instead of whole milk. If you don't drink milk, try fortified soy beverages. Most milk products are high in calcium, riboflavin, protein, and vitamins A and B_{12}.

Meats and Alternatives are to be consumed in moderation. Select lean meat and alternatives prepared with little or no added fat or salt. You can trim visible fat from meats and remove skin on poultry. Try roasting, baking, or poaching instead of frying. Dieticians recommend eating at least two servings of fish each week. Examples include salmon, herring, sardines, and trout. Vegetarian choices for this food group include beans, lentils, and tofu.

As an aid to balancing your diet, the form in Lab 3B enables you to record your daily food intake. (This record is much easier to keep than the complete dietary analysis in Lab 3A.) Make one copy for each day you wish to record. Whenever you have something to eat, record in Figure 3B.1 the food

Phytochemicals Chemical compounds thought to prevent and fight cancer; found in large quantities in fruits and vegetables.

FIGURE 3.9 Fat content of selected foods

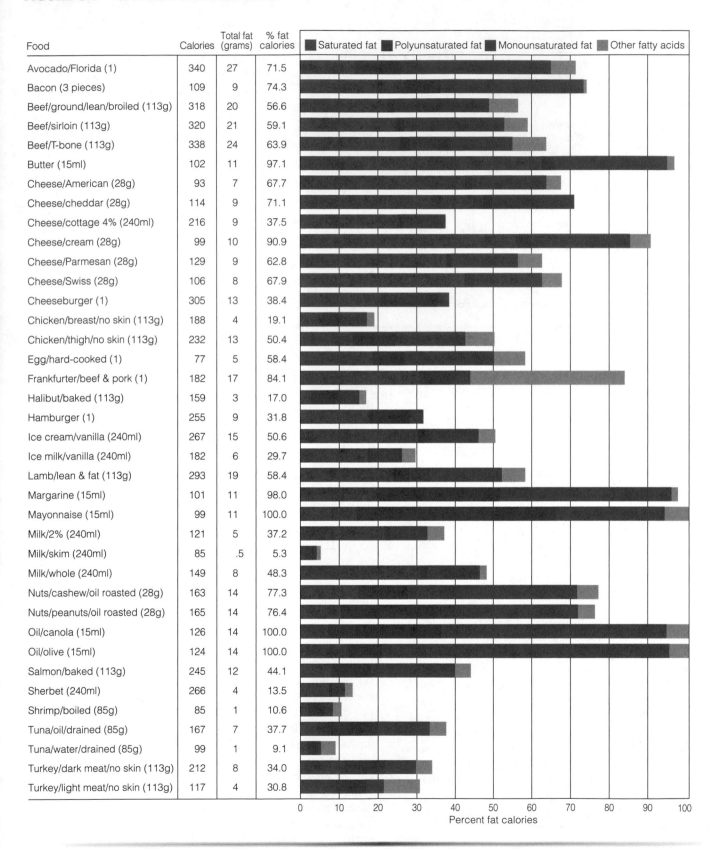

Food	Calories	Total fat (grams)	% fat calories
Avocado/Florida (1)	340	27	71.5
Bacon (3 pieces)	109	9	74.3
Beef/ground/lean/broiled (113g)	318	20	56.6
Beef/sirloin (113g)	320	21	59.1
Beef/T-bone (113g)	338	24	63.9
Butter (15ml)	102	11	97.1
Cheese/American (28g)	93	7	67.7
Cheese/cheddar (28g)	114	9	71.1
Cheese/cottage 4% (240ml)	216	9	37.5
Cheese/cream (28g)	99	10	90.9
Cheese/Parmesan (28g)	129	9	62.8
Cheese/Swiss (28g)	106	8	67.9
Cheeseburger (1)	305	13	38.4
Chicken/breast/no skin (113g)	188	4	19.1
Chicken/thigh/no skin (113g)	232	13	50.4
Egg/hard-cooked (1)	77	5	58.4
Frankfurter/beef & pork (1)	182	17	84.1
Halibut/baked (113g)	159	3	17.0
Hamburger (1)	255	9	31.8
Ice cream/vanilla (240ml)	267	15	50.6
Ice milk/vanilla (240ml)	182	6	29.7
Lamb/lean & fat (113g)	293	19	58.4
Margarine (15ml)	101	11	98.0
Mayonnaise (15ml)	99	11	100.0
Milk/2% (240ml)	121	5	37.2
Milk/skim (240ml)	85	.5	5.3
Milk/whole (240ml)	149	8	48.3
Nuts/cashew/oil roasted (28g)	163	14	77.3
Nuts/peanuts/oil roasted (28g)	165	14	76.4
Oil/canola (15ml)	126	14	100.0
Oil/olive (15ml)	124	14	100.0
Salmon/baked (113g)	245	12	44.1
Sherbet (240ml)	266	4	13.5
Shrimp/boiled (85g)	85	1	10.6
Tuna/oil/drained (85g)	167	7	37.7
Tuna/water/drained (85g)	99	1	9.1
Turkey/dark meat/no skin (113g)	212	8	34.0
Turkey/light meat/no skin (113g)	117	4	30.8

Legend: ■ Saturated fat ■ Polyunsaturated fat ■ Monounsaturated fat ■ Other fatty acids

Percent fat calories (0–100)

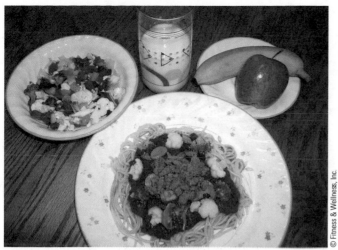

You can restructure your meals so that rice, pasta, beans, breads, and vegetables constitute the major portion of your meal; meats are added primarily for flavouring; fruits are used for desserts; and low- or nonfat milk products are used.

The following "super" foods that fight disease and promote health should be included often in the diet.

- Avocados
- Bananas
- Beans
- Beets
- Blueberries
- Broccoli
- Butternut squash
- Carrots
- Grapes
- Kale
- Kiwifruit
- Flaxseeds
- Nuts (Brazil, walnuts)

- Salmon (wild)
- Soy
- Oats and oatmeal
- Olives and olive oil
- Onions
- Oranges
- Peppers
- Strawberries
- Spinach
- Tea (green, black, red)
- Tomatoes
- Yogurt

and the amount eaten. Do this immediately after each meal so you will be able to keep track of your actual food intake more easily.

If you eat twice the amount of a standard serving, double the number of servings you write down. Evaluate your diet by checking whether you ate the minimum required servings for each food group. If you meet the minimum required servings at the end of each day, you are doing well in balancing your diet.

Once you have completed the nutrient analysis (Lab 3A), you may conduct a self-evaluation of your current nutritional habits. In Lab 3B, you can also assess your current stage of change regarding healthy nutrition and list strategies to help you improve your diet.

Vegetarianism

More than 900,000 people (4 percent of the population) in Canada follow vegetarian diets. **Vegetarians** rely primarily on foods from the bread, cereal, rice, pasta, and fruit and vegetable groups and avoid most foods from animal sources in the dairy and protein groups. The five basic types of vegetarians are as follows:

1. **Vegans** eat no animal products at all.
2. **Ovovegetarians** allow eggs in the diet.
3. **Lactovegetarians** allow foods from the milk group.
4. **Ovolactovegetarians** include egg and milk products in the diet.
5. **Semivegetarians** do not eat red meat, but do include fish and poultry in addition to milk products and eggs in their diet.

Vegetarian diets can be healthful and consistent with the Dietary Guidelines for Canadians and can

meet the DRIs for nutrients. However, vegetarians who do not select their food combinations properly can develop nutritional deficiencies of protein, vitamins, minerals, and even calories. Even greater attention should be paid when planning vegetarian diets for infants and children. Unless carefully planned, a strict plant-based diet will prevent proper growth and development.

Nutrient Concerns

Protein deficiency can be a concern in some vegetarian diets. Vegans in particular must be careful to eat foods that provide a balanced distribution of essential amino acids, such as grain products and legumes. Strict vegans also need a supplement of vitamin B_{12}. This vitamin is not found in plant foods; its only source is animal foods. Deficiency of this vitamin can lead to anemia and nerve damage.

The key to a healthful vegetarian diet is to eat foods that possess complementary proteins. Most plant-based products lack one or more essential amino acids in adequate amounts. For example, both grains and legumes are good protein sources, but neither provides all the essential amino acids. Grains

Vegetarians Individuals whose diet is of vegetable or plant origin.

Vegans Vegetarians who eat no animal products at all.

Ovovegetarians Vegetarians who allow eggs in their diet.

Lactovegetarians Vegetarians who eat foods from the milk group.

Ovolactovegetarians Vegetarians who include eggs and milk products in their diet.

Semivegetarians Vegetarians who include milk products, eggs, and fish and poultry in the diet.

and cereals are low in the amino acid lysine, and legumes lack methionine. Foods from these two groups—such as combinations of tortillas and beans, rice and beans, rice and soybeans, or wheat bread and peanuts—complement each other and provide all required protein nutrients. These complementary proteins may be consumed over the course of one day, but it is best if they are consumed during the same meal.

Other nutrients likely to be deficient in vegetarian diets—and ways to overcome them—are as follows:

- Vitamin D can be obtained from moderate exposure to the sun or by taking a supplement.
- Riboflavin can be found in green leafy vegetables, whole grains, and legumes.
- Calcium can be obtained from fortified soybean milk or fortified orange juice, calcium-rich tofu, and selected cereals. A calcium supplement is also an option.
- Iron can be found in whole grains, dried fruits and nuts, and legumes. To enhance iron absorption, a good source of vitamin C should be consumed with these foods (calcium and iron are the most difficult nutrients to consume in sufficient amounts in a strict vegan diet).
- Zinc can be obtained from whole grains, wheat germ, beans, nuts, and seeds.

Most vegetarians today consume dairy products and eggs. Those who are interested in vegetarian diets are encouraged to consult additional resources, because special vegetarian diet planning cannot be covered adequately in a few paragraphs.

Nuts

Consumption of nuts, commonly used in vegetarian diets, has received considerable attention in recent years. A few years ago, most people regarded nuts as especially high in fat and calories. Although they are 70 to 90 percent fat, most of it is unsaturated fat. And research indicates that people who eat nuts several times a week have a lower incidence of heart disease. Eating 55 to 85 g of almonds, walnuts, or macadamia nuts a day may decrease high blood cholesterol by about 10 percent. Nuts can even enhance the cholesterol-lowering effects of the **Mediterranean diet** (discussed in the next section).

Heart-health benefits are attributed not only to the unsaturated fats, but to other nutrients found in nuts, such as vitamin E and folic acid. And nuts are also packed with additional B vitamins, calcium, copper, potassium, magnesium, fibre, and phytochemicals. Many of these nutrients are cancer- and

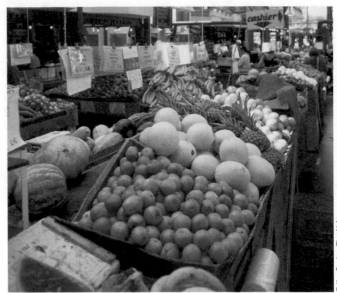

Most fruits and vegetables contain large amounts of cancer-preventing phytochemicals.

cardio-protective, help lower homocysteine levels, and act as antioxidants, discussed in "Antioxidants" (page 73) and "Folate" (page 76).

Nuts do have a drawback: They are high in calories. A handful of nuts provides as many calories as a piece of cake, so nuts should be avoided as a snack. Excessive weight gain is a risk factor for cardiovascular disease. Nuts are recommended for use in place of high-protein foods such as meats, bacon, eggs, or as part of a meal in fruit or vegetable salads, homemade bread, pancakes, casseroles, yogurt, and oatmeal. Peanut butter is also healthier than cheese or some cold cuts in sandwiches.

Soy Products

The increased popularity of soy foods, including use in vegetarian diets, is attributed primarily to Asian research that points to less heart disease, lower cholesterol levels, and fewer hormone-related cancers in people who regularly consume soy foods. The benefits of soy lie in its high protein content and plant chemicals, known as *isoflavones*, that act as antioxidants and may protect against estrogen-related cancers (breast, ovarian, and endometrial). The compound *genistein*, one of many phytochemicals in soy, helps to reduce the risk for breast cancer, and soy consumption also has been linked to a lower risk for prostate cancer.

In addition, soy proteins can lower blood cholesterol to a greater extent than would be expected just from its low-fat and high-fibre content. Approximately 475 millilitres soy milk, 120 millilitres of tofu,

20 grams of soy protein isolate, or 60 millilitres soy flour provide about 10 grams of soy protein.

Mediterranean Diet

Much attention has been given recently to the Mediterranean diet, because people in that region have notably lower rates of diet-linked diseases and a longer life expectancy. The diet focuses on olive oil, grains (whole, not refined), legumes, vegetables, fruits, and, in moderation, fish, red wine, nuts, and dairy products. Although it is a semivegetarian diet, up to 40 percent of the total daily caloric intake may come from fat—mostly monounsaturated fat from olive oil. Moderate intake of red wine is included with meals. The dietary plan also encourages regular physical activity (see Figure 3.10).

More than a "diet," the Mediterranean diet is a dietary pattern that has existed for centuries. According to the largest and most comprehensive research on this dietary pattern, the health benefits and decreased mortality are not linked to any specific component of the diet (such as olive oil or red wine) but are achieved through the interaction of all the components of the pattern.[7] Those who adhere most closely to the dietary pattern had a lower incidence of heart disease (33 percent) and deaths from cancer (24 percent). While most people focus on the olive oil component of the diet, olive oil is used mainly as a means to increase consumption of vegetables because sautéed vegetables in oil taste better than steamed vegetables.

Ethnic Diets

As people migrate, they take their dietary practices with them. Many ethnic diets are healthier than the typical North American diet, because they emphasize consumption of complex carbohydrates and limit fat intake. Unfortunately, the generally healthier ethnic diets quickly become North Americanized. Often, these newcomers cut back on vegetables and add meats and salt to their diet in conformity with the North American consumer.

Ethnic dishes, nonetheless, can be prepared at home. They are easy to make and much healthier when using the typical (original) variety of vegetables, corn, rice, spices, and condiments. Ethnic health recommendations also encourage daily physical activity and suggest no more than two alcoholic drinks per day.

The African American diet (soul food) is based on the regional cuisine of the American South. Soul food includes yams, black-eyed peas, okra, and peanuts. The latter have been combined with American foods such as corn products and pork. Today, most people think of soul food as meat, fried chicken, sweet potatoes, and chitterling.

Hispanic dishes arrived with the Spanish and evolved through combinations with other ethnic diets and local foods available in Latin America. The Hispanic diet incorporates a wide variety of foods, including red meat, but the staple still includes rice, corn, and beans.

Asian-American diets are characteristically rich in vegetables and use minimal meat and fat. The Okinawan diet in Japan, where some of the healthiest and oldest people in the world live, is high in fresh (versus pickled) vegetables, high in fibre, and low in fat and salt. The Chinese cuisine includes more than 200 vegetables, and fat-free sauces and seasoning are used to enhance flavour. The Chinese diet varies somewhat within regions of China. The lowest in fat is that of southern China, with most meals containing fish, seafood, and stir-fried vegetables. Chinese food in North American restaurants contains a much higher percentage of fat and protein than the traditional Chinese cuisine.

FIGURE 3.10 The traditional healthy Mediterranean diet pyramid

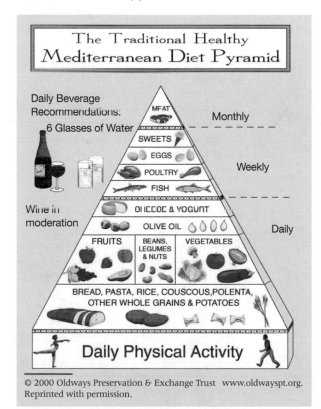

Mediterranean diet Typical diet of people around the Mediterranean region that focuses on olive oil, red wine, grains, legumes, vegetables, and fruits, with limited amounts of meat, fish, milk, and cheese.

Table 3.8 provides a list of healthier foods to choose from when dining at selected ethnic restaurants.

All healthy diets have similar characteristics: They are high in fruits, vegetables, and grains, and low in fat and saturated fat. Healthy diets also use low-fat or fat-free dairy products, and they emphasize portion control—essential in a healthy diet plan.

Many people now think that if a food item is labelled "low-fat" or "fat-free," they can consume it in large quantities. "Low-fat" or "fat-free" does not imply "calorie-free." Many people who consume low-fat diets eat more (and thus increase their caloric intake), which in the long term leads to obesity and its associated health problems.

Nutrient Supplementation

A significant percentage (46 percent of women and 33 percent of men) of all adults in Canada take daily nutrient **supplements**. Nutrient requirements for the body normally can be met by consuming as few as 1,200 Calories per day, as long as the diet contains the recommended servings from the five food groups in Canada's Food Guide. Still, many people consider it necessary to take vitamin supplements.

It's true that our bodies cannot retain water-soluble vitamins as long as fat-soluble vitamins. The body excretes excessive intakes readily, although the body can retain small amounts for weeks or months in various organs and tissues. Fat-soluble vitamins, by contrast, are stored in fatty tissue. Therefore, daily intake of these vitamins is not as crucial. Too much vitamin A and vitamin D actually can be detrimental to health.

People should not take **megadoses** of vitamins and minerals. For some nutrients, a dose of five times the RDA taken over several months may create problems. For other nutrients, it may not pose a threat to human health. Vitamin and mineral doses should not exceed the ULs. For nutrients that do not have an established UL, a person should take a dose no higher than twice the RDA.

Iron deficiency (determined through blood testing) is more common in women than men. Iron supplementation is frequently recommended for women who have heavy menstrual flow. Some pregnant and lactating women also may require supplements. The average pregnant woman who eats an adequate amount of a variety of foods should take a low dose of iron supplement daily. Women who are pregnant with more than one baby may need additional supplements. Folate supplements also are encouraged prior to and during pregnancy to prevent certain birth defects (see following discussions

TABLE 3.8 Ethnic Eating Guide

	Choose Often	Choose Less Often
Chinese	Beef with broccoli Chinese greens Steamed rice, brown or white Steamed beef with pea pods Stir-fry dishes Teriyaki beef or chicken Wonton soup	Crispy duck Egg rolls Fried rice Kung pao chicken (fried) Peking duck Pork spareribs
Japanese	Chiri nabe (fish stew) Grilled scallops Sushi, sashimi (raw fish) Teriyaki Yakitori (grilled chicken)	Tempura (fried chicken, shrimp, or vegetables) Tonkatsu (fried pork)
Italian	Cioppino (seafood stew) Minestrone (vegetarian soup) Pasta with marinara sauce Pasta primavera (pasta with vegetables) Steamed clams	Antipasto Cannelloni, ravioli Fettuccini alfredo Garlic bread White clam sauce
Middle Eastern	Tandoori chicken Curry (yogurt-based) Rice pilaf Lentil soup Shish kebab	Falafel
French	Poached salmon Spinach salad Consommé Salad niçoise	Beef Wellington Escargot French onion soup Sauces in general
Soul Food	Baked chicken Baked fish Roasted pork (not smothered or "etouffe") Sauteed okra Baked sweet potato	Fried chicken Fried fish Smothered pork tenderloin Okra in gumbo Sweet potato casserole or pie
Greek	Gyros Pita Lentil soup	Baklava Moussaka
Mexican	Beans and rice Black bean/vegetable soup Burritos, bean Chili Enchiladas, bean Fajitas Gazpacho Taco salad Tamales Tortillas, steamed	Chili rellenos Chimichangas Enchiladas, beef or cheese Flautas Guacamole Nachos Quesadillas Tostadas Sour cream (as topping)

Source: Adapted from P. A. Floyd, S. E. Mimms, and C. Yelding-Howard. *Personal Health: Perspectives & Lifestyles* (Belmont, CA: Wadsworth/Thomson Learning, 1998).

of antioxidants and folates). In the above instances, supplements should be taken under a physician's supervision.

Other people who may benefit from supplementation are those with nutrient deficiencies (including low calcium intake), alcoholics and street-drug users who do not have a balanced diet, smokers, vegans (strict vegetarians), individuals on extremely low-calorie diets (fewer than 1,200 Calories per day), older adults who don't eat balanced meals regularly, newborn infants (who usually are given a single dose of vitamin K to prevent abnormal bleeding), and people with disease-related disorders or who are taking medications that interfere with proper nutrient absorption.

Although some supplements are encouraged (see discussion that follows), most supplements do not seem to provide additional benefits for healthy people who eat a balanced diet. They do not help people run faster, jump higher, relieve stress, improve sexual prowess, cure a common cold, or boost energy levels.

Antioxidants

Much research is being done to study the effectiveness of **antioxidants** in thwarting several chronic diseases. Although foods probably contain more than 4,000 antioxidants, the four more studied antioxidants are vitamins C, E, and beta-carotene (a precursor to vitamin A), and the mineral selenium (see Table 3.9).

Oxygen is used during metabolism to change carbohydrates and fats into energy. During this process, oxygen is transformed into stable forms of water and carbon dioxide. A small amount of oxygen, however, ends up in an unstable form, referred to as **oxygen free radicals**.

A free radical molecule has a normal proton nucleus with a single unpaired electron. Having only one electron makes the free radical extremely reactive, and it looks constantly to pair its electron with one from another molecule. When a free

radical steals a second electron from another molecule, that other molecule in turn becomes a free radical. This chain reaction goes on until two free radicals meet to form a stable molecule.

Free radicals attack and damage proteins and lipids, in particular cell membranes and DNA. This damage is thought to contribute to the development of conditions such as cardiovascular disease, cancer, emphysema, cataracts, Parkinson's disease, and premature aging. Solar radiation, cigarette smoke, air pollution, radiation, some drugs, injury, infection, chemicals (such as pesticides), and other environmental factors also seem to encourage the formation of free radicals. Antioxidants are thought to offer protection by absorbing free radicals before they can cause damage and also by interrupting the sequence of reactions once damage has begun, thwarting certain chronic diseases (see Figure 3.11).

The body's own defence systems typically neutralize free radicals so they don't cause any damage. When free radicals are produced faster than the body can neutralize them, however, they can damage the cells.

Antioxidants are found abundantly in food, especially in fruits and vegetables. Unfortunately, most people do not eat the minimum seven daily servings of fruits and vegetables (seven to ten is the recommendation in Canada's Food Guide).

Supplements Tablets, pills, capsules, liquids, or powders that contain vitamins, minerals, amino acids, herbs, or fibre that are taken to increase the intake of these nutrients.

Megadoses For most vitamins, 10 times the RDA or more; for vitamins A and D, 5 and 2 times the RDA, respectively.

Antioxidants Compounds such as vitamins C and E, beta-carotene, and selenium that prevent oxygen from combining with other substances in the body to form harmful compounds.

Oxygen free radicals Substances formed during metabolism that attack and damage proteins and lipids, in particular the cell membrane and DNA, leading to diseases such as heart disease, cancer, and emphysema.

TABLE 3.9 Antioxidant Nutrients, Sources, and Functions

Nutrient	Good Sources	Antioxidant Effect
Vitamin C	Citrus fruit, kiwi fruit, cantaloupe, strawberries, broccoli, green or red peppers, cauliflower, cabbage	Appears to deactivate oxygen free radicals.
Vitamin E	Vegetable oils, yellow and green leafy vegetables, margarine, wheat germ, oatmeal, almonds, whole-grain breads, cereals	Protects lipids from oxidation.
Beta-carotene	Carrots, squash, pumpkin, sweet potatoes, broccoli, green leafy vegetables	Soaks up oxygen free radicals.
Selenium	Seafood, Brazil nuts, meat, whole grains	Helps prevent damage to cell structures.

FIGURE 3.11 Antioxidant protection: blocking and absorbing oxygen free radicals to prevent chronic disease

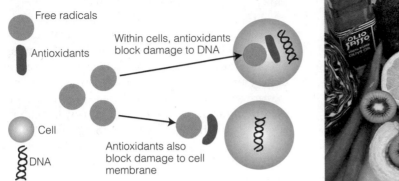

Free radicals

Antioxidants

Within cells, antioxidants block damage to DNA

Cell

DNA

Antioxidants also block damage to cell membrane

© Fitness & Wellness, Inc.

The benefits of antioxidants are obtained primarily from food sources themselves, and controversy surrounds the benefits of antioxidants taken in supplement form.

Some researchers believe that taking antioxidant supplements further prevents free-radical damage. For example, in 2001, the editorial board of the *University of California at Berkeley Wellness Letter* updated its daily antioxidant nutrient intake recommendations to include[8]

■ 250 to 500 mg of vitamin C
■ 200 to 400 **IU (international units)** of vitamin E (look for natural vitamin E, because the body does not use synthetic forms well).

Vitamin C

Based on the above recommendations, people who consume five or more daily servings of fresh fruits and vegetables can get their daily vitamin C requirements through the diet alone. Studies have shown that vitamin C offers benefits against heart disease, cancer, cataracts, and several other health disorders.

Vitamin C is water-soluble, and the body eliminates it in about 12 hours. For best results, consume vitamin C-rich foods twice a day or divide your vitamin C supplement in half and take it twice a day. High intake of a vitamin C supplement (above 500 mg per day) is no longer recommended. More than 500 daily mg is unnecessary, given that research at the National Institutes of Health showed that the body absorbs very little vitamin C beyond the first 200 mg per serving or dose.

Selenium may interfere with the body's absorption of vitamin C, so the two should be taken separately. Wait about an hour following vitamin C intake before taking selenium.

Vitamin E

Vitamin E belongs to a group of eight compounds (four tocopherols and four tocotrienols) of which alpha-tocopherol is the most active form. The antioxidant recommendation for vitamin E is much higher than the RDA (15 mg or 22 IU). To obtain the daily recommended guideline for vitamin E through diet alone, however, is practically impossible. Vitamin E is found primarily in oil-rich seeds and vegetable oils. As shown in Table 3.10, vitamin E is not easily found in large quantities in foods typically consumed in the diet.

Among the benefits of Vitamin E, it may help prevent atherosclerosis in healthy people and diabetics, it seems to lower the risk of stroke, and it improves immune function. Some evidence has suggested that supplemental intake of vitamin E reduces the risk of heart disease, but it may not offer additional protection to people who already have the disease. Healthy people who take vitamin E may have fewer heart problems, and the vitamin seems to slow the progression of plaque (atherosclerosis) in the arteries. Other research, however, has questioned the health benefits of vitamin E supplementation. Thus, controversy exists regarding the benefits of supplementation, and additional research is necessary before final recommendations can be made concerning vitamin E supplementation.

Vitamin E supplements from natural sources contain d-alpha tocopherol, which is better absorbed by the body than dl-alpha tocopherol, a synthetic form composed of a variety of E compounds. Because vitamin E is fat-soluble, it should be taken with a meal that has some fat in it. Vitamin E also enhances the effects of selenium, so these should be taken together for best results. Antioxidant nutrients often work in conjunction with other nutrients in food that may further enhance their beneficial actions.

TABLE 3.10 Antioxidant Content of Selected Foods

Beta-Carotene	IU
Apricot (1 medium)	675
Broccoli (115 g, frozen)	1,740
Broccoli (115 g, raw)	680
Cantaloupe (230 g)	5,160
Carrot (1 medium, raw)	20,255
Green peas (115 g, frozen)	535
Mango (1 medium)	8,060
Mustard greens (115 g, frozen)	3,350
Papaya (1 medium)	6,120
Spinach (115 g, frozen)	7,395
Sweet potato (1 medium, baked)	24,875
Tomato (1 medium)	1,395
Turnip greens (115 g, boiled)	3,960

Vitamin C	mg
Acerola (230 g raw)	1,640
Acerola juice (250 ml)	3,864
Cantaloupe (½ melon, medium)	90
Cranberry juice (250 ml)	90
Grapefruit (½, medium, white)	52
Grapefruit juice (250 ml)	92
Guava (1 medium)	165
Kiwi (1 medium)	75
Lemon juice (250 mL)	110
Orange (1 medium)	66
Orange juice (250 mL)	120
Papaya (1 medium)	85
Pepper (115 g, red, chopped, raw)	95
Strawberries (230 g, raw)	88

Vitamin E	IU	mg*
Almond oil (15 mL)		5.3
Almonds (30 g)	10.1	
Canola oil (15 mL)		9.0
Cottonseed oil (15 mL)		5.2
Hazelnuts (30 g)	4.4	
Kale (230 g)	15.0	
Margarine (15 mL)		2.0
Peanuts (30 g)	3.0	
Shrimp (85 g)	3.1	
Sunflower seeds (30 g, dry)	14.2	
Sunflower seed oil (15 mL)		6.9
Sweet potato (1 medium, baked)	7.2	
Wheat germ oil (15 mL)		20.0

Selenium	mcg
Brazil nuts (1)	100
Bread, whole wheat enriched (1 slice)	15
Beef (85 g)	33
Cereals (100 g)	20
Chicken breast, roasted, no skin (85 g)	24
Cod, baked (85 g)	57
Egg, hard boiled (1 large)	15
Fruits (100 g)	1
Noodles, enriched, boiled (230 g)	50
Oatmeal, cooked (230 g)	23
Red snapper (85 g)	150
Rice, long grain, cooked (230 g)	20
Salmon, baked (85 g)	35
Spaghetti w/meat sauce (230 g)	36
Tuna, canned, water, drained (85 g)	68
Turkey breast, roasted, no skin (85 g)	28
Walnuts, black, chopped (57.5 g)	5
Vegetables (100 g)	1

* Vitamin E values for oils are commonly expressed in milligrams (mg). One mg is almost equal to 1 IU (international unit).

Beta-carotene

Beta-carotene supplementation was encouraged in the early 1990s. It is better, however, to obtain the daily recommended dose of beta-carotene (20,000 IU) from food sources rather than supplements. Clinical trials have found that beta-carotene supplements offered no protection against heart disease and cancer or provided any other health benefits.[9] Therefore, it is recommended that you "skip the pill and eat the carrot." One medium raw carrot contains about 20,000 IU of beta-carotene.

Selenium

Adequate intake of the mineral selenium is encouraged. Studies indicate that individuals who take 200 micrograms (mcg) of selenium daily decreased their risk of prostate cancer by 63 percent, colorectal cancer by 58 percent, and lung cancer by 46 percent.[10] Data also point to decreased risk of breast, liver, and digestive tract cancers. According to Dr. Edward Giovannucci of the Harvard Medical School, the evidence for the benefits of selenium in reducing prostate cancer risk is so strong that public health officials should recommend that people increase their selenium intake.

One Brazil nut (unshelled) that you crack yourself provides about 100 mcg of selenium. Shelled nuts found in supermarkets average only about 20 mcg each. Based on the current body of

International unit (IU) Measure of nutrients in foods.

research, a dose of 100 to 200 mcg per day seems to provide the necessary amount of antioxidant for this nutrient. There is no reason to take more than 200 mcg daily. In fact, the UL for selenium has been set at 400 mcg. Too much selenium can damage cells rather than protect them. If you choose to take supplements, take an organic form of selenium from yeast and not selenium selenite. The selenium content of various foods is provided in Table 3.10.

Although much interest has been generated by the previously mentioned supplements, multivitamins are still the preferred supplement of North Americans. A multivitamin complex that provides 100 percent of the DV for most nutrients can help fill in certain dietary deficiencies.[11] Some evidence suggests that regular intake decreases the risk for heart disease and stroke.

Multivitamins, however, are not magic pills. They can help, but they don't provide a licence to eat carelessly. Multivitamins don't provide energy, fibre, phytochemicals, or the recommended daily dose of vitamin C (250 to 500 mg) and vitamin E (200 to 400 IU).

Folate

Although it is not an antioxidant, 400 mcg of **folate** (a B vitamin) is recommended for all pre-menopausal women. Folate helps prevent certain birth defects and seems to offer protection against colon and cervical cancers. Women who might become pregnant should plan on taking a folate supplement, because studies have shown that folate intake (400 mcg per day) during early pregnancy can prevent serious birth defects.

Increasing evidence also indicates that taking 400 mcg of folate along with vitamins B_6 and B_{12} prevents heart attacks by reducing homocysteine levels in the blood (see Chapter 11). High concentrations of homocysteine accelerate the process of plaque formation (atherosclerosis) in the arteries. Five servings of fruits and vegetables per day usually meet the needs for these nutrients. Currently, many people do not obtain the recommended 400 mcg of folate per day. Because of the critical role of folate in preventing heart disease, some experts recommend a daily vitamin B complex that includes 400 mcg of folate.

Side Effects

Toxic effects from antioxidant supplements are rare when they are taken in the recommended amounts. The daily UL for adults 19 to 70 years of age for vitamin C has been set at 2,000 mg, for vitamin E at 1,000 mg, and for selenium at 400 mcg. If any of the following side effects arise, you should stop supplementation and check with your physician:

- Vitamin E: gastrointestinal disturbances, increase in blood lipids (determined through blood tests)
- Vitamin C: nausea, diarrhea, abdominal cramps, kidney stones, liver problems
- Selenium: nausea, vomiting, diarrhea, irritability, fatigue, flu-like symptoms, lesions of the skin and nervous tissue, loss of hair and nails, respiratory failure, liver damage

Substantial supplementation of vitamin E is not recommended for individuals on **anticoagulant** therapy. Vitamin E is an anticoagulant in itself. Therefore, if you are on such therapy, check with your physician. Pregnant women need a physician's approval prior to beta-carotene supplementation. Vitamin E also may be unsafe if taken with alcohol or by people who drink more than 125 mL of pure alcohol per day (the equivalent of eight beers).

Benefits of Foods

Even though you may consider taking some supplements, fruits and vegetables are the richest sources of antioxidants and phytochemicals. Researchers at the U.S. Department of Agriculture compared the antioxidant effects of vitamins C and E with those of various common fruits and vegetables. The results indicated that 175 g of cooked kale (which contains only 11 IU of vitamin E and 76 mg of vitamin C) neutralized as many free radicals as approximately 800 IU of vitamin E or 600 mg of vitamin C. Other excellent sources of antioxidants found by these researchers include blueberries, strawberries, spinach, Brussels sprouts, plums, broccoli, beets, oranges, and grapes. A list of top antioxidant foods is presented in Figure 3.12.

Many people who regularly eat foods high in fat content or too many sweets think they need supplementation to balance their diet. This is another fallacy about nutrition. The problem here is not necessarily a lack of vitamins and minerals, but a diet too high in calories, fat, and sodium. Vitamin, mineral, and fibre supplements do not supply all of the nutrients and other beneficial substances present in food and needed for good health. Supplements will provide added health benefits, but by no means will they replace a well-balanced diet.

Wholesome foods contain vitamins, minerals, carbohydrates, fibre, proteins, fats, phytochemicals, and other substances not yet discovered. Researchers do not know if the protective effects are caused by the antioxidants alone, or in combination with other nutrients (such as phytochemicals), or by some other nutrients in food that have not been

FIGURE 3.12 Top antioxidant foods

Top Antioxidant Foods [ORAC* units per 100 grams**]			
Fruits		**Vegetables**	
Prunes	5770	Kale	1770
Raisins	2830	Spinach	1260
Blueberries	2400	Brussels sprouts	980
Blackberries	2036	Alfalfa sprouts	930
Strawberries	1540	Broccoli florets	890
Raspberries	1220	Beets	840
Plums	949	Red bell peppers	710
Oranges	750	Onions	450
Red grapes	739	Corn	400
Cherries	670	Eggplant	390
* Oxygen Radical Absorbance Capacity		** About 3.5 ounces	

USDA, Agricultural Research Service, Food & Nutrition Research Briefs, April 1999. www.ars.usda.gov/is/np/fnrb/fnrb499.htm.

investigated yet. Many nutrients work in **synergy**, enhancing chemical processes in the body.

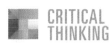

CRITICAL THINKING

Do you take supplements? If so, for what purposes are you taking them—and do you think you could restructure your diet so you could do without them?

Supplementation will not offset poor eating habits. Pills are no substitute for common sense.

If you think your diet is not balanced, you first need to conduct a nutrient analysis (see Lab 3A) to determine which nutrients you lack in sufficient amounts. Eat more of them, as well as foods that are high in antioxidants and phytochemicals. Following a nutrient assessment, a **registered dietitian** can help you decide what supplement(s) might be necessary. You can also access information about the Reference Values for vitamins from Health Canada's website and information about the health benefits of selected minerals from the Canadian Family Physician's website. See the Internet Connections feature at the end of the chapter for the web addresses.

Functional Foods

Functional foods are any food or food ingredient that offers specific health benefits beyond those supplied by the nutrients it contains. Many functional foods come in their natural form. A tomato, for example, is a functional food because it contains the phytochemical lycopene, thought to reduce the risk for prostate cancer. Other examples of functional foods are kale, broccoli, blueberries, red grapes, and green tea.

The term *functional food*, however, has been used primarily as a marketing tool by the food industry to attract consumers. Unlike **fortified foods**, which have been modified to help prevent nutrient deficiencies, the food industry is creating functional foods by adding ingredients aimed at treating or preventing symptoms or disease. In functional foods, the added ingredient(s) is often not typically found in the particular food item in its natural form but is added to allow manufacturers to make appealing health claims.

In most cases, only one extra ingredient is added (a vitamin, mineral, phytochemical, or herb). An example is calcium added to orange juice to make the claim that this brand offers protection against osteoporosis. Food manufacturers now offer cholesterol-lowering margarines (enhanced with plant stanol), cancer-protective (lycopene-fortified) ketchup, memory-boosting (ginkgo-added) candy, calcium-fortified chips, and corn chips containing kava-kava (to enhance relaxation).

Folate One of the B vitamins.

Anticoagulant Any substance that inhibits blood clotting.

Synergy A reaction in which the result is greater than the sum of its two parts.

Registered dietitian (RD) A person with a college degree in dietetics who meets all certification and continuing education requirements of the American Dietetic Association or Dietitians of Canada.

Functional foods Foods or food ingredients containing physiologically active substances that provide specific health benefits beyond those supplied by basic nutrition.

Fortified foods Foods that have added nutrients that either were not present or were present in insignificant amounts with the intent of preventing nutrient deficiencies.

The use of some functional foods, however, may undermine good nutrition. Margarines still may contain saturated fats or partially hydrogenated oils. Regular ketchup consumption on top of large orders of fries adds many calories and fat to the diet. Sweets are also high in calories and sugar. Chips are high in calories, salt, and fat. In all of these cases, the consumer would be better off taking the specific ingredient in a supplement form rather than consuming the functional food with its extra calories, sugar, salt, and/or fat.

Functional foods can provide added benefits, however, if used in conjunction with a healthful diet. You may use nutrient-dense functional foods in your overall wellness plan as an adjunct to health-promoting strategies and treatments.

Genetically Modified Crops

A genetically modified organism (GMO) is one whose DNA (or basic genetic material) is manipulated to obtain certain results. This is done by inserting genes with desirable traits from one plant, animal, or microorganism into another one to either introduce new traits or enhance existing ones.

Crops are genetically modified to make them better resist disease and extreme environmental conditions (such as heat and frost), require fewer fertilizers and pesticides, last longer, and improve their nutrient content and taste. Such crops could help save billions of dollars by producing more crops and helping to feed other people in developing countries around the world.

Concerns over the safety of **genetically modified foods** (GM foods) have created heated public debates in Europe and more recently in Canada. The concern is that genetic modifications create "transgenic" organisms that have not previously existed and that have potentially unpredictable effects on the environment and on humans. Also, there is some concern that GM foods may cause illness or allergies in humans and that cross-pollination may destroy other plants or create "superweeds" with herbicide-resistant genes.

Genetically modified crops were first approved in Canada in 1994. This technology is moving forward very rapidly, and the Canadian Food and Inspection Agency (CFIA) and the Canadian General Standards Board are developing a standard for voluntary labelling of GM products. Labelling of GM products to date is necessary only if the modification has resulted in potential health or safety concerns, such as a nutritional or compositional change or an increase in potential allergenicity. You can find out more about the labelling of GM products in a report prepared for the Canadian Biotechnology Advisory Committee at www.cbac-ccb.ca.

At this point, conclusive evidence that GM products are harmful is not availble, but there is compelling evidence guarantees that they are safe, either. Many questions remain, and much research is required in this field. As a consumer, you need to continue educating yourself as more evidence becomes available in the next few years.

Energy Substrates for Physical Activity

The two main fuels that supply energy for physical activity are glucose (sugar) and fat (fatty acids). The body uses amino acids, derived from proteins, as an energy substrate when glucose is low, such as during fasting, prolonged aerobic exercise, or a low-carbohydrate diet.

Glucose is derived from foods high in carbohydrates such as breads, cereals, grains, pasta, beans, fruits, vegetables, and sweets in general. Glucose is stored as glycogen in muscles and the liver. Fatty acids (discussed on pages 56–58) are the product of the breakdown of fats. Unlike glucose, an almost unlimited supply of fatty acids, stored as fat in the body, can be used during exercise.

Energy (ATP) Production

The energy derived from food is not used directly by the cells. It is first transformed into **adenosine triphosphate (ATP)**. The subsequent breakdown of this compound provides the energy used by all energy-requiring processes of the body (also see Figure 3.13). ATP must be recycled continually to sustain life and work. ATP can be resynthesized in three ways:

1. *ATP and ATP-CP system*. The body stores small amounts of ATP and creatine phosphate (CP). These stores are used during all-out activities such as sprinting, long jumping, and weight lifting. The amount of stored ATP provides energy for just one or two seconds. During brief all-out efforts, ATP is resynthesized from CP, another high-energy phosphate compound. This is the ATP-CP, or phosphagen, system.

   Depending on the amount of physical training, the concentration of CP stored in cells is sufficient to allow maximum exertion for up to 10 seconds. Once the CP stores are depleted, the person is forced to slow down or rest to allow ATP to form through anaerobic and aerobic pathways.

2. *Anaerobic or* **lactic acid** *system*. During maximal-intensity exercise that is sustained between 10 and 180 seconds, ATP is replenished from the breakdown of glucose through a series of chemical reactions that do not require oxygen (hence "anaerobic"). In the process, though, lactic acid is produced. As lactic acid accumulates, it leads to muscular fatigue.

   Because of the accumulation of lactic acid with high-intensity exercise, the formation of ATP during anaerobic activities is limited to about three minutes. A recovery period is then necessary to allow for the removal of lactic acid. Formation of ATP through the anaerobic system requires glucose (carbohydrates).

3. *Aerobic system*. The production of energy during slow-sustained exercise is derived primarily through aerobic metabolism. Glucose (carbohydrates), fatty acids (fat), and oxygen (hence "aerobic") are required to form ATP using this process and, under steady-state exercise conditions, lactic acid accumulation is minimal.

   Because oxygen is required, a person's capacity to utilize oxygen is crucial for successful athletic performance in aerobic events. The higher one's maximal oxygen uptake (VO$_2$max), the greater one's capacity to generate ATP through the aerobic system—and the better the athletic performance in long-distance events.

From the previous discussion, it becomes evident that, for optimal performance, both recreational and highly competitive athletes make the required nutrients a part of their diet.

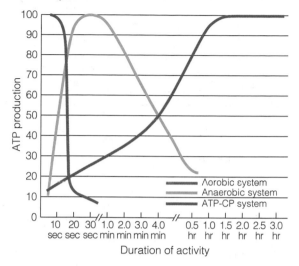

FIGURE 3.13 Contributions of the energy formation mechanisms during various forms of physical activity

Nutrition for Athletes

During resting conditions, fat supplies about two-thirds of the energy to sustain the body's vital processes. During exercise, the body uses both glucose (glycogen) and fat in combination to supply the energy demands. The proportion of fat to glucose changes with the intensity of exercise. When a person is exercising below 60 percent of his or her maximal work capacity (VO$_2$max), fat is used as the primary energy substrate. As the intensity of exercise increases, so does the percentage of glucose utilization—up to 100 percent during maximal work that can be sustained for only two to three minutes.

In general, athletes do not require special supplementation or any other special type of diet. Unless the diet is deficient in basic nutrients, no special secret or magic diet will help people perform better or develop faster as a result of what they eat. As long as the diet is balanced—that is, based on a large variety of nutrients from all basic food groups—athletes do not require additional supplements. Even in strength training and body building, protein in excess of 20 percent of total

Genetically modified foods (GM foods) Foods whose basic genetic material (DNA) is manipulated by inserting genes with desirable traits from one plant, animal, or microorganism into another one either to introduce new traits or to enhance existing ones.

Adenosine triphosphate (ATP) A high-energy chemical compound that the body uses for immediate energy.

Lactic acid End product of anaerobic glycolysis (metabolism).

TABLE 3.11 Recommended Daily Protein Intake

Activity level	Intake in grams per kg of body weight
Sedentary	0.8
Lightly active	0.9
Moderately active	1.1
Very active	1.3
Extremely active	1.5

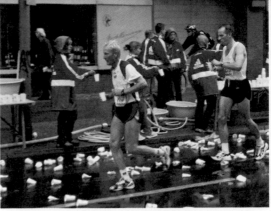

Fluid and carbohydrate replenishment during exercise are essential when participating in long-distance aerobic endurance events, such as a marathon or a triathlon.

daily caloric intake is not necessary. The recommended daily protein intake ranges from 0.8 g/kg of body weight for sedentary people to 1.5 g/kg for extremely active individuals (see Table 3.11).

The main difference between a sensible diet for a sedentary person and a sensible diet for a highly active individual is the total number of calories required daily and the amount of carbohydrate intake needed during prolonged physical activity. People in training consume more calories because of their greater energy expenditure—which is required as a result of intense physical training.

Carbohydrate Loading

On a regular diet, the body is able to store between 1,500 and 2,000 Calories in the form of glycogen. About 75 percent of this glycogen is stored in muscle tissue. This amount, however, can be increased greatly through **carbohydrate loading**.

A regular diet should be altered during several days of heavy aerobic training or when a person is going to participate in a long-distance event of more than 90 minutes (for example, marathon, triathlon, or road cycling). For events shorter than 90 minutes, carbohydrate loading does not seem to enhance performance.

During prolonged exercise, glycogen is broken down into glucose, which then is readily available to the muscles for energy production. In comparison to fat, glucose frequently is referred to as the "high-octane fuel," because it provides about 6 percent more energy per unit of oxygen consumed.

Heavy training over several consecutive days leads to depletion of glycogen faster than it can be replaced through the diet. Glycogen depletion with heavy training is common in athletes. Signs of depletion include chronic fatigue, difficulty in maintaining accustomed exercise intensity, and lower performance.

On consecutive days of exhaustive physical training (this means several hours daily), a carbohydrate-rich diet—70 percent of total daily caloric intake or 8 grams of carbohydrate per kilogram of body weight—is recommended. This diet often restores glycogen

levels in 24 hours. Along with the high-carbohydrate diet, a day of rest often is needed to allow the muscles to recover from glycogen depletion following days of intense training. For people who exercise less than an hour a day, a 60 percent carbohydrate diet or 6 grams of carbohydrate per kilogram of body weight is enough to replenish glycogen stores.

Following an exhaustive workout, eating a combination of carbohydrates and protein (such as a tuna sandwich) within 30 minutes of exercise seems to speed up glycogen storage even more. Protein intake increases insulin activity, thereby enhancing glycogen replenishment. A 70 percent carbohydrate intake then should be maintained throughout the rest of the day.

By following a special diet and exercise regimen five days before a long-distance event, highly (aerobically) trained individuals are capable of storing two to three times the amount of glycogen found in the average person. Athletic performance may be enhanced for long-distance events of more than 90 minutes by eating a regular balanced diet (50 to 60 percent carbohydrates) along with intensive physical training the fifth and fourth days before the event, followed by a diet high in carbohydrates (about 70 percent) and a gradual decrease in training intensity over the last three days before the event.

The amount of glycogen stored as a result of a carbohydrate-rich diet does not seem to be affected by the proportion of complex and simple carbohydrates. Intake of simple carbohydrates (sugars) can be raised while on a 70 percent carbohydrate diet, as long as they don't exceed 25 percent of the total calories. Complex carbohydrates provide more nutrients and fibre making them a better choice for a healthier diet.

On the day of the long-distance event, carbohydrates are still the recommended choice of substrate. As a general rule, athletes should consume 1 gram of carbohydrate for each kilogram of body weight 1 hour prior to exercise. If the pre-event meal is eaten earlier, the amount of carbohydrate can be increased to 2, 3, or 4 g/kg of weight 2, 3, or 4 hours, respectively, before exercise.

During the long-distance event, researchers recommend that 30 to 60 g of carbohydrates (120 to 240 Calories) be consumed every hour. This is best accomplished by drinking 250 mL of a 6 to 8 percent–carbohydrate sports drink every 15 minutes (check labels to ensure proper carbohydrate concentration). This also lessens the chance of dehydration during exercise, which hinders performance and endangers health. The percentage of the carbohydrate drink is determined by dividing the amount of carbohydrate (in grams) by the amount of fluid (in mL) and then multiplying by 100. For example, 18 g of carbohydrate in 240 mL of fluid yields a drink that is 7.5 percent ($18 \div 240 \times 100$) carbohydrate.

Creatine Supplementation

Creatine is an organic compound obtained in the diet primarily from meat and fish. In the human body, creatine combines with inorganic phosphate and forms the high-energy compound **creatine phosphate (CP).** CP is then used to resynthesize ATP during short bursts of all-out physical activity. Individuals on a normal mixed diet consume an average of 1 gram of creatine per day. Each day, 1 additional gram is synthesized from various amino acids. Half a kilogram of meat or fish provides approximately 2 g of creatine.

Creatine supplementation has become popular in recent years among individuals who want to increase muscle mass and improve athletic performance. Creatine monohydrate—a white, tasteless powder that is mixed with fluids prior to ingestion—is the form most popular among people who use the supplement. Supplementation can result in an approximate 20 percent increase in the amount of creatine that is stored in muscles. Most of this creatine binds to phosphate to form CP, and 30 to 40 percent remains as free creatine in the muscle. Increased creatine storage is believed to enable individuals to train more intensely—thus building more muscle mass and enhancing performance in all-out activities of very short duration (less than 30 seconds).

Creatine supplementation has two phases: the *loading phase* and the *maintenance phase*. During the loading phase, the person consumes between 20 and 25 g of creatine per day for 5 to 6 days, divided into 4 or 5 dosages of 5 g each throughout the day (this amount represents the equivalent of consuming 5 or more kilograms of meat per day). Research also suggests that the amount of creatine stored in muscle is enhanced by taking creatine in combination with a high-carbohydrate food. Once the loading phase is complete, taking 2 g per day seems to be sufficient to maintain the increased muscle stores.

To date, no serious side effects have been documented in people who take up to 25 g of creatine per day for five days. Stomach distress and cramping have been reported only in rare instances. The 2 grams taken per day during the maintenance phase is just slightly above the average intake in our daily diet. Long-term effects of creatine supplementation on health, however, have not been established.

A frequently documented result following five to six days of creatine loading is an increase of 1 to 1.5 kg in body weight. This increase appears to be related to increased water retention necessary to maintain the additional creatine stored in muscles. Some data, however, suggest that the increase in stored water and CP stimulates protein synthesis, leading to an increase in lean body mass.

The benefits of elevated creatine stores may be limited to high-intensity/short-duration activities such as sprinting, strength training (weight lifting), and sprint cycling. Supplementation is most beneficial during exercise training itself, rather than as an aid to enhance athletic performance a few days before competition.

Enhanced creatine stores do not benefit athletes competing in aerobic endurance events, because CP is not used in energy production for long-distance events. In fact, the additional weight can be detrimental in long-distance running and swimming events, because the athlete must expend more energy to carry the extra weight during competition.

Amino Acid Supplements

A myth regarding athletic performance is that protein (amino acid) supplements will increase muscle mass. The claims and safety of these products have not been proven scientifically. The RDA for protein is .8 grams per kilogram of body weight per day. That is, if you weigh 70 kg, you should consume 56 g ($70 \times .8$) of protein.

Most athletes, including weight lifters and body builders, increase their caloric intake automatically during intense training. As caloric intake increases, so does the intake of protein, often approaching 2 or more grams per kilogram of body weight. This amount is more than enough to build and repair muscle tissue. Typically, athletes in strength training consume between 3 and 4 g/kg of body weight. In response, supplement manufacturers have created expensive "free-amino acid supplements."

Carbohydrate loading Increasing intake of carbohydrates during heavy aerobic training or prior to aerobic endurance events that last longer than 90 minutes.

Creatine An organic compound derived from meat, fish, and amino acids that combines with inorganic phosphate to form creatine phosphate.

Creatine phosphate (CP) A high-energy compound that the cells use to resynthesize ATP during all-out activities of very short duration.

People who buy costly free-amino acid supplements are led to believe that these contribute to the development of muscle mass. The human body, however, cannot distinguish between amino acids obtained from food or through supplements. Excess protein either is used for energy or is turned into fat. With amino acid supplements, each capsule provides up to 500 milligrams of amino acids and no additional nutrients. In contrast, 85 g of meat or fish provide more than 20,000 mg of amino acids, along with other essential nutrients such as iron, niacin, and thiamin. The benefits of natural foods to health and budget are clear.

Proponents of free-amino acid supplements further claim that only a small amount of amino acids in food is absorbed and that free-amino acids are absorbed more readily than are protein foods. Neither claim is correct. The human body absorbs and utilizes between 85 and 99 percent of all protein from food intake. The body handles whole, natural proteins better than single amino acids that have been predigested in the laboratory setting.

Amino acid supplementation can even be dangerous: An excess of a single amino acid or a group of chemically similar amino acids often prevents the absorption of other amino acids. Needed amino acids then pass through the body unabsorbed, potentially causing critical imbalances and toxicities. Long-term risks associated with amino acid supplementation have not been determined.

The advertised rate of absorption provides no additional benefit, because building muscle takes hours, not minutes. Muscle overload through heavy training, not supplementation, builds muscle. Expensive protein supplements benefit only those who sell them.

Special Nutrient Needs of Women

Three considerations specific to women are bone health, hormone replacement therapy beginning at menopause, and iron supplementation to offset the iron lost through menstruation.

Bone Health and Osteoporosis

Osteoporosis, literally meaning "porous bones," is a condition in which bones lack the minerals required to keep them strong. In osteoporosis, bones —primarily of the hip, wrist, and spine—become so weak and brittle that they fracture readily. The process begins slowly in the third and fourth decades of life. Women are especially susceptible after menopause because of the accompanying loss of **estrogen**, which increases the rate at which bone mass is broken down.

Approximately 1.4 million Canadians have osteoporosis and many don't even know that they have the disease. Osteoporosis is the leading cause of serious morbidity and functional loss in the elderly population. Approximately one in four women and one in eight men over the age of 50 years will be diagnosed with osteoporosis.[12] The chances of a post-menopausal woman developing osteoporosis is much greater than her chances of developing breast cancer or suffering a heart attack or stroke.

Osteoporosis increases the chances of hip fractures, and according to Stanford University researchers, up to 20 percent of people who have a hip fracture die within a year because of complications related to the fracture. As alarming as these figures are, they do not convey the pain and loss of quality of life in people who suffer the crippling effects of osteoporotic fractures. Although osteoporosis is viewed primarily as a women's disease, 20 to 30 percent of osteoporotic fractures in Canada occur in men.

Despite the strong genetic component, osteoporosis is preventable. Maximizing bone density at a young age and subsequently decreasing the rate of bone loss later in life are critical factors in preventing osteoporosis.

Normal hormone levels prior to menopause and adequate calcium intake and physical activity throughout life cannot be overemphasized. These factors are all crucial to preventing osteoporosis. The absence of any one of these three factors leads to bone loss for which the other two factors never completely compensate. Smoking, excessive use of alcohol, and corticosteroid drugs also accelerate the rate of bone loss in women and men alike. Osteoporosis is also more common in whites, Asians, and people with small frames. Figure 3.14 depicts these variables.

Bone health begins at a young age. Some experts have called osteoporosis a "pediatric disease." Bone density can be promoted early in life by making sure the diet has sufficient calcium and participating in weight-bearing activities. Adequate calcium intake in both women and men is also associated with a reduced risk for colon cancer.[13] The RDA for calcium is between 1,000 and 1,300 mg per day, but leading researchers in this area recommend higher intakes (see Table 3.12). Although the recommended daily intakes can be met easily through diet alone, some experts recommend calcium supplements even for children before puberty.

To obtain your daily calcium requirement, get as much calcium as possible from calcium-rich

FIGURE 3.14 Threats to bone health (osteoporosis)

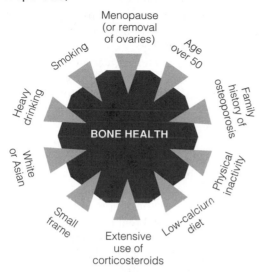

Menopause (or removal of ovaries)

Smoking

Age over 50

Heavy drinking

Family history of osteoporosis

White or Asian

Physical inactivity

BONE HEALTH

Small frame

Low-calcium diet

Extensive use of corticosteroids

TABLE 3.12 Recommended Daily Calcium Intake

Age	Amount (mg)
1–8	800
9–24	1,300
25–50	1,000
Women over 50	1,500
Men 51–65	1,200
Men over 65	1,500

foods, including calcium-fortified foods. If you don't get enough (most people don't), take calcium supplements.

Supplemental calcium can be obtained in the form of calcium citrate and calcium carbonate. Calcium citrate seems to be equally well absorbed with or without food, whereas calcium carbonate is not well absorbed without food. Thus, if your supplement contains calcium carbonate, always take the supplement with meals. Do not take more than 500 mg at a time, because larger amounts are not well absorbed. And don't forget vitamin D, which is vital for calcium absorption.

Avoid taking calcium supplements with an iron-rich meal or in conjunction with an iron-containing multivitamin. Unfortunately, calcium interferes with iron absorption, thus it is best to separate the intake of these two minerals. The benefit of taking your calcium supplement without food (calcium citrate) is that, in a young menstruating woman who needs iron, calcium won't interfere with the absorption of iron.

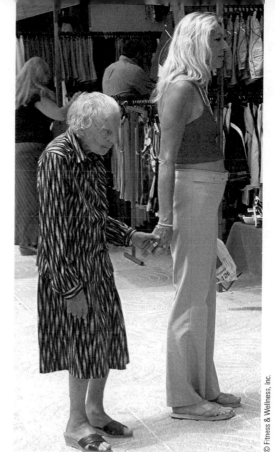

Osteoporosis is a leading cause of morbidity and functional loss in older adults.

Table 3.13 provides a list of selected foods and their calcium content. Along with having an adequate calcium intake, taking 400 to 800 IU of vitamin D daily is recommended for optimal calcium absorption. People over age 50 may require 800 to 1,000 IU. About 40 percent of these adults are deficient in vitamin D.[14]

Excessive protein intake also may affect the body's absorption of calcium. The more protein that is eaten, the higher is the calcium content in the urine (that is, the more calcium excreted). This might be the reason that countries with a high protein intake, including Canada, also have the highest rates of osteoporosis. Aim to achieve the RDA for protein, nonetheless, because people who consume too little protein (less than 35 g per day) lose more bone mass than those who eat too much (more than 100 g per day). The RDA for protein is about 50 g per day for women and 63 for men.

Soft drinks, coffee, and alcoholic beverages can also contribute to a loss in bone density if consumed

Osteoporosis Softening, deterioration, or loss of bone mineral density that leads to disability, bone fractures, and even death from medical complications.

Estrogen Female sex hormone essential for bone formation and conservation of bone density.

TABLE 3.13 Low-Fat Calcium-Rich Foods

Food	Amount	Calcium (mg)	Calories
Beans, red kidney, cooked	230 g	70	218
Beet, greens, cooked	115 g	82	19
Bok choy (Chinese cabbage)	230 g	158	20
Broccoli, cooked, drained	230 g	72	44
Burrito, bean (no cheese)	1	57	225
Cottage cheese, 2% low-fat	125 mL	78	103
Ice milk (vanilla)	125 mL	102	100
Instant breakfast, nonfat milk	240 mL	407	216
Kale, cooked, drained	230 g	94	36
Milk, nonfat, powdered	15 mL	52	15
Milk, skim	240 mL	296	88
Oatmeal, instant, fortified, plain	115 g	109	70
Okra, cooked, drained	115 g	74	23
Orange juice, fortified	240 mL	300	110
Soy milk, fortified, fat free	240 mL	400	110
Spinach, raw	230 g	56	12
Turnip greens, cooked	230 g	197	29
Tofu (some types)	115 g	138	76
Yogurt, fruit	240 mL	372	250
Yogurt, low-fat, plain	240 mL	448	155

in large quantities. They may not cause the damage directly but, rather, because they take the place of dairy products in the diet.

Exercise plays a key role in preventing osteoporosis by decreasing the rate of bone loss following the onset of menopause. Active people are able to maintain bone density much more effectively than their inactive counterparts. A combination of weight-bearing exercises, such as walking or jogging and weight training, is especially helpful.

The benefits of exercise go beyond maintaining bone density. Exercise strengthens muscles, ligaments, and tendons—all of which provide support to the bones (skeleton). Exercise also improves balance and coordination, which can help prevent falls and injuries.

Current studies indicate that people who are active have denser bone mineral than inactive people do. Similar to other benefits of participating in exercise, there is no such thing as "bone in the bank." To have good bone health, people need to participate in a regular lifetime exercise program.

Prevailing research also tells us that estrogen is the most important factor in preventing bone loss. Lumbar bone density in women who have always had regular menstrual cycles exceeds that of women with a history of **oligomenorrhea**

(infrequent or light menstrual periods) and **amenorrhea** (absence of a menstrual period) interspersed with regular cycles. Furthermore, the lumbar density of these two groups of women is higher than that of women who have never had regular menstrual cycles.

For instance, athletes with amenorrhea (who have lower estrogen levels) have lower bone mineral density than even nonathletes with normal estrogen levels. Studies have shown that amenorrheic athletes at age 25 have the bones of women older than 50. Over the last few years, it has become clear that sedentary women with normal estrogen levels have better bone mineral density than active amenorrheic athletes. Many experts believe the best predictor of bone mineral content is the history of menstrual regularity.

As a baseline, women age 65 and older should have a bone density test to establish the risk for osteoporosis. Younger women who are at risk for osteoporosis should discuss a bone density test with their physician at menopause. The test also can be used to monitor changes in bone mass over time and to predict the risk of future fractures. The bone density test is a painless scan requiring only a small amount of radiation to determine bone mass of the spine, hip, wrist, heel, or fingers. The amount of radiation is so low that technicians administering the test can sit right next to the person receiving it. The procedure often takes less than 10 minutes.

Following menopause, every woman should consider some type of therapy to prevent bone loss. The various therapy modalities available should be discussed with a physician.

Adequate Iron Intake

Iron is a key element of **hemoglobin** in blood. The RDA of iron for adult women is between 15 and 18 mg per day (8 to 11 mg for men). Inadequate iron intake is often seen in children, teenagers, women of childbearing age, and endurance athletes. If iron absorption does not compensate for losses or dietary intake is low, iron deficiency develops. Many women suffer from iron deficiency. Over time, excessive depletion of iron stores in the body leads to iron-deficiency anemia, a condition in which the concentration of hemoglobin in the red blood cells is lower than it should be.

Physically active individuals, in particular women, have a greater-than-average need for iron. Heavy training creates a demand for iron that is higher than the recommended intake because small amounts of iron are lost through sweat, urine, and

TABLE 3.14 Iron-Rich Foods

Food	Amount	Iron (mg)	Calories	Cholesterol	% Calories From Fat
Beans, red kidney, cooked	230 g	3.2	218	0	4
Beef, ground lean (21% fat)	85 g	2.1	237	86	57
Beef, sirloin, lean only	85 g	2.9	171	76	36
Beef, liver, fried	85 g	5.3	184	409	33
Beet, greens, cooked	115 g	1.4	19	0	—
Broccoli, cooked, drained	230 g	1.3	44	0	—
Burrito, bean (no cheese)	1	2.3	225	2	28
Egg, hard-cooked	1	.7	77	212	58
Farina (Cream of Wheat), cooked	125 mL	5.2	65	0	—
Instant breakfast, nonfat milk	240 mL	4.8	216	9	4
Peas, frozen, cooked, drained	115 g	1.3	62	0	—
Shrimp, boiled	85 g	2.7	87	172	10
Spinach, raw	230 g	1.5	12	0	—
Vegetables, mixed, cooked	230 g	1.5	108	0	—

stools. Mechanical trauma, caused by the pounding of the feet on the pavement during extensive jogging, may also lead to destruction of iron-containing red blood cells.

A large percentage of female endurance athletes are reported to have iron deficiency. The blood **ferritin** levels of women who participate in intense physical training should be checked frequently.

The rates of iron absorption and iron loss vary from person to person. In most cases, though, people can get enough iron by eating more iron-rich foods such as beans, peas, green leafy vegetables, enriched grain products, egg yolk, fish, and lean meats. Although organ meats, such as liver, are especially good sources, they also are high in cholesterol. A list of foods high in iron is given in Table 3.14.

Proper Nutrition: A Lifetime Prescription for Healthy Living

The three factors that do the most for health, longevity, and quality of life are proper nutrition, a sound exercise program, and quitting (or never starting) smoking. Achieving and maintaining a balanced diet is not as difficult as most people think. If parents were to do a better job of teaching and reinforcing proper nutrition habits in early youth, the current magnitude of nutrition-related health problems would be much smaller. Although treatment of obesity is important, we should place far greater emphasis on preventing obesity in youths and adults in the first place.

Children tend to eat the way their parents do. If parents adopt a healthy diet, children most likely will follow. The difficult part for most people is retraining themselves to follow a lifetime healthy nutrition plan—a diet that includes lots of grains, legumes, fruits, vegetables, and low-fat dairy products, with moderate use of animal protein, junk food, sodium, and alcohol.

In spite of the ample scientific evidence linking poor dietary habits to early disease and mortality rates, many people remain precontemplators: They are not willing to change their eating patterns. Even when faced with obesity, elevated blood lipids, hypertension, and other nutrition-related conditions, people do not change. The motivating factor to change one's eating habits seems to be a major health breakdown, such as a heart attack, a stroke, or cancer—by which time the damage has been done already. In many cases it is irreversible and, for some, fatal.

A gram of prevention is worth a kilogram of cure. The sooner you implement the dietary guidelines presented in this chapter, the better are your chances of preventing chronic diseases and reaching a higher state of wellness.

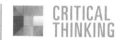

CRITICAL THINKING

What factors in your life and the environment have contributed to your current dietary habits? Do you need to make changes? What may prevent you from doing so?

Oligomenorrhea Irregular menstrual cycles.

Amenorrhea Cessation of regular menstrual flow.

Hemoglobin Protein–iron compound in red blood cells that transports oxygen in the blood.

Ferritin Iron stored in the body.

NEL

NUTRITION FOR WELLNESS 85

ASSESS YOUR KNOWLEDGE

1. The science of nutrition studies the relationship of
   a. vitamins and minerals to health.
   b. foods to optimal health and performance.
   c. carbohydrates, fats, and proteins to the development and maintenance of good health.
   d. the macronutrients and micronutrients to physical performance.
   e. kilocalories to calories in food items.

2. Faulty nutrition often plays a crucial role in the development and progression of which disease?
   a. cardiovascular disease
   b. cancer
   c. osteoporosis
   d. diabetes
   e. All are correct choices.

3. According to Canada's Food Guide how many servings of fruits and vegetables should an adult male consume daily?
   a. 8–10
   b. 2–4
   c. 3–5
   d. 2–3
   e. 1–3

4. The amount of fibre that most adult Canadians receive daily
   a. is largely obtained from meats.
   b. depends on age but not gender.
   c. is less than 20 percent of what is required.
   d. is above what is required.

5. Unhealthy fats include
   a. unsaturated fatty acids.
   b. monounsaturated fats.
   c. polyunsaturated fatty acids.
   d. saturated fats.
   e. alpha-linolenic acid.

6. The daily recommended carbohydrate intake is:
   a. 45 to 65 percent of the total calories.
   b. 10 to 35 percent of the total calories.
   c. 20 to 35 percent of the total calories.
   d. 60 to 75 percent of the total calories.
   e. 35 to 50 percent of the total calories.

7. The amount of a nutrient that is estimated to meet the nutrient requirement of half the healthy people in specific age and gender groups is known as the
   a. Estimated Average Requirement.
   b. Recommended Dietary Allowance.
   c. Daily Values.
   d. Adequate Intake.
   e. Dietary Reference Intakes.

8. The percent fat intake for an individual who on a given day consumes 2,385 Calories with 106 g of fat is
   a. 44 percent of total calories.
   b. 17.7 percent of total calories.
   c. 40 percent of total calories.
   d. 31 percent of total calories.
   e. 22.5 percent of total calories.

9. Carbohydrate loading is beneficial for
   a. endurance athletes.
   b. diabetics.
   c. strength athletes.
   d. sprinters.
   e. all of the above.

10. Osteoporosis is
    a. a crippling disease.
    b. more prevalent in women.
    c. higher in people who were calcium-deficient at a young age.
    d. linked to heavy drinking and smoking.
    e. All are correct choices.

Correct answers can be found at the back of the book.

MEDIA MENU

INTERNET CONNECTIONS

■ Dietitians of Canada. This comprehensive site features daily food tips, frequently asked questions, nutrition resources, and links to other reliable websites on nutrition.

   http://www.dietitians.ca

■ Canadian Council of Food and Nutrition (CCFN). This science-based organization on food and nutrition policy and information aims to be a catalyst in advancing nutritional health and well-being of Canadians. This site comes in handy for those doing a diet and activity assessment.

   http://www.ccfn.ca/

■ Health Canada. Health Canada provides a detailed table of Dietary Reference Intakes at its website. It covers all ages, as well as separate sections for pregnant and lactating women.

   http://www.hc-sc.gc.ca/fn-an/nutrition/reference/ table/ref_vitam_tbl_e.html

■ The Nutrition Facts Table. Most pre-packaged food in Canada is required to carry nutrition information. This new labelling system has been put in place to help Canadians make informed food choices. It also makes it easier to compare products. Information about the table is available at the website.

   http://www.hc-sc.gc.ca/fn-an/label-etiquet/ nutrition/cons/interactive-eng.php

■ College of Family Physicians of Canada. The college publishes a journal, *Canadian Family Physician*, which includes articles about nutrition. One article, "Health

Benefits of Selected Minerals," can be found at the following address.

http://www.cfpc.ca/cfp/2005/May/vol51-may-clinical-3.asp

■ EATracker. The Dietitians of Canada lets you track your daily food and your activity choices on its website. You can compare your food intake and physical activity to Canada's Food Guide and Physical Activity Guide for Healthy Active Living.

http://www.dietitians.ca/public/content/ eat_well_live_well/english/eatracker/

■ Cyberkitchen. This interactive site helps you discover how much you are really eating with an activity on comparing standard serving sizes vs. real serving sizes. You can also provide personal information regarding your age, gender, height, weight, and activity level, and the Cyberkitchen will provide you with a healthy diet plan to meet your weight management goals. It's fun and educational.

http://www.nhlbi.nih.gov/chd/Tipsheets/cyberkit.htm

Notes

1. Health Canada, "Food and Nutrition: Provincial Nutrition Surveys." New Brunswick Nutrition Survey, 2005. Retrieved January 11, 2008, from http://www. hc-sc.gc.ca/fn-an/surveill/nutrition/prov/index_e.html.

2. U.S. Department of Agriculture, Agricultural Research Service. 2005. USDA National Nutrient Database for Standard Reference, Release 18. Nutrient Data Laboratory Home Page, http://www.nal.usda.gov/fnic/ foodcomp.

3. "Is There Flaxseed in Your Fridge Yet?" *Tufts University Health & Nutrition Letter*, September 2002.

4. P. E. Bowen, "Evaluating the Health Claim of Flaxseed and Cancer Prevention," *Nutrition Today* 36 (2001): 144–158.

5. National Academy of Sciences, Institute of Medicine. *Dietary Reference Intakes for Energy, Carbohydrates, Fiber, Fat, Protein and Amino Acids (Macronutrients)* (Washington, DC: National Academy Press, 2002).

6. American College of Sports Medicine, American Dietetic Association, and Dietitians of Canada "Nutrition and Athletic Performance: Joint Position Statement," *Medicine and Science in Sports and Exercise* 32 (2000): 2130–2145.

7. A. Trichopoulou et al., "Adherence to a Mediterranean Diet and Survival in a Greek Population," *New England Journal of Medicine* 348 (2003): 2599–2608.

8. "Should You Take Vitamin C and E Supplements?" *University of California at Berkeley Wellness Letter*. (June 2001).

9. W. G. Christen, J. E. Buring, J. E. Manson, and C. H. Hennekens, "Beta-carotene Supplementation: A Good Thing, a Bad Thing, or Nothing?" *Current Opinion in Lipidology* 10 (1999): 29–34.

10. L. C. Clark et al., "Effects of Selenium Supplementation for Cancer Prevention in Patients with Carcinoma of the Skin: A Randomized Controlled Trial," *Journal of the American Medical Association* 276 (1996): 1957–1963.

11. "The Merits of Multivitamins: EN's Guide to Choosing a Supplement," *Environmental Nutrition* 24 (2001): 1.

12. "Preventing Osteoporosis: Progress in Prevention," Canadian Fitness and Lifestyle Research Institute. Bulletin no. 21. ISSN 1205–7029.

13. M. T. Goodman et al., "Association of Dairy Products, Lactose, and Calcium with the Risk of Ovarian Cancer," *American Journal of Epidemiology* 156 (2002): 148–157.

14. "How to Build Better Bones: Overview of All the New Osteoporosis Options," *Environmental Nutrition* 24, no. 9 (2001): 1, 4–5.

Suggested Readings

American College of Sports Medicine, American Dietetic Association, and Dietitians of Canada. "Joint Position Statement: Nutrition and Athletic Performance." *Medicine and Science in Sports and Exercise* 32 (2000): 2130–2145.

Clark, N. *Nancy Clark's Sports Nutrition Guidebook*. Champaign, IL: Human Kinetics, 2003.

Coleman, E. *Eating for Endurance*. Palo Alto, CA: Bull Publishing, 2003.

Institute of Medicine. *DRI Dietary Reference Intakes: Applications in Dietary Assessment*. Washington, DC: National Academies Press, 2001.

Lau D. C., et al. "Canadian Clinical Practice Guidelines on the Management and Prevention of Obesity in Adults and Children [Summary]." *Canadian Medical Association Journal* 176 (2006): S1–13.

McArdle, W. D., F. I. Katch, and V. L. Katch. *Sports & Exercise Nutrition*. Baltimore: Lippincott Williams & Wilkins, 1999.

National Academy of Sciences, Institute of Medicine. *Dietary Reference Intakes*. Washington, DC: National Academy Press, 1998.

National Academy of Sciences, Institute of Medicine. *Dietary Reference Intakes for Energy, Carbohydrates, Fiber, Fat, Protein and Amino Acids (Macronutrients)*. Washington, DC: National Academy Press, 2002.

Sizer, F. S., E. N. Whitney, and L. Piché. *Nutrition: Concepts and Controversies* (1st Canadian edition). Toronto: Nelson/Thomson Learning, 2009.

Whitney, E. N., and S. R. Rolfes. *Understanding Nutrition*. Belmont, CA: Wadsworth/Thomson Learning, 2005.

Lab 3A

NUTRIENT ANALYSIS

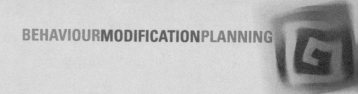

Name: _____ Date: _____ Grade: _____

Instructor: _____ Course: _____ Section: _____

Necessary Lab Equipment

Internet access to the web-based Nutrition tool EATracker, from Dietitians of Canada (http://www.eatracker.ca). Optional: List of Nutrient Value of Some Common Foods from Health Canada, Food and Nutrition, Nutrition and Healthy Eating (http://www.hc-sc.gc.ca/fn-an/nutrition/fiche-nutri-data/index_e.html)

Objective

To track and evaluate your daily food intake and physical activity choice for seven days and compare them to Canada's Food Guide and Physical Activity Guide.

Instructions

- Log on to EATracker at http://www.eatracker.ca.
- Take the Eating and Activity Assessment.
  a. You will be provided with an assessment of your current eating and activity habits based on information you will submit.
  b. Respond to the questions asked and click on Results when you are finished.
- Sign up for EATracker once you have completed the assessment.
  a. You will be asked to enter your e-mail address and a personal password.
  b. Your personal information will be protected. Dietitians of Canada (DC) is committed to protecting individual privacy on the Internet.

- Follow the five steps below to get started.
  1. Go to Calendar and click on the day you are beginning this lab.
  2. Complete the Eating Diary.
     a. List all the foods, beverages, and supplements you consumed that day.
     b. Print out your Daily Menu.
  3. Complete the Physical Activity Diary.
     a. Select the activities you did this day. You can choose from a list of low, moderate, or high-level effort activities.
  4. Review Your Daily Assessment. You will be provided with feedback based on your food and activity choices for each day you enter in your data.
     a. Check out your personal food guide serving intake to the recommended number of food guide servings.
     b. Learn about your calorie intake and estimated energy requirements.
     c. Check out the Nutrient Feedback Chart to determine the amount of protein, fat, and carbohydrates you consumed.
     d. Find out about your fibre, vitamin, and nutrient intake in table and bar graph form.
     e. Review your activity level and compare your score with Canada's Physical Activity Guide to Healthy Living.
  5. Review a summary of your scores.

Lab 3B

HEALTHY DIET PLAN

HOMEWORK ASSIGNMENT

Name: _____ Date: _____ Grade: _____

Instructor: _____ Course: _____ Section: _____

Assignment

This laboratory experience should be carried out as a homework assignment to be completed over the next seven days.

Objective

To meet the minimum daily required servings of the basic food groups and monitor total daily fat intake.

Lab Resources

"Canada's Food Guide" (Figure 3.1, page 52) and list of "Nutritive Value of Selected Foods" (Appendix).

I. Instructions

Keep a seven-day record of your food consumption using Canada's Food Guide and the form given in Figure 3B.1 (make additional copies of this form as needed—at least three days are recommended). Whenever you have something to eat, record the food from the Nutritive Value of Selected Foods list contained in Appendix, the number of calories, grams of fat, and the servings in the corresponding spaces provided for each food group. If a food item is not listed in the Nutritive Value of Selected Foods list, the information can be obtained from the food container itself.

Record all information immediately after each meal, because it will be easier to keep track of foods and amounts eaten. If twice the amount of a particular serving is eaten, the calories and grams of fat must be doubled and two servings should be recorded under the respective food group.

At the end of the day, evaluate the diet by checking whether the minimum required servings for each food group were met, and by the total amount of fat consumed. If you meet the required servings, you are well on your way to achieving a well-balanced diet. In addition, fat intake should not exceed 30 percent of the total daily caloric consumption. If you are on a diet, you may want to reduce fat intake to less than 20 percent of total daily calories (see Table 5.4, page 141)

II. Nutrition Stage of Change

Using Figure 2.4 (page 41) and Table 2.3 (page 41) identify your current stage of change for nutrition (healthy diet):

_____

III. What I Learned and What I Can Do to Improve My Nutrition

Based on the nutrient analysis conducted in Lab 3A and your daily diet analysis conducted in this lab, explain what these experiences have taught you and list specific changes and strategies that you can use to improve your present nutrition habits. Use an extra blank sheet of paper as needed.

I have learned the following about myself/my current diet: _____

_____

_____

Specific changes I plan to make: _____

_____

_____

Strategies I will use: _____

_____

_____

FIGURE 3B.1 Daily diet record form

Name: _____

No.	Food*	Amount	Calories	Fat (gm)	Food Groups (servings)				
					Bread, Cereal, Rice, and Pasta	Vegetable	Fruit	Milk, Yogurt, and Cheese	Meat, Poultry, Fish, Dry Beans, Eggs, and Nuts
1									
2									
3									
4									
5									
6									
7									
8									
9									
10									
11									
12									
13									
14									
15									
16									
17									
18									
19									
20									
21									
22									
23									
24									
25									
26									
27									
28									
29									
30									
Totals									
Deficiencies*									

*See "List of Nutritive Value of Selected Foods" in Appendix.

Chapter 4

Body Composition

Objectives

- Define body composition and understand its relationship to assessment of recommended body weight.

- Explain the difference between essential fat and storage fat.

- Describe various techniques used to assess body composition.

- Be able to assess body composition using hydrostatic weighing, skinfold thickness, and girth measurement techniques.

- Understand the importance of body mass index (BMI) and waist circumference in the assessment of risk for disease.

- Be able to determine recommended weight according to recommended percent body fat values.

Body composition consists of fat and nonfat components. The fat component is usually called fat mass or **percent body fat**. The non-fat component is termed **lean body mass**. It should be noted that when discussing body composition, the terms "weight" and "mass" are often used interchangeably. Although the term "mass" is technically correct, both terms will be used.

For many years people relied on simple height/weight charts to determine their **recommended body weight**. We know, however, that these tables can be highly inaccurate and fail to identify critical fat values associated with higher risk for disease. The proper way to determine recommended weight is to find out what percent of total body weight is fat and what amount is lean tissue—in other words, to determine body composition. Body composition should be assessed by a well-trained technician who understands the procedure that is being used.

Once the fat percentage is known, recommended body weight can be calculated from recommended body fat. Recommended body weight, also called "healthy weight," implies the absence of any medical condition that would improve with weight loss and a fat distribution pattern that is not associated with higher risk for illness.

Although various techniques for determining percent body fat were developed years ago, many people still are unaware of these procedures and continue to depend on height/weight charts to find out their recommended body weight. The standard height/weight tables, first published in 1912, were based on average weights (including shoes and clothing) for men and women who obtained life insurance policies between 1888 and 1905—a notably unrepresentative population. The recommended body weight on these tables is obtained according to sex, height, and frame size. Because no scientific guidelines are given to determine frame size, most people choose their frame size based on the column in which the weight comes closest to their own!

To determine whether people are truly **overweight** or falsely at recommended body weight, body composition must be established. **Obesity** is an excess of body fat. If body weight is the only criterion, an individual might easily appear to be overweight according to height/weight charts, yet not have too much body fat. Typical examples are football players, body builders, weight lifters, and other athletes with large muscle size. Some athletes who appear to be 10 or 15 kg overweight really have little body fat.

The inaccuracy of height/weight charts was illustrated clearly when a young man who weighed about 100 kg applied to join a city police force but was turned down without having been granted an interview. The reason? He was "too fat," according to the height/weight charts. When this young man's

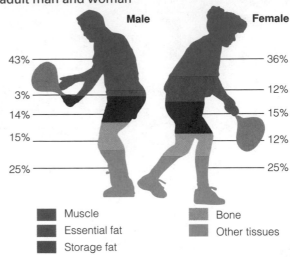

FIGURE 4.1 Typical body composition of an adult man and woman

Male
Female

43% — 36%
3% — 12%
14% — 15%
15% — 12%
25% — 25%

- Muscle
- Essential fat
- Storage fat
- Bone
- Other tissues

body composition was assessed at a preventive medicine clinic, it was determined that only 5 percent of his total body weight was in the form of fat—considerably lower than the recommended standard. In the words of the director of the clinic, "The only way this fellow could come down to the chart's target weight would have been through surgical removal of a large amount of his muscle tissue."

At the other end of the spectrum, some people who weigh very little (and may be viewed as skinny or underweight) can actually be classified as obese because of their high body fat content. People who weigh as little as 55 kg but are more than 30 percent fat (about one-third of their total body weight) are not uncommon. These cases are found more readily in the sedentary population and among people who are always dieting. Physical inactivity and a constant negative caloric balance both lead to a loss in lean body mass (see Chapter 5). These examples illustrate that body weight alone clearly does not tell the whole story.

Essential and Storage Fat

Total fat in the human body is classified into two types: **essential fat** and **storage fat**. Essential fat is needed for normal physiological function. Without it, human health and physical performance deteriorate. This type of fat is found within tissues such as muscles, nerve cells, bone marrow, intestines, heart, liver, and lungs. This essential fat constitutes about 3 percent of the total weight in men and 12 percent in women (see Figure 4.1). The percentage is higher in women because it includes sex-specific fat, such as that found in the breast tissue, the uterus, and other sex-related fat deposits.

Storage fat is the fat stored in adipose tissue, mostly just beneath the skin (subcutaneous fat) and around major organs in the body. This fat serves three basic functions:

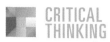

CRITICAL THINKING

Mary is a cross-country runner whose coach has asked her to decrease her total body fat to 7 percent. Can Mary's performance increase at this lower percent body fat? How would you respond to this coach?

1. As an insulator to retain body heat.
2. As energy substrate for metabolism.
3. As padding against physical trauma to the body.

The amount of storage fat does not differ between men and women, except that men tend to store fat around the waist and women around the hips and thighs.

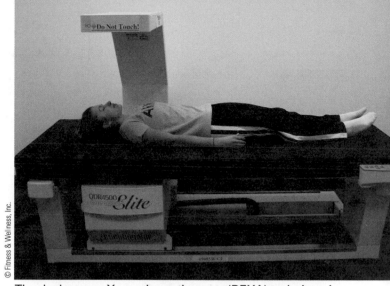

The dual energy X-ray absorptiometry (DEXA) technique is used to assess body composition and bone density.

© Fitness & Wellness, Inc.

Techniques to Assess Body Composition

Body composition can be determined through several procedures. These are described in the following pages.

Dual Energy X-Ray Absorptiometry (DEXA)

Dual energy X-ray absorptiometry (DEXA) is a method to assess body composition that is used most frequently in research and by medical facilities. A radiographic technique, DEXA uses very low-dose beams of X-ray energy (hundreds of times lower than a typical body X-ray) to measure total body fat mass, fat distribution pattern (see waist circumference on page 107), and bone density. Bone density is measured to assess the risk for osteoporosis. The procedure itself is simple and takes only about 15 minutes to administer. Many exercise scientists consider DEXA to be the standard technique to assess body composition.

Because DEXA is not readily available to most fitness participants, other methods to estimate body composition are used. The most common of these are:

1. hydrostatic or underwater weighing
2. air displacement
3. skinfold thickness
4. girth measurements
5. bioelectrical impedance

Because these procedures yield estimates of body fat, each technique may yield slightly different values. Therefore, when assessing changes in body composition, be sure to use the same technique for pre- and post-test comparisons.

Hydrostatic weighing and air displacement are the two most accurate techniques presently available in fitness laboratories. Other techniques to assess body composition are available, but the equipment is costly and not easily accessible to the general population. In addition to percentages of lean tissue and body fat, some of these methods also provide information on total body water and bone mass. Besides DEXA, these techniques include magnetic resonance imaging (MRI), computed tomography (CT), and total body electrical conductivity (TOBEC). With regard to predicting percent body fat, these techniques do not seem to be more accurate than hydrostatic weighing or air displacement.

Body composition The fat and non-fat components of the human body; important in assessing recommended body weight.

Percent body fat Proportional amount of fat in the body based on the person's total weight; includes both essential fat and storage fat; also termed fat mass.

Lean body mass Body weight without body fat.

Recommended body weight Body weight at which there seems to be no harm to human health; healthy weight.

Overweight An excess amount of weight against a given standard, such as height or recommended percent body fat.

Obesity An excessive accumulation of body fat, usually at least 30 percent above recommended body weight.

Essential fat Minimal amount of body fat needed for normal physiological functions; constitutes about 3 percent of total weight in men and 12 percent in women.

Storage fat Body fat in excess of essential fat; stored in adipose tissue.

Dual energy X-ray absorptiometry (DEXA) Method to assess body composition that uses very low-dose beams of X-ray energy to measure total body fat mass, fat distribution pattern, and bone density.

FIGURE 4.2 Hydrostatic weighing procedure

A small tank or pool, an autopsy scale, and a submersible chair are needed. The scale should measure up to about 10 kg and should be readable to the nearest .01 kg. The chair is suspended from the scale and submerged in a tank of water or pool measuring at least 1.5 × 1.5 × 1.5 m. A swimming pool can be used in place of the tank.

The procedure for the technician is

1. Ask the person to be weighed to fast for approximately six to eight hours and to have a bladder and bowel movement prior to underwater weighing.
2. Measure the individual's residual lung volume (RV, or amount of air left in the lungs following complete exhalation). If no equipment (spirometer) is available to measure the residual volume, estimate it using the following predicting equations*

   Men: RV = [(0.027 × height in centimetres) + (0.017 × age)] − 3.447

   Women: RV = [(0.032 × height in centimetres) + (0.009 × age)] − 3.9

3. Have the person remove all jewellery prior to weighing. Weigh the person on land in a swimsuit and subtract the weight of the suit.
4. Record the water temperature in the tank in degrees Celsius. Use that temperature to obtain the water density factor

provided below, which is required in the formula to compute body density.

Temp (°C)	Water Density (gr/ml)	Temp (°C)	Water Density (gr/ml)
28	0.99626	35	0.99406
29	0.99595	36	0.99371
30	0.99567	37	0.99336
31	0.99537	38	0.99299
32	0.99505	39	0.99262
33	0.99473	40	0.99224
34	0.99440		

5. After the person is dressed in the swimsuit, have him or her enter the tank and completely wipe off all air clinging to the skin. Have the person sit in the chair with the water at chin level (raise or lower the chair as needed). Make sure the water and scale remain as still as possible during the entire procedure, because this allows for a more accurate reading. (During underwater weighing, you can decrease scale movement by holding and slowly releasing the neck of the scale until the subject is floating freely in the water.)

Hydrostatic Weighing

For decades, **hydrostatic weighing** has been the most common technique used in determining body composition in exercise physiology laboratories. In essence, a person's "regular" weight is compared with a weight taken underwater. Because fat is more buoyant than lean tissue, comparing the two weights can determine a person's percent of fat. Almost all other indirect techniques to assess body composition have been validated against hydrostatic weighing. The procedure requires a considerable amount of time, skill, space, and equipment and must be administered by a well-trained technician.

This technique has several drawbacks. First, because each individual assessment can take as long

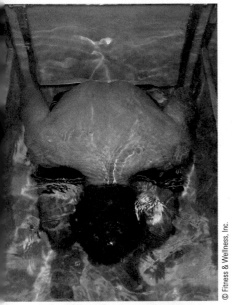

Hydrostatic or underwater weighing technique.

© Fitness & Wellness, Inc.

as 30 minutes, hydrostatic weighing is not feasible when testing a lot of people. Furthermore, the person's residual lung volume (amount of air left in the lungs following complete forceful exhalation) should be measured before testing. If residual volume cannot be measured, as is the case in some laboratories and health/fitness centres, it is estimated using the predicting equations—which may decrease the accuracy of hydrostatic weighing. Also, the requirement of being completely under water makes hydrostatic weighing difficult to administer to **aquaphobic** people. For accurate results, the individual must be able to perform the test properly.

As described in Figure 4.2 and in Lab 4A, for each underwater weighing trial, the person has to (a) force out all the air in the lungs, (b) lean forward and completely submerge underwater for about 5 to 10 seconds (long enough to get the underwater weight), and (c) remain as calm as possible (chair movement makes reading the scale difficult). This procedure is repeated eight to ten times.

Forcing all the air out of the lungs is not easy for everyone but is important for an accurate reading. Leaving additional air (beyond residual volume) in the lungs makes a person more buoyant. Because fat is less dense than water, overweight individuals weigh less in water. Additional air in the lungs makes

6. Place a clip on the person's nose and have him or her forcefully exhale all of the air out of the lungs. The individual then totally submerges underwater. Make sure that all the air is exhaled from the lungs prior to submerging. Record the reading on the scale. Repeat this procedure 8 to 10 times, because practice and experience increase the accuracy of the underwater weight. Use the average of the three heaviest underwater weights as the gross underwater weight.

7. Because tare weight (the weight of the chair and chain or rope used to suspend the chair) accounts for part of the gross underwater weight, subtract this weight to obtain the person's net underwater weight. To determine tare weight, place a clothespin on the chain or rope at the water level when the person is submerged completely. After the person comes out of the water, lower the chair into the water to the pin level. Now record tare weight. Determine the net underwater weight by subtracting the tare weight from the gross underwater weight.

8. Compute body density and percent fat using the following equations:

$$\text{Body density} = \frac{BW}{\dfrac{BW - UW}{WD} - RV - .1}$$

$$\text{Percent fat**} = \frac{495}{BD} - 450$$

WHERE:

BW = body weight in kilograms
UW = net underwater weight
WD = water density (determined by water temperature)
RV = residual volume
BD = body density

A sample computation for body fat assessment according to hydrostatic weighing is provided in Lab 4A.

---

* From: H. L. Goldman and M. R. Becklake, "Respiratory Function Tests: Normal Values at Medium Altitudes and the Prediction of Normal Results," in *American Review of Tuberculosis* 79 (1959): 457–467.

** From W. E. Siri, *Body Composition from Fluid Spaces and Density* (Berkeley: University of California, Donner Laboratory of Medical Physics, March 19, 1956).

---

a person lighter in water, yielding a false, higher body fat percentage.

Air Displacement

Air displacement is a new technique that holds considerable promise. With this method, an individual sits inside a small chamber, commercially known as the **Bod Pod**. Computerized pressure sensors determine the amount of air displaced by the person inside the chamber. Body volume is calculated by subtracting the air volume with the person inside the chamber from the volume of the empty chamber. The amount of air in the person's lungs is also taken into consideration when determining the actual body volume. Body density and percent body fat are then calculated from the obtained body volume.

Initial research has shown that this technique compares very favourably with hydrostatic weighing and it is less cumbersome to administer. The procedure takes only about five minutes. Additional research is needed, however, to determine its accuracy among different age groups, ethnic backgrounds, and athletic populations. Administering this assessment is a relatively easy procedure, but because of the high cost, the Bod Pod is not readily available in fitness centres and exercise laboratories.

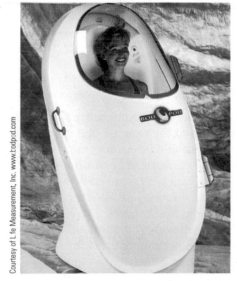

Courtesy of Life Measurement, Inc. www.bodpod.com

The Bod Pod, used for assessment of body composition.

Hydrostatic weighing Underwater technique to assess body composition; considered the most accurate of the body composition assessment techniques.

Aquaphobic Having a fear of water.

Air displacement Technique to assess body composition by calculating the body volume from the air displaced by an individual sitting inside a small chamber.

Bod Pod Commercial name of the equipment used for the assessment of body composition through the air displacement technique.

FIGURE 4.3 Anatomical landmarks for skinfold measurements

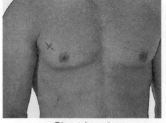
Chest (men)

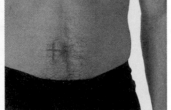
Abdomen (men)

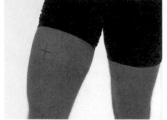
Thigh (men and women)

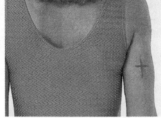
Triceps (women)

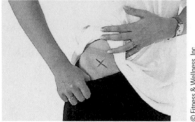
Suprailium (women)

© Fitness & Wellness, Inc.

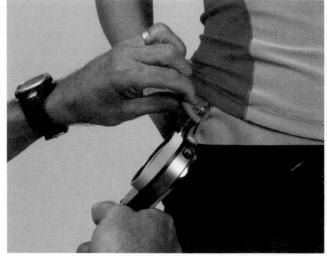
Skinfold thickness technique.

© Fitness & Wellness, Inc.

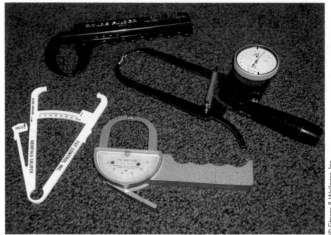
Various types of calipers used to assess skinfold thickness.

© Fitness & Wellness, Inc.

Skinfold Thickness

Because of the cost, time, and complexity of hydrostatic weighing and the expense of Bod Pod equipment, most health and fitness programs use **anthropometric measurement techniques**, which correlate quite well with hydrostatic weighing. These techniques, primarily skinfold thickness and girth measurements, allow quick, simple, and inexpensive estimates of body composition.

Assessing body composition using **skinfold thickness** is based on the principle that approximately half of the body's fatty tissue is directly beneath the skin. Valid and reliable measurements of this tissue give a good indication of percent body fat.

The skinfold test is done with the aid of pressure calipers. Several sites must be measured to reflect the total percentage of fat (see Figure 4.3):

women: triceps, suprailium, and thigh skinfolds

men: chest, abdomen, and thigh.

All measurements should be taken on the right side of the body.

Even with the skinfold technique, experience is necessary to obtain accurate measurements. In addition, different technicians may produce slightly different measurements of the same person. Therefore, the same technician should take pre-test and post-test measurements.

Measurements should be done at the same time of the day—preferably in the morning—because changes in water hydration from activity and exercise can affect skinfold girth. The procedure is given in Figure 4.4. If skinfold calipers are available, you may assess your percent body fat with the help of your instructor or an experienced technician (also see Lab 4B). Then locate the percent fat estimates on the appropriate Table 4.1, 4.2, or 4.3.

FIGURE 4.4 Procedure for body fat assessment using skinfold thickness technique

1. Select the proper anatomical sites. For men, use chest, abdomen, and thigh skinfolds. For women, use triceps, suprailium, and thigh skinfolds. Take all measurements on the right side of the body with the person standing. The correct anatomical landmarks for skinfolds are

   Chest: a diagonal fold halfway between the shoulder crease and the nipple.

   Abdomen: a vertical fold taken about 2.5 centimetres to the right of the umbilicus.

   Triceps: a vertical fold on the back of the upper arm, halfway between the shoulder and the elbow.

   Thigh: a vertical fold on the front of the thigh, midway between the knee and the hip.

   Suprailium: a diagonal fold above the crest of the ilium (on the side of the hip).

2. Measure each site by grasping a double thickness of skin firmly with the thumb and forefinger, pulling the fold slightly away from the muscular tissue. Hold the calipers perpendicular to the fold and take the measurement 1 cm below the finger hold. Measure each site three times and read the values to the nearest .1 to .5 mm. Record the average of the two closest readings as the final value. Take the readings without delay to avoid excessive compression of the skinfold. Releasing and refolding the skinfold is required between readings.

3. When doing pre- and post-assessments, conduct the measurement at the same time of day. The best time is early in the morning to avoid hydration changes resulting from activity or exercise.

4. Obtain percent fat by adding the three skinfold measurements and looking up the respective values on Table 4.1 for women, Table 4.2 for men under age 40, and Table 4.3 for men over 40.

For example, if the skinfold measurements for an 18-year-old female are (a) triceps = 16, (b) suprailium = 4, and (c) thigh = 30 (total = 50), the percent body fat is 20.6%.

Anthropometric measurement techniques Measurement of body girths at different sites.

Skinfold thickness Technique to assess body composition by measuring a double thickness of skin at specific body sites.

TABLE 4.1 Scoring of Body Composition: Males

BMI (kg/m²)	Points Column A	WC (cm)	Points Column B	S05S (mm)	Points Column C
< 18.5	3	All Girths	3	< 25	3
				25–54	4
				55–77	3
				> 77	2
18.5–24.9	4	< 94	4	< 54	4
		94–101	3	54–77	3
		> 101	1	> 77	2
25.0–29.9	3	< 94	4	< 54	4
		94–101	3	54–77	3
		< 101	1	> 77	2
30.0–32.4	2	< 94	4	< 54	4
		94–101	2	54–77	3
		> 101	0	> 77	2
32.5–35.0	1	< 94	4	< 54	4
		94–101	2	54–77	2
		> 101	0	> 77	1
> 35.0	0	< 94	4	< 54	4
		94–101	2	54–77	2
		> 101	0	> 77	0

Scoring of Body Composition: Females

BMI (kg/m²)	Points Column A	WC (cm)	Points Column B	S05S (mm)	Points Column C
< 18.5	3	All Girths	3	< 46	3
				46–83	4
				84–113	3
				> 113	2
18.5–24.9	4	< 80	4	< 83	4
		80–87	3	83–113	3
		> 87	1	> 113	2
25.0–29.9	3	< 80	4	< 83	4
		80–87	3	83–113	3
		> 87	1	> 113	2
30.0–32.4	2	< 80	4	< 83	4
		80–87	2	83–113	3
		> 87	0	> 113	2
32.5–35.0	1	< 80	4	< 83	4
		80–87	2	83–113	2
		> 87	0	> 113	1
> 35.0	0	< 80	4	< 83	4
		80–87	2	83–113	2
		> 87	0	> 113	0

Source: *The Canadian Physical Activity, Fitness & Lifestyle Approach: CSEP-Health & Fitness Program's Health-Related Appraisal and Counselling Strategy*, 3rd edition, © 2003, Reprinted with permission of the Canadian Society for Exercise Physiology.

TABLE 4.2 Healthy Body Composition—Conversion Between Health Benefit Ratings and Scores

Health Benefit Rating	Symbol	Score
Excellent	E	4
Very Good	VG	3
Good	G	2
Fair	F	1
Needs Improvement	NI	0

Source: *The Canadian Physical Activity, Fitness & Lifestyle Approach: CSEP-Health & Fitness Program's Health-Related Appraisal and Counselling Strategy*, 3rd edition, © 2003, Reprinted with permission of the Canadian Society for Exercise Physiology.

TABLE 4.3 Health Benefit Zones for Body Composition

Health Benefit Zone

Excellent	Your body composition falls within a range that is generally associated with optimal health benefits.
Very Good	Your body composition falls within a range that is generally associated with considerable health benefits.
Good	Your body composition falls within a range that is generally associated with many health benefits.
Fair	Your body composition falls within a range that is generally associated with some health risk. Continuing to progress from here into the GOOD zone will further increase the health benefits associated with your body composition.
Needs Improvement	Your body composition falls within a range that is generally associated with considerable health risk.

Source: *The Canadian Physical Activity, Fitness & Lifestyle Approach: CSEP-Health & Fitness Program's Health-Related Appraisal and Counselling Strategy*, 3rd edition, © 2003, Reprinted with permission of the Canadian Society for Exercise Physiology.

Health Benefit Zones

While percent body fat is a common way to assess healthy body composition, determining your Health Benefit Zone is another. The protocol for this particular assessment has been developed by the Canadian Society for Exercise Physiology (CSEP) using mortality and morbidity data to estimate these zones. Points are awarded for different combinations of healthy and unhealthy estimates of Body Mass Index (BMI), the sum of five skinfolds (triceps, biceps, subscapular, iliac crest, and the medial calf), your waist girth, and the sum of two skinfolds (subscapular and iliac crest). Figure 4.5 outlines the procedures for taking

these measures. (Note the different sites compared to Figure 4.4.)

Refer to Tables 4.4, 4.5, and 4.6 for the point scoring system.

Labs 4B and 4C will assist you in determining your Body Fat Percentage and your Health Benefit Zone.

Circumference Measurements

A simpler method to determine body fat is by measuring circumferences at various body sites. This technique requires only a standard measuring tape. Good accuracy can be achieved with little practice. The limitation is that it may not be valid for athletic individuals (men or women) who participate actively in strenuous physical activity or for people who can be classified visually as thin or obese. Measurements for women are the upper arm, hip, and wrist; for men, the waist and wrist (see Tables 4.7 and 4.8).

Bioelectrical Impedance

The **bioelectrical impedance** technique is much simpler to administer, but its accuracy is questionable. In this technique, several sensors are applied to the skin and a weak (totally painless) electrical current is run through the body to estimate body fat, lean body mass, and body water. The technique is based on the principle that fat tissue is a less efficient conductor of electrical current than lean tissue. The easier the conductance, the leaner the individual. Body weight scales with sensors on the surface are also available to perform this procedure.

The accuracy of equations used to estimate percent body fat with this technique is questionable. Research has shown that it does not approach the accuracy of hydrostatic weighing, air displacement, skinfold thickness, or circumference measurement techniques. Following all manufacturers' instructions will ensure the most accurate result, but even then percent body fat may be off by as much as 10 percentage points (or even more on some scales).

Body Mass Index

Another technique to determine thinness and excessive fatness is the **body mass index** (**BMI**), which incorporates height and weight to estimate

Body mass index (BMI) A technique to determine thinness and excessive fatness that incorporates height and weight to estimate critical fat values at which the risk for disease increases.

FIGURE 4.5 Procedure for anthropometric measurement

1. Select the proper anatomical sites. They include the tricep, the bicep, the subscapular, the iliac crest, and the medial calf. Take all measurements on the right side of the body with the person standing. The correct anatomical landmarks for the skinfolds for determining the Health Benefit Zones are

   Triceps skinfold: Bend the upper arm at a right angle then measure from the tip of the acromion process or shoulder to the tip of the olecranon process or elbow to find the midpoint of the right arm. Mark the midpoint. Then extend the arm and raise a skinfold along the midline of the back arm.

   Biceps skinfold: Extend the right arm. Put the palm face forward. Then raise a fold of skin at the midpoint of the midarm. The skinfold should run vertically along the midline of the front of the arm.

   Subscapular skinfold: Relax the shoulders. Extend the arms along the side of the body. The subscapular skinfold runs downward and outward at a 45° angle to the spine. You can raise the subscapular skinfold 1 centimetre below the inferior angle of the right scapula.

   Iliac crest skinfold: Have the client raise his or her right arm so that the right hand touches the right shoulder. The client should be in a standing position. To measure the iliac crest skinfold, move to 3 cm above the right ilium at the midline (also called the mid-axillary line) of the body. The skinfold will run forward and downward.

   Medial calf skinfold: Place the right foot on an elevated surface such as a step or box. The knee should be at a 90° angle. Look for the point of the greatest calf muscle. Raise the medial calf skinfold so that it runs vertically along the midline of the calf.

Skin Fold Measuring Procedure

1. Measure each site by grasping a double thickness of skin firmly with the thumb and forefinger, pulling the fold slightly away from the muscular tissue. Hold the calipers perpendicular to the fold and take the measurement 1 cm below the finger hold. Measure each site once. Then repeat the test. Record the average of the two closest readings as the final value. If you find a difference greater than 0.4 mm, you should take one more measurement at that site. If three measurements are taken, the median value instead of the average should be used. Take the readings without delay to avoid excessive compression of the skinfold. Releasing and refolding the skinfold is required between readings.

2. When doing pre- and post-assessments, conduct the measurement at the same time of day. The best time is early in the morning to avoid hydration changes resulting from activity or exercise.

3. Obtain percent body fat by adding the five skinfold measurements and looking up the respective values on Tables 4.1 to 4.6.

---

critical fat values at which the risk for disease increases. Scientific evidence indicates that there is a significant increase in the risk for disease when BMI exceeds 25.[1]

BMI is calculated by dividing the weight in kilograms by the square of the height in metres. For example, the BMI for an individual who weighs 78 kg and is 1.7 m tall would be 27: $78 \div (1.7)^2$. You can also look up your BMI in Table 4.9 according to your height and weight; then see Table 4.10 for your resultant risk for disease.

In Canada, four general categories of BMI ranges are recognized: underweight (BMI less than 18.5), normal weight (BMI between 18.5 to 24.9), overweight (25 to 29.9), and obese (BMI 30 and over). The last category can be further subdivided (see Tables 4.10 and 4.11). Both too low a BMI (underweight) score or too high a BMI score are associated with health problems. A low BMI (less than 18.5) is associated with osteoporosis, undernutrition, and eating disorders, while too high a BMI

(greater than 25) increases one's risk of developing diabetes, heart disease, high blood pressure, gallbladder disease, and some forms of cancer. It should be noted that since BMI does not distinguish between the quantity and quality of body mass, some very muscular adults (athletes) who may also have a low percentage of body fat may be included in the overweight category. For this reason, the use of BMI is not appropriate with some groups for whom the classification system may underestimate or overestimate health risks. BMI is a calculation that can be used for healthy Canadian adults who are between 20 and 65 years of age. BMI does not apply to infants, children, adolescents, and pregnant or lactating women. BMI is just one tool that can be used to assess one's health risks. For best results, it should be used in conjunction with other tools or considered with other factors.

Bioelecrical impedance Technique to assess body composition by running a weak electrical current through the body.

TABLE 4.4 Health Benefit Zones by Age and Sex*

15–19 Years of Age

Sum of 5 Skinfolds (mm)**		Sum of 2 Trunk Skinfolds (mm)***	
Male	Female	Male	Female
25	36	11	13
27	40	12	14
28	43	13	16
29	46	13	17
31	49	14	18
32	51	15	19
33	54	15	20
35	56	16	21
36	58	17	22
38	61	17	23
40	63	18	24
42	66	19	26
44	69	21	27
47	72	22	29
51	77	24	31
54	83	27	33
61	89	28	37
69	97	32	42
82	116	42	49

30–39 Years of Age

Sum of 5 Skinfolds (mm)**		Sum of 2 Trunk Skinfolds (mm)***	
Male	Female	Male	Female
28	40	14	14
32	45	17	15
35	48	19	17
38	52	20	18
41	55	22	20
44	58	24	21
46	61	26	23
49	63	27	24
52	66	29	25
55	69	31	27
58	72	33	28
60	76	35	30
63	79	37	32
67	83	39	34
71	88	42	36
76	93	45	39
82	99	48	43
89	109	53	48
101	128	59	59

20–29 Years of Age

Sum of 5 Skinfolds (mm)**		Sum of 2 Trunk Skinfolds (mm)***	
Male	Female	Male	Female
26	37	13	13
29	40	14	14
30	43	16	16
32	46	17	17
34	49	18	18
36	51	19	19
38	53	20	20
40	56	21	21
43	58	23	22
46	60	25	23
49	63	27	24
52	65	28	26
55	69	30	27
58	72	32	29
62	76	35	31
68	81	38	33
74	86	41	36
82	95	46	42
94	111	54	48

40–49 Years of Age

Sum of 5 Skinfolds (mm)**		Sum of 2 Trunk Skinfolds (mm)***	
Male	Female	Male	Female
28	42	15	14
37	48	20	16
40	51	22	18
44	56	24	20
46	59	26	21
48	62	27	23
51	66	29	25
53	69	31	26
56	73	32	28
58	77	34	29
60	81	35	32
63	86	36	34
66	90	38	37
69	94	40	40
72	98	42	43
75	105	44	46
79	113	47	50
86	125	50	56
97	150	56	65

(continued)

TABLE 4.4 (Continued)

	50–59 Years of Age				60–69 Years of Age			
Sum of 5 Skinfolds (mm)**		**Sum of 2 Trunk Skinfolds (mm)*****			**Sum of 5 Skinfolds (mm)****		**Sum of 2 Trunk Skinfolds (mm)*****	
Male	**Female**	**Male**	**Female**		**Male**	**Female**	**Male**	**Female**
31	48	17	16		33	45	17	16
36	54	20	19		38	54	21	18
40	60	22	22		41	61	23	22
44	65	24	24		45	65	25	24
46	69	26	26		48	67	27	25
48	73	27	28		50	70	28	28
51	75	29	29		52	72	29	29
53	78	30	30		54	76	31	31
55	81	32	31		56	80	32	33
58	84	33	33		58	82	33	34
60	87	35	35		59	85	34	36
62	90	36	37		61	87	35	38
65	93	38	39		63	93	37	40
68	97	40	41		65	98	38	42
71	101	43	44		69	100	40	44
74	106	45	46		72	103	42	46
77	112	47	49		76	112	45	49
81	121	49	53		81	123	48	54
88	138	54	60		91	139	55	60

* Based on data from Canada Fitness Survey, 1981
** Sum of 5 skinfolds (mm) = Triceps + biceps + subscapular + iliac crest + medial calf
*** Sum of 2 trunk skinfolds (mm) = subscapular + iliac crest

Source: *The Canadian Physical Activity, Fitness & Lifestyle Approach: CSEP-Health & Fitness Program's Health-Related Appraisal and Counselling Strategy*, 3rd edition, © 2003, Reprinted with permission of the Canadian Society for Exercise Physiology.

TABLE 4.5 Body Composition Assessment Scoring

BMI healthy and SO5S healthy	8 points
BMI unhealthy and SO5 healthy	8 points
BMI healthy and SOS unhealthy	3 points
BMI healthy and SO5S unhealthy	0 points
WG healthy and SO2S healthy	8 points
WG healthy and SO2S unhealthy	4 points
WG unhealthy and SO2S healthy	2 points
WG unhealthy and SO2S unhealthy	0 points

Health Benefits Zones for Healthy Body Composition

16 points	Excellent
12 points	Very good
7–11 points	Good
4–5 points	Fair
0–3 points	Needs improvement

Source: *The Canadian Physical Activity, Fitness & Lifestyle Approach: CSEP-Health & Fitness Program's Health-Related Appraisal and Counselling Strategy*, 3rd edition, © 2003, Reprinted with permission of the Canadian Society for Exercise Physiology.

TABLE 4.6 Description of Health Benefit Zones

Health Benefit Zone	
Excellent	Your body composition falls within a range that is generally associated with optimal health benefits
Very Good	Your body composition falls within a range that is generally associated with considerable health benefits
Good	Your body composition falls within a range that is generally associated with many health benefits.
Fair	Your body composition falls within a range that is generally associated with some health benefits but also some health risks. *Progressing from here into the GOOD zone is a very significant step to increasing the health benefits associated with your body composition*
Needs Improvement	Your body composition falls within a range that is generally associated with considerable health risks. *Try to achieve and maintain a healthy body composition by enjoying regular physical activity and healthy eating*

Source: *The Canadian Physical Activity, Fitness & Lifestyle Approach: CSEP-Health & Fitness Program's Health-Related Appraisal and Counselling Strategy*, 3rd edition, © 2003, Reprinted with permission of the Canadian Society for Exercise Physiology.

TABLE 4.7 Circumference Measurement Technique: Conversion Constants to Calculate Body Density for Women

Upper Arm (cm)	Constant A	Age	Constant B	Hip (cm)	Constant C	Hip (cm)	Constant C	Wrist (cm)	Constant D
20.5	1.0966	17	.0086	79	.0957	114.5	.1388	13.0	.0819
21	1.0954	18	.0091	79.5	.0963	115	.1394	13.2	.0832
21.5	1.0942	19	.0096	80	.0970	115.5	.1400	13.4	.0845
22	1.0930	20	.0102	80.5	.0976	116	.1406	13.6	.0857
22.5	1.0919	21	.0107	81	.0982	116.5	.1412	13.8	.0870
23	1.0907	22	.0112	81.5	.0988	117	.1418	14.0	.0882
23.5	1.0895	23	.0117	82	.0994	117.5	.1424	14.2	.0895
24	1.0883	24	.0122	82.5	.1000	118	.1430	14.4	.0908
24.5	1.0871	25	.0127	83	.1006	118.5	.1436	14.6	.0920
25	1.0860	26	.0132	83.5	.1012	119	.1442	14.8	.0933
25.5	1.0848	27	.0137	84	.1018	119.5	.1448	15.0	.0946
26	1.0836	28	.0142	84.5	.1024	120	.1454	15.2	.0958
26.5	1.0824	29	.0147	85	.1030	120.5	.1460	15.4	.0971
27	1.0813	30	.0152	85.5	.1036	121	.1466	15.6	.0983
27.5	1.0801	31	.0157	86	.1042	121.5	.1472	15.8	.0996
28	1.0789	32	.0162	86.5	.1048	122	.1479	16.0	.1009
28.5	1.0777	33	.0168	87	.1054	122.5	.1485	16.2	.1021
29	1.0775	34	.0173	87.5	.1060	123	.1491	16.4	.1034
29.5	1.0754	35	.0178	88	.1066	123.5	.1497	16.6	.1046
30	1.0742	36	.0183	88.5	.1072	124	.1503	16.8	.1059
30.5	1.0730	37	.0188	89	.1079	124.5	.1509	17.0	.1072
31	1.0718	38	.0193	89.5	.1085	125	.1515	17.2	.1084
31.5	1.0707	39	.0198	90	.1091	125.5	.1521	17.4	.1097
32	1.0695	40	.0203	90.5	.1097	126	.1527	17.6	.1109
32.5	1.0683	41	.0208	91	.1103	126.5	.1533	17.8	.1122
33	1.0671	42	.0213	91.5	.1109	127	.1539	18.0	.1135
33.5	1.0666	43	.0218	92	.1115	127.5	.1545	18.2	.1147
34	1.0648	44	.0223	92.5	.1121	128	.1551	18.4	.1160
34.5	1.0636	45	.0228	93	.1127	128.5	.1558	18.6	.1172
35	1.0624	46	.0234	93.5	.1133	129	.1563		
35.5	1.0612	47	.0239	94	.1139	129.5	.1569		
36	1.0601	48	.0244	94.5	.1145	130	.1575		
36.5	1.0589	49	.0249	95	.1151	130.5	.1581		
37	1.0577	50	.0254	95.5	.1157	131	.1587		
37.5	1.0565	51	.0259	96	.1163	131.5	.1593		
38	1.0554	52	.0264	96.5	.1169	132	.1600		
38.5	1.0542	53	.0269	97	.1176	132.5	.1606		
39	1.0530	54	.0274	97.5	.1182	133	.1612		
39.5	1.0518	55	.0279	98	.1188	133.5	.1618		
40	1.0506	56	.0284	98.5	.1194	134	.1624		
40.5	1.0495	57	.0289	99	.1200	134.5	.1630		
41	1.0483	58	.0294	99.5	.1206	135	.1636		
41.5	1.0471	59	.0300	100	.1212	135.5	.1642		
42	1.0459	60	.0305	100.5	.1218	136	.1648		
42.5	1.0448	61	.0310	101	.1224	136.5	.1654		
43	1.0434	62	.0315	101.5	.1230	137	.1660		
43.5	1.0424	63	.0320	102	.1236	137.5	.1666		
44	1.0412	64	.0325	102.5	.1242	138	.1672		
		65	.0330	103	.1248	138.5	.1678		
		66	.0335	103.5	.1254	139	.1685		
		67	.0340	104	.1260	139.5	.1691		
		68	.0345	104.5	.1266	140	.1697		
		69	.0350	105	.1272	140.5	.1703		
		70	.0355	105.5	.1278	141	.1709		
		71	.0360	106	.1285	141.5	.1715		
		72	.0366	106.5	.1291	142	.1721		

(continued)

TABLE 4.7 (Continued)

Upper Arm (cm)	Constant A	Age	Constant B	Hip (cm)	Constant C	Hip (cm)	Constant C	Wrist (cm)	Constant D
		73	.0371	107	.1297	142.5	.1728		
		74	.0376	107.5	.1303	143	.1733		
		75	.0381	108	.1309	143.5	.1739		
				108.5	.1315	144	.1745		
				109	.1321	144.5	.1751		
				109.5	.1327	145	.1757		
				110	.1333	145.5	.1763		
				110.5	.1339	146	.1769		
				111	.1345	146.5	.1775		
				111.5	.1351	147	.1781		
				112	.1357	147.5	.1787		
				112.5	.1363	148	.1794		
				113	.1369	148.5	.1800		
				113.5	.1375	149	.1806		
				114	.1382	149.5	.1812		
						150	.1818		

FIGURE 4.6 Procedure for body fat assessment according to circumference measurements

Circumference Measurements for Women[*]

1. Using a regular tape measure, determine the following circumference measurements in centimetres (cm):

   Upper arm: Take the measure halfway between the shoulder and the elbow.

   Hip: Measure at the point of largest circumference.

   Wrist: Take the circumference in front of the bones where the wrist bends.

2. Obtain the person's age.
3. Using Table 4.4, find the subject's age and circumference measurement for each site in the left column below, then look up the constant values for each. These values will allow you to derive body density (BD) by substituting the constants in the following formula:

   $$BD = A - B - C + D$$

4. Using the derived body density, calculate percent body fat (%F) according to the following equation:

   $$\%F = (495 \div BD) - 450 **$$

Example. Jane is 20 years old, and the following circumference measurements were taken: biceps = 27 cm, hip = 99.5 cm, wrist = 15.4 cm.

Data		Constant		
Upper arm	= 27 cm	A	=	1.0813
Age	= 20	B	=	.0102
Hip	= 99.5 cm	C	=	.1206
Wrist	= 15.4 cm	D	=	.0971

$BD = A - B - C + D$
$BD = 1.0813 - .0102 - .1206 + .0971 = 1.0476$

$\%F = (495 \div BD) - 450$
$\%F = (495 \div 1.0476) - 450 = 22.5$

Circumference Measurements for Men[***]

1. Using a regular tape measure, determine the following circumference measurements in inches (the men's measurements are taken in inches, as opposed to centimetres for women):

   Waist: Measure at the umbilicus (belly button).

   Wrist: Measure in front of the bones where the wrist bends.

2. Subtract the wrist from the waist measurement.
3. Obtain the weight of the subject in kilograms.
4. Look up the percent body fat (%F) in Table 4.5 by using the difference obtained in number 2 above and the person's body weight.

Example: John weighs 72.7 kg, and his waist and wrist circumference measurements are 36.5 and 7.5 inches, respectively.

Waist circumference = 92.7 cm
Wrist circumference = 19 cm
Difference = 73.7 cm
Body weight = 72.7 kg
%F = 22

(handwritten annotations: 72.4; 33 83.82; 7 17.78; 66.04; 77.4)

[*] From R. B. Lambson, "Generalized Body Density Prediction Equations for Women Using Simple Anthropometric Measurements." Unpublished doctoral dissertation, Brigham Young University, Provo, UT, August 1987.

[**] From W. E. Siri, *Body Composition from Fluid Spaces and Density* (Berkeley: University of California, Donner Laboratory of Medical Physics, 1956).

[***] From A. G. Fisher and P. E. Allsen, *Jogging*, Dubuque, IA: Wm. C. Brown, 1987. This table was developed according to "Generalized Body Composition Equation for Men Using Simple Measurement Techniques," by K. W. Penrouse, A. G Nelson, and A G. Fisher, *Medicine and Science in Sports and Exercise* 17, no. 2 (1985): 189. © American College of Sports Medicine, 1985.

TABLE 4.8 Circumference Measurement Technique: Estimated Percent Body Fat for Men

Waist Minus Wrist Circumference Measurement (cm)

Body Weight (kg)	55.9	57.2	58.4	59.7	61	62.2	63.5	64.8	66	67.3	68.6	69.9	71.1	72.4	73.7	74.9	76.2	77.5	78.7	80	81.3	82.6	83.8	85.1	86.4	87.6	88.9	90.2	91.4	92.7	94	95.3	96.5	97.8	99.1	100	102	103	104	105	107	108	109	110	112	113	114	116	117	118	119	121	122	123	124	126	127
54.5	4	4	8	10	12	14	16	18	20	20	23	25	27	29	31	33	35	37	39	41	43	45	47	49	50	52	54	56	58																												
56.8	4	4	7	9	11	13	15	17	18	20	22	24	26	28	29	31	33	35	37	39	41	43	45	46	48	50	52	54	56	58																											
59.1	3	5	7	9	11	12	15	16	18	20	21	23	25	27	28	30	32	34	36	37	39	41	43	44	46	48	50	52	53	55	57																									
61.4	3	5	7	8	10	12	14	16	17	19	20	22	24	26	27	29	31	32	34	36	38	39	41	43	44	46	48	50	51	53	55	56																								
63.6	3	5	6	8	10	11	13	15	17	18	20	21	23	24	26	28	29	31	33	34	36	38	39	41	43	44	46	48	49	51	53	54	56																						
65.9	3	4	6	8	9	11	12	14	16	17	19	20	22	23	25	27	28	30	31	33	35	36	38	39	41	43	44	46	47	49	51	52	54	55																					
68.2	2	4	6	7	9	10	12	13	15	17	18	20	21	23	24	26	27	29	30	32	33	35	36	38	40	41	43	44	46	47	49	50	52	53	55																			
70.5	2	4	5	7	8	10	11	13	14	16	17	19	20	22	23	25	26	28	29	31	32	34	35	37	38	40	41	43	44	46	47	49	50	52	53	55																		
72.7	2	4	5	6	8	9	11	12	14	15	17	18	20	21	22	24	25	27	28	30	31	33	34	35	37	38	40	41	43	44	46	47	48	50	51	53	54																	
75	2	4	5	6	7	9	10	12	13	15	16	17	19	20	22	23	25	26	27	29	30	32	33	34	36	37	39	40	41	43	44	45	47	48	49	51	52	54																
77.3	2	3	4	6	7	9	10	11	13	14	16	17	18	20	21	22	24	25	26	28	29	31	32	33	34	36	37	39	40	42	43	44	46	47	48	49	51	52	54															
79.5	2	3	4	5	7	8	10	11	12	14	15	16	18	19	20	22	23	24	26	27	28	29	31	32	33	35	36	37	39	40	41	43	44	45	47	48	49	51	52	53														
81.8	2	3	4	5	6	8	9	10	12	13	14	16	17	18	19	21	22	23	25	26	27	28	30	31	32	34	35	36	37	39	40	41	43	44	45	46	48	49	50	52	53													
84.1		3	4	5	6	7	9	10	11	13	14	15	16	18	19	20	21	23	24	25	26	28	29	30	31	33	34	35	36	38	39	40	41	43	44	45	46	48	49	50	51	53												
86.4		2	3	4	6	7	8	9	11	12	13	15	16	17	18	20	21	22	23	25	26	27	28	29	31	32	33	34	36	37	38	39	41	42	43	44	45	46	48	49	50	51	52											
88.6		2	3	4	5	7	8	9	10	11	13	14	15	16	18	19	20	21	22	24	25	26	27	28	30	31	32	33	35	36	37	38	40	41	42	43	44	45	46	48	49	50	51	52										
90.9		2	3	4	5	6	8	9	10	11	12	14	15	16	17	18	19	21	22	23	24	25	26	28	29	30	31	32	34	35	36	37	39	40	41	42	43	44	45	47	48	49	50	51	52									
93.2		2	3	4	5	6	7	8	10	11	12	13	14	16	17	18	19	20	21	23	24	25	26	27	28	29	31	32	33	34	35	36	38	39	40	41	42	43	44	46	47	48	49	51	51	52								
95.5		2	3	4	4	6	7	8	9	11	12	13	14	15	16	17	18	20	21	22	23	24	25	26	27	29	30	31	32	33	35	36	37	38	39	40	41	42	43	45	46	47	48	49	51	51	52							
97.7		2	3	4	4	5	6	7	9	10	11	12	13	15	16	17	18	19	20	21	23	24	25	26	27	28	29	30	31	32	34	35	36	37	38	39	40	41	44	44	45	46	47	49	49	50	51	52						
100			2	3	4	4	6	7	8	9	10	11	12	14	15	16	17	18	19	20	22	23	24	25	26	27	28	29	30	31	33	34	35	36	37	38	39	40	41	43	44	45	46	48	48	49	50	51	52					
102			2	3	4	4	5	6	8	9	10	11	12	13	14	15	16	17	18	19	21	22	23	24	25	26	27	28	29	30	32	33	34	35	36	37	38	39	40	42	43	44	45	47	47	48	49	50	51	51				
105			2	3	3	4	5	6	7	8	9	10	11	13	14	15	16	17	18	19	20	21	23	23	24	25	26	27	28	29	31	32	33	34	35	36	37	38	39	41	42	43	44	45	46	47	48	49	50	51	51			
107			2	3	3	4	5	6	7	8	9	10	11	12	13	14	15	16	18	18	19	20	21	22	23	24	25	26	28	28	30	31	32	33	34	35	36	37	38	39	41	41	42	43	44	45	46	47	48	49	50	51		
109			2	3	3	4	5	6	7	8	9	9	11	11	13	14	15	16	17	18	19	20	21	22	23	24	25	26	26	28	29	30	31	32	33	34	35	36	37	38	39	40	41	42	43	44	45	46	47	48	49	50	50	
111			2	3	3	4	4	6	6	8	9	9	10	11	12	13	14	16	16	18	18	19	20	21	22	23	24	25	26	27	28	29	30	31	32	33	34	35	36	37	38	39	40	41	42	43	44	45	46	47	48	49	49	50
114				2	3	3	4	5	6	7	8	9	10	11	12	13	14	15	16	17	18	19	20	21	22	22	23	24	25	26	27	28	29	30	31	32	33	34	35	36	37	38	39	40	41	42	43	44	45	46	47	48	49	49
116				2	3	3	4	5	6	7	8	8	10	10	12	13	14	14	16	16	18	18	19	20	21	22	23	24	25	26	26	27	28	29	30	31	32	33	34	35	36	37	38	39	40	41	42	43	44	45	46	47	48	48
118					2	3	4	5	5	7	7	8	9	11	11	12	13	14	15	16	17	18	19	20	20	21	22	23	24	25	26	27	28	29	30	31	32	33	34	35	36	37	38	39	40	41	42	43	44	44	45	46	47	48
120					2	3	4	4	5	6	7	8	9	10	11	12	13	13	15	15	17	17	18	19	20	21	22	23	23	24	25	26	27	28	29	30	31	32	33	34	35	36	37	38	39	40	41	42	43	44	45	46	47	48
123					2	3	3	4	5	6	7	8	9	10	10	11	12	13	14	15	16	17	18	18	19	20	21	22	23	24	25	26	26	27	28	29	30	31	32	33	34	35	36	37	38	39	40	41	42	43	44	45	46	47
125					2	3	3	4	5	6	7	7	8	9	10	11	12	13	14	14	16	16	17	18	19	20	20	21	22	23	24	25	26	27	27	28	29	30	31	32	33	34	35	36	37	38	39	40	41	42	43	44	45	46
127					2	3	3	4	5	6	6	7	8	9	10	11	11	12	13	14	15	16	17	18	18	19	20	21	22	23	23	24	25	26	27	28	29	29	30	31	32	33	34	35	36	37	38	39	40	41	42	43	44	45
130					2	3	3	4	5	5	6	7	8	9	9	10	11	12	13	14	15	15	16	17	18	19	20	20	21	22	23	24	24	25	26	27	28	29	30	30	31	32	33	34	35	36	37	38	39	39	40	41	42	43
132					2	3	3	4	4	5	6	7	8	9	9	10	11	12	12	14	14	15	16	17	17	18	19	20	21	21	22	23	24	25	25	26	27	28	29	30	31	31	32	33	34	35	36	37	38	38	39	40	41	42
134					2	3	3	4	4	5	6	7	7	8	9	10	11	11	12	14	14	15	16	16	17	18	19	19	20	21	22	23	23	24	25	26	26	27	28	29	30	31	31	32	33	34	35	36	37	38	39	39	40	41
136					2	3	3	4	4	5	6	6	7	8	9	10	10	11	12	13	14	15	16	16	17	17	18	19	20	21	21	22	23	24	24	25	26	27	28	28	29	30	31	32	32	33	34	35	36	37	38	38	39	40

TABLE 4.9 Determination of Body Mass Index (BMI)

Determine your BMI by looking up the number where your weight and height intersect on the table. According to your results, look up your disease risk in Table 4.10.

Height (cm)	50	52	54	56	58	60	62	64	66	68	70	72	74	76	78	80	82	84	86	88	90	92	94	96	98	100	102	104	106	108	110
150	22.2	23.1	24	24.9	25.8	26.7	27.6	28.4	29.3	30.2	31.1	32	32.9	33.8	34.7	35.6	36.4	37.3	38.2	39.1	40	40.9	41.8	42.7	43.6	44.4	45.3	46.2	47.1	48	48.9
152.5	21.5	22.4	23.2	24.1	24.9	25.8	26.7	27.5	28.4	29.2	30.1	31	31.8	32.7	33.5	34.4	35.3	36.1	37	37.8	38.7	39.6	40.4	41.3	42.1	43	43.9	44.7	45.6	46.4	47.3
155	20.8	21.6	22.5	23.3	24.1	25	25.8	26.6	27.5	28.3	29.1	30	30.8	31.6	32.5	33.3	34.1	35	35.8	36.6	37.5	38.3	39.1	40	40.8	41.6	42.5	43.3	44.1	45	45.8
157.5	20.2	21	21.8	22.6	23.4	24.2	25	25.8	26.6	27.4	28.2	29	29.8	30.6	31.4	32.2	33.1	33.9	34.7	35.5	36.3	37.1	37.9	38.7	39.5	40.3	41.1	41.9	42.7	43.5	44.3
160	19.5	20.3	21.1	21.9	22.7	23.4	24.2	25	25.8	26.6	27.3	28.1	28.9	29.7	30.5	31.3	32	32.8	33.6	34.4	35.2	35.9	36.7	37.5	38.3	39.1	39.8	40.6	41.4	42.2	43
162.5	18.9	19.7	20.4	21.2	22	22.7	23.5	24.2	25	25.8	26.5	27.3	28	28.8	29.5	30.3	31.1	31.8	32.6	33.3	34.1	34.8	35.6	36.4	37.1	37.9	38.6	39.4	40.1	40.9	41.7
165	18.4	19.1	19.8	20.6	21.3	22	22.8	23.5	24.2	25	25.7	26.4	27.2	27.9	28.7	29.4	30.1	30.9	31.6	32.3	33.1	33.8	34.5	35.3	36	36.7	37.5	38.2	38.9	39.7	40.4
167.5	17.8	18.5	19.2	20	20.7	21.4	22.1	22.8	23.5	24.2	24.9	25.7	26.4	27.1	27.8	28.5	29.2	29.9	30.7	31.4	32.1	32.8	33.5	34.2	34.9	35.6	36.4	37.1	37.8	38.5	39.2
170	17.3	18	18.7	19.4	20.1	20.8	21.5	22.1	22.8	23.5	24.2	24.9	25.6	26.3	27	27.7	28.4	29.1	29.8	30.4	31.1	31.8	32.5	33.2	33.9	34.6	35.3	36	36.7	37.4	38.1
170.5	17.2	17.9	18.6	19.3	20	20.6	21.3	22	22.7	23.4	24.1	24.8	25.5	26.1	26.8	27.5	28.2	28.9	29.6	30.3	31	31.6	32.3	33	33.7	34.4	35.1	35.8	36.5	37.2	37.8
175	16.3	17	17.6	18.3	18.9	19.6	20.2	20.9	21.6	22.2	22.9	23.5	24.2	24.8	25.5	26.1	26.8	27.4	28.1	28.7	29.4	30	30.7	31.3	32	32.7	33.3	34	34.6	35.3	35.9
177.5	15.9	16.5	17.1	17.8	18.4	19	19.7	20.3	20.9	21.6	22.2	22.9	23.5	24.1	24.8	25.4	26	26.7	27.3	27.9	28.6	29.2	29.8	30.5	31.1	31.7	32.4	33	33.6	34.3	34.9
180	15.4	16	16.7	17.3	17.9	18.5	19.1	19.8	20.4	21	21.6	22.2	22.8	23.5	24.1	24.7	25.3	25.9	26.5	27.2	27.8	28.4	29	29.6	30.2	30.9	31.5	32.1	32.7	33.3	34
182.5	15	15.6	16.2	16.8	17.4	18	18.6	19.2	19.8	20.4	21	21.6	22.2	22.8	23.4	24	24.6	25.2	25.8	26.4	27	27.6	28.2	28.8	29.4	30	30.6	31.2	31.8	32.4	33
185	14.6	15.2	15.8	16.4	16.9	17.5	18.1	18.7	19.3	19.9	20.5	21	21.6	22.2	22.8	23.4	24	24.5	25.1	25.7	26.3	26.9	27.5	28	28.6	29.2	29.8	30.4	31	31.6	32.1
187.5	14.2	14.8	15.4	15.9	16.5	17.1	17.6	18.2	18.8	19.3	19.9	20.5	21	21.6	22.2	22.8	23.3	23.9	24.5	25	25.6	26.2	26.7	27.3	27.9	28.4	29	29.6	30.2	30.7	31.3
190	13.9	14.4	15	15.5	16.1	16.6	17.2	17.7	18.3	18.8	19.4	19.9	20.5	21.1	21.6	22.2	22.7	23.3	23.8	24.4	24.9	25.5	26	26.6	27.1	27.7	28.3	28.8	29.4	29.9	30.5
192.5	13.5	14	14.6	15.1	15.7	16.2	16.7	17.3	17.8	18.4	18.9	19.4	20	20.5	21	21.6	22.1	22.7	23.2	23.7	24.3	24.8	25.4	25.9	26.4	27	27.5	28.1	28.6	29.1	29.7
195	13.1	13.7	14.2	14.7	15.3	15.8	16.3	16.8	17.4	17.9	18.4	18.9	19.5	20	20.5	21	21.6	22.1	22.6	23.1	23.7	24.2	24.7	25.2	25.8	26.3	26.8	27.4	27.9	28.4	28.9

TABLE 4.10 Disease Risk According to Body Mass Index (BMI)

BMI	Disease Risk	Classification
<18.5	Increased	Underweight
18.5–24.9	Least	Normal weight
25–29.9	Increased	Overweight
>30–34.9	High	Obese class I
>35–39.9	Very High	Obese class II
≥40	Extremely High	Obese class III

Canadian Guidelines for Body Weight Classification in Adults, Health Canada, 2003 © Her Majesty the Queen in Right of Canada (2003), pg. 3. © Reproduced with the permission of the Minister of Public Works and Government Services Canada, 2008. Available from http://www.hc-sc.gc.ca/fn-an/alt_formats/hpfb-dgpsa/pdf/nutrition/weight_book-livres_des_poids_e.pdf

In research studies and surveys, BMI is the most widely used measure to determine overweight and obesity. For most people, though, percent body fat techniques are not readily available, nor do technicians have the necessary training and dependability to administer these procedures.

BMI is a useful tool to screen the general population, but its one weakness (similar to the original height/weight charts) is that it fails to differentiate fat from lean body mass or note where most of the fat is located (waist circumference—see discussion that follows). Using BMI, athletes with a large amount of muscle mass (such as body builders and football players) can easily fall in the moderate- or even high-risk categories.

Waist Circumference

Scientific evidence suggests that the way people store fat affects their risk for disease. The total amount of body fat is not what increases the risk for disease but, rather, the location of the body fat. Some individuals tend to store fat in the abdominal area (which produces the "apple" shape). Others store it mainly around the hips and thighs,

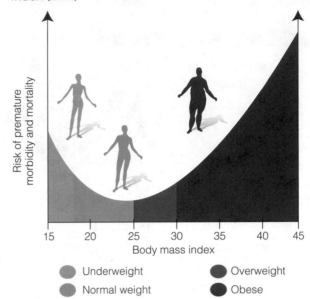

FIGURE 4.7 Mortality risk versus body bass index (BMI)

in gluteal and femoral fat (which creates the "pear" shape).

Research data show that obese individuals with a lot of abdominal fat are clearly at higher risk for heart disease, hypertension, type 2 diabetes (also called "adult-onset" or "non-insulin-dependent" diabetes), and stroke than are obese people with similar amounts of total body fat stored primarily in the hips and thighs.[2] Evidence also indicates that, among individuals with a lot of abdominal fat, those whose fat deposits are located around internal organs (intra-abdominal or visceral fat) have an even greater risk for disease than those with fat mainly just beneath the skin (subcutaneous fat).[3]

Complex scanning techniques to identify individuals at risk because of high intra-abdominal fatness are costly, so a simple waist circumference (WC) measure is used to assess this risk.[4] WC seems to predict abdominal visceral fat as accurately as the DEXA technique.[5] You are at increased risk of developing health problems such as type 2 diabetes, heart disease, and high blood pressure if your waist circumference is

- More than 102 cm (40.2 inches) for Caucasian men or 90 cm (35.4 inches) for Asian men
- More than 88 cm (35 inches) for Caucasian women or 80 cm (31.5 inches) for Asian women

CRITICAL THINKING

Do you think you have a weight problem? Do your body composition results make you feel any different about the way you perceive your current body weight and image?

The Heart and Stroke Foundation of Canada has a waist circumference calculator you can use to determine your health risk level. Access this site at: http://ww2.heartandstroke.ca/page_asp?PageID=1185. Weight loss is encouraged when individuals exceed these measurements. One study concluded that WC might be a better predictor of the risk for disease than BMI.[6]

A second procedure used for years to identify health risk based on the pattern of fat distribution is the **waist-to-hip ratio (WHR)** test. The waist measurement is taken at the umbilicus (belly button), and the hip measurement is taken at the point of greatest circumference. The waist measurement is then divided by the hip measurement.

The WHR differentiates the "apples" from the "pears." Men tend to be apples, and women tend to be pears. Men need to lose weight if the WHR is 1.0 or higher (that is, if the waist is even slightly larger than the hips). Women need to lose weight if the WHR is .85 or higher (see Table 4.12). For example, the WHR for a man with a 100 cm (40 inch) waist and a 95 cm (38 inch) hip would be 1.05 (100 ÷ 95)—which may indicate higher risk for disease.

During the last few years, several studies have found that WC is a better indicator than WHR of abdominal visceral obesity.[7] Thus, a combination of BMI and WC, rather than WHR, is now recommended by health care professionals to assess potential risk for disease.

TABLE 4.11 Percentage Distribution of BMI by Sex, Household Population aged 18 or older, Canada, 2004

	Both sexes		Men		Women	
	'000	%	'000	%	'000	%
Underweight	471	2.0	170[2]	1.4[1,2]	302	2.5
Normal weight	9,328	38.9	3,986	33.6[1]	5,343	44.1
Overweight	8,647	36.1	4,984	42.0[1]	3,663	30.2
Obese Class I	3,656	15.2	1,959	16.5	1,697	14.0
Obese Class II	1,231	5.1	568	4.8	663	5.5
Obese Class III	651	2.7	194	1.6[1]	457	3.8
Overweight and obese (BMI ≥ 25)	14,185	59.1	7,706	65.0[1]	6,480	53.4
Obese (BMI ≥ 30)	5,539	23.1	2,722	22.9	2,817	23.2

[1] Significantly different from estimate for women (p < 0.05)
[2] Coefficient of variation between 16.6% and 33.3% (interpret with caution)

Source. Adapted from Statistics Canada publication *Nutrition: Findings from the Canadian Community Health Survey,* Catalogue 82-620 MWE. Issue 1, http:// www.statcan.ca/english/research/82-620-MIE/2005001/tables/adults/ table1.htm

Determining Recommended Body Weight

After finding out your percent body fat, you can determine your current body composition classification by consulting Table 4.13, which presents percentages of fat according to both the health fitness standard and the high physical fitness standard (see discussion in Chapter 1).

For example, the recommended health fitness fat percentage for a 20-year-old female is 28 percent or less. Although there are no clearly identified percent body fat levels at which the disease risk definitely increases (as is the case with BMI), the health fitness standard in Table 4.13 is currently the best estimate of the point at which there seems to be no harm to health.

According to Table 4.13, the high physical fitness range for this same 20-year-old woman would be between 18 and 23 percent. The high physical fitness standard does not mean you cannot be somewhat below this number. Many highly trained male athletes are as low as 3 percent, and some female distance runners have been measured at 6 percent body fat (which may not be healthy).

Although people generally agree that the mortality rate is higher for obese people, some evidence indicates that the same is true for underweight people. "Underweight" and "thin" do not necessarily mean the same thing. The body fat of a healthy thin person is around the high physical fitness standard,

TABLE 4.12 Disease Risk According to Waist-to-Hip Ratio

Waist-to-Hip Ratio		
Men	Women	Disease Risk
≤0.95	≤0.80	Very Low
0.96–0.99	0.81–0.84	Low
≥1.00	≥0.85	High

whereas an underweight person has extremely low body fat, even to the point of compromising the essential fat.

The 3 percent essential fat for men and 12 percent for women seem to be the lower limits for people to maintain good health. Below these percentages, normal physiological functions can be seriously impaired. Some experts point out that a little storage fat (in addition to the essential fat) is better than none at all. As a result, the health and high fitness standards for percent fat in Table 4.13 are set higher than the minimum essential fat requirements, at a point beneficial to optimal health and well-being. Finally, because lean tissue decreases with age, one extra percentage point is allowed for every additional decade of life.

Your recommended body weight is computed based on the selected health or high fitness fat percentage for your age and sex. Your decision to select a "desired" fat percentage should be based on your current percent body fat and your personal health/fitness objectives. Following are steps to compute your own recommended body weight:

1. Determine the kilograms of body weight that are fat (FW) by multiplying your body weight (BW) by the current percent fat (%F) expressed in decimal form (FW = BW × %F).
2. Determine lean body mass (LBM) by subtracting the weight in fat from the total body weight (LBM = BW − FW). (Anything that is not fat must be part of the lean component.)
3. Select a desired body fat percentage (DFP) based on the health or high fitness standards given in Table 4.13.

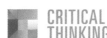

CRITICAL THINKING

How do you feel about your current body weight and what influence does society have on the way you perceive yourself with regard to your weight? Do your body composition results make you feel any different about the way you see your current body weight and image?

Waist-to-hip ratio (WHR) A measurement to assess potential risk for disease based on distribution of body fat.

TABLE 4.13 Body Composition Classification According to Percent Body Fat

MEN

Age	Underweight	Excellent	Good	Moderate	Overweight	Significantly Overweight
≤19	<3	12.0	12.1–17.0	17.1–22.0	22.1–27.0	≥27.1
20–29	<3	13.0	13.1–18.0	18.1–23.0	23.1–28.0	≥28.1
30–39	<3	14.0	14.1–19.0	19.1–24.0	24.1–29.0	≥29.1
40–49	<3	15.0	15.1–20.0	20.1–25.0	25.1–30.0	≥30.1
≥50	<3	16.0	16.1–21.0	21.1–26.0	26.1–31.0	≥31.1

WOMEN

Age	Underweight	Excellent	Good	Moderate	Overweight	Significantly Overweight
≤19	<12	17.0	17.1–22.0	22.1–27.0	27.1–32.0	≥32.1
20–29	<12	18.0	18.1–23.0	23.1–28.0	28.1–33.0	≥33.1
30–39	<12	19.0	19.1–24.0	24.1–29.0	29.1–34.0	≥34.1
40–49	<12	20.0	20.1–25.0	25.1–30.0	30.1–35.0	≥35.1
≥50	<12	21.0	21.1–26.0	26.1–31.0	31.1–36.0	≥36.1

☐ High physical fitness standard   ☐ Health fitness standard

4. Compute recommended body weight (RBW) according to the formula RBW = LBM ÷ (1.0 − DFP).

As an example of these computations, a 19-year-old female who weighs 72.7 kg pounds and is 30 percent fat would like to know what her recommended body weight would be at 22 percent:

Sex: female
Age: 19
BW: 72.7 kg
%F: 30% (.30 in decimal form)
1. FW = BW × %F
   FW = 72.7 × .30 = 21.7 kg
2. LBM = BW − FW
   LBM = 72.7 − 21.7 = 51 kg
3. DFP: 22% (.22 in decimal form)
4. RBW = LBM ÷ (1.0 − .DFP)
   RBW = 51 kg ÷ (1.0 − .22)
   RBW = 51 kg ÷ .78 = 65.4 kg

In Labs 4A and 4B, you will have the opportunity to determine your own body composition, recommended body weight, and disease risk according to waist-to-hip ratio and BMI. A second column is provided in both labs for a follow-up assessment at a future date.

Other than hydrostatic weighing and air displacement, skinfold thickness seems to be the most practical and valid technique to estimate body fat. If skinfold calipers are available, use this technique to assess your percent body fat. If calipers are not available, estimate your percent fat according to the circumference measurements technique or another technique available to you. You may also wish to use several techniques and compare the results.

Importance of Regular Body Composition Assessment

Children do not start with a weight problem. Although a small number struggle with weight throughout life, most are not overweight in the early years of life.

Trends indicate that, starting at age 25, the average person gains about 0.5 kg of weight per year. Thus, by age 65, the average person will have gained 20 kg. Because of the typical reduction in physical activity in our society, however, the average person also loses 0.25 kg of lean tissue each year. Therefore, this span of 40 years has produced an actual fat gain of 30 kg accompanied by a 10 kg loss of lean body mass[8] (see Figure 4.8). These changes cannot be detected unless body composition is assessed periodically.

If you are on a diet/exercise program, you should repeat your percent body fat assessment and recommended weight computations about once a month.

FIGURE 4.8 Obesity rates by age group, household population aged 18 or older, Canada, 1978–1979 and 2004

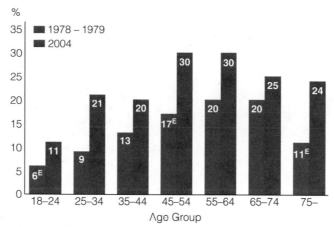

*Significantly higher than estimate for 1978-1979 (p < 0.05)
ECoefficient of variation 15.6% to 33.3% (interpret with caution)

Source: Adapted from Statistics Canada publication *Nutrition: Findings from the Canadian Community Health Survey*, Catalogue 82-620 MWE. Issue 1, Chart 1, http://www.statcan.ca/english/research/82-620-MIE/2005001/charts/adults/chart1.htm

FIGURE 4.9 Effects of a 6-week aerobics exercise program on body composition

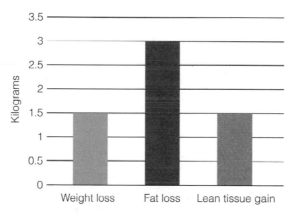

*W.W.K. Hoeger, data collected at the University of Texas of the Permian Basin, 1985.

This is important because lean body mass is affected by weight-reduction programs and amount of physical activity. As lean body mass changes, so will your recommended body weight. To make valid comparisons, use the same technique for both pre- and post-program assessments. Knowing your percent body fat also is useful to identify fad diets that promote water loss and lean body mass, especially muscle mass (also see Diet Crazes in Chapter 5, page 125).

Changes in body composition resulting from a weight control/exercise program were illustrated in a co-ed aerobic dance course taught during a six-week summer term. Students participated in a 60-minute aerobics routine four times a week. On the first and last days of class, several physiological parameters, including body composition, were assessed. Students also were given information on diet and nutrition, but they followed their own dietary program.

At the end of the six weeks, the average weight loss for the entire class was 1.4 kg (see Figure 4.9). But, because body composition was assessed, class members were surprised to find that the average fat loss was actually 2.8 kg, accompanied by a 1.4 kg increase in lean body mass.

When dieting, have your body composition reassessed periodically because of the effects of negative caloric balance on lean body mass. As discussed in Chapter 5, dieting does decrease lean body mass. This loss of lean body mass can be offset or eliminated by combining a sensible diet with exercise.

ASSESS YOUR KNOWLEDGE

1. Body composition incorporates
   a. a fat component.
   b. a non-fat component.
   c. percent body fat.
   d. lean body mass.
   e. all of the four components above.

2. The best way to determine recommended body weight is through
   a. height/weight charts.
   b. body composition analysis.
   c. lean body mass assessment.
   d. hip-to-waist ratio.
   e. body mass index.

3. Essential fat in women is
   a. 3 percent.
   b. 5 percent.
   c. 10 percent.
   d. 12 percent.
   e. 17 percent.

4. Which of the following is *not* a technique used in the assessment of body fat?
   a. body mass index
   b. skinfold thickness
   c. hydrostatic weighing
   d. circumference measurements
   e. air displacement

5. Which of the following sites is used in the assessment of percent body fat according to skinfold thickness in men?
   a. suprailium
   b. chest
   c. scapular
   d. triceps
   e. All four sites are used.

6. Which variable is *not* used in the assessment of percent body fat in women according to girth measurements?
   a. age
   b. hip
   c. wrist
   d. upper arm
   e. height

7. The waist-to-hip ratio is used to
   a. determine percent body fat.
   b. assess risk for disease.
   c. measure lean body mass.
   d. identify underweight people.
   e. do all of the above.

8. An acceptable BMI is between
   a. 15 and 19.99.
   b. 20 and 24.99.
   c. 25 and 29.99.
   d. 30 and 34.99.
   e. 35 and 39.99.

9. The health fitness percent body fat for women of various ages is in the range of
   a. 3 to 7 percent.
   b. 7 to 12 percent.
   c. 12 to 20 percent.
   d. 20 to 27 percent.
   e. 27 to 31 percent.

10. When a previously inactive individual starts an exercise program, the person may
    a. lose weight.
    b. gain weight.
    c. improve body composition.
    d. lose more fat pounds than total weight pounds.
    e. do all of the above.

Correct answers can be found at the back of the book.

MEDIA MENU

INTERNET CONNECTIONS

- The Canadian Institute for Health Information (CIHI). CIHI is an independent, not-for-profit organization that provides essential data and analysis on Canada's health system and the health of Canadians. The institute's data and reports focus on health care services, health spending, health human resources, and population health.

  http://www.cihi.ca

- Health Canada. Learn about the Canadian guidelines for body weight classification in adults, with questions and answers for the public, at this site.

  http://www.hc-sc.gc.ca/fn-an/nutrition/

  weights-poids/guide-ld-adult/qa-qr-pub-e.html#2/

- The Heart and Stroke Foundation of Canada. This site has numerous research articles and interactive health tools that support the promotion of healthy living.

  http://www.heartandstroke.ca/

Notes

1. J. Stevens, J. Cai, E. R. Pamuk, D. F. Williamson, M. J. Thun, and J. L. Wood, "The Effect of Age on the Association Between Body Mass Index and Mortality," *New England Journal of Medicine* 338 (1998): 1–7.

2. "Comparing Apples and Pears," *University of California at Berkeley Wellness Letter* (Palm Coast, FL: The Editors, March 2004).

3. C. Bouchard, G. A. Bray, and V. S. Hubbard, "Basic and Clinical Aspects of Regional Fat Distribution," *American Journal of Clinical Nutrition* 52 (1990): 946–950.

   J. P. Després, I. Lemieux, and D. Prudhomme, "Treatment of Obesity: Need to Focus on High Risk Abdominally Obese Patients," *British Medical Journal* 322 (2001): 716–720.

   M. C. Pouliot et al., "Waist Circumference and Abdominal Sagittal Diameter: Best Simple Anthropometric Indexes of Abdominal Visceral Adipose Tissue Accumulation and Related Cardiovascular Risk in Men and Women," *American Journal of Cardiology* 73 (1994): 460–468.

4. National Heart, Lung, and Blood Institute, National Institutes of Health, *The Practical Guide: Identification, Evaluation, and Treatment of Overweight and Obesity in Adults* (NIH Publication no. 00–4084) (Washington DC: Government Printing Office, 2000).

5. M. B. Snijder, et al., "The Prediction of Visceral Fat by Dual-Energy X-ray Absorptiometry in the Elderly: A Comparison with Computed Tomography and Anthropometry," *International Journal of Obesity* 26 (2002): 984–993.

6. I. Janssen, P. T. Katzmarzyk, and R. Ross, "Waist Circumference and Not Body Mass Index Explains Obesity-Related Health Risk," *American Journal of Clinical Nutrition* 79 (2004): 379–384.

7. P. M. Ribisl, "Toxic 'Waist' Dump: Our Abdominal Visceral Fat," *ACSM's Health & Fitness Journal* 8, no. 4 (2004): 22–25.

8. J. H. Wilmore, "Exercise and Weight Control: Myths, Misconceptions, and Quackery," lecture given at annual meeting of American College of Sports Medicine, Indianapolis, June 1994.

Suggested Readings

Alberta Centre for Active Living. "Healthy Measures." http://www.healthymeasures.ca/.

Health Canada. "Canadian Guidelines for Body Weight Classification in Adults." Cat. No. H49-179/2003E. Publication ID: 4645.

Heyward, V. H., and D. Wagner. *Applied Body Composition Assessment.* Champaign, IL: Human Kinetics, 2004.

Katzmarzyk P. T., and C. K. Mason. "Prevalence of Class I, II and III Obesity in Canada." *Canadian Medical Association Journal* 174 (2006): 156–57.

"Prevention in Progress: Body Mass Index." Canadian Lifestyles and Fitness Research Institute. Bulletin no. 15. June 1997.

Roche, A. F., T. G. Lohman, and S. B. Heymsfield. *Human Body Composition.* Champaign, IL: Human Kinetics, 1996.

Sokar-Todd H. B., and A. M. S. Sharma. "Obesity Research in Canada: Literature Overview of the Last Three Decades." *Obesity Research* 12 (2004): 1547–553.

Stevens, J., J. E. McLain, and K. P. Truesdale. "Commentary: Obesity Claims and Controversies." *International Journal of Epidemiology* 35: 77–78. Available online at http://ije.oxfordjournals.org/cgi/reprint/35/1/77.

World Health Organization. "Global Strategy on Diet, Physical Activity and Health." Available online at http://www.who.int/hpr/NPH/docs/gs_obesity.pdf.

Lab 4A

HYDROSTATIC WEIGHING FOR BODY COMPOSITION ASSESSMENT

Name: _____   Date: _____   Grade: _____

Instructor: _____   Course: _____   Section: _____

Necessary Lab Equipment

Hydrostatic or underwater weighing tank and residual volume spirometer (if no spirometer is available, predicting equations can be used to determine this volume—see Figure 4.2, pages 96–97).

Objective

To determine body density and percent body fat.

Lab Preparation

Bring a swimsuit and towel to this lab. A six- to eight-hour fast and bladder and bowel movements are recommended prior to underwater weighing.

Instructions

Follow the procedure outlined in Figure 4.2. If time is a factor, assess only the body composition of one or two participants in the course and compute the results using the form provided below. A sample of the computations is provided on the back of this page.

I. Hydrostatic Weighing

Name: _____   Age: _____   Weight: _____ kg

Height: _____ cm   Water temperature: _____ °C   Water density (WD): _____ gr/ml

Residual volume (RV): _____ lt   (See Figure 4.2)

BW in kg = _____

Gross underwater weights:

1. _____ kg   2. _____ kg   3. _____ kg   4. _____ kg   5. _____ kg

6. _____ kg   7. _____ kg   8. _____ kg   9. _____ kg   10. _____ kg

Average of three heaviest underwater weights (AUW): _____ kg

Tare weight (TW): _____ kg

Net underwater weight (UW) = AUW − TW

Net underwater weight (UW) = _____ − _____ = _____ kg

Body density (BD):

$$BD = \frac{BW}{\frac{BW - UW}{WD} - RV - .1} \qquad BD = \frac{\rule{2cm}{0.4pt}}{\frac{\rule{1.5cm}{0.4pt}}{\rule{1cm}{0.4pt}} - \rule{1cm}{0.4pt} - .1} = \rule{2cm}{0.4pt}$$

Percent body fat (%Fat):

$$\%Fat = \frac{495}{BD} - 450 = \frac{495}{\rule{2cm}{0.4pt}} - 450 = \rule{1.5cm}{0.4pt} \%$$ **Follow-up** percent body fat: _____ %

FIGURE 4A.1 Sample computation for percent body fat according to hydrostatic weighing

Name: Jane Doe   Age: 20   Weight: 67.36 kg

Height: 170.2 cm   Water temperature: 33 °C   Water density (WD): .99473 gr/ml

Residual volume (RV): 1.73 lt   See Figure 4.2.

BW in kg = 67.36 kg

Gross underwater weights:

1. 6.15 kg   2. 6.12 kg   3. 6.24 kg   4. 6.26 kg   5. 6.21 kg

6. 6.26 kg   7. 6.29 kg   8. 6.28 kg   9. 6.24 kg   10. 6.27 kg

Average of three heaviest underwater weights (AUW): 6.28 kg

Tare weight (TW): 5.154 kg

Net underwater weight (UW) = AUW − TW

Net underwater weight (UW) = 6.28 − 5.154 = 1.126 kg

Body density (BD):

$$BD = \frac{BW}{\dfrac{BW - UW}{WD} - RV - .1} \qquad BD = \frac{67.36}{\dfrac{67.36 - 1.126}{.99473} - 1.73 - .1} = 1.0402301$$

Percent body fat (%Fat):

$$\%Fat = \frac{495}{BD} - 450 = \frac{495}{1.0402301} - 450 = 25.9 \%$$ **Follow-up** percent body fat: ____ %

II. What I learned from the underwater weighing procedure.

Describe the experience of being weighed underwater. Do you feel that the results of the test were accurate?

_____

_____

_____

_____

_____

_____

_____

_____

_____

_____

_____

_____

Lab 4C

DETERMINING YOUR HEALTH BENEFIT ZONE

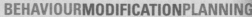

Name:		Date:		Grade:	
Instructor:		Course:		Section:	

Necessary Lab Equipment

Weigh scale, skinfold calipers, standard measuring tape and metre stick.

Objective

To measure weight, height, and Body Mass Index. To determine Health Benefit Zones by measuring skinfold thicknesses and waist girth (circumference).

Instructions

To measure weight, use weigh scale.

To measure height, use standard measuring tape or metre stick.

To determine Body Mass Index, use formula below.

Measure skinfolds as described in Figure 4.5, page 101.

To measure Waist Girth (circumference):

- Clear your abdominal area of clothing.
- Stand upright with your feet shoulder width apart and your stomach relaxed. Wrap the measuring tape around your waist.
- Find the uppermost edge of your hipbones, using the borders of your hands. The hipbone located toward the front of your body is not the top of the hip bone. Follow this spot upward and back toward the side of your body to find the true top of your hip.
- Align the bottom edge of the measuring tape with the top of the hipbones on both sides of your body.
- Make sure the tape is parallel to the floor. Do not let the tape measure twist.
- Relax. Take two normal breaths. Then tighten the tape around your waist. The tape should fit comfortably, but feel snug. Your stomach should be relaxed.
- Take the reading on the tape.

I. Weight (kg)

II. Height (m)

III. Sum of the 5 Skinfolds (SO5S)

Men			Women	
Triceps (mm):			Triceps (mm):	
Bicep (mm):			Bicep (mm):	
Subscapular (mm):			Subscapular (mm):	
Iliac Crest (mm):			Iliac Crest (mm):	
Medical calf (mm):			Medical calf (mm):	
Total			Total	

Refer to Tables 4.4 to 4.6. Check to see if your SO5S is in the shaded zone for Estimated Health Benefit Zone according to trends in morbidity and mortality data.

IV. Sum of the 2 Skinfolds (SO2S)

Men		**Women**	
Subscapular (mm):		Subscapular (mm):	
lliac Crest (mm):		lliac Crest (mm):	
Total (mm):		Total (mm):	

In healthy zone? yes ☐   no ☐

Refer to Tables 4.4 to 4.6. Check to see if your SO2S is in the shaded zone for Estimated Health Benefit Zone according to trends in morbidity and mortality data.

V. Body Mass Index   (BMI)

Calculate your BMI. $\dfrac{\text{Weight (kg)} =}{\text{Height (m)}^2 =}$

VI. Waist Girth (circumference) (cm) _____

Scoring of Body Composition Assessments

BMI health and SO5S healthy _____ 8 points

BMI unhealthy and SO5S healthy _____ 8 points

BMI healthy and SO5S unhealthy _____ 3 points

BMI unhealthy and SO5S unhealthy _____ 0 points

WG healthy and SO2S healthy _____ 8 points

WG healthy and SO2S unhealthy _____ 4 points

WG unhealthy and SO2S healthy _____ 2 points

WG unhealthy and SO2S unhealthy _____ 0 points

Corresponding Health Benefit Zones for Healthy Body Composition

16 points   _____ Excellent

12 points   _____ Very Good

7 – 11 points   _____ Good

4 – 5 points   _____ Fair

0 – 3 points   _____ Needs improvement

Source: *The Canadian Physical Activity, Fitness & Lifestyle Approach: CSEP-Health & Fitness Program's Health-Related Appraisal and Counselling Strategy,* 3rd edition, © 2003, Reprinted with permission of the Canadian Society for Exercise Physiology.

Chapter 5

Weight Management

© Workbook Stock/Jupiter Images

Objectives

- Describe the health consequences of obesity.
- Expose some popular fad diets and myths and fallacies regarding weight control.
- Describe eating disorders and their associated medical problems and behaviour patterns, and the need for professional help in treating these conditions.
- Explain the physiology of weight loss, including setpoint theory and the effects of diet on basal metabolic rate.
- Explain the role of a lifetime exercise program as the key to a successful weight loss and weight maintenance program.
- Be able to implement a physiologically sound weight reduction and weight maintenance program.
- Describe behaviour modification techniques that help a person adhere to a lifetime weight maintenance program.

Two terms commonly used to describe the condition of weighing more than recommended are *overweight* and *obesity*. The obesity level is the point at which excess body fat can lead to serious health problems. Obesity is a health hazard of epidemic proportions in most developed countries around the world. According to the World Health Organization, an estimated 35 percent of the adult population in industrialized nations is obese. **Obesity** has been defined as a body mass index (BMI) of 30 or higher.

Over the past few decades there has been an increase in the number of Canadians who have become overweight and/or obese. This increase is likely the result of both inactivity and poor dietary habits. According to Statistics Canada, between 1996 and 2005 the average weight gain for adult females and males (aged 18 to 56 years) was over 3.0 and 4.0 kg, respectively. Although both men and women tend to gain weight each year, the rate of weight gain has slowed down significantly in recent years.

In the early 1970s, roughly 47 percent of Canadian men and 33.9 percent of Canadian women were either overweight or obese. By the late 1970s, the percentage had increased to 56 percent and 42 percent for men and women, respectively. By the early 1990s, the numbers remained similar for men (58 percent) but slightly decreased for women (41 percent).[1] However, that plateau was short lived as obesity rates have again risen. During the period from 1978 to 2004, the prevalence of obesity rose in almost all adult age groups with the greatest increases in people younger than 35 and older than 75 years. Canadian adults between the ages of 25 and 34 years showed a doubling (from 8.5 percent to 20.5 percent) as did those over 75 (from 10.6 percent to 23.6). Interestingly, obesity was lowest in those aged 18 to 24 where only 10.7 percent of men and 12.1 percent of women were considered obese.[2] As can be seen in Figure 5.1, Health Canada reports the percentage of adults who are obese (both males and females) by province as estimated in 2004. The consequences of these increases, both medical and economic, will be realized shortly.

Overweight Versus Obesity

Overweight and obesity are not the same thing. Many overweight people (people who weigh about 5 to 10 kg pounds over the recommended weight) are not obese. Although a kilogram or so of excess weight may not be harmful to most people, this is not always the case. People with excessive body fat who have type 2 diabetes and other cardiovascular risk factors (elevated blood lipids, high blood pressure, physical inactivity, and poor eating habits) benefit from weight loss. People who have a few extra kilograms of weight but who are otherwise healthy and physically active, exercise regularly, and eat a healthy diet may

HEALTH CONSEQUENCES OF EXCESSIVE BODY WEIGHT

Being overweight or obese increases the risk for

- high blood pressure
- elevated blood lipids (high blood cholesterol and triglycerides)
- type 2 (non-insulin-dependent) diabetes
- insulin resistance, glucose intolerance
- coronary heart disease
- angina pectoris
- congestive heart failure
- stroke
- gallbladder disease
- gout
- osteoarthritis
- obstructive sleep apnea and respiratory problems
- some types of cancer (endometrial, breast, prostate, and colon)
- complications of pregnancy (gestational diabetes, gestational hypertension, preeclampsia, and complications during C-sections)
- poor female reproductive health (menstrual irregularities, infertility, irregular ovulation)
- bladder control problems (stress incontinence)
- psychological disorders (depression, eating disorders, distorted body image, discrimination, and low self-esteem)
- shortened life expectancy
- decreased quality of life

Source: Centers for Disease Control and Prevention, 2004.

FIGURE 5.1 Measured body mass index—percentage of adults who are obese (both males and females) (2004)

Province	Estimate
Newfoundland & Labrador	34.7
Prince Edward Island	26.8
Nova Scotia	24.6
New Brunswick	29.1
Quebec	21.9
Ontario	22.6
Manitoba	28.1
Saskatchewan	30.6
Alberta	25.2
British Columbia	19.3
All of Canada	23.1

Source: *Food and Nutrition. Map of Obesity According to Measured Body Mass Index (BMI) in Adults in Canada (both males and females)—Canada's Nutrition and Health Atlas.* Health Canada, 2004. © Reproduced with the permission of the Minister of Public Works and Government Services Canada, 2008. Retrieved May 24, 2008. http://www.hc-sc.gc.ca/fn-an/surveill/atlas/map-carte/mass_adult_obes_mf-hf_e.html.

FIGURE 5.2 Obesity Trends* among Canadian Adults, 1985–1998

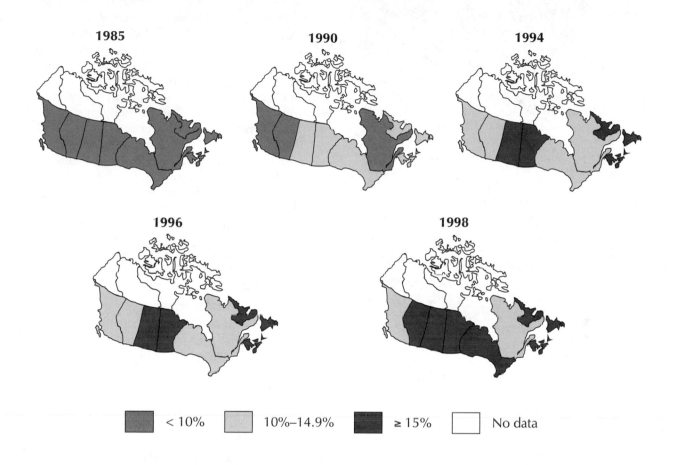

1985   1990   1994

1996   1998

< 10%   10%–14.9%   ≥ 15%   No data

* BMI ≥ 30, or ~30 lbs overweight for 5'4" woman.

Source: "The Canadian obesity epidemic, 1985–1998." CMAJ, 16-Apr-02; 166(8), pp. 1039–1040, Fig. 1, pg. 1039, by permission of the publisher. © 2002 Canadian Medical Association.

not be at greater risk for early death. Such is not the case, however, with obese individuals.

Research data indicate that individuals who are 15 or more kilograms overweight during middle age (30 to 49 years of age) lose about seven years of life, whereas being 5 to 15 kg overweight decreases lifespan by about three years.[3] These decreases are similar to those seen with tobacco use. Severe obesity (BMI greater than 45) at a young age, nonetheless, may cut up to 20 years off one's life.[4]

Although the loss of years of life is significant, the decreased life expectancy doesn't even begin to address the loss in quality of life and increased illness and disability throughout the years. Even a modest reduction of 5 to 10 percent can reduce the risk for chronic diseases including heart disease, high blood pressure, high cholesterol, and diabetes.[5]

A primary objective to achieve overall physical fitness and enhanced quality of life is to attain recommended body composition. Individuals at recommended body weight are able to participate in a wide variety of moderate-to-vigorous activities without functional limitations. These people have the freedom to enjoy most of life's recreational activities to their fullest potential. Excessive body weight does not afford an individual the fitness level to enjoy many lifetime activities such as

Obesity A chronic disease characterized by body mass index (BMI) 30 or higher.

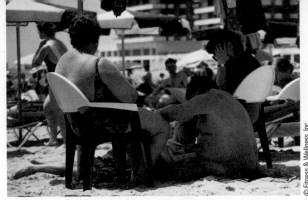

Obesity is a health hazard of epidemic proportions in industrialized nations.

achieve these unrealistic figures. Failure to attain a "perfect body" may lead to eating disorders in some individuals.

When people set their own target weight, they should be realistic. Attaining the "Excellent" percent of body fat shown in Table 4.13 (page 110) is extremely difficult for some. It is even more difficult to maintain over time, unless the person makes a commitment to a vigorous lifetime exercise program and permanent dietary changes. Few people are willing to do that. The "Moderate" percent body fat category may be more realistic for many people.

The question you should ask yourself is: Am I happy with my weight? Part of enjoying a higher quality of life is being happy with yourself. If you are not, you either need to do something about it or learn to live with it.

If your percent of body fat is higher than those in the Moderate category of Table 4.13 (page 110), you should try to reduce it and stay in this category, for health reasons. This is the category that seems to pose no detriment to health.

If you are in the Moderate category but would like to reduce your percent of body fat further, you need to ask yourself a second question: How badly do I want it? Do I want it badly enough to implement lifetime exercise and dietary changes? If you are not willing to change, you should stop worrying about your weight and deem the Moderate category "tolerable" for you.

The Weight Loss Dilemma

Yo-yo dieting carries as great a health risk as being overweight and remaining overweight in the first place. Epidemiological data show that frequent fluctuations in weight (up or down) markedly increase the risk of dying of cardiovascular disease.

Based on the findings that constant losses and regains can be hazardous to health, quick-fix diets should be replaced by a slow but permanent weight-loss program (as described under "Losing Weight the Sound and Sensible Way"). Individuals reap the benefits of recommended body weight when they get to that weight and stay there throughout life.

Unfortunately, only about 10 percent of all people who begin a traditional weight-loss program without exercise are able to lose the desired weight. Worse, only 5 in 100 are able to keep the weight off. The body is highly resistant to permanent weight changes through caloric restrictions alone.

Traditional diets have failed because few of them incorporate lifetime changes in food selection and an overall increase in physical activity and exercise as fundamental to successful weight loss

basketball, soccer, racquetball, surfing, mountain cycling, or mountain climbing. Maintaining high fitness and recommended body weight gives a person a degree of independence throughout life that most people in developed nations no longer enjoy.

Scientific evidence also recognizes problems with being underweight. Although the social pressure to be thin has declined slightly in recent years, the pressure to attain model-like thinness is still with us and contributes to the gradual increase in the number of people who develop eating disorders (anorexia nervosa and bulimia, discussed under "Eating Disorders" on pages 128–130).

Extreme weight loss can lead to medical conditions such as heart damage, gastrointestinal problems, shrinkage of internal organs, immune system abnormalities, disorders of the reproductive system, loss of muscle tissue, damage to the nervous system, and even death.

CRITICAL THINKING

Do you consider yourself overweight? If so, how long have you had a weight problem, what attempts have you made to lose weight, and what has worked best for you?

Tolerable Weight

Many people want to lose weight so they will look better. That's a noteworthy goal. The problem, however, is that they have a distorted image of what they would really look like if they were to reduce to what they think is their ideal weight. Hereditary factors play a big role, and only a small fraction of the population has the genes for a "perfect body."

The media have the greatest influence on people's perception of what constitutes ideal body weight. Most people use fashion, fitness, and beauty magazines to determine what they should look like. The "ideal" body shapes, physiques, and proportions seen in these magazines are rare and are achieved mainly through airbrushing and medical reconstruction.[6] Many individuals, primarily young women, go to extremes in an attempt to and weight maintenance. When the diet stops, weight gain begins. The $40-billion diet industry tries to capitalize on the false idea that weight can be lost quickly without considering the consequences of fast weight loss or the importance of lifetime behavioural changes to ensure proper weight loss and maintenance.

In addition, various studies indicate that most people, especially obese people, underestimate their energy intake. Those who try to lose weight but apparently fail to do so are often described as "diet-resistant." One study found that, while on a "diet," a group of obese individuals with a self-reported history of diet resistance underreported their average daily caloric intake by almost 50 percent (1,028 self-reported versus 2,081 actual calories—see Figure 5.3).[7] These individuals also overestimated their amount of daily physical activity by about 25 percent (1,022 self-reported versus 771 actual calories). These differences represent an additional 1,304 calories of energy per day unaccounted for by the subjects in the study. The findings indicate that failing to lose weight often is related to misreports of actual food intake and level of physical activity.

Diet Crazes

Capitalizing on hopes that the latest diet to hit the market will really work this time, fad diets continue to appeal to people of all shapes and sizes. These diets may work for a while, but their success is usually short-lived. Regarding the effectiveness of these diets, Dr. Kelly Brownell, a foremost researcher in the field of weight management, has stated: "When I get the latest diet fad, I imagine a trick birthday cake candle that keeps lighting up and we have to keep blowing it out."

Fad diets deceive people and claim that dieters will lose weight by following all instructions. Most diets are very low in calories and deprive the body of certain nutrients, generating a metabolic imbalance. Under these conditions, a lot of the weight lost is in the form of water and protein, and not fat.

On a crash diet, close to half the weight loss is in lean (protein) tissue. When the body uses protein instead of a combination of fats and carbohydrates as a source of energy, weight is lost as much as 10 times faster. This is because a gram of protein produces half the amount of energy that fat does. In the case of muscle protein, one-fifth of protein is mixed with four-fifths water. Therefore, each 0.5 kg of muscle yields only one-tenth the amount of energy of a 0.5 kg of fat. As a result, most of the weight lost is in the form of water, which on the scale, of course, looks good.

Low-Carb Diets

Among the most popular diets on the market today are the low-carbohydrate/high-protein (LCHP) diet plans. Although small variations exist among them, in general, "low-carb" diets limit the intake of carbohydrate-rich foods—bread, potatoes, rice, pasta, cereals, crackers, juices, sodas, sweets (candy, cake, cookies), and even fruits and vegetables. Dieters are allowed to eat all the protein-rich foods they desire, including steak, ham, chicken, fish, bacon, eggs, nuts, cheese, tofu, high-fat salad dressings, butter, and small amounts of a few fruits and vegetables. Typically, these diets are also high in fat content. Examples of these diets are the Atkins Diet, The Zone, Protein Power, the Scarsdale Diet, The Carb Addict's Diet, South Beach Diet (initially low-carb), and Sugar Busters.

During digestion, carbohydrates are converted into glucose, a basic fuel used by every cell in the body. As blood glucose rises, insulin is released from the pancreas. Insulin is a hormone that facilitates the entry of glucose into the cells, thereby lowering the glucose level in the bloodstream. If the cells don't soon use the glucose for normal cell functions or to fuel physical activity, glucose is converted to, and stored as, body fat.

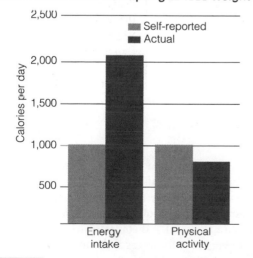

FIGURE 5.3 Differences between self-reported and actual daily caloric intake and exercise in obese individuals attempting to lose weight

Source: Adapted from S.W. Lichtman et al., "Discrepancy Between Self-Reported and Actual Caloric Intake and Exercise in Obese Subjects," *New England Journal of Medicine* 327 (1992), pp.1893–1898.

Yo-yo dieting Constantly losing and gaining weight.

ARE LOW-CARB/HIGH-PROTEIN DIETS MORE EFFECTIVE?

A few studies suggest that, at least over the short term, low-carb/high-protein (LCHP) diets are more effective in producing weight loss than carbohydrate-based diets. These results are preliminary and controversial. In LCHP diets:

■ A large amount of weight loss is water and muscle protein, not body fat. Some of this weight is quickly regained when regular dietary habits are resumed.

■ Few people are able to stay with LCHP diets for more than a few weeks at a time. The majority stop dieting before the targeted program completion.

■ LCHP dieters are rarely found in a national weight-loss registry of people who have lost 15 kg and kept them off for a minimum of six years.

■ Food choices are severely restricted in LCHP diets. With less variety, individuals tend to eat less (800 to 1,200 calories/day) and thus lose more weight.

■ LCHP diets may promote heart disease and cancer and increase the risk for osteoporosis.

■ LCHP diets are fundamentally high in fat (about 60 percent fat calories).

■ LCHP diets are not recommended for people with diabetes, high blood pressure, heart disease, or kidney disease.

■ LCHP diets do not promote long-term healthy eating patterns.

HOW TO RECOGNIZE FAD DIETS

Fad diets share common characteristics. These diets typically

■ are nutritionally unbalanced.
■ are based on testimonials.
■ were developed according to "confidential research."
■ promote rapid and "painless" weight loss.
■ promise miraculous results.
■ restrict food selection.
■ require the use of selected products.
■ use liquid formulas instead of foods.
■ misrepresent salespeople as individuals qualified to provide nutrition counselling.
■ fail to provide information on risks associated with weight loss and diet use.
■ do not involve physical activity.
■ do not encourage healthy behavioural changes.
■ are not supported by the scientific community or national health organizations.
■ fail to provide information for weight maintenance upon completion of diet phase.

TABLE 5.1 Glycemic Index of Selected Foods

Food Item	Index	Food Item	Index
Glucose	100	Muesli	56
Carrots	92	Frosted Flakes	55
Honey	87	Fruit cocktail	55
Baked potatoes	85	Sweet corn	55
Jelly beans	80	Sweet potato	51
White rice	72	Peas	51
White bread	69	White pasta	50
Whole-wheat bread	69	Whole-wheat pasta	42
Pineapple	66	Spaghetti	41
Table sugar	65	Oranges	40
Bananas	62	Apples	39
Boiled potatoes	62	Low-fat yogurt	33
Corn	59	Fructose	20
Oatmeal	59	Peanuts	13

Not all carbohydrates cause a similar rise in blood glucose. The rise in glucose is based on the speed of digestion, which depends on a number of factors, including the size of the food particles. Small-particle carbohydrates break down rapidly and cause a quick, sharp rise in blood glucose. Thus, to gauge a food's effect on blood glucose, carbohydrates are classified by their **glycemic index**.

A high glycemic index signifies a food that causes a quick rise in blood glucose. At the top of the 100-point scale is glucose itself. This index is not directly related to simple and complex carbohydrates, and the glycemic values are not always what one might expect. Rather, the index is based on the actual laboratory-measured speed of absorption. Processed foods generally have a high glycemic index, whereas high-fibre foods tend to have a lower index (see Table 5.1).

The body functions best when blood sugar remains at a constant level. Although this is best accomplished with low-glycemic index foods, elimination of all high-glycemic index foods from the diet is not necessary (foods with a high glycemic index are especially useful to replenish depleted glycogen stores following prolonged or exhaustive exercise). Combining high- with low-glycemic index items or with some fat and protein brings the average index down. Regular consumption of high-glycemic foods, nonetheless, can increase the risk of cardiovascular disease, especially in people at risk for diabetes.

Proponents of LCHP diets indicate that if a person eats fewer carbohydrates and more protein, the pancreas will produce less insulin, and as insulin drops, the body will turn to its own fat deposits for energy. There is no scientific proof, however, that high levels of insulin lead to weight

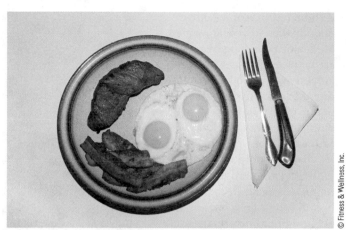

High-protein/low-carb diets create nutritional deficiencies and contribute to the development of cardiovascular disease, cancer, and osteoporosis.

gain. None of the authors of these diets have published any studies that validate their claims. Yet these authors base their diets on the faulty premise that high insulin leads to obesity. In fact, we know the opposite to be true: Excessive body fat causes insulin levels to rise, thereby increasing the risk for developing diabetes.

The reason for rapid weight loss during LCHP diets is that a low carbohydrate intake forces the liver to produce glucose. The source for most of this glucose is body proteins—your lean body mass, including muscle. As indicated earlier, protein is mostly water; thus, weight is lost rapidly. When a person terminates the diet, the body rebuilds some of the protein tissue and quickly regains some weight.

A study in the *New England Journal of Medicine* indicated that individuals on a LCHP (Atkins) diet for 12 months lost about twice as much weight as those on a low-fat diet at the midpoint of the study.[8] The effectiveness of the diet, however, seemed to dwindle over time. At 12 months into the diet, the LCHP diet participants had regained more weight than those on the low-fat diet plan.

Years of research will be required to determine the extent to which long-term adherence to LCHP diets increase the risk for heart disease, cancer, and kidney or bone damage. Low-carb diets are contrary to the nutrition advice of most national leading health organizations (which recommend a diet low in animal fat and saturated fat and high in complex carbohydrates). Without fruits, vegetables, and whole grains, high-protein diets lack many vitamins, minerals, and fibre—all dietary factors that protect against an array of ailments and diseases.

The major risk associated with long-term adherence to LCHP diets could be the increased risk of heart disease because high-protein foods are also high in fat content (see Chapter 11). A low

carbohydrate intake also produces a loss of vitamin B, calcium, and potassium. Potential bone loss can further accentuate the risk for osteoporosis. Side effects commonly associated with these diets include weakness, nausea, bad breath, constipation, irritability, lightheadedness, and fatigue. Long-term adherence to a LCHP diet also can increase the risk of cancer. Phytochemicals found in fruits, vegetables, and whole grains protect against certain types of cancer. If you choose to go on a LCHP diet for longer than a few weeks, let your physician know so he or she may monitor your blood lipids, bone density, and kidney function.

Combo Diets

In addition to the low-carb diets, "combo diets" such as the Schwarzbein and Suzanne Sommers diets are also popular of late. The Schwarzbein diet claims that eating proteins and nonstarchy carbohydrates together will keep the food from being stored as fat. The Suzanne Sommers diet doesn't allow you to eat proteins within three hours of carbohydrates, and if fruits are eaten, the dieter must wait at least 20 minutes before eating other carbohydrate foods. Both of these diets allow consumption of high-protein/high-fat food items, which can increase the risk for heart disease.

If people only would realize that no magic foods will provide all of the necessary nutrients, that a person has to eat a variety of foods to be well-nourished, the diet industry would not be as successful. Most of these diets create a nutritional deficiency, which at times may be fatal.

The reason many of these diets succeed is that they restrict a large number of foods. Thus, people tend to eat less food overall. With the extraordinary variety of foods available to us, it is unrealistic to think that people will adhere to these diets for very long. People eventually get tired of eating the same thing day in and day out and start eating less, leading to weight loss. If they happen to achieve the lower weight but do not make permanent dietary changes, they regain the weight quickly once they go back to their previous eating habits.

A few diets recommend exercise along with caloric restrictions—the best method for weight reduction, of course. People who adhere to these programs will succeed, so the diet has achieved its purpose. Unfortunately, if the people do not change their food selection and activity level permanently,

Glycemic index An index that is used to rate the plasma glucose response of carbohydrate-containing foods with the response produced by the same amount of carbohydrate from a standard source, usually glucose or white bread.

BEHAVIOUR MODIFICATION PLANNING

EPHEDRA AND WEIGHT LOSS

A very popular and controversial weight-loss supplement now taken off the market was the herbal supplement ma huang, more commonly known as ephedra. Ma huang contains ephedra alkaloids, whose actions are similar to those of sympathetic nervous system hormones. In 2002, Health Canada requested a voluntary recall of certain products containing ephedra after research concluded that these products posed a serious risk to the health of Canadians. Some of the health issues that concerned medical experts were an increased risk of stroke, heart attacks, heart rate irregularities, seizures, psychoses, and even death. Individuals suffering from heart conditions, high blood pressure, and diabetes were at even a higher risk. Products that have a dose unit of more than 8 mg of ephedrine or recommend more than an 8 mg dose or 32 mg/day were targeted with this recall. Products that contained caffeine and ephedrine were also recalled.[9]

they gain back the weight once they discontinue dieting and exercise.

Also, let's not forget that we eat for pleasure and for health. Two of the most essential components of a wellness lifestyle are healthy eating and regular physical activity, and they provide the best weight-management program available today.

Eating Disorders

Eating disorders are medical illnesses that involve critical disturbances in eating behaviours thought to stem from some combination of environmental pressures. These disorders are characterized by an intense fear of becoming fat, which does not disappear even when losing extreme amounts of weight. The two most common types of eating disorders are **anorexia nervosa** and **bulimia nervosa**. A third condition, binge-eating disorder, also known as compulsive overeating, is also recognized as an eating disorder.

Most people who have eating disorders are afflicted by significant family and social problems. They may lack fulfillment in many areas of their lives. The eating disorder then becomes the coping mechanism to avoid dealing with these problems. Taking control over their own body weight helps them feel that they are restoring some sense of control over their lives.

Anorexia nervosa and bulimia nervosa are common in industrialized nations where society encourages low-calorie diets and thinness. The female role in society is changing rapidly, which makes women more susceptible to eating disorders.

Although the disorders are frequently seen in young women, the majority seeking treatment are between the ages of 25 and 50. Surveys, nonetheless, indicate that as many as 40 percent of university- and college-age women are struggling with an eating disorder.

Eating disorders are not limited to women. Every one in nine cases exists in men. But because the role of men in society and their body image are viewed differently, these cases often go unreported.

Although genetics may play a role in the development of eating disorders, most cases are environmentally related. Individuals who have clinical depression and obsessive compulsive behaviour are more susceptible. About half of all people with eating disorders have some sort of chemical dependency (alcohol and drugs), and a majority of them come from families with alcohol and drug-related problems. Of reported cases of eating disorders, a large number are individuals who are, or have been, victims of sexual molestation.

Eating disorders develop in stages. Typically, individuals who are already dealing with significant issues in life start a diet. At first they feel in control and are happy about the weight loss even if they are not overweight. Encouraged by the prospect of weight loss and the control they can exert over their own weight, the dieting becomes extreme and often is combined with exhaustive exercise and the overuse of laxatives and diuretics.

Although a genetic predisposition may contribute, the syndrome typically emerges following emotional issues or a stressful life event and the uncertainty about the ability to cope efficiently. Life experiences that can trigger the syndrome might be gaining weight, starting the menstrual period, beginning university or college, losing a boyfriend, having poor self-esteem, being socially rejected, starting a professional career, or becoming a wife or a mother.

The eating disorder now takes on a life of its own and becomes the primary focus of attention for the individuals afflicted with it. Self-worth revolves around what the scale reads every day, their relationship with food, and their perception of how they look each day.

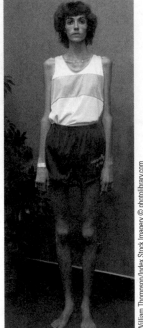

Society's unrealistic view of what constitutes recommended weight and "ideal" body image contributes to the development of eating disorders.

Anorexia Nervosa

Over 38,000 Canadian women suffer from anorexia nervosa. Anorexic individuals seem to fear weight gain more than death from starvation. Furthermore, they have a distorted image of their body and think of themselves as being fat even when they are emaciated.

Anorexics commonly develop obsessive and compulsive behaviours and emphatically deny their condition. They are preoccupied with food, meal planning, and grocery shopping, and they have unusual eating habits. As they lose weight and their health begins to deteriorate, anorexics feel weak and tired. They might realize they have a problem, but they will not stop the starvation and refuse to consider the behaviour as abnormal.

Once they have lost a lot of weight and malnutrition sets in, physical changes become more visible. Typical changes are amenorrhea (stopping menstruation), digestive problems, extreme sensitivity to cold, hair and skin problems, fluid and electrolyte abnormalities (which may lead to an irregular heartbeat and sudden stopping of the heart), injuries to nerves and tendons, abnormalities of immune function, anemia, growth of fine body hair, mental confusion, inability to concentrate, lethargy, depression, dry skin, lower skin and body temperature, and osteoporosis.

Diagnostic criteria for anorexia nervosa are:[10]

- Refusal to maintain body weight over a minimal normal weight for age and height (weight loss leading to maintenance of body weight less than 85 percent of that expected or failure to make expected weight gain during periods of growth, leading to body weight less than 85 percent of that expected).
- Intense fear of gaining weight or becoming fat, even though underweight.
- Disturbance in the way in which one's body weight, size, or shape is perceived, undue influences of body weight or shape on self-evaluation, or denial of the seriousness of the current low body weight.
- In postmenarcheal females, amenorrhea (absence of at least three consecutive menstrual cycles). (A woman is considered to have amenorrhea if her periods occur only following estrogen therapy.)

Many of the changes induced by anorexia nervosa can be reversed. Individuals with this condition can get better with professional therapy, turn to bulimia nervosa, or die from the disorder. Twenty percent of anorexics die as a result of their condition. Anorexia nervosa has the highest mortality rate of all psychosomatic illnesses today. The disorder, however, is 100 percent curable. But treatment

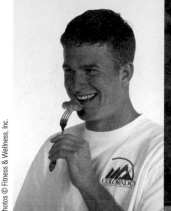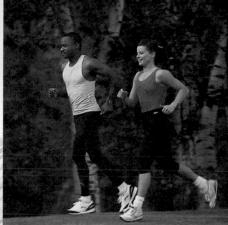

Photos © Fitness & Wellness, Inc.

Achieving and maintaining a high physical fitness percent body fat standard requires a lifetime commitment to regular physical activity and proper nutrition.

almost always requires professional help, and the sooner it is started, the better are the chances for reversibility and cure.

Therapy consists of a combination of medical and psychological techniques to restore proper nutrition, prevent medical complications, and modify the environment or events that triggered the syndrome.

Seldom can anorexics overcome the problem by themselves. They strongly deny their condition. They are able to hide it and deceive friends and relatives. Based on their behaviour, many of them meet all of the characteristics of anorexia nervosa, but it goes undetected because both thinness and dieting are socially acceptable. Only a well-trained clinician is able to diagnose anorexia nervosa.

Bulimia Nervosa

Bulimia nervosa is more prevalent than anorexia nervosa. As many as one in every five women on college campuses may be bulimic, according to some estimates. Bulimia nervosa also is more prevalent than anorexia nervosa in males, although bulimia is still much more prevalent in females.

Bulimics usually are healthy-looking people, well-educated, and near recommended body weight. They seem to enjoy food and often socialize around it. In actuality, they are emotionally insecure, rely on others, and lack self-confidence and self-esteem. Recommended weight and food are important to them.

Anorexia nervosa An eating disorder characterized by self-imposed starvation to lose and maintain very low body weight.

Bulimia nervosa An eating disorder characterized by a pattern of binge eating and purging in an attempt to lose weight and maintain low body weight.

WEIGHT MANAGEMENT

The binge–purge cycle usually occurs in stages. As a result of stressful life events or the simple compulsion to eat, bulimics engage periodically in binge eating that may last an hour or longer.

With some apprehension, bulimics anticipate and plan the cycle. Next they feel an urgency to begin, followed by large and uncontrollable food consumption, during which they may eat several thousand calories (up to 10,000 calories in extreme cases). After a short period of relief and satisfaction, feelings of deep guilt, shame, and intense fear of gaining weight ensue. Purging seems to be an easy answer, as the binging cycle can continue without fear of gaining weight.

The diagnostic criteria for bulimia nervosa are:[11]

■ Recurrent episodes of binge eating. An episode of binge eating is characterized by both of the following:
   ■ Eating in a discrete period of time (for example, within any two-hour period), an amount of food that is definitely more than most people would eat during a similar period and under similar circumstances.
   ■ A sense of lack of control over eating during the episode (a feeling that one cannot stop eating or control what or how much one is eating).
■ Recurring inappropriate compensatory behaviours to prevent weight gain, such as self-induced vomiting; misuse of laxatives, diuretics, enemas, or other medications; fasting; or excessive exercise.
■ The binge eating and inappropriate compensatory behaviours both occur, on average, at least twice a week for three months.
■ Self-evaluation is unduly influenced by body shape and weight.

The most typical form of purging is self-induced vomiting. Bulimics, too, frequently ingest strong laxatives and emetics. Near-fasting diets and strenuous bouts of exercise are common. Medical problems associated with bulimia nervosa include cardiac arrhythmias, amenorrhea, kidney and bladder damage, ulcers, colitis, tearing of the esophagus or stomach, tooth erosion, gum damage, and general muscular weakness.

Unlike anorexics, bulimics realize their behaviour is abnormal and feel great shame about it. Fearing social rejection, they pursue the binge–purge cycle in secrecy and at unusual hours of the day.

Bulimia nervosa can be treated successfully when the person realizes that this destructive behaviour is not the solution to life's problems. A change in attitude can prevent permanent damage or death.

Binge-Eating Disorder

Binge-eating disorder (BED) is probably the most common of the three eating disorders. It generally does not involve vomiting or excessive exercise, and individuals with BED are often obese. Although most people think they overeat from time to time, eating more than one should now and then does not mean the individual has a binge-eating disorder. The disorder is slightly more common in women than in men as three women for every two men have this disorder.

Binge-eating disorder is characterized by uncontrollable episodes of eating excessive amounts of food within a relatively short time. The causes of binge-eating disorder are unknown, although depression, anger, sadness, boredom, and worry can trigger an episode. Unlike bulimics, binge eaters do not purge; thus, most people with this disorder are either overweight or obese. Typical symptoms of binge-eating disorder include:

■ Eating what most people think is an unusually large amount of food
■ Eating until uncomfortably full
■ Eating out of control
■ Eating much faster than usual during binge episodes
■ Eating alone because of embarrassment of how much food is being consumed
■ Feeling disgusted, depressed, or guilty after overeating.

Treatment

Treatment for eating disorders is available on most school campuses through the school's counselling centre or the health centre. Local hospitals also offer treatment for these conditions. Many communities have support groups, frequently led by professional personnel and often free of charge. All information and the identity of the individual are kept confidential so the person need not fear embarrassment or repercussion when seeking professional help.

Physiology of Weight Loss

Traditional concepts related to weight control have centred on three assumptions:

1. Balancing food intake against output allows a person to achieve recommended weight.
2. All fat people just eat too much.
3. The human body doesn't care how much (or little) fat it stores.

Although these statements contain some truth, they are open to much debate and research. We now know that the causes of obesity are complex, including a combination of genetics, behaviour, and lifestyle factors.

Energy-Balancing Equation

The principle embodied in the **energy-balancing equation** is simple: As long as caloric input equals caloric output, the person will not gain or lose weight. If caloric intake exceeds output, the person gains weight; when output exceeds input, the person loses weight. If daily energy requirements could be determined accurately, caloric intake could be balanced against output. This is not always the case, though, because genetic and lifestyle-related individual differences determine the number of calories required to maintain or lose body weight.

Table 5.3 (page 141) offers some general guidelines to determine the estimated energy requirement (EER) in calories per day according to lifestyle patterns. This is only an estimated figure and (as discussed under "Losing Weight the Sound and Sensible Way," pages 138–142) serves only as a starting point from which individual adjustments have to be made.

The total daily energy requirement has three basic components (see Figure 5.4):

1. Resting metabolic rate (RMR)
2. The thermic effect of food (TEF)
3. Physical activity

The **resting metabolic rate**—the energy requirement to maintain the body's vital processes in the resting state—accounts for approximately 60 percent to 70 percent of the total daily energy requirement. The thermic effect of food, the energy required to digest, absorb, and store food, accounts for about 5 percent to 10 percent of the total daily requirement. Physical activity accounts for 15 percent to 30 percent of the daily total requirement.

One kilogram of fat is the equivalent of 7,700 calories. If a person's **estimated energy requirement (EER)** is 2,500 Calories and that person were to decrease intake by 500 Calories per day, it should result in a loss of 0.45 kg of fat in 7 days (500 × 7 = 3,500). But research has shown—and many people have experienced—that even when dieters carefully balance caloric input against caloric output, weight loss does not always happen as predicted. Furthermore, two people with similar measured caloric intake and output seldom lose weight at the same rate.

The most common explanation for individual differences in weight loss and weight gain has been the variation in human metabolism from one person to another. We are all familiar with people who can eat "all day long" and not gain any weight while others cannot even "dream about food" without gaining weight. Because experts did not believe that human metabolism alone could account for such extreme differences, they developed several theories that might better explain these individual variations.

Setpoint Theory

Results of several research studies point toward a **weight-regulating mechanism (WRM)** that has a **setpoint** for controlling both appetite and the amount of fat stored. Setpoint is hypothesized to work like a thermostat for body fat, maintaining fairly constant body weight, because it "knows" at all times the exact amount of adipose tissue stored in the fat cells. Some people have high settings; others have low settings.

If body weight decreases (as in dieting), the setpoint senses this change and triggers the WRM to increase the person's appetite or make the body conserve energy to maintain the "set" weight. The

Binge-eating disorder An eating disorder characterized by uncontrollable episodes of eating excessive amounts of food within a relatively short time.

Energy-balancing equation A principle holding that as long as caloric input equals caloric output, the person will not gain or lose weight. If caloric intake exceeds output, the person gains weight; when output exceeds input, the person loses weight.

Resting metabolic rate (RMR) The energy requirement to maintain the body's vital processes in the resting state.

Estimated energy requirement (EER) The average dietary energy (caloric) intake that is predicted to maintain energy balance in a healthy adult of defined age, gender, weight, height, and level of physical activity, consistent with good health.

Weight-regulating mechanism (WRM) A feature of the hypothalamus of the brain that controls how much the body should weigh.

Setpoint Weight control theory that the body has an established weight and strongly attempts to maintain that weight.

FIGURE 5.4 Components of total daily energy requirement

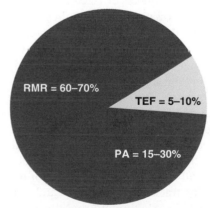

RMR = resting metabolic rate
TEF = thermic effect of food
PA = physical activity

opposite also may be true. Some people have a hard time gaining weight. In this case, the WRM decreases appetite or causes the body to waste energy to maintain the lower weight.

SETPOINT AND CALORIC INPUT

Every person has his or her own certain body fat percentage (as established by the setpoint) that the body attempts to maintain. The genetic instinct to survive tells the body that fat storage is vital, and therefore it sets an acceptable fat level. This level may remain somewhat constant or may climb gradually because of poor lifestyle habits.

For instance, under strict calorie reduction, the body may make extreme metabolic adjustments in an effort to maintain its setpoint for fat. The **basal metabolic rate (BMR)**, the lowest level of caloric intake necessary to sustain life, may drop dramatically when operating under a consistent negative caloric balance, and that person's weight loss may plateau for days or even weeks. A low metabolic rate compounds a person's problems in maintaining recommended body weight.

These findings were substantiated by research conducted at Rockefeller University in New York.[12] The authors showed that the body resists maintaining altered weight. Obese and lifetime non-obese individuals were used in the investigation. Following a 10 percent weight loss, in an attempt to regain the lost weight, the body compensated by burning up to 15 percent fewer calories than expected for the new reduced weight (after accounting for the 10 percent loss). The effects were similar in the obese and non-obese participants. These results imply that after a 10 percent weight loss, a person would have to eat even less or exercise even more to compensate for the estimated 15 percent slowdown (a difference of about 200 to 300 Calories).

In this same study, when the participants were allowed to increase their weight to 10 percent above their "normal" body (pre-weight loss) weight, the body burned 10 to 15 percent *more* calories than expected—attempting to waste energy and maintain the pre-set weight. This is another indication that the body is highly resistant to weight changes unless additional lifestyle changes are incorporated to ensure successful weight management. (These methods are discussed under "Losing Weight the Sound and Sensible Way," pages 138–142.)

Dietary restriction alone will not lower the setpoint, even though the person may lose weight and fat. When the dieter goes back to the normal or even below-normal caloric intake (at which the weight may have been stable for a long time), he or she quickly regains the lost fat as the body strives to regain a comfortable fat store.

Let's use a practical illustration. A person would like to lose some body fat and assumes that his or her current, stable body weight has been reached at an average daily caloric intake of 1,800 Calories (no weight gain or loss occurs at this daily intake). In an attempt to lose weight rapidly, this person now goes on a **very low-calorie diet** (defined as fewer than 800 Calories per day) or, even worse, a near-fasting diet. This immediately activates the body's survival mechanism and readjusts the metabolism to a lower caloric balance. After a few weeks of dieting at fewer than 800 Calories per day, the body can now maintain its normal functions at 1,300 Calories per day. This new figure (1,300) represents a drop of 500 Calories per day in the metabolic rate.

Having lost the desired weight, the person terminates the diet, but realizes that the original intake of 1,800 Calories per day will have to be lower to maintain the new lower weight. To adjust to the new lower body weight, the person restricts intake to about 1,600 Calories per day. The individual is surprised to find that, even at this lower daily intake (200 fewer Calories), weight comes back at a rate of 0.5 kg every one to two weeks. After the diet is over, this new lowered metabolic rate may take several months to kick back up to its normal level.

Based on this explanation, individuals clearly should not go on very low-calorie diets. Not only will this slow down resting metabolic rate, but it will also deprive the body of basic daily nutrients required for normal function. Very low-calorie diets should be used only in conjunction with dietary supplements and under proper medical supervision.[13] Furthermore, people who use very low-calorie diets are not as effective in keeping the weight off once the diet is terminated.

Daily caloric intakes of 1,200 to 1,500 Calories provide the necessary nutrients if they are distributed properly over the basic food groups (meeting the daily required servings from each group). Of course, the individual will have to learn which foods meet the requirements and yet are low in fat and sugar.

Under no circumstances should a person go on a diet that calls for fewer than 1,200 Calories for women or 1,500 Calories for men. Weight (fat) is gained over months and years, not overnight. Likewise, weight loss should be gradual, not abrupt.

A second way in which the setpoint may work is by keeping track of the nutrients and calories consumed daily. It is thought that the body, like a cash register, records the daily food intake and that the brain will not feel satisfied until the calories and nutrients have been "registered."

 CRITICAL THINKING

Is there a difference in the amount of food that you are now able to eat compared with the amount that you ate in your mid- to late-teen years? If so, to what do you attribute these differences? What actions are you taking to account for the difference?

This setpoint for calories and nutrients seems to operate even when people participate in moderately intense exercise. Some evidence suggests that people do not become hungrier with moderate physical activity. Therefore, people can choose to lose weight either by going hungry or by combining a sensible calorie-restricted diet with an increase in daily physical activity. Burning more calories through physical activity helps to lower body fat.

LOWERING THE SETPOINT

The most common question regarding the setpoint is how it can be lowered so the body will feel comfortable at a reduced fat percentage. These factors seem to affect the setpoint directly by lowering the fat thermostat:

1. Exercise
2. A diet high in complex carbohydrates
3. Nicotine
4. Amphetamines

The last two are more destructive than the extra fat weight, so they are not reasonable alternatives (as far as the extra strain on the heart is concerned, smoking one pack of cigarettes per day is said to be the equivalent of carrying 20 to 30 kg of excess body fat).

On the other hand, a diet high in fats and refined carbohydrates, near-fasting diets, and perhaps even artificial sweeteners seem to raise the setpoint. Therefore, the only practical and sensible way to lower the setpoint and lose fat weight is a combination of exercise and a diet high in complex carbohydrates and only moderate amounts of fat.

Because of the effects of proper food management on the body's setpoint, most of the successful dieter's effort should be spent in re-forming eating habits, increasing the intake of complex carbohydrates and high-fibre foods, and decreasing the consumption of processed foods that are high in refined carbohydrates (sugars) and fats. This change in eating habits will bring about a decrease in total daily caloric intake. Because 1 gram of carbohydrates provides only 4 Calories, as opposed to 9 Calories per gram of fat, you could eat twice the volume of food (by weight) when substituting carbohydrates for fat. Some fat, however, is recommended in the diet. Preferably use polyunsaturated and monounsaturated fats. These so-called good

fats do more than help protect the heart; they help delay hunger pangs.

A "diet" should not be viewed as a temporary tool to aid in weight loss but, instead, as a permanent change in eating behaviours to ensure weight management and better health. The role of increased physical activity also must be considered, because successful weight loss, maintenance, and recommended body composition seldom are attained without a moderate reduction in caloric intake combined with a regular exercise program.

Diet and Metabolism

Fat can be lost by selecting the proper foods, exercising, or restricting calories. When a person tries to lose weight by dietary restrictions alone, lean body mass (muscle protein, along with vital organ protein) always decreases. The amount of lean body mass lost depends entirely on caloric limitation.

When people go on a near-fasting diet, up to half of the weight loss is lean body mass and the other half is actual fat loss (see Figure 5.5).[14] When diet is combined with exercise, close to 100 percent of the weight loss is in the form of fat, and lean tissue actually may increase. Loss of lean body mass is never good, because it weakens the organs and muscles and slows metabolism. Large losses in lean tissue can cause disturbances in heart function and damage to other organs. Equally important is not to overindulge (binge) following a very low-calorie diet as this may cause changes in metabolic rate and electrolyte balance, which could trigger fatal cardiac arrhythmias.

Contrary to some beliefs, aging is not the main reason for the lower metabolic rate. It is not so much

FIGURE 5.5 Outcome of three forms of diet on fat loss

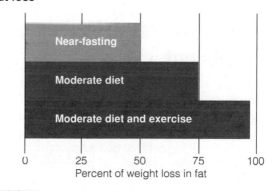

Adapted from R. J. Shephard, *Alive Man: The Physiology of Physical Activity.* (Springfield, IL: Charles C. Thomas, 1975): 484–488.

Basal metabolic rate (BMR) The lowest level of caloric intake necessary to sustain life.

Very low-calorie diet A diet that only allows an energy intake (consumption) of 800 or fewer calories per day.

that metabolism slows down as that people slow down. As people age, they tend to rely more on the amenities of life (remote controls, cell phones, intercoms, single-level homes, riding lawnmowers) that lull a person into sedentary living.

Basal metabolism is related directly to lean body weight. The more lean tissue, the higher is the metabolic rate. As a consequence of sedentary living and less physical activity, the lean component decreases and fat tissue increases. The human body requires a certain amount of oxygen per 0.5 kg of lean body mass. Given that fat is considered metabolically inert from the point of view of caloric use, the lean tissue uses most of the oxygen, even at rest. As muscle and organ mass (lean body mass) decrease, so do the energy requirements at rest.

Diets with caloric intakes below 1,200 to 1,500 Calories cannot guarantee the retention of lean body mass. Even at this intake level, some loss is inevitable, unless the diet is combined with exercise. Despite the claims of many diets that they do not alter the lean component, the simple truth is that, regardless of what nutrients may be added to the diet, severe caloric restrictions always prompt the loss of lean tissue. Too many people go on very low-calorie diets constantly. Every time they do, their metabolic rate slows down as more lean tissue is lost.

People in their 40s and older who weigh the same as they did when they were 20 tend to think they are at recommended body weight. During this span of 20 years or more, they may have dieted many times without participating in an exercise program. After they terminate each diet, they regain the weight, and much of that gain is additional body fat. Maybe at age 20 they weighed 65 kg, of which only 15 percent was fat. Now at age 40, even though they still weigh 65 kg, they might be 30 percent fat (see Figure 5.6). At recommended body weight, they wonder why they are eating very little and still having trouble staying at that weight.

Exercise: The Key to Weight Management

A more effective way to tilt the energy-balancing equation in your favour is by burning calories through physical activity. Research shows that the combination of diet and exercise leads to greater weight loss. Further, maintenance of exercise appears to be the best predictor of long-term weight loss maintenance.[15]

Exercise seems to exert control over how much a person weighs. On the average, starting at age 25, a person gains 0.5 to 1 kg of weight per

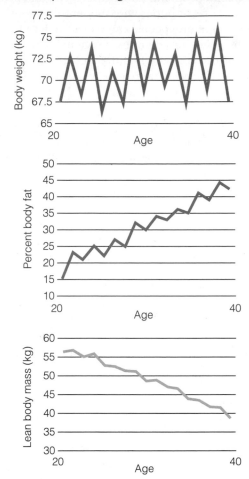

FIGURE 5.6 Body composition changes as a result of frequent dieting without exercise

year. A 0.5 kg weight gain represents a simple energy surplus of under 10 Calories per day. The additional weight accumulated in middle age comes from people becoming less physically active and increasing caloric intake.

Exercise enhances the rate of weight loss and is vital in maintaining the weight loss. Not only will exercise maintain lean tissue, but advocates of the setpoint theory say that exercise resets the fat thermostat to a new, lower level. This change may be rapid, or it may take time. Although a few individuals lose weight by participating in 30 minutes of exercise per day, many overweight people need 60 minutes of daily exercise to see significant weight loss. People with a "sticky" setpoint have to be patient and persistent.

If a person is trying to lose weight, a combination of aerobic and strength-training exercises works best. Aerobic exercise is the best to offset the setpoint, and the continuity and duration of these types of activities cause many calories to be burned in the process. The role of aerobic exercise in successful lifetime weight management cannot be overestimated. Strength training is critical in helping maintain lean body mass. Unfortunately, of those individuals who are attempting to lose weight, only 19 percent of women and 22 percent of men decrease their caloric intake and exercise above an average of 25 or more minutes per day.[16]

As illustrated in Figure 5.7, greater weight loss is achieved by combining a diet with an exercise program. Of even greater significance, only the individuals who remain physically active for 60 minutes or longer per day are able to keep the weight off[17] (see Figure 5.8). Those who are active for less than 60 minutes per day gradually regain lost weight, whereas individuals who completely stop physical activity regain almost 100 percent of the lost weight within 18 months of discontinuing the weight loss program. Thus, it appears that only those who remain physically active for about an hour per day are able to successfully maintain weight loss.

Weight loss might be more rapid when aerobic exercise is combined with a strength-training program. Each additional kilogram of muscle tissue may raise the basal metabolic rate by as many as 77 Calories per day.[18] Thus, an individual who adds

2 kg of muscle tissue as a result of strength training could increase the basal metabolic rate by 154 Calories per day (77 × 2), which burns up the equivalent of 56,210 Calories per year (154 × 365) eliminating the equivalent of 7.3 kg of fat (56,210 ÷ 7,700).

Strength training is suggested especially for people who think they are at their recommended body weight, yet their body fat percentage is higher than recommended. The number of calories burned during a typical hour-long strength-training session is much less than during an hour of aerobic exercise. Because of the high intensity of strength training, the person needs frequent rest intervals to recover from each set of exercises. The average person actually lifts weights only 10 to 12 minutes during each hour of exercise. In the long run, however, the person enjoys the benefits of gains in lean tissue. Guidelines for developing aerobic and strength-training programs are given in Chapters 7 and 8.

Although size (centimetres) and percent body fat both decrease when sedentary individuals begin an exercise program, body weight often remains the same or may even increase during the first couple of weeks of the program. Exercise helps to increase muscle tissue, connective tissue, blood volume (as much as 500 mL, or the equivalent of 0.5 kg, following the first week of aerobic exercise), enzymes and other structures within the cell, and glycogen (which binds water). All of these changes lead to a higher functional capacity of the human body. With

FIGURE 5.7 The roles of diet and exercise in weight loss

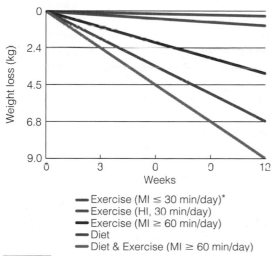

* Exercise with no change in daily caloric intake
 MI = moderate intensity
 HI = high intensity
Diet: 1,200–1,500 calories/day   © Fitness & Wellness, Inc.

Based on data from American College of Sports Medicine, "Position Stand: Appropriate Intervention Strategies for Weight Loss and Prevention for Weight Regain for Adults," *Medicine and Science in Sports and Exercise* 33 (2001): 2145–2156. Used with permission.

FIGURE 5.8 Effects of different amounts of daily energy expenditure on weight maintenance following a weight reduction program

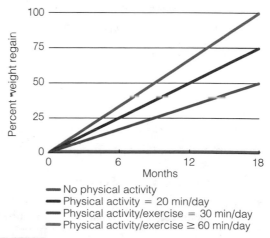

Based on data from American College of Sports Medicine, "Position Stand: Appropriate Intervention Strategies for Weight Loss and Prevention for Weight Regain for Adults," *Medicine and Science in Sports and Exercise* 33 (2001): 2145–2156. Used with permission.

exercise, most of the weight loss becomes apparent after a few weeks of training, when the lean component has stabilized.

Although we know that a negative caloric balance of 7,700 Calories does not always result in a loss of exactly 1 kg of fat, the role of exercise in achieving a negative balance by burning additional calories is significant in weight reduction and maintenance programs. Sadly, some individuals claim that the number of calories burned during exercise is hardly worth the effort. They think that cutting their daily intake by some 300 Calories is easier than participating in some sort of exercise that would burn the same amount of calories. The problem is that the willpower to cut those 300 Calories lasts only a few weeks, and then the person goes right back to the old eating patterns.

If a person gets into the habit of exercising regularly, say three times a week, jogging 5 km per exercise session (about 300 Calories burned), this represents 900 Calories in one week, about 3,600 calories in one month, or 46,800 Calories per year. This minimal amount of exercise represents as many as 6 extra kilograms of fat in one year, 12 in two, and so on.

We tend to forget that our weight creeps up gradually over the years, not just overnight. Hardly worth the effort? And we have not even taken into consideration the increase in lean tissue, possible resetting of the setpoint, benefits to the cardiovascular system, and, most important, the improved quality of life. The fundamental reasons for overfatness and obesity, few could argue, are sedentary living and lack of a regular exercise program.

With regard to preventing disease, many of the health benefits people try to achieve by losing weight are reaped through exercise alone, even without weight loss. Exercise offers protection against premature morbidity and mortality for everyone, including people who already have risk factors for disease.

Low-Intensity Versus High-Intensity Exercise for Weight Loss

Some individuals promote low-intensity exercise over high-intensity for weight loss purposes. Compared with high intensity, a greater proportion of calories burned during low-intensity exercise are derived from fat. The lower the intensity of exercise, the higher the percentage of fat utilization as an energy source. In theory, if you are trying to lose fat, this principle makes sense, but in reality it is misleading. The bottom line when you are trying to lose weight is to burn more calories. When your daily caloric expenditure exceeds your intake, weight is lost. The more calories you burn, the more fat is lost.

During low-intensity exercise, up to 50 percent of the calories burned may be derived from fat (the other 50 percent from glucose [carbohydrates]). With intense exercise, only 30 to 40 percent of the caloric expenditure comes from fat. Overall, however, you can burn twice as many calories during high-intensity exercise and, subsequently, more fat as well.

Let's look at a practical illustration (also see Table 5.2). If you exercise for 30 to 40 minutes at moderate intensity and burn 200 Calories, about 100 of those calories (50 percent) would come from fat. If you exercise at high intensity during those same 30 to 40 minutes, you can burn 400 Calories with 120 to 160 of the calories (30 to 40 percent) coming from fat. Thus, even though it is true that the percentage of fat used is greater during low-intensity exercise, the overall amount of fat used is still less during low-intensity exercise. Plus, if you were to exercise at a low intensity, you would have to do so twice as long to burn the same amount of calories. Another benefit is that the metabolic rate remains at a slightly higher level longer after high-intensity exercise, so you continue to burn a few extra calories following exercise.

Moreover, high-intensity exercise by itself appears to trigger greater fat loss than low-intensity

TABLE 5.2 Comparison of Energy Expenditure Between 30–40 Minutes of Low-Intensity vs. High-Intensity Exercise

Exercise Intensity	Total Energy Expenditure (Calories)	Percent Calories From Fat	Total Fat Calories	Percent Calories From CHO*	Total CHO Calories	Calories Burned Per Minute	Calories Per kg Per Minute
Low Intensity	200	50%	100	50%	100	6.67	0.099
High Intensity	400	30%	120	70%	280	13.5	0.198

* CHO = Carbohydrates

exercise. Research conducted at Laval University in Quebec, showed that subjects who performed a high-intensity intermittent-training program lost more body fat than participants in a low- to moderate-intensity continuous aerobic endurance group.[19] Even more surprisingly, this finding occurred despite the fact that the high-intensity group burned fewer total calories per exercise session. The results support the notion that vigorous exercise is more conducive to weight loss than low- to moderate-intensity exercise.

Before you start high-intensity exercise sessions, a word of caution is in order: Be sure that it is medically safe for you to participate in such activities and that you build up gradually to that level. If you are cleared to participate in high-intensity exercise, do not attempt to do too much too quickly, because you may incur injuries and become discouraged. You must allow your body a proper conditioning period of 8 to 12 weeks, or even longer for people with a moderate to serious weight problem. High intensity also does not mean high impact. High-impact activities are the most common cause of exercise-related injuries. Additional information on these topics is presented in Chapter 6.

The previous discussion on high- versus low-intensity exercise does not mean that low intensity is ineffective. Low-intensity exercise provides substantial health benefits, and people who initiate exercise programs are more willing to participate and stay with low-intensity programs. Low-intensity exercise does promote weight loss, but it is not as effective. You will need to exercise longer to obtain the same results.

Healthy Weight Gain

"Skinny" people, too, should realize that the only healthy way to gain weight is through exercise (mainly strength-training exercises) and a slight increase in caloric intake. Attempting to gain weight just by overeating will raise the fat component and not the lean component—which is not the path to better health. Exercise is the best solution to weight (fat) reduction and weight (lean) gain alike.

A strength-training program such as the one outlined in Chapter 7 is the best approach to add body weight. The training program should include at least two exercises of three sets for each major body part. Each set should consist of about 8 to 12 repetitions maximum.

Even though the metabolic cost of synthesizing 500 g of muscle tissue is still unclear, consuming an estimated 500 additional calories per day is recommended to gain an average of 500 g of muscle tissue per week. Your diet should include a daily total intake of about 1.5 g of protein per kilogram of body weight. If your daily protein intake already exceeds 1.5 g per day, the extra 500 calories should be primarily in the form of complex carbohydrates. The higher caloric intake must be accompanied by a strength-training program, otherwise, the increase in body weight will be in the form of fat, not muscle tissue.

Strength Training, Diet, and Muscle Mass

The time of day when carbohydrates and protein are consumed in relation to the strength-training workout also plays a role in promoting muscle growth. Studies suggest that consuming a pre-exercise snack consisting of a combination of carbohydrates and protein is beneficial to muscle development. The carbohydrates supply energy for training, and the availability of amino acids (the building blocks of protein) in the blood during training enhances the muscle building process. A peanut butter, turkey, or tuna fish sandwich; milk or yogurt and fruit; or nuts and fruit consumed 30 to 60 minutes before training are excellent choices for a pre-workout snack.

The consumption of a carbohydrate/protein snack immediately following strength training, as well as an hour thereafter, further promotes muscle growth and strength development. Post-exercise carbohydrates help restore muscle glycogen depleted during training, and, in combination with protein, induce an increase in blood insulin and growth hormone levels. These hormones are essential to the muscle-building process.

Muscle fibres also absorb a greater amount of amino acids up to 48 hours following strength-training. The first hour, nonetheless, seems to be the most critical. A higher level of circulating amino acids in the bloodstream immediately after training is believed to increase protein synthesis to a greater extent than amino acids made available later in the day. A ratio of 3-to-1 g of carbohydrates to protein is recommended for a post-exercise snack.

Weight-Loss Myths

Cellulite and **spot reducing** are mythical concepts. **Cellulite** is nothing but enlarged fat cells that bulge out from accumulated body fat.

Spot reducing Fallacious theory that exercising a specific body part will result in significant fat reduction in that area.

Cellulite Term frequently used in reference to fat deposits that "bulge out"; these deposits are nothing but enlarged fat cells from excessive accumulation of body fat.

Doing several sets of daily sit-ups will not get rid of fat in the midsection of the body. When fat comes off, it does so throughout the entire body, not just the exercised area. The greatest proportion of fat may come off the biggest fat deposits, but the caloric output of a few sets of sit-ups has practically no effect on reducing total body fat. A person has to exercise much longer to really see results.

Other touted means of quick weight loss, such as rubberized sweatsuits, steam baths, and mechanical vibrators, are misleading. When a person wears a sweatsuit or steps into a sauna, the weight lost is not fat, but merely a significant amount of water. Sure, it looks nice when you step on the scale immediately afterward, but this represents a false loss of weight. As soon as you replace body fluids, you gain back the weight quickly.

Wearing rubberized sweatsuits hastens the rate of body fluid that is lost—fluid that is vital during prolonged exercise—and raises core temperature at the same time. This combination puts a person in danger of dehydration, which impairs cellular function and, in extreme cases, can even cause death.

Similarly, mechanical vibrators are worthless in a weight-control program. Vibrating belts and turning rollers may feel good, but they require no effort whatsoever. Fat cannot be shaken off. It is lost primarily by burning it in muscle tissue.

Losing Weight the Sound and Sensible Way

Dieting never has been fun and never will be. People who are overweight and are serious about losing weight, however, have to include regular exercise in their lives along with proper food management and a sensible reduction in caloric intake.

Because excessive body fat is a risk factor for cardiovascular disease, some precautions are in order. Depending on the extent of the weight problem, a medical examination, and possibly a stress ECG (see "Abnormal Electrocardiograms" in Chapter 11), may be a good idea before undertaking the exercise program. A physician should be consulted in this regard.

Significantly overweight individuals may have to choose activities in which they will not have to support their own body weight but that still will be effective in burning calories. Injuries to joints and muscles are common in excessively overweight individuals who participate in weight-bearing exercises such as walking, jogging, and aerobics.

Swimming may not be a good weight loss exercise either. More body fat makes a person more buoyant, and many people are not at the skill level required to swim fast enough to get the best training effect, thus limiting the number of calories burned as well as the benefits to the cardiorespiratory system.

Better alternatives during the initial stages of exercise include riding a bicycle (either road or stationary), walking in a shallow pool, doing water aerobics, or running in place in deep water (treading water). The latter forms of water exercise are gaining popularity and have proven to be effective in reducing weight without fear of injuries.

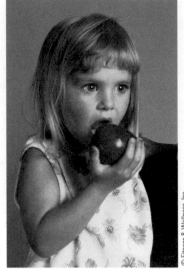

Establishing healthy eating patterns should start at a young age.

How long should each exercise session last? The amount of exercise for successful weight loss and weight loss maintenance is different from the amount for improving fitness. For health fitness, accumulating 30 minutes of physical activity on most days of the week is recommended. To develop and maintain cardiorespiratory fitness, 20 to 30 minutes of exercise at the recommended target rate, three to five times per week, is suggested (see Chapter 6). For successful weight loss, however, 60 minutes of physical activity five to six times a week is recommended.

A person should not try to do too much too fast. Unconditioned beginners should start with about 15 minutes of aerobic activity three times a week, and during the next three to four weeks gradually increase the duration by approximately five minutes per week and the frequency by one day per week.

One final benefit of long-duration exercise for weight control is that it allows fat to be burned more efficiently. Carbohydrates and fats are both sources of energy. When the glucose levels begin to drop during prolonged exercise, more fat is used as energy substrate.

Equally important is that fat-burning enzymes increase with aerobic training. Fat is lost primarily by burning it in muscle. Therefore, as the concentration of the enzymes increases, so does the ability to burn fat.

In addition to exercise and adequate food management, a sensible reduction in caloric intake, and careful monitoring of this intake, are recommended. Most research finds that a negative caloric balance is required to lose weight because:

1. Most people underestimate their caloric intake and are eating more than they should be eating.

2. Developing new behaviours takes time, and most people have trouble changing and adjusting to new eating habits.
3. Many individuals are in such poor physical condition that they take a long time to increase their activity level enough to offset the setpoint and burn enough calories to aid in loss of body fat.
4. Most successful dieters carefully monitor their daily caloric intake.
5. A few people simply will not alter their food selection. For those who will not (which will still increase their risk for chronic diseases), the only solution to lose weight successfully is a large increase in physical activity, a negative caloric balance, or a combination of the two.

Perhaps the only exception to a decrease in caloric intake for weight loss purposes occurs in people who already are eating too few calories. A nutrient analysis (see Chapter 3) often reveals that long-term dieters are not consuming enough calories. These people actually need to increase their daily caloric intake and combine that with an exercise program to get their metabolism to kick back up to a normal level.

You must also learn to make wise food choices. Think in terms of long-term benefits (weight management) as opposed to instant gratification (unhealthy eating and subsequent weight gain). Making healthful choices allows you to eat a greater amount of food, more nutritious food, and ingest fewer calories. For example, instead of eating a high-fat, 700-Calorie scone, you could eat as much as 1 orange, 250 mL of grapes, a hard-boiled egg, 2 slices of whole-wheat toast, 2 spoons of jam, 125 mL of honey-sweetened oatmeal, and 1 glass of skim milk (see Figure 5.9).

You can estimate your daily energy (caloric) requirement by consulting Tables 5.3 and 5.4 and completing Lab 5A. Given that this is only an estimated value, individual adjustments related to many of the factors discussed in this chapter may be necessary to establish a more precise value. Nevertheless, the estimated value does offer a beginning guideline for weight control or reduction.

The estimated energy requirement without exercise is based on typical lifestyle patterns, total body weight, and gender. Individuals who hold jobs that require heavy manual labour burn more calories during the day than those who have sedentary jobs (such as working behind a desk). To find your activity level, refer to Table 5.3 and rate yourself accordingly. The number given in Table 5.3 is per kilogram of body weight, so you multiply your current weight by that number. For example, the estimated energy requirement to maintain body weight for a moderately active male who weighs 72 kg is 2,376 Calories (72 kg $\times$ 33 Cal/kg).

To determine the average number of calories you burn daily as a result of exercise, figure out the total number of minutes you exercise weekly, then figure the daily average exercise time. For instance, a person cycling at 16 km per hour five times a week, 60 minutes each time, exercises 300 minutes per week (5×60). The average daily exercise time is therefore 42 minutes ($300 \div 7$, rounded off to the lowest unit).

Next, from Table 5.4, find the energy expenditure for the activity (or activities) chosen for the exercise program. In the case of cycling (16 km per hour), the expenditure is 0.1 calories per kilogram of body weight per minute of activity (cal/kg/min). With a body weight of 72 kg, this man would burn 7.2 Calories each minute (body weight $\times$ 0.1, or 72×0.1). In 42 minutes he burns approximately 345 Calories (42×7.2).

Now you can obtain the daily energy requirement, with exercise, needed to maintain body weight. To do this, add the estimated energy requirement (without exercise) obtained from Table 5.3 and the average calories burned through exercise. In our example, it is 2,721 Calories ($2,376 + 345$).

If a negative caloric balance is recommended to lose weight, this person has to consume fewer than 2,721 Calories daily to achieve the objective. Because of the many factors that play a role in weight control, this 2,721-Calorie value is only an estimated daily requirement. Furthermore, we cannot predict that you will lose exactly 500 g of fat in 1 week if you cut your daily intake by 500 Calories ($500 \times 7 = 3,500$ Calories, or the equivalent of 500 g of fat).

The daily energy requirement figure is only a target guideline for weight control. Periodic readjustments are necessary because individuals differ, and the daily requirement changes as you lose weight and modify your exercise habits.

To determine the target caloric intake to lose weight, multiply your current weight by 11 and subtract this amount from the total daily energy requirement (2,721 in our example) with exercise. For our moderately active male example, this would mean 1,929 Calories per day to lose weight ($72 \times 11 = 792$ and $2,721 - 792 = 1,929$ Calories).

This final caloric intake to lose weight should never be below 1,200 Calories for women and 1,500 for men. If distributed properly over the various food groups, these figures are the lowest caloric intakes that provide the necessary nutrients the body needs. As far as percentages of total calories, the daily distribution should be approximately 60 percent carbohydrates (mostly complex carbohydrates), less than 30 percent fat, and about 12 percent protein.

Many experts believe that a person can take off weight more efficiently by reducing the amount of daily fat intake to about 20 percent of the total daily

FIGURE 5.9 Making wise food choices

These illustrations provide a comparison of how much more food you can eat when you make healthy choices. You also get more vitamins, minerals, phytochemicals, antioxidants, and fibre by making healthy choices.

Breakfast

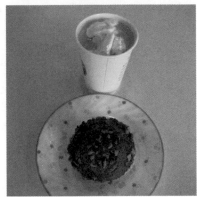

1 banana nut muffin, 1 cafe mocha
Calories: 940
Percent fat calories: 48%

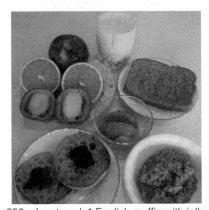

250 mL oatmeal, 1 English muffin with jelly,
1 slice whole wheat bread with honey,
125 mL peaches, 1 kiwi fruit, 1 orange,
1 apple, 250 mL skim milk
Calories: 900
Percent fat calories: 5%

Lunch

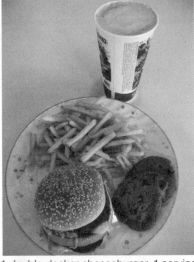

1 double-decker cheeseburger, 1 serving
medium French fries, 2 chocolate chip
cookies, 1 medium strawberry milkshake
Calories: 1790
Percent fat calories: 37%

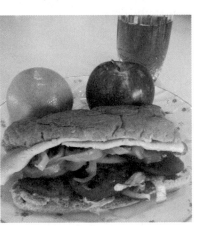

6-inch turkey breast/vegetable sandwich,
1 apple, 1 orange,
250 mL sweetened green tea
Calories: 500
Percent fat calories: 10%

Dinner

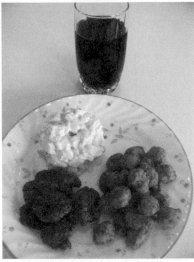

170 g popcorn chicken, 85 g barbecue
chicken wings, 250 mL potato salad,
1 355 mL cola drink
Calories: 1250
Percent fat calories: 42%

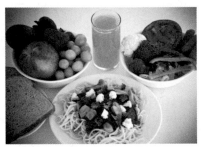

460 g spaghetti with tomato sauce
and vegetables, a 460 g salad bowl
with 30 mL Italian dressing,
2 slices whole wheat bread, 225 g
grapes, 3 large strawberries, 1 kiwi fruit,
1 peach, 1 355 mL fruit juice drink
Calories: 1240
Percent fat calories: 14%

caloric intake. Because 1 g of fat supplies more than twice the amount of calories that carbohydrates and protein do, the general tendency when someone eats less fat is to consume fewer calories. With fat intake at 20 percent of total calories, the individual will have sufficient fat in the diet to feel satisfied and avoid frequent hunger pangs.

Further, it takes only 3 to 5 percent of ingested calories to store fat as fat, whereas it takes approxi-mately 25 percent of ingested calories to convert carbohydrates to fat. Some evidence indicates that if people eat the same number of calories as carbohy-drate or as fat, those on the fat diet will store more fat. Long-term successful weight-loss and weight-management programs are low in fat content.

Many people have trouble adhering to a low-fat-calorie diet. During times of weight loss, how-ever, you are strongly encouraged to do so. Refer

TABLE 5.3 Estimated Energy Requirement (EER) per Kilogram of Body Weight Based on Lifestyle Patterns and Gender

	Calories Per Kilogram	
	Men	Women*
Sedentary—limited physical activity	28.6	26.4
Moderate physical activity	33	29.7
Hard labour—strenuous physical effort	37.4	33

* Pregnant or lactating women add 3 Calories to these values.

TABLE 5.4 Caloric Expenditure of Selected Physical Activities

Activity*	Cal/kg/min	Activity*	Cal/kg/min
Aerobics		4.4 min/km	0.224
Moderate	0.143	3.75 min/km	0.251
Vigorous	0.209	Deep water**	0.220
Step aerobics	0.154	Skating (moderate)	0.084
Archery	0.068	Skiing	
Badminton		Downhill	0.132
Recreation	0.084	Level (8 km/h)	0.172
Competition	0.143	Soccer	0.129
Baseball	0.068	Stairmaster	
Basketball		Moderate	0.154
Moderate	0.101	Vigorous	0.198
Competition	0.139	Stationary Cycling	
Bowling	0.066	Moderate	0.121
Calisthenics	0.073	Vigorous	0.154
Cycling (on a level surface)		Strength Training	0.110
8.8 km/h	0.073	Swimming (crawl)	
16 km/h	0.110	20 m/min	0.068
20.8 km/h	0.156	25 m/min	0.088
Dance		45 m/min	0.125
Moderate	0.066	50 m/min	0.154
Vigorous	0.121	Table Tennis	0.066
Golf	0.066	Tennis	
Gymnastics		Moderate	0.099
Light	0.066	Competition	0.141
Heavy	0.123	Volleyball	0.066
Handball	0.141	Walking	
Hiking	0.088	7.2 km/h	0.099
Judo/Karate	0.189	Shallow pool	0.198
Racquetball	0.143	Water Aerobics	
Rope Jumping	0.132	Moderate	0.110
Rowing (vigorous)	0.198	Vigorous	0.154
Running (on a level surface)		Wrestling	0.187
7 min/km	0.154		
5.3 min/km	0.198		

*Values are for actual time engaged in the activity.
**Treading water

Adapted from:
P. E. Allsen, J. M. Harrison, and B. Vance, *Fitness for Life: An Individualized Approach* (Dubuque, IA: Wm. C. Brown, 1989).
C. A. Bucher and W. E. Prentice, *Fitness for College and Life* (St. Louis: Times Mirror/Mosby College Publishing, 1989).
C. F. Consolazio, R. E. Johnson, and L. J. Pecora, *Physiological Measurements of Metabolic Functions in Man* (New York: McGraw-Hill, 1963).
R. V. Hockey, *Physical Fitness: The Pathway to Healthful Living* (St. Louis: Times Mirror/Mosby College Publishing, 1989).
W. W. K. Hoeger et al., Research conducted at Boise State University, 1986–1993.

to Table 5.5 to aid you in determining the grams of fat at 20 percent of the total calories for selected energy intakes. Also, use the form provided in Lab 3B (Chapter 3, page 92) to monitor your daily fat intake. For weight maintenance, data from the U.S. National Weight Control Registry shows that individuals who have been successful in maintaining an average weight loss of about 14 kg for more than five years are consuming about 24 percent of calories from fat, 56 percent from carbohydrates, and 20 percent from protein.[20]

The time of day when food is consumed also may play a part in weight reduction. When a person is attempting to lose weight, intake should consist of a minimum of 25 percent of the total daily calories for breakfast, 50 percent for lunch, and 25 percent or less at dinner. Breakfast, in particular, is a critical meal. Many people skip breakfast because it's the easiest meal to skip. Evidence, however, indicates that people who skip breakfast are hungrier later in the day and end up consuming more total daily calories than those who eat breakfast. Furthermore, regular breakfast eaters have less of a weight problem, lose weight more effectively, and have less difficulty maintaining lost weight.

If most of the daily calories are consumed during one meal (as in the typical evening meal), the body may perceive that something is wrong and will slow down the metabolism so it can store more calories in the form of fat. Also, eating most of the calories during one meal causes a person to go hungry the rest of the day, making it more difficult to adhere to the diet.

Consuming most of the calories earlier in the day seems helpful in losing weight and also in managing atherosclerosis. The time of day when most of the fats and cholesterol are consumed can influence blood lipids and coronary heart disease. Peak digestion

time following a heavy meal is about seven hours after that meal. If most lipids are consumed during the evening meal, digestion peaks while the person is sound asleep, when the metabolism is at its lowest

WEIGHT MANAGEMENT

TABLE 5.5 Grams of Fat at 10%, 20%, and 30% of Total Calories for Selected Energy Intakes

Caloric Intake	Grams of Fat		
	10%	20%	30%
1,200	13	27	40
1,300	14	29	43
1,400	16	31	47
1,500	17	33	50
1,600	18	36	53
1,700	19	38	57
1,800	20	40	60
1,900	21	42	63
2,000	22	44	67
2,100	23	47	70
2,200	24	49	73
2,300	26	51	77
2,400	27	53	80
2,500	28	56	83
2,600	29	58	87
2,700	30	60	90
2,800	31	62	93
2,900	32	64	97
3,000	33	67	100

rate. Consequently, the body may not metabolize fats and cholesterol as well, leading to a higher blood lipid count and increasing the risk for atherosclerosis and coronary heart disease.

Before you proceed with the development of a thorough weight-loss program, take a moment to identify, in Section II of Lab 5A, your current stage of change as it pertains to your recommended body weight. If applicable—that is, if you are not at recommended weight—list also the processes and techniques for change that you will use to accomplish your goal. In Section III of this lab, you can outline your exercise program for weight management.

Monitoring Your Diet with Daily Food Logs

To help you monitor and adhere to a weight-loss program, use the daily food logs provided in Lab 5B. If the goal is to maintain or increase body weight, use Lab 5C.

Evidence indicates that people who monitor daily caloric intake are more successful at weight loss than those who don't self-monitor. Before using the forms in Lab 5B, make a master copy for your files so you can make future copies as needed. Guidelines are provided for 1,200-, 1,500-, 1,800-, and 2,000-Calorie

diet plans. These plans have been developed based on Canada's Food Guide and the Dietary Guidelines to meet the Recommended Dietary Allowances.[21] The objective is to meet (not exceed) the number of servings allowed for each diet plan. Each time you eat a serving of a certain food, record it in the appropriate box.

To lose weight, you should use the diet plan that most closely approximates your target caloric intake. The plan is based on the following caloric allowances for each food group:

■ Bread, cereal, rice, and pasta group: 80 Calories per serving.
■ Fruit group: 60 Calories per serving.
■ Vegetable group: 25 Calories per serving.
■ Milk, yogurt, and cheese group (use low-fat products): 120 Calories per serving.
■ Meat, poultry, fish, dry beans, eggs, and nuts group: Use low-fat (300 Calories per serving) frozen

entrées or an equivalent amount if you prepare your own main dish (see the following discussion).

As you start your diet plan, pay particular attention to food serving sizes. To find out what counts as one serving, refer to the Food Guide (see Figure 3.1, page 52). Take care with cup and glass sizes. A standard cup is 250 mL, but most glasses nowadays contain between 350 and 470 mL. If you drink 350 mL of fruit juice, in essence you are getting two servings of fruit because a standard serving is ¾ cup of juice.

Read food labels carefully to compare the caloric value of the serving listed on the label with the caloric guidelines provided above. Here are some examples:

- One slice of standard white bread has about 80 Calories. A plain bagel may have 200 to 350 Calories. Although it is low in fat, a 350-Calorie bagel is equivalent to almost four servings in the bread, cereal, rice, and pasta group.
- The standard serving size listed on the food label for most cereals is 250 mL. As you read the nutrition information, however, you will find that for the same amount of cereal, one type of cereal has 120 Calories and another cereal has 200 Calories. Because a standard serving in the bread, cereal, rice, and pasta group is 80 Calories, the first cereal would be 1½ servings and the second one 2½ servings.
- A medium-size fruit is usually considered to be 1 serving. A large fruit could provide as many as 2 or more servings.
- In the milk, yogurt, and cheese groups, 1 serving represents 120 Calories. Two hundred and fifty millilitres of whole milk has about 160 Calories, compared to 250 mL of skim milk, which contains 88 Calories. Two hundred and fifty millilitres of whole milk, therefore, would provide 1⅓ servings in this food group.

Preparing Low-Fat Entrées

Making a commitment to managing your weight might mean learning how to prepare low-fat entrées for meals. You can prepare many nutritional meals using about 85 g of lean meat, poultry, or fish and additional vegetables, rice, or pasta, which will provide 300 Calories with fewer than 6 grams of fat per dish.

In your daily logs, be sure to record the amount of each serving. You can use EATracker to verify your caloric intake and food distribution pattern (percent of total calories from carbohydrate, fat and protein).

Behaviour Modification and Adherence to a Weight Management Program

Achieving and maintaining recommended body composition is by no means impossible, but it does require desire and commitment. If weight management is to become a priority in life, people must realize that they have to transform their behaviour to some extent.

Modifying old habits and developing new, positive behaviours take time. Individuals who apply the management techniques provided in the Behaviour Modification box (on page 144) are more successful at changing detrimental behaviour and adhering to a positive lifetime weight-control program. In developing a retraining program, people are not expected to incorporate all the strategies given, but should note the ones that apply to them. The form provided in Lab 5D will allow you to evaluate and monitor your own weight management behaviours.

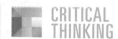

CRITICAL THINKING

What behavioural strategies have you used to properly manage your body weight? How do you think those strategies would work for others?

The Simple Truth

There is no quick and easy way to take off excess body fat and keep it off for good. Weight management is accomplished by making a lifetime commitment to physical activity and proper food selection. When taking part in a weight (fat) reduction program, people also have to decrease their caloric intake moderately, be physically active, and implement strategies to modify unhealthy eating behaviours.

During the process, relapses into past negative behaviours are almost inevitable. The three most common reasons for relapse are:

1. Stress-related factors (such as major life changes, depression, job changes, illness).
2. Social reasons (entertaining, eating out, business travel).
3. Self-enticing behaviours (placing yourself in a situation to see how much you can get away with: "One small taste won't hurt" leads to "I'll eat just one slice" and finally to "I haven't done well, so I might as well eat some more").

Making mistakes is human and does not necessarily mean failure. Failure comes to those who give up and do not use previous experiences to build upon and, in turn, develop skills that will prevent self-defeating behaviours in the future. Where there's a will, there's a way, and those who persist will reap the rewards.

WEIGHT LOSS STRATEGIES

1. Make a commitment to change. The first necessary ingredient is the desire to modify your behaviour. You need to stop precontemplating or contemplating change and get going! Sincere commitment increases your chances for success.

2. Set realistic goals. The weight problem developed over several years. Similarly, new lifetime eating and exercise habits both take time to develop. A realistic long-term goal will also include short-term objectives that allow for regular evaluation and help maintain motivation and renewed commitment to attain the long-term goal.

3. Incorporate exercise into the program. Choosing enjoyable activities, places, times, equipment, and people to work out with will help you adhere to an exercise program. (See Chapters 6, 7, 8, and 9.)

4. Differentiate hunger and appetite. Hunger is the actual physical need for food. Appetite is a desire for food, usually triggered by factors such as stress, habit, boredom, depression, availability of food, or just the thought of food itself. Developing and sticking to a regular meal pattern will help control hunger.

5. Eat less fat. Each gram of fat provides 9 Calories, and protein and carbohydrates provide only 4. In essence, you can eat more food on a low-fat diet because you consume fewer calories with each meal.

6. Pay attention to calories. Just because food is labelled "low-fat" does not mean you can eat as much as you want. When reading food labels—and when eating—don't just look at the fat content but pay attention to calories as well.

7. Cut unnecessary items from your diet. Substituting water for a daily can of pop would cut 51,100 (140 × 365) Calories yearly from the diet—the equivalent of 6.6 kg (51,000 ÷ 7,700) of fat.

8. Maintain daily intake of calcium-rich foods, especially low-fat or non-fat dairy products.

9. Add to your diet foods that reduce cravings, such as eggs; small amounts of red meat, fish, poultry, tofu, oils, fats; and nonstarchy vegetables such as lettuce, green beans, peppers, asparagus, broccoli, mushrooms, and Brussels sprouts. Consuming only carbohydrates increases cravings.

10. Avoid automatic eating. Many people associate certain daily activities with eating, for example, cooking, watching television, or reading. Most foods consumed in these situations lack nutritional value or are high in sugar and fat.

11. Stay busy. People tend to eat more when they sit around and do nothing. Occupying the mind and body with activities not associated with eating helps take away the desire to eat. Some options are walking; cycling; playing sports; gardening; sewing; or visiting a library, a museum, or a park. You might also develop other skills and interests not associated with food.

12. Plan meals and shop sensibly. Always shop on a full stomach, because hungry shoppers tend to buy unhealthy foods impulsively—and then snack on the way home. Always use a shopping list, which should include whole-grain breads and cereals, fruits and vegetables, low-fat milk and dairy products, lean meats, fish, and poultry.

13. Cook wisely:

    ■ Use less fat and fewer refined foods in food preparation.
    ■ Trim all visible fat from meats and remove skin from poultry before cooking.
    ■ Skim the fat off gravies and soups.
    ■ Bake, broil, boil, or steam instead of frying.
    ■ Sparingly use butter, cream, mayonnaise, and salad dressings.
    ■ Avoid coconut oil, palm oil, and cocoa butter.
    ■ Prepare plenty of foods that contain fibre.
    ■ Include whole-grain breads and cereals, vegetables, and legumes in most meals.
    ■ Eat fruits for dessert.
    ■ Stay away from pop, fruit juices, and fruit-flavoured drinks.
    ■ Use less sugar and cut down on other refined carbohydrates, such as corn syrup, malt sugar, dextrose, and fructose.
    ■ Drink plenty of water—at least six glasses a day.

14. Do not serve more food than you should eat. Measure the food in portions and keep serving dishes away from the table. Do not force yourself or anyone else to "clean the plate" after they are satisfied (including children after they already have had a healthy, nutritious serving).

15. Try "junior size" instead of "super size." People who are served larger portions eat more, whether they are hungry or not. Use smaller plates, bowls, cups, and glasses. Try eating half as much food as you commonly eat. Watch for portion sizes at restaurants as well: Supersized foods create supersized people.

16. Eat out infrequently. The more often people eat out, the more body fat they have. People who eat out six or more times per week consume an average of about 300 extra calories per day and 30 percent more fat than those who eat out less often.

17. Eat slowly and at the table only. Eating on the run promotes overeating because the body doesn't have enough time to "register" consumption, and people overeat before the body perceives the fullness signal. Eating at the table encourages people to take time out to eat and deters snacking between meals. After eating, do not sit around the table but, rather, clean up and put away the food to avoid snacking.

18. Avoid social binges. Social gatherings tend to entice self-defeating behaviour. Use visual imagery to plan ahead. Do not feel pressured to eat or drink and don't rationalize in these situations. Choose low-calorie foods and entertain yourself with other activities, such as dancing and talking.

19. Do not place unhealthy foods within easy reach. Ideally, avoid bringing high-calorie, high-sugar, or high-fat foods into the house. If they are there already, store them where they are hard to get to or see—perhaps the garage or basement.

20. Avoid evening food raids. Most people do really well during the day but then "lose it" at night. Take control. Stop and think. To avoid excessive nighttime snacking, stay busy after your evening meal. Go for a short walk; floss and brush your teeth, and get to bed earlier.

21. Practise stress management techniques (discussed in Chapter 10). Many people snack and increase food consumption in stressful situations.

22. Get support. People who receive support from friends, relatives, and formal support groups are much more likely to lose weight and maintain weight loss than those without such support. The more support you receive, the better off you will be.

23. Monitor changes and reward accomplishments. Being able to exercise without interruption for 15, 20, 30, or 60 minutes; swimming a certain distance; running a kilometre—all these accomplishments deserve recognition. Create rewards that are not related to eating: new clothing, a tennis racquet, a bicycle, exercise shoes, or something else that is special and you would not have acquired otherwise.

24. Prepare for slips. Most people will slip and occasionally splurge. Do not despair and give up. Reevaluate and continue with your efforts. An occasional slip will not make much difference in the long run.

25. Think positive. Avoid negative thoughts about how difficult changing past behaviours might be. Instead, think of the benefits you will reap, such as feeling, looking, and functioning better, plus enjoying better health and improving the quality of life. Avoid negative environments and unsupportive people.

ASSESS YOUR KNOWLEDGE

1. During the last decade, the rate of obesity in Canada has
   a. been on the decline.
   b. increased at an alarming rate.
   c. increased slightly.
   d. remained steady.
   e. increased in men and decreased in women.

2. Obesity is defined as a body mass index equal to or above
   a. 10.
   b. 25.
   c. 30.
   d. 45.
   e. 50.

3. Obesity increases the risk for
   a. hypertension.
   b. congestive heart failure.
   c. atherosclerosis.
   d. type 2 diabetes.
   e. all of the above.

4. Tolerable weight is a body weight
   a. that is not ideal but one that you can live with.
   b. that will tolerate the increased risk of chronic diseases.
   c. with a BMI range between 25 and 30.
   d. that meets both ideal values for percent body weight and BMI.
   e. All are correct choices.

5. When the body uses protein instead of a combination of fats and carbohydrates as a source of energy
   a. weight loss is very slow.
   b. a large amount of weight loss is in the form of water.
   c. muscle turns into fat.
   d. fat is lost very rapidly.
   e. fat cannot be lost.

6. Eating disorders
   a. are characterized by an intense fear of becoming fat.
   b. are physical and emotional conditions.
   c. almost always require professional help for successful treatment of the disease.
   d. are common in societies that encourage thinness.
   e. All are correct choices.

7. The mechanism that seems to regulate how much a person weighs is known as
   a. setpoint.
   b. weight factor.
   c. basal metabolic rate.
   d. metabolism.
   e. energy-balancing equation.

8. The key to successful weight loss maintenance is
   a. frequent dieting.
   b. very low-calorie diets when "normal" dieting doesn't work.
   c. a lifetime exercise program.
   d. regular high protein/low carbohydrate meals.
   e. All are correct choices.

9. The daily amount of physical activity recommended for weight-loss purposes is
   a. 15 to 20 minutes.
   b. 20 to 30 minutes.
   c. 30 to 40 minutes.
   d. 45 to 60 minutes.
   e. Any amount is sufficient as long as it is done daily.

10. A daily energy expenditure of 300 calories through physical activity is the equivalent of approximately _____ kilograms of fat per year.
    a. 6
    b. 10
    c. 14
    d. 18
    e. 22

Correct answers can be found at the back of the book.

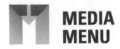

MEDIA MENU

INTERNET CONNECTIONS

■ Canadian Fitness and Lifestyle Research Institute. The institute's site provides Canadian data on topics related to physical activity.

http://www.cflri.ca

■ The Canadian Obesity Network (CON). At this site the expertise and dedication of researchers, clinicians, allied health care providers, and other professionals with an interest in obesity come together in a unified effort to reduce the mental, physical, and economic burden of obesity on Canadians.

http://www.obesitynetwork.ca

■ Active Healthy Kids Canada. This organization is an advocate for high-quality, accessible, and enjoyable physical activity for children and youth. On its website, it publishes annual "report cards" that rate the physical activity of Canadian children.

http://www.activehealthykids.ca

■ National Eating Disorder Centre (NEDIC). This Canadian, non-profit organization has a resource library on its site complete with many informational articles on eating disorders. The site also offers more valuable information and resources for individuals dealing with eating disorders and those who are attempting to help others.

http://www.nedic.ca/

■ Eating Disorders. This award-winning site, by Mental Health Net, features links describing symptoms, possible causes, consequences, treatment, online resources, organizations, online support, and research.

http://eatingdisorders.mentalhelp.net

■ Mayo Clinic Food & Nutrition Centre. This site features a wealth of reliable nutrition information including information on different food pyramids and the benefits and dangers of herbs, vitamins, and mineral supplements.

http://www.mayoclinic.com

Notes

1. "Overweight and Obesity in Canada: A Population Health Perspective."*Canadian Institute for Health Information*. 2004

2. Statistics Canada, "Health Reports."Adult Obesity. Vol. 17 no. 3. Aug. 2006, p. 9–25.

3. Peters, et al. (2003). Obesity in adulthood and its consequences for life expectancy: A life-table analysis. *Annals of Internal Medicine*. 138, 2432.

4. Fontaine, K.R., et al.(2003). Years of life lost due to obesity. *Journal of the American Medical Association*. 289, 187–193.

5. Wing, R.R., Venditti, E., Jakicic, J.M., Polley, A., & Lang, W. (1998). Lifestyle intervention in overweight individuals with a family history of diabetes. *Diabetes care*. 21, 350–359.

6. Thomsen, S. (2003). A steady diet of images. *BYU Magazine*. 57, (3), 20–21.

7. Lichtman, S., et al. (1992). Discrepancy between self-reported and actual caloric intake and exercise in obese subjects. *New England Journal of Medicine*. 327, 1893–1898.

8. Foster, G.D., et al. (2003). Randomized trial of a low-carbohydrate diet for obesity. *New England Journal of Medicine*. 348, 2082–2090.

9. Health Canada. Advisory. Health Canada requests recall of certain products containing Ephedra/ephedrine. January 9, 2002. Retrieved on January 20, 2008 at: http://www.hc-sc.gc.ca/ahc-asc/media/advisories-avis/_2002/2002_01_e.html

10. American Psychiatric Association, Diagnostic and Statistical Manual of Mental Disoders (Washington, DC: APA, 1994).

11. See note 10.

12. Liebel, R.L., Rosenbaum, M., and Hirsh, J. (1995). Changes IN Energy expenditure resulting from altered body weight. *New England Journal of Medicine*. 332, 621–628.

13. American College of Sports Medicine. (2001). Position stand: appropriate interventions strategies for weight loss and prevention for weight regain for adults. *Medicine and Science in Sports and Exercise*. 33, 2145–2156

14. Shepard, R.J. (1975). Alive man: the physiology of physical activity. Springfield, IL: Charles C Thomas. 484–488.

15. Miller, W.C., Koceja, D.M., and Hamilton, E.J. (1997). Meta-analysis of the past 25 years of weight loss reseach using diet, exercise, or diet plus exercise intervention. *International Journal of Obesity*. 21, 941–947.

16. M. K. Serdula et al., "Prevalence of Attempting Weight Loss and Strategies for Controlling Weight," *Journal of the American Medical Association* 282 (1999): 1353–1358.

17. National Academy of Sciences, Institute of Medicine, dietary Reference Intakes for Energy, Carbohydrates, Fibre, Fat, Protein and Amino Acids (Macronutrients). Washington, DC: National Academy Press, 2002.

18. Campbell, W.W., Crim, M.C., and Evans, W.J. (1994). Increased energy requirements and changes in body composition with resistance training in older adults. *American Journal of Clinical Nutrition*. 60, 167–175.

19. Tremblay, A., Simoneau, J.A., and Bouchard, C. Impact of exercise intensity on body fatness and skeletal muscle metabolism. *Metabolism*. 43, 814–818.

20. Klem, M.L., Wing, R.R., McGuire, M.T., Seagle, H.M., and Hill, J.O. A descriptive study of individuals successful at long-term maintenance of substantial weight loss. *American Journal of Clinical Nutrition*. 66, 239–246.

21. U.S. Department of Health and Human Services, Department of Agriculture, Nutrition and Your Health: Dietary Guidelines for Americans (Home and Garden Bulletin 232), 2000.

Suggested Readings

American College of Sports Medicine. "Effective Weight Management." *ACSM Fit Society Page* (http://acsm.org/health+fitness/fit_society.htm), Summer 2004.

American College of Sports Medicine. "Position Stand: Appropriate Intervention Strategies for Weight Loss and Prevention for Weight Regain for Adults." *Medicine and Science in Sports and Exercise* 33 (2001): 2145–2156.

American Diabetes Association and American Dietetic Association. *Exchange Lists for Meal Planning*. Chicago: American Dietetic Association and American Diabetes Association, 1995.

Brien, S.E., Katzmarzyk, P.T., Craig, C.L., Gauvin, L. Physical activity, cardiorespiratory fitness and body mass index as predictors of substantial weight gain and obesity: the Canadian physical activity longitudinal study. *Canadian Journal of Public Health*. 98(2):121–4, 2007.

Brownell, K. *The Learn Program for Weight Control*. Dallas: American Health Publishing, 1997.

Clarkson, P. M. "The Skinny on Weight Loss Supplements and Drugs: Winning the War against Fat." *ACSM's Health and Fitness Journal* (1998): 18.

Katzmarzyk, P.T. The Canadian obesity epidemic: an historical perspective. *Obesity*. 10(7):666–74, 2002.

Katzmarzyk, P.T. The Canadian obesity epidemic, 1985–1998. *Canadian Medical Association Journal*. 166(8):1039–40, 2002.

Lau, D.C.W., Douketis, J.D., Morrison, K.M., Hramiak, I.M., Sharma, A.M., Ur, Ehud for members of the Obesity Canada Clinical Practice Guidelines Expert Panel. (2006). 2006 Canadian clinical practice guidelines on the management and prevention of obesity in adults and children. *Canadian Medical Association Journal*, 176(8), Supplement S1–S13.

McDonald, S.D. Management and prevention of obesity in adults and children. *Canadian Medical Association Journal*. 176(8):1109–10, 2007.

Mokdad, A. H., et al. "The Spread of the Obesity Epidemic in the United States, 1991–1998." *Journal of the American Medical Association* 282 (1999): 1519–1522.

National Academy of Sciences, Institute of Medicine. *Dietary Reference Intakes for Energy, Carbohydrates, Fibre, Fat, Protein and Amino Acids (Macronutrients)*. Washington, DC: National Academy Press, 2002.

National Institutes of Health. *Clinical Guidelines on the Identification, Evaluation, and Treatment of Overweight and Obesity in Adults* (NIH Publication No. 98-4083). Washington, DC: NIH, 1998.

Lab 5B

CALORIE-RESTRICTED DIET PLANS

Name: _____   Date: _____   Grade: _____

Instructor: _____   Course: _____   Section: _____

Necessary Lab Equipment

Nutrient Value of Some Common Foods (Appendix) and Eating Well With Canada's Food Guide.

Lab Preparation

Read Chapter 5 prior to this lab.

Objective

To help you implement a calorie-restricted diet plan according to your target caloric intake obtained in Lab 5A.

1,200-Calorie Diet Plan

Instructions:

The objective of the diet plan is to meet (not exceed) the number of servings for the food groups listed. Each time that you eat a particular food, record it in the space provided for each group along with the amount you ate. Refer to Canada's Food Guide to determine what counts as one serving for each group listed.

Vegetables and Fruits (480 Calories) Females (19–50) 7–8 servings Males (19–50) 8–10 servings

1. _____
2. _____
3. _____
4. _____
5. _____
6. _____
7. _____
8. _____
9. _____
10. _____

Grain Products (480 Calories) Females (19–50) 6–7 servings Males (19–50) 8 servings

1. _____
2. _____
3. _____
4. _____
5. _____

6

7

8

Milk and Alternatives (120 Calories)   Females (19–50) 2 servings   Males (19–50) 2 servings

1

2

Meat and Alternatives (120 Calories)   Females (19–50) 2 servings   Males (19–50) 2 servings

1

2

Today's physical activity:

1,500-Calorie Diet Plan

Instructions:

The objective of the diet plan is to meet (not exceed) the number of servings for the food groups listed. Each time that you eat a particular food, record it in the space provided for each group along with the amount you ate. Refer to the Canada Food Guide to determine what counts as one serving for each group listed.

Vegetables and Fruits (600 Calories)   Females (19–50) 7–8 servings   Males (19–50) 8–10 servings

1
2
3
4
5
6
7
8
9
10

Grain Products (600 Calories)   Females (19–50) 6–7 servings   Males (19–50) 8 servings

1
2
3
4
5
6
7
8

Milk and Alternatives (150 Calories)   Females (19–50) 2 servings   Males (19–50) 2 servings

1
2

Meat and Alternatives (150 Calories)   Females (19–50) 2 servings   Males (19–50) 2 servings

1
2

Today's physical activity:

1,800-Calorie Diet Plan

Instructions:
The objective of the diet plan is to meet (not exceed) the number of servings for the food groups listed. Each time that you eat a particular food, record it in the space provided for each group along with the amount you ate. Refer to the Canada Food Guide to determine what counts as one serving for each group listed.

Vegetables and Fruits (720 Calories)   Females (19–50) 7–8 servings   Males (19–50) 8–10 servings

1

2

3

4

5

6

7

8

9

10

Grain Products (720 Calories)   Females (19–50) 6–7 servings   Males (19–50) 8 servings

1

2

3

4

5

6

7

8

Milk and Alternatives (180 Calories)   Females (19–50) 2 servings   Males (19–50) 2 servings

1

2

Meat and Alternatives (180 Calories)   Females (19–50) 2 servings   Males (19–50) 2 servings

1

2

Today's physical activity:

Lab 5C

HEALTHY DIETARY PLAN FOR WEIGHT MAINTENANCE OR WEIGHT GAIN

Name: _____   Date: _____   Grade: _____

Instructor: _____   Course: _____   Section: _____

Necessary Lab Equipment
None.

Lab Preparation
Read Chapters 3, 4, and 5 prior to this lab.

Objective
To design a sample daily healthy diet plan to maintain current body weight or increase body weight.

I. Daily Caloric Requirement

A. Current body weight in kilograms .... _____

B. Current percent body fat .... _____

C. Current body composition classification (Table 4.13, page 110) .... _____

D. Total daily energy requirement with exercise to maintain body weight (use item L from Lab 5A).
   Use this figure and stop further computations if the goal is to maintain body weight .... _____

E. Target body weight to increase body weight .... _____

F. Number of additional daily calories to increase body weight (combine this increased caloric intake
   with a strength-training program, see Chapter 7) 500

G. Total daily energy (caloric) requirement with exercise to increase body weight (D + 500) .... _____

II. Strength-Training Program

For weight gain purposes, indicate three days during the week and the time when you will engage in a strength-training program.

_____

_____

III. Healthy Diet Plan

Design a sample healthy daily diet plan according to the total daily energy requirement computed in D (maintenance) or G (weight gain) above. Using Appendix, list all individual food items that you can consume on that day, along with their caloric, carbohydrate, fat, protein content. Be sure that the diet meets the recommended number of servings from the four food groups.

Breakfast

	Food item	Serving Size	Calories	Carbohydrates (g)	Fat (g)	Protein (g)
1.						
2.						
3.						
4.						
5.						

Breakfast

	Food item	Serving Size	Calories	Carbohydrates (g)	Fat (g)	Protein (g)
6.						
7.						
8.						

Lunch

1.						
2.						
3.						
4.						
5.						
6.						
7.						
8.						

Snack

1.						

Dinner

1.						
2.						
3.						
4.						
5.						
6.						
7.						
8.						
	Totals:					

IV. Percent of Macronutrients

Determine the percent of total calories that are derived from carbohydrates, fat, and protein.

A. Total calories = _____

B. Grams of carbohydrates _____ $\times$ 4 $\div$ _____ (total calories) = _____ %

C. Grams of fat _____ $\times$ 9 $\div$ _____ (total calories) = _____ %

D. Grams of protein _____ $\times$ 4 $\div$ _____ (total calories) = _____ %

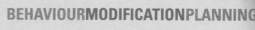

Lab 5D
BEHAVIOURAL GOALS FOR WEIGHT MANAGEMENT

Name: _____ Date: _____ Grade: _____

Instructor: _____ Course: _____ Section: _____

Necessary Lab Equipment
None.

Lab Preparation
Read Chapters 2, 3, 4, and 5 prior to this lab.

Objective
To prepare and monitor behavioural changes for weight management.

I. Please answer all the following:

1. State your own feelings regarding your current body weight, your target body composition, and a completion date for this goal.

_____

_____

_____

_____

Completion date: _____

2. Do you have an eating disorder? If so, express your feelings about it. Can your instructor help you find professional advice so that you can work toward resolving this problem?

_____

_____

_____

_____

_____

3. Is your present diet adequate according to the nutrient analysis?   Yes [ ]   No [ ]

4. State dietary changes necessary to achieve a balanced diet and/or to lose weight (increase or decrease caloric intake, decrease fat intake, increase intake of complex carbohydrates, etc.). List specific foods that will help you improve in areas where you may have deficiencies and food items to avoid or consume in moderation to help you achieve better nutrition.

Changes to make: _____

_____

Foods that will help: _____

_____

Foods to avoid: _____

_____

II. Behaviour Modification Progress Form

Instructions: Read the section on tips for behaviour modification and adherence to a weight management program (page 143–145). On a weekly or bi-weekly basis, go through the list of strategies and provide a "Yes" or "No" answer to each statement. If you are able to answer "Yes" to most questions, you have been successful in implementing positive weight management behaviours. (Make additional copies of this page as needed.)

Strategy Date						
1. I have made a commitment to change.						
2. I set realistic goals.						
3. I exercise regularly.						
4. I have healthy eating patterns.						
5. I exercise control over my appetite.						
6. I am consuming less fat in my diet.						
7. I pay attention to the number of calories in food.						
8. I have eliminated unnecessary food items from my diet.						
9. I use craving-reducing foods in my diet.						
10. I avoid automatic eating.						
11. I stay busy.						
12. I plan meals ahead of time.						
13. I cook wisely.						
14. I do not serve more food than I should eat.						
15. I use portion control in my diet.						
16. I eat slowly and at the table only.						
17. I avoid social binges.						
18. I avoid food raids.						
19. I do not eat out more than once per week. When I do, I eat low-fat meals.						
20. I practise stress management.						
21. I have a strong support group.						
22. I monitor behaviour changes.						
23. I prepare for lapses/relapses.						
24. I reward my accomplishments.						
25. I think positive.						

Chapter 6

Cardiorespiratory Endurance

Exercise is the closest thing we'll ever get to the miracle pill that everyone is seeking. It brings weight loss, appetite control, improved mood and self-esteem, an energy kick, and longer life by decreasing the risk of heart disease, diabetes, stroke, osteoporosis, and chronic disabilities.[1]

© Digital Vision/Getty Images

Objectives

■ Define cardiorespiratory endurance and describe the benefits of cardiorespiratory endurance training in maintaining health and well-being.

■ Define aerobic and anaerobic exercise, and give examples.

■ Be able to assess cardiorespiratory fitness through five different test protocols (2.4 km Run Test, 1.6 km Walk Test, Step Test, Astrand-Ryhming Test, and 12-Minute Swim Test).

■ Be able to interpret cardiorespiratory endurance assessment test results according to health fitness and physical fitness standards.

■ Be able to estimate oxygen uptake and caloric expenditure from walking and jogging.

■ Determine your readiness to start an exercise program.

■ Explain the principles that govern cardiorespiratory exercise prescription: intensity, type, mode, duration, and frequency.

■ Learn some ways to foster adherence to exercise.

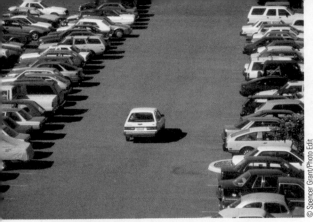

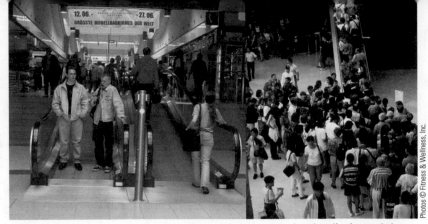

The epitome of physical inactivity: driving around a parking lot for several minutes in search of a parking spot 20 metres closer to the store's entrance.

Advances in modern technology have almost completely eliminated the need for physical activity, significantly enhancing the deterioration rate of the human body.

The single most important component of health-related physical fitness is **cardiorespiratory endurance**. The exception occurs among older adults, for whom muscular strength is particularly important. A person does need a certain amount of muscular strength and flexibility to engage in normal daily activities. Nevertheless, one can get by without high levels of strength and flexibility but cannot do without a good cardiorespiratory system.

Aerobic exercise is especially important in preventing cardiovascular disease. A poorly conditioned heart, which has to pump more often just to keep a person alive, is subject to more wear and tear than a well-conditioned heart. In situations that place strenuous demands on the heart, such as doing yardwork, lifting heavy objects or weights, or running to catch a bus, the unconditioned heart may not be able to sustain the strain. Regular participation in cardiorespiratory endurance activities also helps a person achieve and maintain recommended body weight, the fourth component of health-related physical fitness.

Physical activity, unfortunately, is no longer a natural part of our existence. Technological developments have driven most people in developed countries into sedentary lifestyles. For instance, when many people go to a store only a couple of blocks away, most drive their automobiles and then spend a couple of minutes driving around the parking lot to find a spot 20 metres closer to the store's entrance.

Similarly, during a visit to a multi-level shopping mall, almost everyone chooses to ride the escalators instead of taking the stairs (which tend to be inaccessible). Automobiles, elevators, escalators, telephones, intercoms, remote controls, electric garage door openers—all are modern-day commodities that minimize the amount of movement and effort required of the human body.

One of the most harmful effects of modern-day technology is an increase in chronic conditions related to a lack of physical activity. These include hypertension, heart disease, chronic low-back pain,

and obesity and are referred to as **hypokinetic diseases**. The term "hypo" means low or little, and "kinetic" implies motion. Lack of adequate physical activity is a fact of modern life that most people can avoid no longer. To enjoy modern-day conveniences and still expect to live life to its fullest, however, one needs to make a personalized lifetime exercise program a part of daily living.

Basic Cardiorespiratory Physiology: A Quick Survey

Before we begin to overhaul our bodies with an exercise program, we should understand the mechanisms that we propose to alter and survey the ways by which to measure their performance.

Cardiorespiratory endurance is a measure of how the pulmonary (lungs), cardiovascular (heart and blood vessels), and muscular systems work together during aerobic activities. As a person breathes, part of the oxygen in the air is taken up by the **alveoli** in the lungs. As blood passes through the alveoli, oxygen is picked up by **hemoglobin** and transported in the blood to the heart. The heart then is responsible for pumping the oxygenated blood through the circulatory system to all organs and tissues of the body.

At the cellular level, oxygen is used to convert food substrates (primarily carbohydrates and fats) through aerobic metabolism into **adenosine triphosphate (ATP)**. This compound provides the energy for physical activity, body functions, and maintenance of a constant internal equilibrium. During physical exertion, more ATP is needed to perform the activity. As a result, the lungs, heart, and blood vessels have to deliver more oxygen to the muscle cells to supply the required energy.

During prolonged exercise, an individual with a high level of cardiorespiratory endurance is able to deliver the required amount of oxygen to the tissues with relative ease. In contrast, the cardiorespiratory

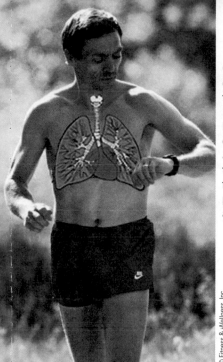

Cardiorespiratory endurance refers to the ability of the lungs, heart, and blood vessels to deliver adequate amounts of oxygen to the cells to meet the demands of prolonged physical activity.

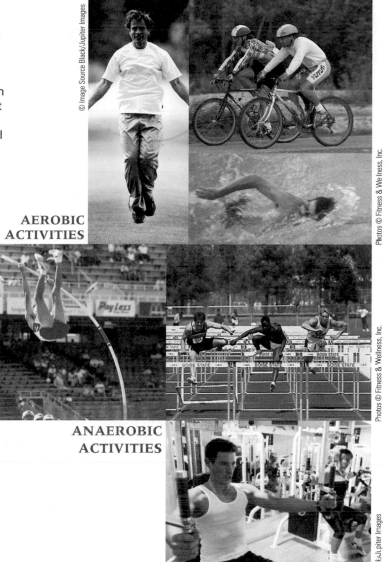

AEROBIC ACTIVITIES

ANAEROBIC ACTIVITIES

system of a person with a low level of endurance has to work much harder, the heart has to work at a higher rate, less oxygen is delivered to the tissues and, consequently, the individual fatigues faster. Hence, a higher capacity to deliver and utilize oxygen—called **oxygen uptake** or **VO₂**—indicates a more efficient cardio-respiratory system. Measuring oxygen uptake is therefore an important way to evaluate our cardiorespiratory health.

Aerobic and Anaerobic Exercise

Cardiorespiratory endurance activities often are called **aerobic** exercises; examples are walking, jogging, swimming, cycling, cross-country skiing, water aerobics, rope skipping, and aerobics. The intensity of **anaerobic** exercise is so high that oxygen cannot be delivered and utilized to produce energy. Because energy production is limited in the absence of oxygen, these activities can be carried out for only short periods—two to three minutes. The higher the intensity of the activity, the shorter the duration.

Good examples of anaerobic activities are the 100, 200, and 400 metres in track and field; the 100 metres in swimming; gymnastics routines; and strength training. Anaerobic activities do not con-tribute much to development of the cardiorespira-tory system. Only aerobic activities will help increase cardiorespiratory endurance. The basic guidelines for cardiorespiratory exercise prescription are set forth later in this chapter.

Cardiorespiratory endurance The ability of the lungs, heart, and blood vessels to deliver adequate amounts of oxygen to the cells to meet the demands of prolonged physical activity.

Hypokinetic diseases "Hypo" denotes "lack of"; therefore, lack of physical activity.

Alveoli Air sacs in the lungs where oxygen is taken up and carbon dioxide (produced by the body) is released from the blood.

Hemoglobin Iron-containing compound, found in red blood cells, that transports oxygen.

Adenosine triphosphate (ATP) A high-energy chemical compound that the body uses for immediate energy.

Oxygen uptake (VO₂) The amount of oxygen used by the human body.

Aerobic Exercise that requires oxygen to produce the necessary energy (ATP) to carry out the activity.

Anaerobic Exercise that does not require oxygen to produce the necessary energy (ATP) to carry out the activity.

TABLE 6.1 Average Resting and Maximal Cardiac Output, Stroke Volume, and Heart Rate for Sedentary, Trained, and Highly Trained Males*

	Resting			Maximal		
	Cardiac Output (L/min)	Stroke Volume (mL)	Heart Rate (bpm)	Cardiac Output (L/min)	Stroke Volume (mL)	Heart Rate (bpm)
Sedentary	5–6	68	74	20	100	200
Trained	5–6	90	56	30	150	200
Highly Trained	5–6	110	45	35	175	200

*Cardiac output and stroke volume in women are about 25 percent lower than in men.

Benefits of Aerobic Training

Everyone who participates in a cardiorespiratory or aerobic exercise program can expect a number of beneficial physiological adaptations from training. Among them are the following:

1. A higher **maximal oxygen uptake (VO$_2$max)**. The amount of oxygen the body is able to use during physical activity increases significantly. This allows the individual to exercise longer and more intensely before becoming fatigued. Depending on the initial fitness level, the increases in maximal oxygen uptake average 15 to 20 percent, although increases greater than 50 percent have been reported in people who have very low initial levels of fitness or who were significantly overweight prior to starting the aerobic exercise program.

2. An increase in the oxygen-carrying capacity of the blood. As a result of training, the red blood cell count goes up. Red blood cells contain hemoglobin, which transports oxygen in the blood.

3. A decrease in **resting heart rate** and an increase in cardiac muscle strength. During resting conditions, the heart ejects between 5 and 6 L of blood per minute. This amount of blood, also referred to as **cardiac output**, meets the body's energy demands in the resting state.

   Like any other muscle, the heart responds to training by increasing in strength and size. As the heart gets stronger, the muscle can produce a more forceful contraction, which helps the heart to eject more blood with each beat. This **stroke volume** yields a lower heart rate. The lower heart rate also allows the heart to rest longer between beats. Average resting and maximal cardiac outputs, stroke volumes, and heart rates for sedentary, trained, and highly trained (elite) individuals are shown in Table 6.1.

Resting heart rates frequently decrease by 10 to 20 beats per minute (bpm) after only 6 to 8 weeks of training. A reduction of 20 bpm saves the heart about 10,483,200 beats per year. The average heart beats between 70 and 80 bpm. As seen in the table, resting heart rates in highly trained athletes are often around 45 bpm.

4. A lower heart rate at given **workloads**. When compared with untrained individuals, a trained person has a lower heart rate response to a given task because of greater efficiency of the cardiorespiratory system. Individuals also are surprised to find that, following several weeks of training, a given workload (let's say a 10-minute kilometre) elicits a much lower heart rate response than the response when they first started training.

5. An increase in the number and size of the **mitochondria**. All energy necessary for cell function is produced in the mitochondria. As their size and numbers increase, so does the potential to produce energy for muscular work.

6. An increase in the number of functional **capillaries**. Capillaries allow for the exchange of oxygen and carbon dioxide between the blood and the cells. As more vessels open up, more gas exchange can take place, delaying the onset of fatigue during prolonged exercise. This increase in capillaries also speeds up the rate at which waste products of cell metabolism can be removed. This increased capillarization also occurs in the heart, which enhances the oxygen delivery capacity to the heart muscle itself.

7. A faster **recovery time**. Trained individuals recover more rapidly after exercising. A fit system is able to more quickly restore any internal equilibrium disrupted during exercise.

8. Lower blood pressure and blood lipids. A regular aerobic exercise program leads to lower blood pressure (thus reducing a major risk factor for stroke) and lower levels of fats (such as

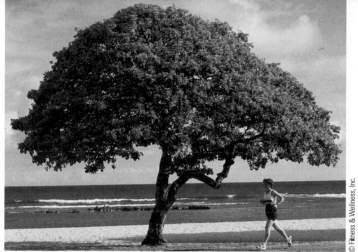
Aerobic fitness leads to better health and a higher quality of life.

cholesterol and triglycerides), all of which have been linked to the formation of atherosclerotic plaque, which obstructs the arteries. This decreases the risk of coronary heart disease (see Chapter 11).

9. An increase in fat-burning enzymes. These enzymes are significant because fat is lost primarily by burning it in muscle. As the concentration of the enzymes increases, so does the ability to burn fat.

Physical Fitness Assessment

The assessment of physical fitness serves several purposes:

- To educate participants regarding their present fitness levels and compare them to health fitness and physical fitness standards.
- To motivate individuals to participate in exercise programs.
- To provide a starting point for individualized exercise prescriptions.
- To evaluate improvements in fitness achieved through exercise programs and make adjustments in exercise prescriptions.
- To monitor changes in fitness throughout the years.

Responders versus Nonresponders

Individuals who follow similar training programs show a wide variation in physiological responses. Heredity plays a crucial role in how each person responds to and improves after beginning an exercise program. Several studies have documented that following exercise training, most individuals, called **responders**, readily show improvements, but a few, **nonresponders**, exhibit small or no improvements at all. This concept is referred to as the **principle of individuality**.

After several months of aerobic training, VO_2max increases are between 15 and 20 percent, on the average, although individual responses can range from 0 percent (in a few selected cases) to more than

BEHAVIOUR MODIFICATION PLANNING

TIPS TO INCREASE DAILY PHYSICAL ACTIVITY

- Walk to nearby places where you usually drive.
- Use a pedometer to count your daily steps.
- At work, walk to nearby offices instead of sending e-mails or using the phone.
- Take stairs as often as possible.
- Ride a bike or walk to work.
- Walk or stretch a few minutes every hour that you are at your desk.
- Learn a new sport or join a sports team.
- Incorporate activity into your lunch break (walk to the restaurant).
- Play outside with children and grandchildren.
- Spend more time playing sports than sitting in front of the TV or the computer.
- Stay in hotels with fitness centres when out of town.
- Avoid carts when golfing.
- Do household tasks.
- Work in the yard or garden.

50 percent improvement, even when all participants follow exactly the same training program. Non-fitness and low-fitness participants, however, should not label themselves as nonresponders based on the previous discussion. Nonresponders constitute less

Maximal oxygen uptake (VO_2max) Maximum amount of oxygen the body is able to utilize per minute of physical activity, commonly expressed in mL/kg/min, the best indicator of cardiorespiratory or aerobic fitness.

Resting heart rate (RHR) Heart rate after a person has been sitting quietly for 15–20 minutes.

Cardiac output Amount of blood pumped by the heart in one minute.

Stroke volume Amount of blood pumped by the heart in one beat.

Workload Load (or intensity) placed on the body during physical activity.

Mitochondria Structures within the cells where energy transformations take place.

Capillaries Smallest blood vessels carrying oxygenated blood to the tissues in the body.

Recovery time Amount of time the body takes to return to resting levels after exercise.

Responders Individuals who exhibit improvements in fitness as a result of exercise training.

Nonresponders Individuals who exhibit small or no improvements in fitness as compared to others who undergo the same training program.

Principle of individuality Training concept that states that genetics plays a major role in individual responses to exercise training and these differences must be considered when designing exercise programs for different people.

than 5 percent of exercise participants. Although additional research is necessary, lack of improvement in cardiorespiratory endurance among nonresponders might be related to low levels of leg strength. By increasing lower body muscle mass, more muscle tissue becomes available to take up and utilize any delivered oxygen, thereby increasing oxygen consumption. A lower body strength-training program has been shown to help these individuals improve VO_2max through aerobic exercise.[2]

Following assessment of cardiorespiratory fitness, if your fitness level is less than adequate, do not let that discourage you, but make it a priority to be physically active every day. In addition to regular exercise, lifestyle behaviours such as walking, taking stairs, cycling to work, parking farther from the office, doing household tasks, gardening, and doing yardwork provide substantial benefits. In this regard, monitoring daily physical activity and exercise habits should be used in conjunction with fitness testing to evaluate compliance among nonresponders. After all, it is through increased daily activity that we reap the health benefits that improve quality of life.

Assessment of Cardiorespiratory Endurance

Cardiorespiratory endurance, cardiorespiratory fitness, or aerobic capacity is determined by the maximal amount of oxygen the human body is able to utilize (the oxygen uptake) per minute of physical activity (VO_2max). This value can be expressed in litres per minute (L/min) or millilitres per kilogram per minute (mL/kg/min). The relative value in mL/kg/min is used most often because it considers total body mass (weight) in kilograms. When comparing two individuals with the same absolute value, the one with the lesser body mass will have a higher relative value, indicating that more oxygen is available to each kilogram of body weight. Because all tissues and organs of the body need oxygen to function, higher oxygen consumption indicates a more efficient cardiorespiratory system.

Components of Oxygen Uptake (VO_2)

The amount of oxygen that the body actually uses at rest or during submaximal (VO_2) or maximal (VO_2max) physical activity is determined by the heart rate, the stroke volume, and the amount of oxygen removed from the vascular system (for use by all organs and tissues of the body, including the muscular system).

HEART RATE

Normal heart rate may range from about 40 bpm during resting conditions in trained athletes to 200 bpm or higher during maximal exercise. The **maximal heart rate** that a person can achieve starts to drop by about one beat per year beginning at about 12 years of age. Maximal heart rate in trained endurance athletes is sometimes slightly lower than in untrained individuals. This adaptation to training is thought to allow the heart more time to effectively fill with blood so as to produce a greater stroke volume.

STROKE VOLUME

Stroke volume ranges from 50 mL per beat (stroke) during resting conditions in untrained individuals to 200 mL at maximum in endurance-trained athletes (see Table 6.1). Following endurance training, stroke volume increases significantly. Some of the increase is the result of a stronger heart muscle, but it is also related to an increase in total blood volume and a greater filling capacity of the ventricles during the resting phase (diastole) of the heart cycle. As more blood enters the heart, a greater amount can be ejected with each heartbeat (systole). The increase in stroke volume is primarily responsible for the increase in VO_2max seen with endurance training.

AMOUNT OF OXYGEN REMOVED FROM BLOOD

The amount of oxygen removed from the vascular system is known as the **arterial-venous oxygen difference (a-$\overline{v}O_2$diff)**. The oxygen content in the arteries at sea level is typically 20 mL of oxygen per 100 cc of blood. (This value decreases at higher altitudes because of the drop in barometric pressure, which affects the amount of oxygen picked up by hemoglobin.) The oxygen content in the veins during a resting state is about 15 mL per 100 cc. Thus, the a-$\overline{v}O_2$diff—that is, the amount of oxygen in the arteries minus the amount in the veins—at rest is 5 mL per 100 cc. The arterial value remains constant during both resting and exercise conditions but, during maximal exercise, the venous oxygen content drops to about 5 mL per 100 cc, yielding an a-$\overline{v}O_2$diff of 15 mL per 100 cc. The latter value may be slightly higher in endurance athletes.

These three factors are used to compute VO_2 using the following equation:

$$VO_2 \text{ in L/min} = (HR \times SV \times \text{a-}\overline{v}O_2\text{diff}) \div 100{,}000$$

where

HR = heart rate
SV = stroke volume

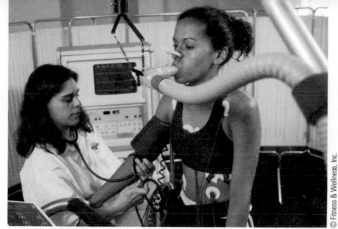
Oxygen uptake, as determined through direct gas analysis.

For example, the resting VO_2 (also known as "resting metabolic rate") of an individual with a resting heart rate of 76 bpm and a stroke volume of 79 mL would be

$$VO_2 \text{ in L/min} = (76 \times 79 \times 5) \div 100,000 = 0.3 \text{ L/min}$$

Likewise, the VO_2max of a person exercising maximally who achieves a heart rate of 190 bpm and a maximal stroke volume of 120 mL would be

$$VO_2\text{max in L/min} = (190 \times 120 \times 15) \div 100,000 = 3.42 \text{ L/min}$$

To convert L/min to mL/kg/min, multiply the L/min value by 1,000 and divide by body weight in kilograms. In the above example, if the person weighed 70 kg, the VO_2max in mL/kg/min would be 48.9 ($3.42 \times 1000 \div 70$).

Because the actual measurement of the stroke volume and the a-$\overline{v}O_2$diff is impractical in the fitness setting, VO_2 is also determined through gas (air) analysis. The person being tested breathes into a metabolic cart that measures the difference in oxygen content between the person's exhaled air and the atmosphere. (The air we breathe contains 21 percent oxygen; thus, VO_2 can be assessed by establishing the difference between 21 percent, the percent of oxygen left in the air the person exhales, and the total amount of air taken into the lungs.) This type of equipment, however, is expensive. Consequently, several alternative methods of estimating VO_2max using limited equipment have been developed. These methods are discussed in the next section.

VO_2max is affected by genetics, training, gender, age, and body composition. Although aerobic training can help people attain good or excellent cardiorespiratory fitness, only those with a strong genetic component are able to reach an "elite" level of aerobic capacity (60 to 80 mL/kg/min). Further, VO_2max is 15 to 30 percent higher in men. This is related to a greater hemoglobin content, lower body fat (see "Essential and Storage Fat" in Chapter 4), and larger heart size in men (a larger heart pumps more blood, thus producing a greater stroke

volume). VO_2max also decreases by about 1 percent per year starting at age 25. This decrease, however, is only 0.5 percent per year in physically active individuals.

Tests to Estimate VO_2max

Even though most cardiorespiratory endurance tests probably are safe to administer to apparently healthy individuals (those with no major coronary risk factors or symptoms), the American College of Sports Medicine recommends that a physician be present for all maximal exercise tests on apparently healthy men over age 45 and women over age 55. A maximal test is any test that requires the participant's all-out or nearly all-out effort. For submaximal exercise tests, a physician should be present when testing higher risk/symptomatic individuals or diseased people, regardless of the participant's current age.

Five exercise tests used to assess cardiorespiratory fitness are introduced in this chapter: the 2.4 km Run Test (commonly known as the 1.5 Mile Run Test), the 1.6 km Walk Test (commonly known as the 1.0 Mile Walk Test), the Step Test, the Astrand–Ryhming Test, and the 12-Minute Swim Test. The test procedures are explained in detail in Figures 6.1, 6.2, 6.3, 6.4, and 6.5, respectively.

Multiple tests are provided in this chapter so you may choose one test depending on time, equipment, and individual physical limitations. For example, people who can't jog or walk could take the bike or swim test. You may perform more than one of these tests, but because these are different tests and they estimate maximal oxygen uptake, they will not necessarily yield the same results. Therefore, to make valid comparisons, you should take the same test when doing pre- and post-assessments. You may record the results of your test(s) in Lab 6A.

2.4 KM RUN TEST
The 2.4 km Run Test is used most frequently to predict maximal oxygen uptake according to the time the person takes to run or walk a 2.4 km course (see Figure 6.1). Maximal oxygen uptake is estimated based on the time the person takes to cover the distance (see Table 6.2).

The only equipment necessary to conduct this test is a stopwatch and a track or premeasured

Maximal heart rate (MHR) Highest heart rate for a person, related primarily to age.

Arterial-venous oxygen difference (a-$\overline{v}O_2$diff) The amount of oxygen removed from the blood as determined by the difference in oxygen content between arterial and venous blood.

FIGURE 6.1 Procedure for the 2.4 km Run Test

1. Make sure you qualify for this test. This test is contra-indicated for unconditioned beginners, individuals with symptoms of heart disease, and those with known heart disease or risk factors.
2. Select the testing site. Find a school track (each lap is 400 m) or a premeasured 2.4 km course.
3. Have a stopwatch available to determine your time.
4. Conduct a few warm-up exercises prior to the test. Do some stretching exercises, some walking, and slow jogging.
5. Initiate the test and try to cover the distance in the fastest time possible (walking or jogging). Time your-self during the run to see how fast you have covered the distance. If any unusual symptoms arise during the

test, do not continue. Stop immediately and retake the test after another six weeks of aerobic training.
6. At the end of the test, cool down by walking or jogging slowly for another three to five minutes. Do not sit or lie down after the test.
7. According to your performance time, look up your esti-mated maximal oxygen uptake(VO_2max) in Table 6.2.

Example: A 20-year-old female runs the 2.4 km course in 12 minutes and 40 seconds. Table 6.2 shows a VO_2max of 39.8 mL/kg/min for a time of 12:40. According to Table 6.8, this VO_2max would place her in the "good" cardiorespiratory fitness category.

TABLE 6.2 Estimated Maximal Oxygen Uptake (VO_2max) for the 2.4 km Run Test

Time	VO_2max (mL/kg/min)	Time	VO_2max (mL/kg/min)	Time	VO_2max (mL/kg/min)
6:10	80.0	10:30	48.6	14:50	34.0
6:20	79.0	10:40	48.0	15:00	33.6
6:30	77.9	10:50	47.4	15:10	33.1
6:40	76.7	11:00	46.6	15:20	32.7
6:50	75.5	11:10	45.8	15:30	32.2
7:00	74.0	11:20	45.1	15:40	31.8
7:10	72.6	11:30	44.4	15:50	31.4
7:20	71.3	11:40	43.7	16:00	30.9
7:30	69.9	11:50	43.2	16:10	30.5
7:40	68.3	12:00	42.3	16:20	30.2
7:50	66.8	12:10	41.7	16:30	29.8
8:00	65.2	12:20	41.0	16:40	29.5
8:10	63.9	12:30	40.4	16:50	29.1
8:20	62.5	12:40	39.8	17:00	28.9
8:30	61.2	12:50	39.2	17:10	28.5
8:40	60.2	13:00	38.6	17:20	28.3
8:50	59.1	13:10	38.1	17:30	28.0
9:00	58.1	13:20	37.8	17:40	27.7
9:10	56.9	13:30	37.2	17:50	27.4
9:20	55.9	13:40	36.8	18:00	27.1
9:30	54.7	13:50	36.3	18:10	26.8
9:40	53.5	14:00	35.9	18:20	26.6
9:50	52.3	14:10	35.5	18:30	26.3
10:00	51.1	14:20	35.1	18:40	26.0
10:10	50.4	14:30	34.7	18:50	25.7
10:20	49.5	14:40	34.3	19:00	25.4

Source: Adapted from K. H. Cooper, "A Means of Assessing Maximal Oxygen Intake," *Journal of the American Medical Association*, 203 (1968): 201–204; M. L. Pollock, J. H. Wilmore, and S. M. Fox III, *Health and Fitness Through Physical Activity* (New York: John Wiley & Sons, 1978); and J. H. Wilmore and D. L. Costill, *Training for Sport and Activity* (Dubuque, IA: Wm. C. Brown Publishers, 1988).

2.4 km course. This perhaps is the easiest test to administer, but a note of caution is in order when conducting the test: Given that the objective is to cover the distance in the shortest time, it is consid-ered a maximal exercise test. The 2.4 km Run Test should be limited to conditioned individuals who have been cleared for exercise. The test is not rec-ommended for unconditioned beginners, men over age 45, and women over age 55 without proper medical clearance, symptomatic individuals, and those with known disease or risk factors for coro-nary heart disease. A program of at least six weeks of aerobic training is recommended before uncondi-tioned individuals take this test.

1.6 KM WALK TEST

This test can be used by individuals who are unable to run because of low fitness levels or injuries. All that is required is a brisk 1.6 km walk that will elicit an exercise heart rate of at least 120 beats per minute at the end of the test.

You will need to know how to take your heart rate by counting your pulse. This can be done by gently placing the middle and index fingers over the radial artery on the wrist (inside the wrist on the side of the thumb) or over the carotid artery in the neck just below the jaw, next to the voice box. The thumb should not be used to check the pulse because it has a strong pulse of its own, which can make you miscount. When checking the carotid pulse, do not press too hard, because it may cause a reflex action that slows the heart. Some exercise leaders recommend that when you check the pulse over the carotid artery, the hand on the same side of the neck (left hand over left carotid artery) be used to avoid excessive pressure

FIGURE 6.2   Procedure for the 1.6 km Walk Test

1. Select the testing site. Use a 400 m track (4 laps = 1600 m) or a premeasured 1.0-km course.
2. Determine your body weight in kilograms prior to the test.
3. Have a stopwatch available to determine total walking time and exercise heart rate.
4. Walk the 1.6 km course at a brisk pace (the exercise heart rate at the end of the test should be above 120 beats per minute).
5. At the end of the 1.6 km walk, check your walking time and immediately count your pulse for 10 seconds. Multiply the 10-second pulse count by 6 to obtain the exercise heart rate in beats per minute.
6. Convert the walking time from minutes and seconds to minute units. Because each minute has 60 seconds, divide the seconds by 60 to obtain the fraction of a minute. For instance, a walking time of 12 minutes and 15 seconds would equal 12 + (15 ÷ 60), or 12.25 minutes.
7. To obtain the estimated maximal oxygen uptake (VO_2max) in mL/kg/min, plug your values in the following equation: VO_2max = 88.768 − (0.0957 × W) + (8.892 × G) − (1.4537 × T) − (0.1194 × HR)

WHERE:

W = Weight in kilograms
G = Gender (use 0 for women and 1 for men)
T = Total time for the 1.6 km walk in minutes (see item 6)
HR = Exercise heart rate in beats per minute at the end of the 1.6 km walk

Example: A 19-year-old female who weighs 140 pounds completed the 1.6 km walk in 14 minutes 39 seconds and with an exercise heart rate of 148 beats per minute. The estimated VO_2max would be:

W = 60 kg
G = 0 (female gender = 0)
T = 14:39 = 14 + (39 ÷ 60) = 14.65 min
HR = 148 bpm
VO_2max = 88.768 − (0.0957 × 60) + (8.892 × 0) − (1.4537 × 14.65) − (0.1194 × 148)
VO_2max = 36.4 mL/kg/min

Source: F. A. Dolgener, L. D. Hensley, J. J. Marsh, and J. K. Fjelstul, "Validation of the Rockport Fitness Walking Test in College Males and Females," *Research Quarterly for Exercise and Sport* 65 (1994): 152–158. Used with permission.

on the artery. With minimum experience, however, you can be accurate using either hand as long as only gentle pressure is applied. If available, heart rate monitors can be used to increase the accuracy of heart rate assessment.

Maximal oxygen uptake is estimated according to a prediction equation that requires the following data: 1.6 km walk time, exercise heart rate at the end of the walk, gender, and body weight in kilograms. The procedure for this test and the equation are given in Figure 6.2.

STEP TEST

The Step Test requires little time and equipment and can be administered to almost anyone, because a submaximal workload is used to estimate maximal oxygen uptake. Symptomatic and diseased individuals should not take this test. Significantly overweight individuals and those with joint problems in the lower extremities may have difficulty performing the test.

The actual test takes only 3 minutes. A 15-second recovery heart rate is taken between 5 and 20 seconds following the test (see Figure 6.3 and Table 6.3). The equipment required consists of a bench or gymnasium bleacher 40 cm high, a stopwatch, and a metronome.

You also will need to know how to take your heart rate by counting your pulse (explained under

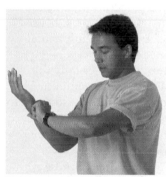

Pulse taken at the radial artery.

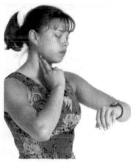

Pulse taken at the carotid artery.

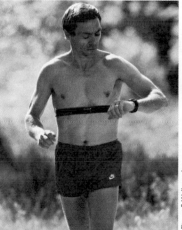

Heart rate monitors increase the accuracy of heart rate assessment.

FIGURE 6.3 Procedure for the Step Test

1. Conduct the test with a bench or gymnasium bleacher 40 cm high.
2. Perform the stepping cycle to a four-step cadence (up-up-down-down). Men should perform 24 complete step-ups per minute, regulated with a metronome set at 96 beats per minute. Women perform 22 step-ups per minute, or 88 beats per minute on the metronome.
3. Allow a brief practice period of 5 to 10 seconds to familiarize yourself with the stepping cadence.
4. Begin the test and perform the step-ups for exactly 3 minutes.
5. Upon completing the 3 minutes, remain standing and take your heart rate for a 15-second interval from 5 to 20 seconds into recovery. Convert recovery heart rate to beats per minute (multiply 15-second heart rate by 4).

6. Maximal oxygen uptake (VO_2max) in mL/kg/min is estimated according to the following equations:
Men:
$$VO_2max = 111.33 - (0.42 \times \text{recovery heart rate in bpm})$$
Women:
$$VO_2max = 65.81 - (0.1847 \times \text{recovery heart rate in bpm})$$

Example: The recovery 15-second heart rate for a male following the 3-minute step test is found to be 39 beats. VO_2max is estimated as follows:

15-second heart rate = 39 beats
Minute heart rate = 39 × 4 = 156 bpm
$VO_2max = 111.33 - (0.42 \times 156) = 45.81$ mL/kg/min
VO_2max also can be obtained according to recovery heart rates in Table 6.3.

Adapted from W.D. McArdle et al., *Exercise Physiology: Energy, Nutrition, and Human Performance* (Philadelphia: Lea & Febiger, 1986).

the 1.6 km Walk Test). Once people learn to take their own heart rate, a large group of people can be tested at once, using gymnasium bleachers for the steps.

ASTRAND–RYHMING TEST

Because of its simplicity and practicality, the Astrand–Ryhming test is one of the most popular tests used to estimate maximal oxygen uptake in the laboratory setting. The test is conducted on a bicycle ergometer, and, similar to the Step Test, it requires only sub-maximal workloads and little time to administer.

The cautions given for the Step Test also apply to the Astrand–Ryhming Test. Nevertheless, because the participant does not have to support his or her own body weight while riding the bicycle, over-weight individuals and those with limited joint problems in the lower extremities can take this test.

The bicycle ergometer to be used for this test should allow for the regulation of workloads (see the test procedure in Figure 6.4). Besides the bicycle ergometer, a stopwatch and an additional technician to monitor the heart rate are needed to conduct the test.

The heart rate is taken every minute for six minutes. At the end of the test, the heart rate should be in the range given for each workload in Table 6.5 (generally between 120 and 170 bpm).

When administering the test to older people, good judgment is essential. Low workloads should

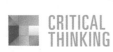

CRITICAL THINKING

Should fitness testing be a part of a fitness program? Why or why not? Are there benefits to pre-participation fitness testing or should fitness testing be done at a later date?

TABLE 6.3 Predicted Maximal Oxygen Uptake for the Step Test

15-Sec Heart Rate	Heart Rate (bpm)	VO₂max (mL/kg/min) Men	VO₂max (mL/kg/min) Women
30	120	60.9	43.6
31	124	59.3	42.9
32	128	57.6	42.2
33	132	55.9	41.4
34	136	54.2	40.7
35	140	52.5	40.0
36	144	50.9	39.2
37	148	49.2	38.5
38	152	47.5	37.7
39	156	45.8	37.0
40	160	44.1	36.3
41	164	42.5	35.5
42	168	40.8	34.8
43	172	39.1	34.0
44	176	37.4	33.3
45	180	35.7	32.6
46	184	34.1	31.8
47	188	32.4	31.1
48	192	30.7	30.3
49	196	29.0	29.6
50	200	27.3	28.9

be used, because if the higher heart rates (around 150 to 170 bpm) are reached, these individuals could be working near or at their maximal capacity, making it an unsafe test without adequate medical supervision. When testing older people, choose workloads so the final exercise heart rates do not exceed 130 to 140 bpm.

FIGURE 6.4 Procedure for the Astrand–Ryhming test

1. Adjust the bike seat so the knees are almost completely extended as the foot goes through the bottom of the pedalling cycle.
2. During the test, keep the speed constant at 50 revolutions per minute. Test duration is 6 minutes.
3. Select the appropriate workload for the bike based on age, weight, health, and estimated fitness level. For unconditioned individuals: women, use 300 kpm (kilopounds per metre) or 450 kpm; men, 300 kpm or 600 kpm. Conditioned adults: women, 450 kpm or 600 kpm; men, 600 kpm or 900 kpm.*
4. Ride the bike for 6 minutes and check the heart rate every minute, during the last 10 seconds of each minute. Determine heart rate by recording the time it takes to count 30 pulse beats and then converting to beats per minute using Table 6.4.
5. Average the final two heart rates (5th and 6th minutes). If these two heart rates are not within 5 beats per minute of each other, continue the test for another few minutes until this is accomplished. If the heart rate continues to climb significantly after the 6th minute, stop the test and rest for 15 to 20 minutes. You may then retest, preferably at a lower workload. The final average heart rate should also fall between the ranges given for each workload in Table 6.5 (men: 300 kpm = 120 to 140 beats per minute; 600 kpm = 120 to 170 beats per minute).

6. Based on the average heart rate of the final 2 minutes and your workload, look up the maximal oxygen uptake (VO_2max) in Table 6.5 (for example: men: 600 kpm and average heart rate = 145, VO_2max = 2.4 litres/minute).
7. Correct VO_2max using the correction factors found in Table 6.6 (if VO_2max = 2.4 and age 35, correction factor = .870. Multiply 2.4 × .870 and final corrected VO_2max = 2.09 L/minute).
8. To obtain VO_2max in mL/kg/min, multiply the VO_2max by 1,000 (to convert litres to millilitres) and divide by body weight in kilograms.

Example: Corrected VO_2max = 2.09 L/minute
Body weight = 60 kg

$$VO_2max \text{ in mL/kg/min} = \frac{2.09 \times 1,000}{60} = 34.8 \text{ mL/kg/min}$$

2,090 divided by 60 = 34.8 mL/kg/min

---

* On the Monarch bicycle ergometer, at a speed of 50 revolutions per minute, a load of 1 kp = 300 kpm, 1.5 kp = 450 kpm, 2 kp = 600 kpm, and so forth, with increases of 150 kpm to each half kp.

TABLE 6.4 Conversion of Time for 30 Pulse Beats to Pulse Rate Per Minute

Sec.	bpm	Sec.	bpm	Sec.	bpm	Sec.	bpm	Sec.	bpm	Sec.	bpm
22.0	82	19.6	92	17.2	105	14.8	122	12.4	145	10.0	180
21.9	82	19.5	92	17.1	105	14.7	122	12.3	146	9.9	182
21.8	83	19.4	93	17.0	106	14.6	123	12.2	148	9.8	184
21.7	83	19.3	93	16.9	107	14.5	124	12.1	149	9.7	186
21.6	83	19.2	94	16.8	107	14.4	125	12.0	150	9.6	188
21.5	84	19.1	94	16.7	108	14.3	126	11.9	151	9.5	189
21.4	84	19.0	95	16.6	108	14.2	127	11.8	153	9.4	191
21.3	85	18.9	95	16.5	109	14.1	128	11.7	154	9.3	194
21.2	85	18.8	96	16.4	110	14.0	129	11.6	155	9.2	196
21.1	85	18.7	96	16.3	110	13.9	129	11.5	157	9.1	198
21.0	86	18.6	97	16.2	111	13.8	130	11.4	158	9.0	200
20.9	86	18.5	97	16.1	112	13.7	131	11.3	159	8.9	202
20.8	87	18.4	98	16.0	113	13.6	132	11.2	161	8.8	205
20.7	87	18.3	98	15.9	113	13.5	133	11.1	162	8.7	207
20.6	87	18.2	99	15.8	114	13.4	134	11.0	164	8.6	209
20.5	88	18.1	99	15.7	115	13.3	135	10.9	165	8.5	212
20.4	88	18.0	100	15.6	115	13.2	136	10.8	167	8.4	214
20.3	89	17.9	101	15.5	116	13.1	137	10.7	168	8.3	217
20.2	89	17.8	101	15.4	117	13.0	138	10.6	170	8.2	220
20.1	90	17.7	102	15.3	118	12.9	140	10.5	171		
20.0	90	17.6	102	15.2	118	12.8	141	10.4	173		
19.9	90	17.5	103	15.1	119	12.7	142	10.3	175		
19.8	91	17.4	103	15.0	120	12.6	143	10.2	176		
19.7	91	17.3	104	14.9	121	12.5	144	10.1	178		

TABLE 6.5 Maximal Oxygen Uptake (VO₂max) Estimates for the Astrand–Ryhming Test

	Men					Women				
	Workload					Workload				
Heart Rate	300	600	900	1200	1500	300	450	600	750	900
120	2.2	3.4	4.8			2.6	3.4	4.1	4.8	
121	2.2	3.4	4.7			2.5	3.3	4.0	4.8	
122	2.2	3.4	4.6			2.5	3.2	3.9	4.7	
123	2.1	3.4	4.6			2.4	3.1	3.9	4.6	
124	2.1	3.3	4.5	6.0		2.4	3.1	3.8	4.5	
125	2.0	3.2	4.4	5.9		2.3	3.0	3.7	4.4	
126	2.0	3.2	4.4	5.8		2.3	3.0	3.6	4.3	
127	2.0	3.1	4.3	5.7		2.2	2.9	3.5	4.2	
128	2.0	3.1	4.2	5.6		2.2	2.8	3.5	4.2	4.8
129	1.9	3.0	4.2	5.6		2.2	2.8	3.4	4.1	4.8
130	1.9	3.0	4.1	5.5		2.1	2.7	3.4	4.0	4.7
131	1.9	2.9	4.0	5.4		2.1	2.7	3.4	4.0	4.6
132	1.8	2.9	4.0	5.3		2.0	2.7	3.3	3.9	4.5
133	1.8	2.8	3.9	5.3		2.0	2.6	3.2	3.8	4.4
134	1.8	2.8	3.9	5.2		2.0	2.6	3.2	3.8	4.4
135	1.7	2.8	3.8	5.1		2.0	2.6	3.1	3.7	4.3
136	1.7	2.7	3.8	5.0		1.9	2.5	3.1	3.6	4.2
137	1.7	2.7	3.7	5.0		1.9	2.5	3.0	3.6	4.2
138	1.6	2.7	3.7	4.9		1.8	2.4	3.0	3.5	4.1
139	1.6	2.6	3.6	4.8		1.8	2.4	2.9	3.5	4.0
140	1.6	2.6	3.6	4.8	6.0	1.8	2.4	2.8	3.4	4.0
141		2.6	3.5	4.7	5.9	1.8	2.3	2.8	3.4	3.9
142		2.5	3.5	4.6	5.8	1.7	2.3	2.8	3.3	3.9
143		2.5	3.4	4.6	5.7	1.7	2.2	2.7	3.3	3.8
144		2.5	3.4	4.5	5.7	1.7	2.2	2.7	3.2	3.8
145		2.4	3.4	4.5	5.6	1.6	2.2	2.7	3.2	3.7
146		2.4	3.3	4.4	5.6	1.6	2.2	2.6	3.2	3.7
147		2.4	3.3	4.4	5.5	1.6	2.1	2.6	3.1	3.6
148		2.4	3.2	4.3	5.4	1.6	2.1	2.6	3.1	3.6
149		2.3	3.2	4.3	5.4		2.1	2.6	3.0	3.5
150		2.3	3.2	4.2	5.3		2.0	2.5	3.0	3.5
151		2.3	3.1	4.2	5.2		2.0	2.5	3.0	3.4
152		2.3	3.1	4.1	5.2		2.0	2.5	2.9	3.4
153		2.2	3.0	4.1	5.1		2.0	2.4	2.9	3.3
154		2.2	3.0	4.0	5.1		2.0	2.4	2.8	3.3
155		2.2	3.0	4.0	5.0		1.9	2.4	2.8	3.2
156		2.2	2.9	4.0	5.0		1.9	2.3	2.8	3.2
157		2.1	2.9	3.9	4.9		1.9	2.3	2.7	3.2
158		2.1	2.9	3.9	4.9		1.8	2.3	2.7	3.1
159		2.1	2.8	3.8	4.8		1.8	2.2	2.7	3.1
160		2.1	2.8	3.8	4.8		1.8	2.2	2.6	3.0
161		2.0	2.8	3.7	4.7		1.8	2.2	2.6	3.0
162		2.0	2.8	3.7	4.6		1.8	2.2	2.6	3.0
163		2.0	2.8	3.7	4.6		1.7	2.2	2.6	2.9
164		2.0	2.7	3.6	4.5		1.7	2.1	2.5	2.9
165		2.0	2.7	3.6	4.5		1.7	2.1	2.5	2.9
166		1.9	2.7	3.6	4.5		1.7	2.1	2.5	2.8
167		1.9	2.6	3.5	4.4		1.6	2.1	2.4	2.8
168		1.9	2.6	3.5	4.4		1.6	2.0	2.4	2.8
169		1.9	2.6	3.5	4.3		1.6	2.0	2.4	2.8
170		1.8	2.6	3.4	4.3		1.6	2.0	2.4	2.7

From Astrand, I. *Acta Physiologica Scandinavica* 49 (1960). Supplementum 169: 45–60. Used with permission of John Wiley & Sons Ltd.

TABLE 6.6 Age-Based Correction Factors for Maximal Oxygen Uptake

Age	Correction Factor	Age	Correction Factor	Age	Correction Factor
14	1.11	32	.909	50	.750
15	1.10	33	.896	51	.742
16	1.09	34	.883	52	.734
17	1.08	35	.870	53	.726
18	1.07	36	.862	54	.718
19	1.06	37	.854	55	.710
20	1.05	38	.846	56	.704
21	1.04	39	.838	57	.698
22	1.03	40	.830	58	.692
23	1.02	41	.820	59	.686
24	1.01	42	.810	60	.680
25	1.00	43	.800	61	.674
26	.987	44	.790	62	.668
27	.974	45	.780	63	.662
28	.961	46	.774	64	.656
29	.948	47	.768	65	.650
30	.935	48	.762		
31	.922	49	.756		

Adapted from Astrand, I. *Acta Physiologica Scandinavica* 49 (1960). Supplementum 169: 45–60. Used with permission of John Wiley & Sons Ltd.

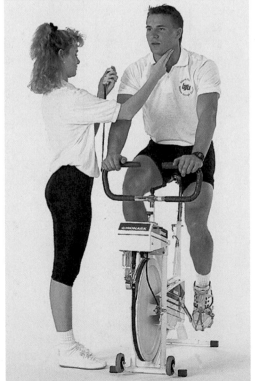

Monitoring heart rate on the carotid artery during the Astrand–Ryhming Test.

FIGURE 6.5 Procedure for the 12-Minute Swim Test

1. Enlist a friend to time the test. The only other requisites are a stopwatch and a swimming pool. Do not attempt to do this test in an unsupervised pool.
2. Warm up by swimming slowly and doing a few stretching exercises before taking the test.
3. Start the test and swim as many laps as possible in 12 minutes. Pace yourself throughout the test and do not swim to the point of complete exhaustion.
4. After completing the test, cool down by swimming another 2 or 3 minutes at a slower pace.
5. Determine the total distance you swam during the test and look up your fitness category in Table 6.7.

TABLE 6.7 12-Minute Swim Test Fitness Categories

Distance (metres)	Fitness Category
≥640	Excellent
460–640	Good
365–460	Average
185–365	Fair
≤185	Poor

Adapted from K. H. Cooper, *The Aerobics Program for Total Well-Being* (New York: Bantam Books, 1982).

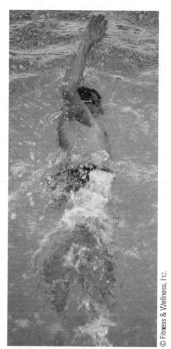

Only those with swimming skill and proper conditioning should take the 12-minute swim test.

12-MINUTE SWIM TEST

Similar to the 2.4 Km Run test, the 12-Minute Swim Test is considered a maximal exercise test, and the same precautions apply. The objective is to swim as far as possible during the 12-minute test.

Unlike land-based tests, predicting maximal oxygen uptake through a swimming test is difficult. A swimming test (Figure 6.5) is practical only for those who are planning to take part in a swimming program or who cannot perform any of the other tests. Differences in skill level, swimming conditioning, and body composition greatly affect the energy requirements (oxygen uptake) of swimming.

Unskilled and unconditioned swimmers can expect lower cardiorespiratory fitness ratings than those obtained with a land-based test. A skilled swimmer is able to swim more efficiently and expend much less energy than an unskilled swimmer. Improper breathing patterns cause premature fatigue. Overweight individuals are more buoyant in the water, and the larger surface area (body size) produces greater friction against movement in the water medium.

Lack of conditioning affects swimming test results as well. An unconditioned skilled swimmer who is in good cardiorespiratory shape because of a regular jogging program will not perform as effectively in a swimming test. Swimming

TABLE 6.8 Cardiorespiratory Fitness Category According to Maximal Oxygen Uptake (VO₂max)

Gender	Age	Poor	Fair	Average	Good	Excellent
		FITNESS CLASSIFICATION (based on VO₂max in mL/kg/min)				
Men	<29	<24.9	25–33.9	34–43.9	44–52.9	>53
	30–39	<22.9	23–30.9	31–41.9	42–49.9	>50
	40–49	<19.9	20–26.9	27–38.9	39–44.9	>45
	50–59	<17.9	18–24.9	25–37.9	38–42.9	>43
	60–69	<15.9	16–22.9	23–35.9	36–40.9	>41
	≥70	≤12.9	13–20.9	21–32.9	33–37.9	≥38
Women	<29	<23.9	24–30.9	31–38.9	39–48.9	>49
	30–39	<19.9	20–27.9	28–36.9	37–44.9	>45
	40–49	<16.9	17–24.9	25–34.9	35–41.9	>42
	50–59	<14.9	15–21.9	22–33.9	34–39.9	>40
	60–69	<12.9	13–20.9	21–32.9	33–36.9	>37
	≥70	≤11.9	12–19.9	20–30.9	31–34.9	≥35

Health fitness standard   High physical fitness standard

See the Chapter 1 discussion on health fitness versus physical fitness.

conditioning is important for adequate performance on this test.

Because of these limitations, maximal oxygen uptake cannot be estimated for a swimming test and the fitness categories given in Table 6.7 are only estimated ratings.

Interpreting Your Maximal Oxygen Uptake Results

After obtaining your maximal oxygen uptake, you can determine your current level of cardiorespiratory fitness by consulting Table 6.8. Locate the maximal oxygen uptake in your age category, and on the top

CRITICAL THINKING

Your relative maximal oxygen uptake can be improved without engaging in an aerobic exercise program. How do you accomplish this? Would you benefit from doing so?

row you will find your present level of cardiorespiratory fitness. For example, a 19-year-old male with a maximal oxygen uptake of 35 mL/kg/min would be classified in the "Average" cardiorespiratory fitness category. After you initiate your personal cardiorespiratory exercise program (see Lab 6D), you may wish to retest yourself periodically to evaluate your progress.

Predicting Oxygen Uptake and Caloric Expenditure from Walking and Jogging

As indicated earlier in the chapter, oxygen uptake can be expressed in litres per minute (L/min) or millilitres per kilogram per minute (mL/kg/min). The latter is used to classify individuals into the various cardiorespiratory fitness categories (see Table 6.8).

Oxygen uptake expressed in L/min is valuable in determining the caloric expenditure of physical activity. The human body burns about 5 Calories for each litre of oxygen consumed. During aerobic exercise the average person trains between 60 and 75 percent of maximal oxygen uptake.[3]

A person with a maximal oxygen uptake of 3.5 L/min who trains at 60 percent of maximum uses 2.1 (3.5 × .60) L of oxygen per minute of physical activity. This indicates that 10.5 Calories are burned each minute of exercise (2.1 × 5). If the activity is carried out for 30 minutes, 315 Calories (10.5 × 30) have been burned.

For individuals concerned about weight management, these computations are valuable in determining energy expenditure. Because a kilogram of body fat represents 7,700 Calories, this individual would have to exercise for a total of 733 minutes (7,700 ÷ 10.5) to burn the equivalent of a kilogram of body fat. At 30 minutes per exercise session, approximately 24 sessions would be required to expend the 7,700 Calories.

Applying the principle of 5 kcals burned per litre of oxygen consumed, you can determine with reasonable accuracy your own caloric output for walking and jogging. Table 6.9 contains the oxygen requirement (uptake) for walking speeds between 50 and 100 m per minute and for jogging speeds in excess of 80 m per minute.

There is a transition period from walking to jogging for speeds in the range of 80 to 134 m per minute. Consequently, the person must be truly jogging at these lower speeds to use the estimated oxygen uptakes for jogging in Table 6.9. Because these uptakes are expressed in mL/kg/min, you will have to convert this figure to L/min to predict caloric output. This is done by multiplying the

TABLE 6.9 Oxygen Requirement Estimates for Selected Walking and Jogging Speeds

Walking		Jogging			
Speed (m/min)	VO$_2$ (mL/kg/min)	Speed (m/min)	VO$_2$ (mL/kg/min)	Speed (m/min)	VO$_2$ (mL/kg/min)
50	8.5	80	19.5	210	45.5
52	8.7	85	20.5	215	46.5
54	8.9	90	21.5	220	47.5
56	9.1	95	22.5	225	48.5
58	9.3	100	23.5	230	49.5
60	9.5	105	24.5	235	50.5
62	9.7	110	25.5	240	51.5
64	9.9	115	26.5	245	52.5
66	10.1	120	27.5	250	53.5
68	10.3	125	28.5	255	54.5
70	10.5	130	29.5	260	55.5
72	10.7	135	30.5	265	56.5
74	10.9	140	31.5	270	57.5
76	11.1	145	32.5	275	58.5
78	11.3	150	33.5	280	59.5
80	11.5	155	34.5		
82	11.7	160	35.5		
84	11.9	165	36.5		
86	12.1	170	37.5		
88	12.3	175	38.5		
90	12.5	180	39.5		
92	12.7	185	40.5		
94	12.9	190	41.5		
96	13.1	195	42.5		
98	13.3	200	43.5		
100	13.5	205	44.5		

m/min = metres per minute

mL/kg/min = millilitres per kilogram per minute

Table developed using the metabolic calculations contained in *Guidelines for Exercise Testing and Exercise Prescription*, by the American College of Sports Medicine (Baltimore: Lippincott Williams & Wilkins, 2005).

oxygen uptake in mL/kg/min by your body weight in kilograms and then dividing by 1,000.

For example, let's estimate the caloric cost for an individual who weighs 66 kg and runs 4.8 km in 21 minutes. Therefore, 4,800 m in 21 minutes represents a pace of 228.6 m per minute (4,800 ÷ 21).

Table 6.9 indicates an oxygen requirement (uptake) of about 49.5 mL/kg/min for a speed of 228.6 m per minute. At a weight of 66 kg, the oxygen uptake in L/min now can be calculated by multiplying the value in mL/kg/min by body weight in kilograms and dividing by 1,000. In our example, it is (49.5 × 66) ÷ 1,000 = 3.3 L/min. This oxygen uptake in 21 minutes represents a total of 347 Calories (3.3 × 5 × 21).

In Lab 6B you have an opportunity to determine your own oxygen uptake and caloric expenditure for walking and jogging. Using your oxygen uptake information in conjunction with exercise heart rates allows you to estimate your caloric expenditure for almost any activity, as long as the heart rate ranges from 110 to 180 beats per minute.

To make an accurate estimate, you have to be skilled in assessing exercise heart rate. Also, as your level of fitness improves, you will need to reassess your exercise heart rate because it will drop (given the same workload) with improved physical condition.

Principles of Cardiorespiratory Exercise Prescription

Before proceeding with the principles of exercise prescription, you should ask yourself if you are willing to give exercise a try. A low percentage of the Canadian population (~33 percent) is truly committed to exercise. Further, more than half of the people who start exercising drop out during the first three to six months of the program. Sports psychologists are trying to find out why some people exercise habitually and many do not. All the benefits of exercise cannot help unless people commit to a lifetime program of physical activity.

Readiness for Exercise

The first step is to answer the question: Am I ready to start an exercise program? The information provided in Lab 6C can help you answer this question. You are evaluated in four categories: mastery (self-control), attitude, health, and commitment. The higher you score in any category—mastery, for example—the more important that reason is for you to exercise.

Scores can vary from 4 to 16. A score of 12 and above is a strong indicator that that factor is important to you, whereas 8 and below is low. If you score 12 or more points in each category, your chances of initiating and sticking to an exercise program are good. If you do not score at least 12 points each in any three categories, your chances of succeeding at exercise may be slim. You need to be better informed about the benefits of exercise, and a retraining process might be helpful. More tips on how you can become committed to exercise are provided in the section "Getting Started and Adhering to a Lifetime Exercise Program" (pages 179–180).

Next, you will have to decide positively that you will try. Using Lab 6C, you can list the advantages and disadvantages of incorporating exercise into your lifestyle. Your list might include advantages such as the following:

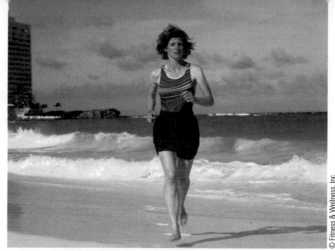

Aerobic exercise promotes cardiorespiratory development and helps decrease the risk for disease.

■ It will make me feel better.
■ I will lose weight.
■ I will have more energy.
■ It will lower my risk for chronic diseases.

Your list of disadvantages might include the following:

■ I don't want to take the time.
■ I'm too out of shape.
■ There's no good place to exercise.
■ I don't have the willpower to do it.

When your reasons for exercising outweigh your reasons for not exercising, you will find it easier to try. In Lab 6C you will also determine your stage of change for aerobic exercise. Using the information learned in Chapter 2, you can outline specific processes and techniques for change.

Guidelines for Cardiorespiratory Exercise Prescription

In spite of numerous government reports on physical inactivity and health and the overwhelming amount of evidence on the benefits of exercise on health and longevity, current estimates indicate that only about 20 percent of adults in Canada are considered active.

Most people are not familiar with the basic principles of cardiorespiratory exercise prescription. Thus, although they exercise regularly, they do not reap significant improvements in cardiorespiratory endurance.

To develop the cardiorespiratory system, the heart muscle has to be overloaded—like any other muscle in the human body. Just as the biceps muscle in the upper arm is developed through strength-training exercises, the heart muscle has to be exercised to increase in size, strength, and efficiency. To better understand how the cardiorespiratory system can be developed, you have to be familiar with the four variables that govern exercise prescription: intensity, mode, duration, and frequency.[4] The acronym FITT is sometimes used to describe these variables: *F*requency, *I*ntensity, *T*ype (mode), and *T*ime (duration).

First, however, you should be aware that the American College of Sports Medicine (ACSM) recommends that a medical exam and a diagnostic exercise stress test be administered prior to **vigorous exercise** to apparently healthy men over age 45 and women over age 55.[5] The ACSM has defined vigorous exercise as an exercise intensity above 60 percent of maximal capacity. For people initiating an exercise program, this intensity is the equivalent of exercise that provides a "substantial challenge" to the participant or one that cannot be maintained for 20 continuous minutes.

Intensity of Exercise

When trying to develop the cardiorespiratory system, many people often ignore **intensity** of exercise. For muscles to develop, they have to be overloaded to a given point. The training stimulus to develop the biceps muscle, for example, can be accomplished with arm curl-up exercises with increasing weights. Likewise, the cardiorespiratory system is stimulated by making the heart pump faster for a specified period.

Cardiorespiratory development occurs when the heart is working between 40 and 85 percent of heart rate reserve (see the section below on calculating intensity).[6] Individuals who are not fit should start at a 40 to 50 percent training intensity. Active and fit people can train at higher intensities. Increases in VO_2max are accelerated when the heart is working closer to 85 percent of **heart rate reserve (HRR)**. For this reason, many experts prescribe exercise between 60 and 85 percent. Intensity of exercise can be calculated easily, and training can be monitored by checking your pulse.

To determine the intensity of exercise or **cardiorespiratory training zone** according to heart rate reserve, follow these steps:

1. Estimate your maximal heart rate (MHR) according to the following formula:

$$MHR = 220 \text{ minus age } (220 - age)$$

2. Check your resting heart rate (RHR) some time after you have been sitting quietly for 15 to 20 minutes. You may take your pulse for 30 seconds and multiply by 2, or take it for a full minute. As explained on pages 166–167, you can check your pulse on the wrist, by placing two or three fingers over the radial artery or in the neck, using the carotid artery.

3. Determine the heart rate reserve (HRR) by subtracting the resting heart rate from the maximal heart rate (HRR = MHR − RHR).
4. Calculate the training intensities (TI) at 40, 50, 60, and 85 percent. Multiply the heart rate reserve by the respective .40, .50, .60, and .85, and then add the resting heart rate to all four of these figures (for example, 85% TI = HRR × .85 + RHR).

Example. The 40, 50, 60, and 85 percent training intensities for a 20-year-old with a resting heart rate of 68 beats per minute (bpm) would be as follows:

MHR: 220 − 20 = 200 bpm

RHR: = 68 bpm

HRR: 200 − 68 = 132 beats

40% TI = (132 × .40) + 68 = 121 bpm

50% TI = (132 × .50) + 68 = 134 bpm

60% TI = (132 × .60) + 68 = 147 bpm

85% TI = (132 × .85) + 68 = 180 bpm

Low-intensity cardiorespiratory training zone: 121 to 134 bpm

Moderate-intensity cardiorespiratory training zone: 134 to 147 bpm

Optimal cardiorespiratory training zone: 147 to 180 bpm

When you exercise to improve the cardiorespiratory system, maintain your heart rate between the 60 and 85 percent training intensities to obtain adequate development (see Figure 6.6). If you have been physically inactive, you should train around the 40 to 60 percent intensity during the first six to eight weeks of the exercise program. After that, you should exercise between 60 and 85 percent training intensity.

Following a few weeks of training, you may have a considerably lower resting heart rate (10 to 20 beats fewer in 8 to 12 weeks). Therefore, you should recompute your target zone periodically. You can compute your own cardiorespiratory training zone using Lab 6D. Once you have reached an ideal level of cardiorespiratory endurance, continued training in the 60 to 85 percent range will allow you to maintain your fitness level.

COUNTING THE PULSE

During the first few weeks of an exercise program, you should monitor your exercise heart rate regularly to make sure you are training in the proper zone. Wait until you are about 5 minutes into the aerobic phase of your exercise session before taking your first reading. When you check your heart rate, count your pulse for 10 seconds, then multiply by 6 to get the per-minute

FIGURE 6.6 Recommended cardiorespiratory or aerobic training pattern

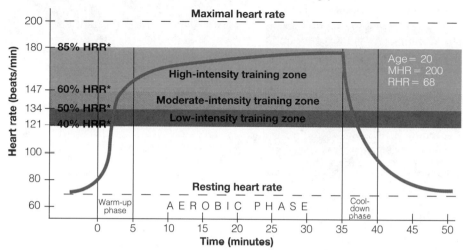

pulse rate. The exercise heart rate will remain at the same level for about 15 seconds following aerobic exercise, then drop rapidly. Do not hesitate to stop during your exercise bout to check your pulse. If the rate is too low, increase the intensity of exercise. If the rate is too high, slow down.

To develop the cardiorespiratory system, you do not have to exercise above the 85 percent rate. From a fitness standpoint, training above this percentage will not give extra benefits and actually may be unsafe for some individuals. Unconditioned people and older adults should train around the 50 percent rate to discourage potential problems associated with high-intensity exercise.

When determining the training intensity for your own program, you need to consider your personal fitness goals. Individuals who exercise at around the 50 percent training intensity will reap significant health benefits—in particular, improvements in the metabolic profile (see "Health Fitness Standards" in Chapter 1). Training at this lower percentage, however, may place you in only the "average" (moderate fitness) category (see Table 6.8 on page 171). Exercising at this lower intensity does lower the risk for cardiovascular mortality (the health fitness standard), but will not allow you to achieve a "good" or "excellent" cardiorespiratory fitness rating (the physical fitness standard). The latter ratings are obtained by exercising closer to the 85 percent threshold.

RATE OF PERCEIVED EXERTION

Because many people do not check their heart rate during exercise, or find it difficult to do so, an

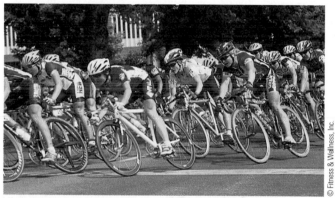

High-intensity exercise is required to achieve the high physical fitness standard (excellent category) for cardiorespiratory endurance.

alternative method of prescribing intensity of exercise, the **Rate of Perceived Exertion (RPE)** scale developed by Dr. Gunnar Borg is often used. Using the scale in Figure 6.7, a person subjectively rates the perceived exertion or difficulty of

Vigorous exercise Cardiorespiratory exercise that requires an intensity level above 60 percent of maximal capacity.

Intensity In cardiorespiratory exercise, how hard a person has to exercise to improve or maintain fitness.

Heart rate reserve (HRR) The difference between the maximal heart rate and the resting heart rate.

Cardiorespiratory training zone The recommended training intensity range, in terms of exercise heart rate, to obtain adequate cardiorespiratory endurance development.

Rate of perceived exertion (RPE) A perception scale to monitor or interpret the intensity of aerobic exercise.

FIGURE 6.7 Rate of perceived exertion (RPE) scale

6	
7	Extremely light
8	
9	Very light
10	
11	Fairly light
12	
13	Somewhat hard
14	
15	Hard
16	
17	Very Hard
18	
19	Very, very hard
20	

Source: Borg-RPE-scale® from G. Borg (1998), *Borg's perceived exertion and pain scales*. Champaign: Il: Human Kinetics. © Gunnar Borg, 1970, 1985, 1994, 1998. Used with permission of Dr. G. Borg. Instructions can be obtained from Borg Perception in Sweden.

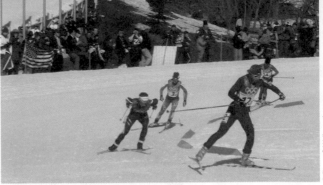

Cross-country skiing uses more oxygen and energy than most other aerobic activities.

exercise when training in the appropriate RPE value. The rating of 6 means no exertion at all and 20 means maximal exertion. Start by choosing a number that best represents or describes your level of physical activity exertion. You can then choose to slow down or increase the level of intensity of your workout to match your exercise goals.

Some individuals perceive less exertion than others when training, therefore you have to associate your own inner perception of the physical activity with the phrases given on the scale. It is your own feeling of exercise effort that is important.

More information about the RPE scale or other scales developed by Dr. Borg are available in his book, *Borg's Perceived Exertion and Pain Scales*, published in 1998 and available from Champaign, IL: Human Kinetics and in an article by Borg, G., & Borg, E., 2001 titled "A new generation of scaling methods: Level-anchored ratio scaling," in *Psycholgica*, volume 28, pages 15–45.

Whether you monitor the intensity of exercise by checking your pulse or through rate of perceived exertion, you should be aware that changes in normal exercise conditions will affect the training zone. For example, exercising on a hot, humid day or at high altitude increases the heart rate response to a given task, requiring adjustments in the intensity of your exercise.

Mode of Exercise

The **mode** of exercise that develops the cardiorespiratory system has to be aerobic in nature. Once you have established your cardiorespiratory training zone, any activity or combination of activities that will get your heart rate up to that training zone and keep it there for as long as you exercise will give you adequate development. Examples of these activities are walking, jogging, aerobics, swimming, water aerobics, cross-country skiing, rope skipping, cycling, racquetball, stair climbing, and stationary running or cycling.

Aerobic exercise has to involve the major muscle groups of the body, and it has to be rhythmic and continuous. As the amount of muscle mass involved during exercise increases, so do the demands on the cardiorespiratory system. The activity you choose should be based on your personal preferences, what you most enjoy doing, and your physical limitations. Low-impact activities greatly reduce the risk for injuries. Most injuries to beginners result from high-impact activities. General strength conditioning (see Chapter 7) is also recommended prior to initiating an aerobic exercise program for individuals who have been inactive. Strength conditioning can significantly reduce the incidence of injuries.

The amount of strength or flexibility you develop through various activities differs. In terms of cardiorespiratory development, though, the heart doesn't know whether you are walking, swimming, or cycling. All the heart knows is that it has to pump at a certain rate, and as long as that rate is in the desired range, your cardiorespiratory fitness will improve. From a health fitness point of view, training in the lower end of the cardiorespiratory zone will yield optimal health benefits. The closer the heart rate is to the higher end of the cardiorespiratory training zone, however, the greater will be the improvements in maximal oxygen uptake (high physical fitness).

Duration of Exercise

The general recommendation is that a person train between 20 and 60 minutes per session. The duration of exercise is based on how intensely a person trains. If the training is done at around 85 percent, 20 to 30 minutes are sufficient. At 50 percent intensity, the person should train between 30 and 60 minutes. As mentioned under "Intensity of Exercise" on page 174, unconditioned people and older adults should train at lower percentages; therefore, the activity should be carried out over a longer time.

Although most experts recommend 20 to 30 minutes of aerobic exercise per session, accumulating 30 minutes or more of moderate-intensity physical activity throughout the day does provide substantial health benefits.[7] Three 10-minute exercise sessions per day (separated by at least 4 hours), at approximately 70 percent of maximal heart rate, also produce training benefits.[8] Although the increases in maximal oxygen uptake with the latter program were not as large (57 percent) as those found in a group performing a continuous 30-minute bout of exercise per day, the researchers concluded that moderate-intensity physical activity, conducted for 10 minutes, three times per day, benefits the cardiorespiratory system significantly.

Results of this study are meaningful because people often mention lack of time as the reason for not taking part in an exercise program. Many think they have to exercise at least 20 continuous minutes to get any benefits at all. Even though a duration of 20 to 30 high-intensity minutes is ideal, short, intermittent exercise bouts are beneficial to the cardiorespiratory system.

From a weight management point of view, the National Institute of Medicine recommends that people accumulate 60 minutes of moderate-intensity physical activity most days of the week.[9] This recommendation is based on evidence that people who maintain healthy weight typically accumulate one hour of daily physical activity. If lack of time is a concern, you should exercise at a high intensity for 30 minutes, which can burn as many calories as 60 minutes of moderate intensity (see Low-Intensity Versus High-Intensity Exercise for Weight Loss, Chapter 5, pages 136–137).

Exercise sessions should always be preceded by a five-minute **warm-up** and be followed by a five-minute **cool-down** period (see Figure 6.6, page 175). The warm-up should consist of general calisthenics, stretching exercises, or exercising at a lower intensity level than the actual target zone. In the cool-down, the intensity of exercise is decreased gradually. Stopping abruptly causes blood to pool in the exercised body parts, diminishing the return of blood to the heart. Less blood return can cause dizziness and faintness or even bring on cardiac abnormalities.

FREQUENCY OF EXERCISE

When you start an exercise program, a **frequency** of three to five 20- to 30-minute training sessions per week is recommended to improve maximal oxygen uptake. When training is conducted more than five days a week, further improvements are minimal.

For individuals on a weight-loss program, the recommendation is 60-minute exercise sessions of low to moderate intensity, on most days of the week. Longer exercise sessions increase caloric expenditure for faster weight reduction (see Chapter 5, "Exercise: The Key to Weight Management," pages 134–137). Three 20- to 30-minute training sessions per week, on nonconsecutive days, will maintain cardiorespiratory fitness as long as the heart rate is in the appropriate target zone. Summaries of the cardiorespiratory exercise prescription guidelines according to Health Canada and the American College of Sports Medicine are provided in Figures 6.8 and 6.9, respectively. There are slight differences in the recommended guidelines. The main message is to move a little more a little more often.

Although three exercise sessions per week will maintain cardiorespiratory fitness, the importance of regular physical activity in preventing disease and enhancing quality of life has been pointed out clearly by Canadian and American organizations and researchers. They advocate at least 30 minutes of moderate-intensity physical activity almost daily. This routine has been promoted as an effective way to improve health.

If you want to enjoy better health and fitness, physical activity must be pursued on a regular basis. According to Dr. William Haskell of Stanford University: "Most of the health-related benefits of exercise are relatively short-term, so people should think of exercise as medication and take it on a daily basis."[10] Many of the benefits of exercise and activity diminish within two weeks of substantially decreased physical activity. These benefits are completely lost within two to eight months of inactivity.[11]

To sum up: Ideally, a person should engage in physical activity six to seven times per week. Based on the previous discussion, to reap both the high-

Mode Form or type of exercise.

Warm-up Starting a workout slowly.

Cool-down Tapering off an exercise session slowly.

Frequency How many times per week a person engages in an exercise session.

FIGURE 6.8 Cardiorespiratory exercise prescription guidelines (Health Canada)

Time needed depends on effort

Very Light Effort	Light Effort *60 minutes*	Moderate Effort *30-60 minutes*	Vigorous Effort *20-30 minutes*	Maximum Effort
• Strolling	• Light walking	• Brisk walking	• Aerobics	• Sprinting
• Dusting	• Volleyball	• Biking	• Jogging	• Racing
	• Easy gardening	• Raking leaves	• Hockey	
	• Stretching	• Swimming	• Basketball	
		• Dancing	• Fast swimming	
		• Water aerobics	• Fast dancing	

Range needed to stay healthy

Source: *Canada's Physical Activity Guide to Healthy Active Living* (1998), http://www.phac-aspc.gc.ca/pau-uap/fitness/pdf/handbook_e.pdf, Health Canada. Reproduced with the permission of the Minister of Public Works and Government Services Canada, 2008.

FIGURE 6.9 Cardiorespiratory exercise prescription guidelines (American College of Sports Medicine)

Activity: Aerobic (examples: walking, jogging, cycling, swimming, aerobics, racquetball, soccer, stair climbing)

Intensity: 40/50%–85% of heart rate reserve

Duration: 20–60 minutes of continuous aerobic activity

Frequency: 3 to 5 days per week

Source: Based on American College of Sports Medicine, "Position Stand: The Recommended Quantity and Quality of Exercise for Developing and Maintaining Cardiorespiratory and Muscular Fitness, and Flexibility in Healthy Adults," *Medical Science Sports Exercise*, 30 (1998): 975–991.

fitness and health-fitness benefits of exercise, a person needs to exercise a minimum of three times per week in the appropriate target zone for high fitness maintenance and three to four additional times per week in moderate-intensity activities (see Canada's Physical Activity Guide to Healthy Active Living, p. 12). Depending on the intensity of the activity, all aerobic exercise/activity sessions should last from 20 to 60 minutes.

Fitness Benefits of Aerobic Activities

The contributions of different aerobic activities to the health-related components of fitness vary.

Although an accurate assessment of the contributions to each fitness component is difficult to establish, a summary of likely benefits of several activities is provided in Table 6.10. Instead of a single rating or number, ranges are given for some of the categories. The benefits derived are based on the person's effort while participating in the activity.

The nature of the activity often dictates the potential aerobic development. For example, jogging is much more strenuous than walking. The effort during exercise also affects the amount of physiological development. During a low-impact aerobics routine, accentuating all movements (instead of just going through the motions) increases training benefits by orders of magnitude.

Table 6.10 indicates a starting fitness level for each aerobic activity. Attempting to participate in high-intensity activities without proper conditioning often leads to injuries and discouragement. Beginners should start with low-intensity activities that carry a minimum risk for injuries.

In some cases, such as high-impact aerobics and rope skipping, the risk for injuries remains high even if the participants are adequately conditioned. These activities should be supplemental only and are not recommended as the sole mode of exercise. Most exercise-related injuries occur as a result of high-impact activities, not high intensity of exercise.

Physicians who work with cardiac patients frequently use **METs** as an alternative method of prescribing exercise intensity. One **MET** represents the rate of energy expenditure at rest. METs, short for metabolic equivalents, are used to measure the intensity of physical activity and exercise in multiples of the resting metabolic rate. At an intensity level of 10 METs, the activity requires a tenfold increase in the resting energy requirement (or approximately 35 mL/kg/min). MET levels for a given activity vary according to the effort expended. The MET range for various activities is included in Table 6.10 on page 179. The harder a person exercises, the higher is the MET level.

The effectiveness of various aerobic activities in weight management is also provided in Table 6.10. As a general rule, the greater the muscle mass involved in exercise, the better the results. Rhythmic and continuous activities that involve large amounts of muscle mass are most effective in burning calories.

Higher-intensity activities increase caloric expenditure as well. Exercising longer, however, compensates for lower intensities. If carried

CRITICAL THINKING

Your friend Joe is not physically active and doesn't exercise. He manages to keep his weight down by dieting and tells you that because he feels and looks good, he doesn't need to exercise. How do you respond to your friend?

TABLE 6.10 Ratings for Selected Aerobic Activities

Activity	Recommended Starting Fitness Level[1]	Injury Risk[2]	Potential Cardiorespiratory Endurance Development (VO_2max)[3.5]	Upper Body Strength Development[3]	Lower Body Strength Development[3]	Upper Body Flexibility Development[3]	Lower Body Flexibility Development[3]	Weight Control[3]	MET Level[4,5,6]	Caloric Expenditure (cal/hour)[5,6]
Aerobics										
High-Impact Aerobics	A	H	3–4	2	4	3	2	4	6–12	450–900
Moderate-Impact Aerobics	I	M	2–4	2	3	3	2	3	6–12	450–900
Low-Impact Aerobics	B	L	2–4	2	3	3	2	3	5–10	375–750
Step Aerobics	I	M	2–4	2	3–4	3	2	3–4	5–12	375–900
Cross-Country Skiing	B	M	4–5	4	4	2	2	4–5	10–16	750–1,200
Cross-Training	I	M	3–5	2–3	3–4	2–3	1–2	3–5	6–15	450–1,125
Cycling										
Road	I	M	2–5	1	4	1	1	3	6–12	450–900
Stationary	B	L	2–4	1	4	1	1	3	6–10	450–750
Hiking	B	L	2–4	1	3	1	1	3	6–10	450–750
In-Line Skating	I	M	2–4	2	4	2	2	3	6–10	450–750
Jogging	I	M	3–5	1	3	1	1	5	6–15	450–1,125
Jogging, Deep Water	A	L	3–5	2	2	1	1	5	8–15	600–1,125
Racquet Sports	I	M	2–4	3	3	3	2	3	6–10	450–750
Rope Skipping	I	H	3–5	2	4	1	2	3–5	8–15	600–1,125
Rowing	B	L	3–5	4	2	3	1	4	8–14	600–1,050
Spinning	I	L	4–5	1	4	1	1	4	8–15	600–1,125
Stair Climbing	B	L	3–5	1	4	1	1	4–5	8–15	600–1,125
Swimming (front crawl)	B	L	3–5	4	2	3	1	3	6–12	450–900
Walking	B	L	1–2	1	2	1	1	3	4–6	300–450
Walking, Water, Chest-Deep	I	L	2–4	2	3	1	1	3	6–10	450–750
Water Aerobics	B	L	2–4	3	3	3	2	3	6–12	450–900

[1] B = Beginner, I = Intermediate, A = Advanced
[2] L = Low, M = Moderate, H = High
[3] 1 = Low, 2 = Fair, 3 = Average, 4 = Good, 5 = Excellent
[4] One MET represents the rate of energy expenditure at rest (3.5 mL/kg/min). Each additional MET is a multiple of the resting value.

For example, 5 METs represents an energy expenditure equivalent to five times the resting value, or about 17.5 mL/kg/min.
[5] Varies according to the person's effort (intensity) during exercise.
[6] Varies according to body weight.

out long enough (45 to 60 minutes five to six times per week), even walking is a good exercise mode for weight management. Additional information on a comprehensive weight management program is given in Chapter 5.

Getting Started and Adhering to a Lifetime Exercise Program

Following the guidelines provided in Lab 6D, you may proceed to initiate your cardiorespiratory endurance program. If you have not been exercising regularly, you might begin by attempting to train five or six times a week for 30 minutes at a time. You might find this discouraging, however, and drop out before getting too far, because you will probably develop some muscle soreness and

METs Short for metabolic equivalents, an alternative method of prescribing exercise intensity in multiples of the resting metabolic rate.

MET Represents the rate of resting energy expenditure at rest; MET is the equivalent of 3.5 mL/kg/min.

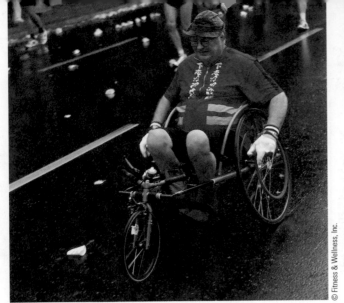

Physically challenged people can participate in and derive health and fitness benefits from a high-intensity exercise program.

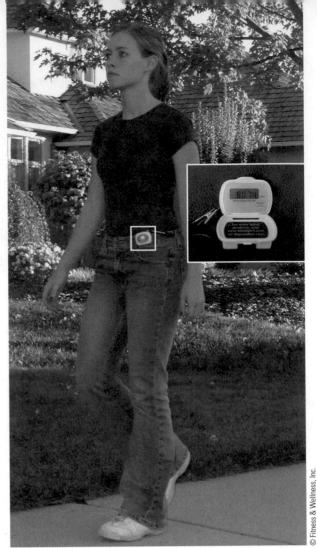

A pedometer can be used to monitor daily physical activity. The recommendation is a total of 10,000 steps daily.

stiffness and possibly incur minor injuries. Muscle soreness and stiffness and the risk for injuries can be lessened or eliminated by increasing the intensity, duration, and frequency of exercise progressively, as outlined in Lab 6D.

Once you have determined your exercise prescription, the difficult part begins: starting and sticking to a lifetime exercise program. Although you may be motivated after reading the benefits to be gained from physical activity, lifelong dedication and perseverance are necessary to reap and maintain good fitness.

The first few weeks will probably be the most difficult, but where there's a will, there's a way. Once you begin to see positive changes, it won't be as hard. Soon you will develop a habit of exercising that will be deeply satisfying and will bring about a sense of self-accomplishment. The suggestions provided in the accompanying Behaviour Modification Planning box have been used successfully to help change behaviour and adhere to a lifetime exercise program.

CRITICAL THINKING

Mary started an exercise program last year as a means to lose weight and enhance her body image. She now runs more than 12 km every day, works out regularly on stair climbers and elliptical machines, strength-trains daily, participates in step-aerobics three times per week, and plays tennis or racquetball twice a week. Will you evaluate her program and make suggestions for improvements?

A Lifetime Commitment to Fitness

The benefits of fitness can be maintained only through a regular lifetime program. Exercise is not like putting money in the bank. It doesn't help much to exercise four or five hours on Saturday and not do anything else the rest of the week. If anything, exercising only once a week is unsafe for unconditioned adults.

Even the greatest athletes on earth, if they were to stop exercising, would be, after just a few years, at a risk for disease similar to someone who never has done any physical activity. Staying with a physical fitness program long enough brings about positive physiological and psychological changes. Once you are there, you will not want to have it any other way.

The time involved in losing the benefits of exercise varies among the different components of physical fitness and also depends on the person's condition before the interruption. In regard to cardiorespiratory endurance, it has been estimated that four weeks of aerobic training are completely reversed in two consecutive weeks of physical inactivity. On the other hand, if you have been exercising regularly for months or years, two weeks of inactivity

1. Set aside a regular time for exercise. If you don't plan ahead, it is a lot easier to skip. On a weekly basis, using red ink, schedule your exercise time into your day planner. Next, hold your exercise hour "sacred." Give exercise priority equal to the most important school or business activity of the day.

   If you are too busy, attempt to accumulate 30 to 60 minutes of daily activity by doing separate 10-minute sessions throughout the day. Try reading the mail while you walk, taking stairs instead of elevators, walking the dog, or riding the stationary bike as you watch the evening news.

2. Exercise early in the day, when you will be less tired and the chances of something interfering with your workout are minimal; thus you will be less likely to skip your exercise session.

3. Select aerobic activities you enjoy. Exercise should be as much fun as your favourite hobby. If you pick an activity you don't enjoy, you will be unmotivated and less likely to keep exercising. Don't be afraid to try out a new activity, even if that means learning new skills.

4. Combine different activities. You can train by doing two or three different activities the same week. This cross-training may reduce the monotony of repeating the same activity every day. Try lifetime sports. Many endurance sports, such as racquetball, basketball, soccer, badminton, roller skating, cross-country skiing, and body surfing (paddling the board), provide a nice break from regular workouts.

5. Use the proper clothing and equipment for exercise. A poor pair of shoes, for example, can make you more prone to injury, discouraging you from the beginning.

6. Find a friend or group of friends to exercise with. Social interaction will make exercise more fulfilling. Besides, it's harder to skip if someone is waiting to go with you.

7. Set goals and share them with others. Quitting is tougher when someone else knows what you are trying to accomplish. When you reach a targeted goal, reward yourself with a new pair of shoes or a jogging suit.

8. Purchase a pedometer (step counter) and build up to 10,000 steps per day. These 10,000 steps may include all forms of daily physical activity combined. Pedometers motivate people toward activity because they track daily activity, provide feedback on activity level, and remind the participant to enhance daily activity.

9. Don't become a chronic exerciser. Overexercising can lead to chronic fatigue and injuries. Exercise should be enjoyable, and in the process you should stop and smell the roses.

10. Exercise in different places and facilities. This will add variety to your workouts.

11. Exercise to music. People who listen to fast-tempo music tend to exercise more vigorously and longer. Using headphones when exercising outdoors, however, can be dangerous. Even indoors, it is preferable not to use headphones, so that you can still be aware of your surroundings.

12. Keep a regular record of your activities. Keeping a record allows you to monitor your progress and compare it against previous months and years (see Figure 6.10, pages 184 and 185).

13. Conduct periodic assessments. Improving to a higher fitness category is often a reward in itself, and creating your own rewards is even more motivating.

14. Listen to your body. Stop exercising if you experience pain or unusual discomfort. Pain and aches are an indication of potential injury. If you do suffer an injury, do not return to your regular workouts until you are fully recovered. You may cross-train using activities that do not aggravate your injury (for instance, swimming instead of jogging).

15. If a health problem arises, see a physician. When in doubt, it's better to be safe than sorry.

will not hurt you as much as it will someone who has exercised only a few weeks. As a rule, after 48 to 72 hours of aerobic inactivity, the cardiorespiratory system starts to lose some of its capacity.

To maintain fitness, you should keep up a regular exercise program, even during vacations. If you have to interrupt your program for reasons beyond your control, you should not attempt to resume training at the same level you left off but, rather, build up gradually again.

ASSESS YOUR KNOWLEDGE

1. Cardiorespiratory endurance is determined by
   a. the amount of oxygen the body is able to utilize per minute of physical activity.
   b. the length of time it takes the heart rate to return to 120 bpm following the 2.4 km run test.
   c. the difference between the maximal heart rate and the resting heart rate.
   d. the product of the heart rate and blood pressure at rest versus exercise.
   e. the time it takes a person to reach a heart rate between 120 and 170 bpm during the Astrand–Ryhming test.

2. Which of the following is not a benefit of aerobic training?
   a. a higher maximal oxygen uptake
   b. an increase in red blood cell count
   c. a decrease in resting heart rate
   d. an increase in heart rate at a given workload
   e. an increase in functional capillaries

3. The oxygen uptake for a person with an exercise heart rate of 130, a stroke volume of 100, and an a-$\overline{v}O_2$diff of 10 is
   a. 130,000 mL/kg/min.
   b. 1300 L/min.
   c. 1.3 L/min.
   d. 130 mL/kg/min.
   e. 13 mL/kg/min.

4. The oxygen uptake in mL/kg/min for a person with a VO_2 of 2.0 L/min who weighs 60 kg is
   a. 120.
   b. 26.5.
   c. 33.3.
   d. 30.
   e. 120,000.

5. The step test estimates maximal oxygen uptake according to
   a. how long a person is able to sustain the proper step test cadence.
   b. the lowest heart rate achieved during the test.
   c. the recovery heart rate following the test.
   d. the difference between the maximal heart rate achieved and the resting heart rate.
   e. the exercise heart rate and the total stepping time.

6. An "excellent" cardiorespiratory fitness rating, in mL/kg/min, for young male adults is about
   a. 10.
   b. 20.
   c. 30.
   d. 40.
   e. 50.

7. A person exercising at 2 L/min burns approximately _____ Calories per minute of physical activity.
   a. 2
   b. 5
   c. 10
   d. 12
   e. 20

8. The optimal or high-intensity cardiorespiratory training zone for a 22-year-old individual with a resting heart rate of 68 bpm is
   a. 120 to 148.
   b. 132 to 156.
   c. 138 to 164.
   d. 146 to 179.
   e. 154 to 188.

9. Which of the following activities does not contribute to the development of cardiorespiratory endurance?
   a. low-impact aerobics
   b. jogging
   c. 400-metre dash
   d. racquetball
   e. All of these activities contribute to its development.

10. The recommended duration for each cardiorespiratory training session is
    a. 10 to 20 minutes.
    b. 15 to 30 minutes.
    c. 20 to 60 minutes.
    d. 45 to 70 minutes.
    e. 60 to 120 minutes.

Correct answers can be found at the back of the book.

MEDIA MENU

INTERNET CONNECTIONS

■ Canadian Society for Exercise Physiology (CSEP). CSEP is a voluntary organization composed of professionals interested and involved in the scientific study of exercise physiology, exercise biochemistry, fitness, and health.

   http://www.csep.ca

■ The Canadian Health Network (CHN). This national, bilingual health promotion program is designed to help Canadians find information on how to stay healthy and prevent disease. The network of health information providers includes the Public Health Agency of Canada, Health Canada and national and provincial/territorial non-profit organizations, as well as universities, hospitals, libraries, and community organizations.

   http://www.canadian-health-network.ca

■ The Healthy Living Unit. This organization has the lead responsibility within the Public Health Agency of Canada for delivering on the federal government's role in physical activity. The work of the unit is based on an approach to partnerships that is multi-sectoral, multi-level, and multi-disciplinary. Its mission is to improve the health and well-being of Canadians through regular physical activity.

   http://www.phac-aspc.gc.ca/
   pau-uap/fitness/index.html

Notes

1. H. Atkinson, "Exercise for Longer Life: The Physician's Perspective," *HealthNews* 7:3 (1997), 3.

2. R. B. O'Hara et al., "Increased Volume Resistance Training: Effects upon Predicted Aerobic Fitness in a Select Group of Air Force Men," *ACSM's Health and Fitness Journal* 8, no. 4 (2004): 16–25.

3. R. K. Dishman, "Prescribing Exercise Intensity for Healthy Adults Using Perceived Exertion," *Medicine and Science in Sports and Exercise* 26 (1994): 1087–1094.

4. American College of Sports Medicine, "Position Stand: The Recommended Quantity and Quality of Exercise for Developing and Maintaining Cardiorespiratory and Muscular Fitness, and Flexibility in Healthy Adults," *Medicine and Science in Sports and Exercise* 30 (1998): 975–991.

5. American College of Sports Medicine, *Guidelines for Exercise Testing and Prescription* (Philadelphia: Lippincott Williams & Wilkins, 2000).

6. American College of Sports Medicine, *Guidelines for Exercise Testing and Prescription* (Philadelphia: Lippincott Williams & Wilkins, 2000).

7. S. Blair, "Surgeon General's Report on Physical Fitness: The Inside Story," *ACSM's Health & Fitness Journal* 1 (1997): 14–18.

8. R. F. DeBusk, U. Stenestrand, M. Sheehan, and W. L. Haskell, "Training Effects of Long Versus Short Bouts of Exercise in Healthy Subjects," *American Journal of Cardiology* 65 (1990): 1010–1013.

9. National Academy of Sciences, Institute of Medicine, *Dietary Reference Intakes for Energy, Carbohydrates, Fiber, Fat, Protein and Amino Acids (Macronutrients)*. Washington, DC: National Academy Press, 2002.

10. "Scanning Sports," *Physician and Sportsmedicine* 21, no. 11 (1993): 34.

11. American College of Sports Medicine, *Guidelines for Exercise Testing and Prescription* (Philadelphia: Lippincott Williams & Wilkins, 2000).

Suggested Readings

ACSM's Guidelines for Exercise Testing and Prescription. Philadelphia: Lippincott Williams & Wilkins, 2000.

ACSM's Resource Manual for Guidelines for Exercise Testing and Prescription. Philadelphia: Lippincott Williams & Wilkins, 2001.

Akalan, C., L. Kravitz, and R. Robergs. "VO$_2$max: Essentials of the Most Widely Used Test in Exercise Physiology." *ACSM's Health & Fitness Journal* 8, no. 3 (2004): 5–9.

Borg, G. "Perceived Exertion: A Note on History and Methods." *Medicine and Science in Sports and Exercise* 5 (1993): 90–93.

Brien S. E., P. T. Katzmarzyk, C. L. Craig, and L. Gauvin. "Physical Activity, Cardiorespiratory Fitness and Body Mass Index as Predictors of Substantial Weight Gain and Obesity: the Canadian Physical Activity Longitudinal Study." *Canadian Journal of Public Health* 98(2007): 121–24.

Hoeger, W. W. K., and S. A. Hoeger. *Lifetime Fitness & Wellness: A Personalized Program*. Belmont, CA: Wadsworth/ Thomson Learning, 2005.

Karvonen, M. J., E. Kentala, and O. Mustala. "The Effects of Training on the Heart Rate, a Longitudinal Study." *Annales Medicinae Experimetalis et Biologiae Fenniae* 35 (1957): 307–315.

McArdle, W. D., F. I. Katch, and V. L. Katch. *Exercise Physiology: Energy, Nutrition, and Human Performance*. Philadelphia: Lippincott Williams & Wilkins, 2004.

Nieman, D. C. *Exercise Testing and Prescription: A Health-Related Approach*. Boston: McGraw–Hill, 2003.

Warburton D. E., C. W. Nicol, S. S. Bredin. Health Benefits of Physical Activity: The Evidence. *Canadian Medical Association Journal* 174(2006): 801–809.

Wilmore, J. H., and D. L. Costill. *Physiology of Sport and Exercise*. Champaign, IL: Human Kinetics, 2004.

FIGURE 6.10 Cardiorespiratory exercise record form

Month _____

Date	Body Weight	Exercise Heart Rate	Type of Exercise	Distance In Kilometres	Time Hrs/Min	RPE*
1						
2						
3						
4						
5						
6						
7						
8						
9						
10						
11						
12						
13						
14						
15						
16						
17						
18						
19						
20						
21						
22						
23						
24						
25						
26						
27						
28						
29						
30						
31						
			Total			

*Rate of perceived exertion.

Month _____

Date	Body Weight	Exercise Heart Rate	Type of Exercise	Distance In Kilometres	Time Hrs/Min	RPE*
1						
2						
3						
4						
5						
6						
7						
8						
9						
10						
11						
12						
13						
14						
15						
16						
17						
18						
19						
20						
21						
22						
23						
24						
25						
26						
27						
28						
29						
30						
31						
			Total			

*Rate of perceived exertion.

FIGURE 6.10 Cardiorespiratory exercise record form

Month _____

Date	Body Weight	Exercise Heart Rate	Type of Exercise	Distance In Kilometres	Time Hrs/Min	RPE*
1						
2						
3						
4						
5						
6						
7						
8						
9						
10						
11						
12						
13						
14						
15						
16						
17						
18						
19						
20						
21						
22						
23						
24						
25						
26						
27						
28						
29						
30						
31						
Total						

*Rate of perceived exertion.

Month _____

Date	Body Weight	Exercise Heart Rate	Type of Exercise	Distance In Kilometres	Time Hrs/Min	RPE*
1						
2						
3						
4						
5						
6						
7						
8						
9						
10						
11						
12						
13						
14						
15						
16						
17						
18						
19						
20						
21						
22						
23						
24						
25						
26						
27						
28						
29						
30						
31						
Total						

*Rate of perceived exertion.

Lab 6D

CARDIORESPIRATORY EXERCISE PRESCRIPTION

Name: _____   Date: _____   Grade: _____

Instructor: _____   Course: _____   Section: _____

Necessary Lab Equipment

None required.

Objective

To write your own cardiorespiratory exercise prescription.

I. Intensity of Exercise

1. Estimate your own maximal heart rate (MHR)

   MHR = 220 minus age (220 − age)

   MHR = 220 − _____ = _____ bpm

2. Resting Heart Rate (RHR) = _____ bpm

3. Heart Rate Reserve (HRR) = MHR − RHR

   HRR = _____ − _____ = _____ beats

4. Training Intensities (TI) = HRR × TI + RHR

   40 Percent TI = _____ × .40 + _____ = _____ bpm

   50 Percent TI = _____ × .50 + _____ − _____ bpm

   60 percent TI = _____ × .60 + _____ = _____ bpm

   85 Percent TI − _____ × .85 + _____ = _____ bpm

5. Cardiorespiratory Training Zone. The optimum cardiorespiratory training zone is found between the 60 percent and 85 percent training intensities. Older adults, individuals who have been physically inactive or are in the poor or fair cardiorespiratory fitness categories, however, should follow a 40 percent to 50 percent training intensity during the first few weeks of the exercise program.

   Cardiorespiratory Training Zone: _____ (60% TI) to _____ (85% TI)

   Rate of Perceived Exertion (see Figure 6.7, page 176): _____ to _____

II. Mode of Exercise

Select any activity or combination of activities that you enjoy doing. The activity has to be continuous in nature and must get your heart rate up to the cardiorespiratory training zone and keep it there for as long as you exercise. Indicate your preferred mode(s) of exercise:

1. _____   2. _____   3. _____

4. _____   5. _____   6. _____

III. Cardiorespiratory Exercise Program

The following is your weekly program for development of cardiorespiratory endurance. If you are in the average, good, or excellent fitness category, you may start at week 5. After completing this 12-week program, for you to maintain your fitness level, you should exercise in the 60 percent to 85 percent training zone for about 20 to 30 minutes, a minimum of three times per week, on non-consecutive days. You should also recompute your target zone periodically because you will experience a significant reduction in resting heart rate with aerobic training (approximately 10 to 20 beats in about 8 to 12 weeks).

Week	Duration (min)	Frequency	Training Intensity	Heart Rate (bpm)		10-Sec Pulse Count*		
1	15	3	Between 40% and 50%		to		to	beats
2	15	4	Between 40% and 50%					
3	20	4	Between 40% and 50%					
4	20	5	Between 40% and 50%					
5	20	4	Between 50% and 60%		to		to	beats
6	20	5	Between 50% and 60%					
7	30	4	Between 50% and 60%					
8	30	5	Between 50% and 60%					
9	30	4	Between 60% and 85%		to		to	beats
10	30	5	Between 60% and 85%					
11	30–40	5	Between 60% and 85%					
12	30–40	5	Between 60% and 85%					

*Fill out your own 10-second pulse count under this column.

IV. Briefly State Your Experiences and Feelings Regarding Aerobic Exercise:

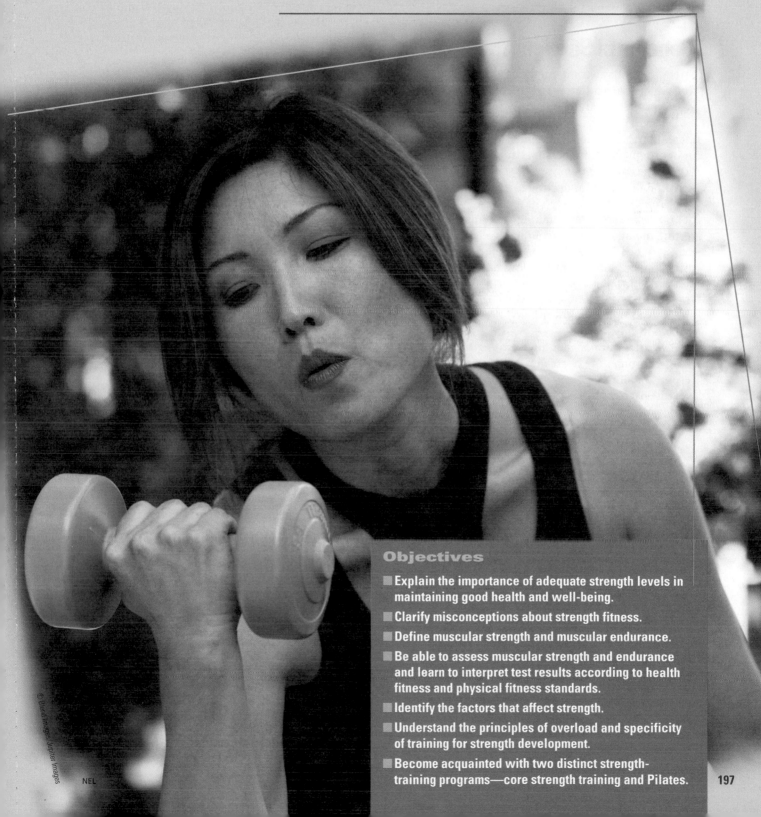

Chapter **7**

Muscular Strength and Endurance

Objectives

- Explain the importance of adequate strength levels in maintaining good health and well-being.
- Clarify misconceptions about strength fitness.
- Define muscular strength and muscular endurance.
- Be able to assess muscular strength and endurance and learn to interpret test results according to health fitness and physical fitness standards.
- Identify the factors that affect strength.
- Understand the principles of overload and specificity of training for strength development.
- Become acquainted with two distinct strength-training programs—core strength training and Pilates.

The benefits of **strength training** (also referred to as resistance training) to enhance health and well-being are well-documented. Some people, nonetheless, have the impression that strength is necessary only for highly trained athletes, fitness enthusiasts, and individuals who have jobs that require heavy muscular work. In fact, a well-planned strength-training program leads to increased muscle strength and endurance, muscle tone, tendon and ligament strength, and bone density—all of which help to improve functional physical capacity.

Benefits of Strength Training

Strength is a basic component of fitness and wellness and is crucial for optimal performance in daily activities such as sitting, walking, running, lifting and carrying objects, doing housework, and enjoying recreational activities. Strength also is of great value in improving posture, personal appearance, and self-image; in developing sports skills; in promoting joint stability; and in meeting certain emergencies in life. From a health standpoint, increasing strength helps to increase or maintain muscle and a higher resting metabolic rate, encourages weight loss and maintenance, lessens the risk for injury, prevents osteoporosis, reduces chronic low-back pain, alleviates arthritic pain, aids in childbearing, improves cholesterol levels, promotes psychological well-being, and may also help to lower blood pressure and control blood sugar.

An important adaptation to strength training is that, with time, the heart rate and blood pressure response to lifting a heavy resistance (that is, a weight) decreases. This adaptation reduces the demands on the cardiovascular system when performing activities such as carrying a child, the groceries, or a suitcase.

Regular strength training also can help control blood sugar. Much of the blood glucose from food consumption goes to the muscles, where it is stored as glycogen. When muscles are not used, muscle cells become insulin-resistant and glucose cannot enter the cells, thus increasing the risk for diabetes. Following 16 weeks of strength training, a group of diabetic men and women improved their blood sugar control, gained strength, increased lean body mass, lost body fat, and lowered blood pressure.[1]

Muscular Strength and Aging

In the older adult population, muscular strength may be the most important health-related component of physical fitness. Though proper cardiorespiratory endurance is necessary to help maintain a healthy heart, good strength contributes more to independent living than any other fitness component. Older adults with good strength levels can successfully perform most **activities of daily living**.

Sarcopenia, or loss of lean body mass, strength, and function, is a common occurrence as people age. How much of this loss is related to the aging process itself or to actual physical inactivity and faulty nutrition is unknown. And while thinning of the bones from osteoporosis renders the bones prone to fractures, the gradual loss of muscle mass and ensuing frailty is what leads to falls and subsequent loss of function in older adults. Strength training helps to slow the age-related loss of muscle function. Protein deficiency, seen in some older adults, also contributes to loss of lean tissue.

More than anything else, older adults want to enjoy good health and to function independently. Many of them, however, are confined to nursing homes because they lack sufficient strength to move about. They cannot walk very far, and many have to be helped in and out of beds, chairs, and tubs.

A strength-training program can enhance quality of life tremendously, and nearly everyone can benefit from it. Only people with advanced heart disease are advised to refrain from strength training. Inactive adults between the ages of 56 and 86 who participated in a 12-week strength-training program increased their lean body mass by about 1.5 kg, lost about 2 kg of fat, and increased their resting metabolic rate by almost 7 percent.[2] In other research, leg strength improved by as much as 200 percent in previously inactive adults over age 90.[3] As strength improves, so does the ability to move about, the capacity for independent living, and enjoyment of life during the "golden years." More specifically, good strength enhances quality of life in the following ways:

- It improves balance and restores mobility.
- It makes lifting and reaching easier.
- It decreases the risk for injuries and falls.
- It stresses the bones and preserves bone mineral density, thus decreasing the risk for osteoporosis.

The Relationship Between Strength and Metabolism

Perhaps one of the most significant benefits of maintaining a good strength level is its relationship to human **metabolism**. A primary outcome of a strength-training program is an increase in muscle mass or size (lean body mass), known as muscle **hypertrophy**.

Muscle tissue uses energy even at rest. By contrast, fatty tissue uses little energy and may be considered metabolically inert from the standpoint of caloric use (that is, your body expends calories to maintain muscle and very few calories to maintain fat). As muscle size increases, so does **resting metabolism**. Even small increases in muscle mass may improve resting metabolism.

Each additional 0.45 kg of muscle tissue increases resting metabolism by as much as 35 Calories per day.[4] All other factors being equal, if two individuals both weigh 70 kg but have different amounts of muscle mass, the one with more muscle mass will have a higher resting metabolic rate, allowing this person to ingest more calories (which will be used to maintain the muscle tissue, not to create fat). Briefly, the higher your metabolic rate, the more you can eat without gaining fat.

Effect of Aging on Metabolism

Loss of lean tissue is also thought to be the main reason for the decrease in metabolism as people grow older. Contrary to some beliefs, metabolism does not have to slow down significantly with aging. It is not so much that metabolism slows down. It's that we slow down.

Lean body mass decreases with sedentary living, which, in turn, slows down the resting metabolic rate. If people continue eating at the same rate, body fat increases. Daily requirements decrease an average of 360 Calories between age 26 and age 60.[5] Hence, participating in a strength-training program is important in preventing and reducing excess body fat.

Gender Differences

One of the most common misconceptions about physical fitness concerns women in strength training. Because of the increase in muscle mass typically seen in men, some women think that a strength-training program will result in their developing large musculature. Even though the quality of muscle in men and women is the same, endocrinological differences do not allow women to achieve the same amount of muscle hypertrophy (size) as men. Men also have more muscle fibres and, because of the sex-specific male hormones, each individual fibre has more potential for hypertrophy. On the average, following six months of training, women can achieve up to a 50 percent increase in strength but only a 10 percent increase in muscle size.

The idea that strength training allows women to develop muscle hypertrophy to the same extent as men do is as false as the notion that playing basketball will turn women into giants. Masculinity and femininity are established by genetic inheritance, not by the amount of physical activity. Variations in the extent of masculinity and femininity are determined by individual differences in hormonal secretions of androgen, testosterone, estrogen, and progesterone. Women with a bigger-than-average build often are

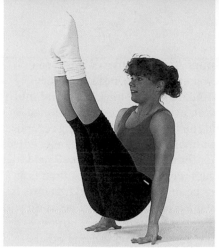

A female gymnast performs a strength skill.

inclined to participate in sports because of their natural physical advantage. As a result, many people have associated women's participation in sports and strength training with large muscle size.

As the number of females who participate in sports increased steadily during the last few years, the myth of strength training in women leading to large increases in muscle size abated somewhat. For example, per kilogram of body weight, female gymnasts are among the strongest athletes in the world. These athletes engage regularly in serious strength-training programs. Yet female gymnasts have some of the most well-toned and graceful figures of all women.

In recent years, improved body appearance has become the rule rather than the exception for women who participate in strength-training programs. Some of the most attractive female movie stars also train with weights to further improve their personal image.

Nonetheless, you may ask, "If weight training does not masculinize women, why do so many women body builders develop such heavy musculature?" In the sport of body building, the athletes follow intense training routines consisting of two or more hours of constant weight lifting with short rest intervals between sets. Many body-building training routines call for back-to-back exercises using the

Strength training A program designed to improve muscular strength and/or endurance through a series of resistance (weight) training exercises that overload the muscular system and cause physiological development.

Activities of daily living Everyday behaviours that people normally do to function in life (cross the street, carry groceries, lift objects, do laundry, sweep floors).

Sarcopenia Age-related loss of lean body mass, strength, and function.

Metabolism All energy and material transformations that occur within living cells; necessary to sustain life.

Hypertrophy An increase in the size of the cell, as in muscle hypertrophy.

Resting metabolism Amount of energy (expressed in millilitres of oxygen per minute or total calories per day) an individual requires during resting conditions to sustain proper body function.

same muscle groups. The objective of this type of training is to pump extra blood into the muscles. This additional fluid makes the muscles appear much bigger than they do in a resting condition. Based on the intensity and the length of the training session, the muscles can remain filled with blood, appearing measurably larger for several hours after completing the training session. Performing such routines is a common practice before competitions. Therefore, in real life, these women are not as muscular as they seem when they are participating in a contest.

In the sport of body building (among others), a big point of controversy is the use of **anabolic steroids** and human growth hormones. These hormones, however, produce detrimental and undesirable side effects in women (such as hypertension, fluid retention, decreased breast size, deepening of the voice, whiskers, and other atypical body hair growth), which some women deem tolerable. Anabolic steroid use in general—except for medical reasons and when carefully monitored by a physician—can lead to serious health consequences.

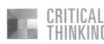

CRITICAL THINKING

What role should strength training have in a fitness program? Should people be motivated for the health fitness benefits, or should they participate to enhance their body image? What are your feelings about individuals (male or female) with large body musculature?

Anabolic steroid use among female body builders and female track and field athletes around the world does occur. These athletes use anabolic steroids to remain competitive at the highest level. During the 2004 Olympic Games in Athens, Greece, two women shot putters, including the gold medal winner (later stripped of the medal), were expelled from the games for steroid use. Women who take steroids undoubtedly will build heavy musculature and, if they take the steroids long enough, the steroids will produce masculinizing effects.

As a result, the International Federation of Body Building instituted a mandatory steroid-testing program for females participating in the Miss Olympia contest. Canadian athletes who are competing on a national or international stage are subjected to testing by the Canadian Centre for Ethics in Sport (CCES), which has adopted the World Anti-Doping code developed in 2000. The CCES has the only International Olympic Committee (IOC) accredited lab in Canada. It is now the athlete's responsibility to be aware of and comply with the anti-doping rules of each organization they belong to.[6]

The Canadian Body Building Federation (CBBF) also has adopted a doping control policy that follows the CCES policy. The CBBF accesses the CCES lab for drug testing of competitors.[7] When drugs are not used to promote development,

SELECTED DETRIMENTAL EFFECTS OF ANABOLIC STEROID USE

- Liver tumours
- Hepatitis
- Hypertension
- Reduction of high-density lipoprotein (HDL) cholesterol
- Elevation of low-density lipoprotein (LDL) cholesterol
- Hyperinsulinism
- Impaired pituitary function
- Impaired thyroid function
- Mood swings
- Aggressive behaviour
- Increased irritability
- Acne
- Fluid retention
- Decreased libido
- HIV infection (via injectable steroids)
- Prostate problems (men)
- Testicular atrophy (men)
- Reduced sperm count (men)
- Clitoral enlargement (women)
- Decreased breast size (women)
- Increased body and facial hair (nonreversible in women)
- Deepening of the voice (nonreversible in women)

improved body image is the rule rather than the exception among females who participate in body building, strength training, or sports in general.

Changes in Body Composition

A benefit of strength training, accentuated even more when combined with aerobic exercise, is a decrease in adipose or fatty tissue around muscle fibres themselves. This decrease is often greater than the amount of muscle hypertrophy (see Figure 7.1). Therefore, losing centimetres but not body weight is common.

Because muscle tissue is more dense than fatty tissue (and despite the fact that centimetres are lost during a combined strength-training and aerobic program), people, especially women, often become discouraged because they cannot see the results readily on the scale. They can offset this discouragement by determining body composition regularly to monitor changes in percent body fat rather than simply measuring changes in total body weight (see Chapter 4).

Assessment of Muscular Strength and Endurance

Although muscular strength and endurance are interrelated, they do differ. **Muscular strength** is the ability to exert maximum force against resistance. **Muscular endurance** is the ability of a muscle to exert submaximal force repeatedly over time.

FIGURE 7.1 Changes in body composition as a result of a combined aerobic and strength-training program

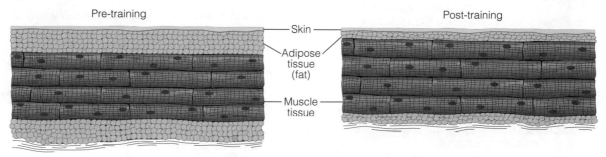

Pre-training   Post-training

Skin — Adipose tissue (fat) — Muscle tissue

Muscular endurance (also referred to as "localized muscular endurance") depends to a large extent on muscular strength. Weak muscles cannot repeat an action several times or sustain it. Based upon these principles, strength tests and training programs have been designed to measure and develop absolute muscular strength, muscular endurance, or a combination of the two.

Muscular strength is usually determined by the maximal amount of resistance (weight)—**one repetition maximum**, or **1 RM**—an individual is able to lift in a single effort. Although this assessment yields a good measure of absolute strength, it does require considerable time, because the 1 RM is determined through trial and error. For example, strength of the chest muscles is frequently measured through the bench press exercise. If an individual has not trained with weights, he may try 50 kg and lift this resistance quite easily. After adding 20 kg, he fails to lift the resistance. The resistance then is decreased by 5 or 10 kg. Finally, after several trials, the 1 RM is established.

Using this method, a true 1 RM might be difficult to obtain the first time an individual is tested, because fatigue becomes a factor. By the time the 1 RM is established, the person has already made several maximal or near-maximal attempts.

Muscular endurance is typically established by the number of repetitions an individual can perform against a submaximal resistance or by the length of time a given contraction can be sustained. For example: How many push-ups can an individual do? Or how many times can a 15 kg resistance be lifted? Or how long can a person hold a chin-up?

If time is a factor and only one test item can be done, the Hand Grip Test, described in Figure 7.2, is commonly used to assess strength. This test, though, provides only a weak correlation with overall body strength. Two additional strength tests are provided in Figures 7.3 and 7.4. Lab 7A also provides the opportunity to assess your own level of muscular strength or endurance with all three tests. You may

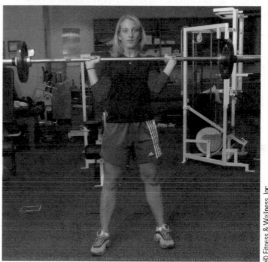

The maximal amount of resistance that an individual is able to lift in one single effort (one repetition maximum or 1 RM) is a measure of absolute strength.

take one or more of these tests according to your time and the facilities available.

Muscular strength and muscular endurance are both highly specific. A high degree of strength or endurance in one body part does not necessarily indicate similarity in other parts. Accordingly, exercises for the strength tests were selected to include the upper body, lower body, and abdominal regions.

In strength testing, several body sites should be assessed. Because different body parts have different

Anabolic steroids Synthetic versions of the male sex hormone testosterone, which promotes muscle development and hypertrophy.

Muscular strength The ability of a muscle to exert maximum force against resistance (for example, 1 repetition maximum [or 1 RM] of the bench press exercise).

Muscular endurance The ability of a muscle to exert submaximal force repeatedly over time.

One repetition maximum (1 RM) The maximum amount of resistance an individual is able to lift in a single effort.

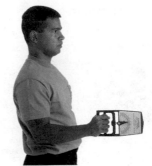

The Hand Grip tests strength.

strength levels, no single strength test provides a good assessment of overall body strength. As a minimum, a strength profile should include the upper body, the lower body, and the abdominal muscles.

Before taking the strength test, you should become familiar with the procedures for the respective tests. For safety reasons, always take at least one friend with you whenever you train with weights or undertake any type of strength assessment. Also, these are different tests, so to make valid comparisons, the same test should be used for pre- and post-assessments. The following are your options.

Muscular Strength: Hand Grip Test

As indicated previously, when time is a factor, the Hand Grip Test can be used to provide a rough estimate of strength. Unlike the next two tests, this is an isometric (static contraction, discussed later in the chapter) test. If the proper grip is used, no finger motion or body movement is visible during the test. The test procedure is given in Figure 7.2, and percentile ranks based on your results are provided in Table 7.1. You can record the results of this test in Lab 7A.

Changes in strength may be more difficult to evaluate with this test. Most strength-training programs are dynamic in nature (body segments are moved through a range of motion, discussed later in the chapter), whereas this test provides an isometric assessment. Further, grip strength exercises are seldom used in strength training, and increases in strength are specific to the body parts exercised. This test, however, also can be used to supplement the following strength tests.

Muscular Endurance Test

Three exercises were selected to assess the endurance of the upper body, lower body, and mid-body muscle groups (see Figure 7.3). The advantage of this test is that it does not require strength-training equipment—only a stopwatch, a metronome,

FIGURE 7.2 Procedure for the Hand Grip Strength Test

1. Adjust the width of the dynamometer* so the middle bones of your fingers rest on the distant end of the dynamometer grip.
2. Use your dominant hand for this test. Place your elbow at a 90° angle and about 5 cm away from the body.

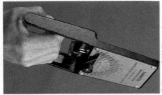

3. Now grip as hard as you can for a few seconds. Do not move any other body part as you perform the test (do not flex or extend the elbow, do not move the elbow away or toward the body, and do not lean forward or backward during the test).
4. Record the dynamometer reading in kilograms.
5. Three trials are allowed for this test. Use the highest reading for your final test score. Look up your percentile rank for this test in Table 7.1.
6. Based on your percentile rank, obtain the hand grip strength fitness category according to the following guidelines:

Percentile Rank	Fitness Category
≥90	Excellent
70–80	Good
50–60	Average
30–40	Fair
≤20	Poor

* A Lafayette model 78010 dynamometer is recommended for this test from NexGen Ergonomics Inc., 6600 Trans Canada Highway, Suite 750, Pointe Claire (Montreal), Quebec; tel.: (514) 685-8593; fax: (514) 685-8687.

TABLE 7.1 Scoring Table for Hand Grip Strength Test

Percentile Rank	Men	Women
99	153	101
95	145	94
90	141	91
80	139	86
70	132	80
60	124	78
50	122	74
40	114	71
30	110	66
20	100	64
10	91	60
5	76	58

▓ High physical fitness standard
░ Health fitness standard

FIGURE 7.3 Muscular Endurance Test

Three exercises are conducted on this test: bench jumps, modified dips (men) or modified push-ups (women), and bent-leg curl-ups or abdominal crunches. All exercises should be conducted with the aid of a partner. The correct procedure for performing each exercise is as follows:

Bench-jump. Using a bench or gymnasium bleacher 40 cm high, attempt to jump up onto and down off of the bench as many times as possible in 1 minute. If you cannot jump the full minute, you may step up and down. A repetition is counted each time both feet return to the floor.

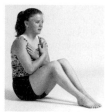

Modified dip. Men only: Using a bench or gymnasium bleacher, place the hands on the bench with the fingers pointing forward. Have a partner hold your feet in front of you. Bend the hips at approximately 90° (you also may use three sturdy chairs: Put your hands on two chairs placed by the sides of your body and place your feet on the third chair in front of you). Lower your body by flexing the elbows until they reach a 90° angle, then return to the starting position (also see Exercise 6, page 223). Perform the repetitions to a two-step cadence (down-up) regulated with a metronome set at 56 beats per minute. Perform as many continuous repetitions as possible. Do not count any more repetitions if you fail to follow the metronome cadence.

Figure 7.3a Bench jump

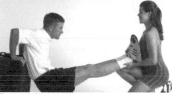

Figure 7.3b Modified dip

Modified push-up. Women: Lie down on the floor (face down), bend the knees (feet up in the air), and place the hands on the floor by the shoulders with the fingers pointing forward. The lower body will be supported at the knees (as opposed to the feet) throughout the test (see Figure 7.3c). The chest must touch the floor on each repetition. As with the modified-dip exercise (above), perform the repetitions to a two-step cadence (up-down) regulated with a metronome set at 56 beats per minute. Perform as many continuous repetitions as possible. Do not count any more repetitions if you fail to follow the metronome cadence.

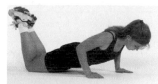

Figure 7.3c Modified push-up

Bent-leg curl-up. Lie down on the floor (face up) and bend both legs at the knees at approximately 100°. The feet should be on the floor, and you must hold them in place yourself throughout the test. Cross the arms in front of the chest, each hand on the opposite shoulder. Now raise the head off the floor, placing the chin against the chest. This is the starting and finishing position for each curl-up (see Figure 7.3d). **The back of the head may not come in contact with the floor, the hands cannot be removed from the shoulders, nor may the feet or hips be raised off the floor at any time during the test. The test is terminated if any of these four conditions occur.**

When you curl up, the upper body must come to an upright position before going back down (see Figure 7.3e). The repetitions are performed to a two-step cadence (up-down)

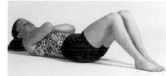

Figure 7.3d Bent-leg curl-up

regulated with the metronome set at 40 beats per minute. For this exercise, you should allow a brief practice period of 5 to 10 seconds to familiarize yourself with the cadence (the *up* movement is initiated with the first beat, then you must wait for the next beat to initiate the *down* movement; one repetition is accomplished every two beats of the metronome). Count as many repetitions as you are able to perform following the proper cadence. The test is also terminated if you fail to maintain the appropriate cadence or if you accomplish 100 repetitions. Have your partner check the angle at the knees throughout the test to make sure to maintain the 100° angle as close as possible.

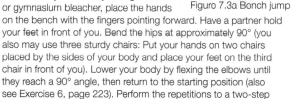

Figure 7.3e Bent-leg curl-up

Abdominal crunch. This test is recommended only for individuals who are unable to perform the bent-leg curl-up test because of susceptibility to low-back injury. Exercise form must be carefully monitored during the test. Several authors and researchers have indicated that proper form during this test is extremely difficult to control. Subjects often slide their bodies, bend their elbows, or shrug their shoulders during the test. Such actions facilitate the performance of the test and misrepresent the actual test results. Biomechanical factors also limit the ability to perform this test. Further, lack of spinal flexibility keeps some individuals from being able to move the full 8 cm range of motion. Others are unable to keep their heels on the floor during the test. The validity of this test as an effective measure of abdominal strength or abdominal endurance has also been questioned through research.

Tape a 8 × 75 cm strip of cardboard onto the floor. Lie down on the floor in a supine position (face up) with the knees bent at approximately 100° and the legs slightly apart. The feet should be on the floor, and you must hold them in place yourself throughout the test. Straighten out your arms and place them on the floor alongside the trunk with the palms down and the fingers fully extended. The fingertips of both hands should barely touch the closest edge of the cardboard (see Figure 7.3f). Bring the head off the floor until the chin is 3 to 5 cm away from your chest. Keep the head in this position during the entire test (do not move the head by flexing or extending the neck). You are now ready to begin the test.

Perform the repetitions to a two-step cadence (up-down) regulated with a metronome set at 60 beats per minute. As you curl up, slide the fingers over the cardboard until the fingertips reach the far edge (8 cm) of the board (see Figure 7.3g), then return to the starting position.

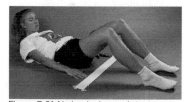

Figure 7.3f Abdominal crunch test

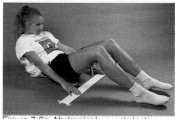

Figure 7.3g Abdominal crunch test

Allow a brief practice period of 5 to 10 seconds to familiarize yourself with the cadence. Initiate the *up* movement with the first beat and the *down* movement with the next beat. Accomplish one repetition every two beats of the metronome. Count as many repetitions as you are able to perform following the proper cadence. You may not count a repetition if the fingertips fail to reach the distant edge of the cardboard.

Terminate the test if you (a) fail to maintain the appropriate cadence, (b) bend the elbows, (c) shrug the shoulders, (d) slide

(Continued)

FIGURE 7.3 (Continued)

the body, (e) lift heels off the floor, (f) raise the chin off the chest, (g) accomplish 100 repetitions, or (h) no longer can perform the test. Have your partner check the angle at the knees throughout the test to make sure that the 100° angle is maintained as closely as possible.

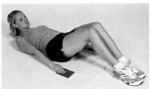
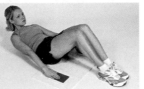

Figure 7.3h   Figure 7.3i
Abdominal crunch test performed with a Crunch-Ster Curl-Up Tester.

For this test you may also use a Crunch-Ster Curl-Up Tester, available from Novel Products.* An illustration of the test performed with this equipment is provided in Figures 7.3h and 7.3i.

According to the results, look up your percentile rank for each exercise in the far left column of Table 7.2 and determine your

muscular endurance fitness category according to the following classification:

Average Score	Fitness Category	Points
≥90	Excellent	5
70–80	Good	4
50–60	Average	3
30–40	Fair	2
≤20	Poor	1

Look up the number of points assigned for each fitness category above. Total the number of points and determine your overall strength endurance fitness category according to the following ratings:

Total Points	Strength Endurance Category
≥13	Excellent
10–12	Good
7–9	Average
4–6	Fair
≤3	Poor

*Novel Products, Inc. Figure Finder Collection, P.O. Box 408, Rockton, IL U.S.A. 61072-0408. 1-800-323-5143, Fax 815-624-4866.

TABLE 7.2   Muscular Endurance Scoring Table

Percentile Rank	Men				Women			
	Bench Jumps	Modified Dips	Bent-Leg Curl-Ups	Abdominal Crunches	Bench Jumps	Modified Push-ups	Bent-Leg Curl-Ups	Abdominal Crunches
99	66	54	100	100	58	95	100	100
95	63	50	81	100	54	70	100	100
90	62	38	65	100	52	50	97	69
80	58	32	51	66	48	41	77	49
70	57	30	44	45	44	38	57	37
60	56	27	31	38	42	33	45	34
50	54	26	28	33	39	30	37	31
40	51	23	25	29	38	28	28	27
30	48	20	22	26	36	25	22	24
20	47	17	17	22	32	21	17	21
10	40	11	10	18	28	18	9	15
5	34	7	3	16	26	15	4	0

▇ High physical fitness standard   ▨ Health fitness standard

a bench or gymnasium bleacher 40 cm high, a cardboard strip 8 cm wide by 75 cm long, and a partner. A percentile rank is given for each exercise according to the number of repetitions performed (see Table 7.2). An overall endurance rating can be obtained by totalling the number of points obtained on each exercise. Record the results of this test in Lab 7A.

Muscular Strength and Endurance Test

In this test you will lift a submaximal resistance as many times as possible using the six strength-training exercises listed in Figure 7.4. The resistance for each lift is determined according to selected percentages of body weight (see Figure 7.4 and Lab 7A).

With this test, if an individual does only a few repetitions, the test will primarily measure absolute strength. For those who are able to do a lot of repetitions, the test will be an indicator of muscular endurance. If you are not familiar with the different lifts, illustrations are provided at the end of this chapter.

A strength/endurance rating is determined according to the maximum number of repetitions you are able to perform on each exercise. Fixed-resistance,

FIGURE 7.4 Muscular Strength and Endurance Test

1. Familiarize yourself with the six lifts used for this test: lat pull-down, leg extension, bench press, bent-leg curl-up or abdominal crunch,* leg curl, and arm curl. Graphic illustrations for each lift are given on pages 229, 230, 226, 222, 228, and 227 respectively. For the leg curl exercise, the knees should be flexed to 90°. A description and illustration of the bent-leg curl-up and the abdominal crunch exercises are provided in Figure 7.3. For the lateral pull-down exercise, use a sitting position and have your partner hold you down by the waist or shoulders. On the leg extension lift, maintain the trunk in an upright position.

2. Determine your body weight in kilograms.

3. Determine the amount of resistance to be used on each lift. To obtain this number, multiply your body weight by the percent given below for each lift.

Lift	Percent of Body Weight	
	Men	**Women**
Lat Pull-Down	.70	.45
Leg Extension	.65	.50
Bench Press	.75	.45
Bent-Leg Curl-Up or Abdominal Crunch*	NA**	NA**
Leg Curl	.32	.25
Arm Curl	.35	.18

* The abdominal crunch exercise should be used only by individuals who suffer or are susceptible to low-back pain.

** NA = not applicable—see Figure 7.3

4. Perform the maximum continuous number of repetitions possible.

5. Based on the number of repetitions performed, look up the percentile rank for each lift in the left column of Table 7.3.

6. The individual strength fitness category is determined according to the following classification:

Percentile Rank	Fitness Category	Points
≥90	Excellent	5
70–80	Good	4
50–60	Average	3
30–40	Fair	2
≤20	Poor	1

7. Look up the number of points assigned for each fitness category under item 6 above. Total the number of points and determine your overall strength fitness category according to the following ratings:

Total Points	Strength Category
≥25	Excellent
19–24	Good
13–18	Average
7–12	Fair
≤6	Poor

8. Record your results in Lab 7A.

Universal Gym units are necessary to administer all but the abdominal curls exercise on this test (see Dynamic Training on page 208 for an explanation of fixed-resistance equipment).

A percentile rank for each exercise is given based on the number of repetitions performed (see Table 7.3). As with the muscular endurance test, an overall muscular strength/endurance rating is obtained by totalling the number of points obtained on each exercise.

If no fixed resistance Universal Gym equipment is available, you can still perform the test using different equipment. In that case, though, the percentile rankings and strength fitness categories may not be completely accurate because a certain resistance (for example, 20 kg) is seldom the same on two different weight machines (for example, Universal Gym versus Nautilus). The industry has no standard calibration procedure for strength equipment. Consequently, if you lift a certain resistance on one machine, you may or may not be able to lift the same amount on a different machine.

Even though the percentile ranks may not be valid when using different equipment, test results can be used to evaluate changes in fitness. For example, you may be able to do 7 repetitions during the initial test, but if you can perform 14 repetitions after 12 weeks of training, that's a measure of improvement. The results for the Muscular Strength and Endurance Test can be recorded in Lab 7A.

Strength-Training Prescription

The capacity of muscle fibres to exert force increases and decreases according to the demands placed upon the muscular system. If muscle fibres are overloaded beyond their normal use, such as in strength-training programs, the fibres increase in size (hypertrophy) and strength. If the demands placed on the muscle fibres decrease, such as in sedentary living or required rest because of illness

TABLE 7.3 Muscular Strength and Endurance Scoring Table

Percentile Rank	Men							Women						
	Lat Pull-Down	Leg Extension	Bench Press	Bent-Leg Curl-Up	Abdom-inal Crunch	Leg Curl	Arm Curl	Lat Pull-Down	Leg Extension	Bench Press	Bent-Leg Curl-Up	Abdom-inal Crunch	Leg Curl	Arm Curl
99	30	25	26	100	100	24	25	30	25	27	100	100	20	25
95	25	20	21	81	100	20	21	25	20	21	100	100	17	21
90	19	19	19	65	100	19	19	21	18	20	97	69	12	20
80	16	15	16	51	66	15	15	16	13	16	77	49	10	16
70	13	14	13	44	45	13	12	13	11	13	57	37	9	14
60	11	13	11	31	38	11	10	11	10	11	45	34	7	12
50	10	12	10	28	33	10	9	10	9	10	37	31	6	10
40	9	10	7	25	29	8	8	9	8	5	28	27	5	8
30	7	9	5	22	26	6	7	7	7	3	22	24	4	7
20	6	7	3	17	22	4	5	6	5	1	17	21	3	6
10	4	5	1	10	18	3	3	3	3	0	9	15	1	3
5	3	3	0	3	16	1	2	2	1	0	4	0	0	2

■ High physical fitness standard   ■ Health fitness standard

or injury, the fibres **atrophy** and lose strength. A good level of muscular strength is important to develop and maintain fitness, health, and total well-being.

Factors That Affect Strength

Several physiological factors combine to create muscle contraction and subsequent strength gains: neural stimulation, type of muscle fibre, overload, and specificity of training. Basic knowledge of these concepts is important to understand the principles involved in strength training.

Neural Stimulation

Within the neuromuscular system, single **motor neurons** branch and attach to multiple muscle fibres. The motor neuron and the fibres it innervates (supplies with nerves) form a **motor unit**. The number of fibres a motor neuron can innervate varies from just a few in muscles that require precise control (eye muscles, for example) to as many as 1,000 or more in large muscles that do not perform refined or precise movements.

Stimulation of a motor neuron causes the muscle fibres to contract maximally or not at all. Variations in the number of fibres innervated and the frequency of their stimulation determine the strength of the muscle contraction. As the number of fibres innervated and frequency of stimulation increases, so does the strength of the muscular contraction.

Types of Muscle Fibre

The human body has two basic types of muscle fibres: (a) slow-twitch or red fibres and (b) fast-twitch or white fibres. **Slow-twitch fibres** have a greater capacity for aerobic work. **Fast-twitch fibres** have a greater capacity for anaerobic work and produce more overall force. The latter are important for quick and powerful movements commonly used in strength-training activities.

The proportion of slow- and fast-twitch fibres is primarily determined genetically and consequently varies from one person to another. Nevertheless, training increases the functional capacity of both types of fibre and, more specifically, strength training increases their ability to exert force.

During muscular contraction, slow-twitch fibres always are recruited first. As the force and speed of muscle contraction increase, the relative importance of the fast-twitch fibres increases. To activate the fast-twitch fibres, an activity must be intense and powerful.

Overload

Strength gains are achieved in two ways:

1. Through increased ability of individual muscle fibres to generate a stronger contraction.
2. By recruiting a greater proportion of the total available fibres for each contraction.

These two factors combine in the **overload principle**. The demands placed on the muscle must be increased systematically and progressively over time, and the resistance must be of a magnitude significant enough to cause physiological adaptation. In simpler terms, just like all other organs and systems of the human body, to increase in physical capacity, muscles have to be taxed repeatedly beyond their accustomed loads. Because of this principle, strength training also is called "progressive resistance training."

Several procedures can be used to overload in strength training:[8]

1. Increasing the resistance.
2. Increasing the number of repetitions.
3. Increasing the speed of the repetitions.
4. Decreasing rest interval for endurance improvements or lengthening the rest interval for strength gains.
5. Increasing volume (sum of the repetitions performed multiplied by the resistance used).
6. Using any combination of the above.

Specificity of Training

The principle of **specificity of training** states that, for a muscle to increase in strength or endurance, the training program must be specific to obtain the desired effects (also see discussion on Resistance on page 210).

The principle of specificity also applies to activity or sport-specific development and is commonly referred to as **SAID training,** or **specific adaptation to imposed demand**. The SAID principle implies that if an individual is attempting to improve specific sport skills, the strength-training exercises performed should resemble as closely as possible the movement patterns encountered in that particular activity or sport.

For example, a soccer player who wishes to become stronger and faster would emphasize exercises that will develop leg strength and power. In contrast, an individual recovering from a lower-limb fracture initially exercises to increase strength and stability, and subsequently muscle endurance. Additional information on the principle of specificity is provided under "Sport-Specific Conditioning" on page 286 in Chapter 9.

Understanding all four concepts (neural stimulation, muscle fibre types, overload, and specificity) is required to design an effective strength-training program.

Principles Involved in Strength Training

Because muscular strength and endurance are important in developing and maintaining overall fitness and well-being, the principles necessary to develop a strength-training program have to be understood, just as in the prescription for cardiorespiratory endurance. These principles are mode, resistance, sets, frequency, and volume of training. The key factor to successful muscular strength development, however, is the individualization of the program according to these principles and the person's goals, as well as the magnitude of the individual's effort during training itself.[9]

Mode of Training

Two types of training methods are used to improve strength: isometric (static) and dynamic (previously called "isotonic"). In isometric training, muscle contractions produce little or no movement, such as pushing or pulling against an immovable object. In dynamic training, the muscle contractions produce movement, such as extending the knees with resistance on the ankles (leg extension). The specificity of training principle applies here, too. To increase isometric versus dynamic strength, an individual must use static instead of dynamic training to achieve the desired results.

ISOMETRIC TRAINING

Isometric training does not require much equipment, but its popularity of several years ago has waned. Because strength gains with isometric training are specific to the angle of muscle contraction,

Atrophy Decrease in the size of a cell.

Motor neurons Nerves connecting the central nervous system to the muscle.

Motor unit The combination of a motor neuron and the muscle fibres that neuron innervates.

Slow-twitch fibres Muscle fibres with greater aerobic potential and slow speed of contraction.

Fast-twitch fibres Muscle fibres with greater anaerobic potential and fast speed of contraction.

Overload principle Training concept that the demands placed on a system (cardiorespiratory or muscular) must be increased systematically and progressively over time to cause physiological adaptation (development or improvement).

Specificity of training Principle that training must be done with the specific muscle the person is attempting to improve.

Specific adaptation to imposed demand (SAID) training Training principle stating that, for improvements to occur in a specific activity, the exercises performed during a strength-training program should resemble as closely as possible the movement patterns encountered in that particular activity.

Isometric training Strength-training method referring to a muscle contraction that produces little or no movement, such as pushing or pulling against an immovable object.

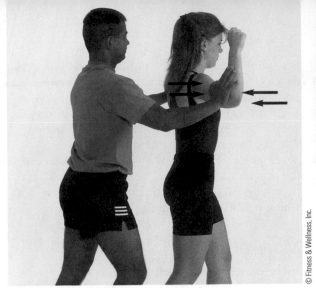

In isometric training, muscle contraction produces little or no movement.

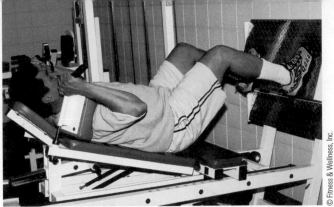

In dynamic training, muscle contraction produces movement in the respective joint.

this type of training is beneficial in a sport such as gymnastics, which requires regular static contractions during routines. As presented in Chapter 8, however, isometric training is a critical component of back health conditioning programs (see Preventing and Rehabilitating Low Back Pain, pages 249–252).

DYNAMIC TRAINING

Dynamic training is the most popular mode for strength training. The primary advantage is that strength is gained through the full **range of motion**. Most daily activities are dynamic in nature. We are constantly lifting, pushing, and pulling objects, and strength is needed through a complete range of motion. Another advantage is that improvements are measured easily by the amount lifted.

Dynamic training consists of two action phases when an exercise is performed: **concentric** or **positive resistance** and **eccentric** or **negative resistance**. In the concentric phase, the muscle shortens as it contracts to overcome the resistance; in the eccentric phase, it lengthens to overcome the resistance. For example, during a bench press exercise, when the person lifts the resistance from the chest to full-arm extension, the triceps muscle on the back of the upper arm shortens to extend the elbow. During the eccentric phase, the same triceps muscle must lengthen to lower the weight during elbow flexion, but the muscle lengthens slowly to avoid dropping the resistance. Both motions work the same muscle against the same resistance.

Eccentric muscle contractions allow us to lower weights in a smooth, gradual, and controlled manner. Without eccentric contractions, weights would be dropped on the way down. Because the same muscles work when you lift and lower a resistance, always be sure to execute both actions in a controlled manner. Failure to do so diminishes the benefits of the training program and increases the risk for injuries.

Dynamic training programs can be conducted without weights, with exercise bands, **free weights**, **fixed-resistance** machines, **variable-resistance** machines, or isokinetic equipment. When you perform dynamic exercises without weights (for example, pull-ups and push-ups), with free weights, or with fixed-resistance machines, you move a constant resistance through a joint's full range of motion. The greatest resistance that can be lifted equals the maximum weight that can be moved at the weakest angle of the joint. This is because of changes in muscle length and angle of pull as the joint moves through its range of motion.

As strength training became more popular, new strength-training machines were developed. This technology brought about **isokinetic training** and variable-resistance training programs, which require special machines equipped with mechanical devices that provide differing amounts of resistance, with the intent of overloading the muscle group maximally through the entire range of motion. A distinction of isokinetic training is that the speed of the muscle contraction is kept constant because the machine provides resistance to match the user's force through the range of motion. The mode of training an individual selects depends mainly on the type of equipment available and the specific objective the training program is attempting to accomplish.

The benefits of isokinetic and variable-resistance training are similar to the other dynamic training methods. Theoretically, strength gains should be better because maximum resistance is applied at all angles. Research, however, has not shown this type of training to be more effective than other modes of dynamic training.

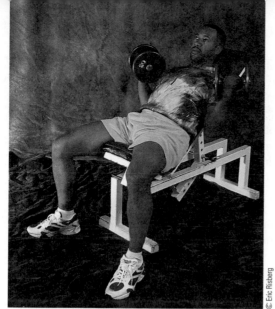

Strength training can be done using free weights.

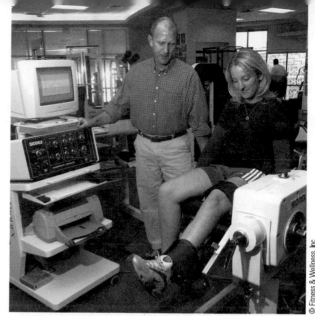

In isokinetic training, the speed of muscle contraction is constant.

FREE WEIGHTS VERSUS MACHINES IN DYNAMIC TRAINING

The most popular weight-training devices available during the first half of the 20th century were plate-loaded barbells (free weights). Strength-training machines were developed in the middle of the century but did not become popular until the 1970s. With subsequent technological improvements to these machines, a stirring debate surfaced over which of the two training modalities was better.

Free weights require that the individual balance the resistance through the entire lifting motion. Thus, one could logically assume that free weights are a better training modality because additional stabilizing muscles are needed to balance the resistance as it is moved through the range of motion. Research, however, has not shown any differences in strength development between the two exercise modalities.[10]

Although each modality has pros and cons, muscles do not know whether the source of a resistance is a barbell, a dumbbell, a Universal Gym machine, a Nautilus machine, or a simple cinder block. What determines the degree of a person's strength development is the quality of the program and the individual's effort during the training program itself—not the type of equipment used.

ADVANTAGES OF FREE WEIGHTS

Following are the advantages of using free weights instead of machines in a strength-training program.

1. *Cost:* Free weights are much less expensive than most exercise machines. On a limited budget, free weights are a better option.
2. *Variety:* A bar and a few plates can be used to perform many exercises to strengthen most muscles in the body.

3. *Portability:* Free weights are portable and can be easily moved from one area or station to another.
4. *Balance:* Free weights require that a person balance the weight through the entire range of motion. This feature involves additional stabilizing muscles to keep the weight moving properly.
5. *One size fits all:* Free weights can be used by people of almost all ages. A drawback of machines is that individuals who are at the extremes in height or limb length often do not fit into the machines. In particular, small women and adolescents are at a disadvantage.

Range of motion Entire arc of movement of a given joint.

Dynamic training Strength-training method referring to a muscle contraction with movement.

Concentric Shortening of a muscle during muscle contraction.

Positive resistance The lifting, pushing, or concentric phase of a repetition during a strength-training exercise.

Eccentric Lengthening of a muscle during muscle contraction.

Negative resistance The lowering or eccentric phase of a repetition during a strength training exercise.

Free weights Barbells and dumbbells.

Fixed resistance Type of exercise in which a constant resistance is moved through a joint's full range of motion.

Variable resistance Training using special machines equipped with mechanical devices that provide differing amounts of resistance through the range of motion.

Isokinetic training Strength-training method in which the speed of the muscle contraction is kept constant because the equipment (machine) provides an accommodating resistance to match the user's force (maximal) through the range of motion.

ADVANTAGES OF MACHINES

Strength training machines have the following advantages over free weights:

1. *Safety*: Machines are safer because spotters are rarely needed to monitor exercises.
2. *Selection*: A few exercises—such as hip flexion, hip abduction, leg curls, lat pulldowns, and neck exercises—can be performed only with machines.
3. *Variable resistance*: Most machines provide variable resistance. Free weights provide only fixed resistance.
4. *Isolation*: Individual muscles are better isolated with machines because stabilizing muscles are not used to balance the weight during the exercise.
5. *Time*: Exercising with machines requires less time because the resistance is quickly set using a selector pin instead of having to manually change dumbbells or weight plates on both sides of a barbell.
6. *Flexibility*: Most machines can provide resistance over a greater range of movement during the exercise, thereby contributing to greater flexibility in the joints. For example, a barbell pullover exercise provides resistance over a range of 100 degrees, whereas a weight machine may allow for as much as 260 degrees.
7. *Rehabilitation*: Machines are more useful during injury rehabilitation. A knee injury, for instance, is practically impossible to rehab using free weights, whereas small loads can be easily selected through a limited range of motion with a weight machine.
8. *Skill acquisition*: Learning a new exercise movement—and performing it correctly—is faster because the machine controls the direction of the movement.

Resistance

Resistance in strength training is the equivalent of intensity in cardiorespiratory exercise prescription. The amount of resistance, load, or weight lifted depends on whether the individual is trying to develop muscular strength or muscular endurance.

To stimulate strength development, a resistance of approximately 80 percent of the maximum capacity (1 RM) is recommended.[11] For example, a person with a 1 RM of 65 kg should work with at least 52 kg (65 $\times$ .80). Less than 80 percent will help increase muscular endurance rather than strength.

Because of the time factor involved in constantly determining the 1 RM on each lift to ensure that the person is indeed working above 80 percent,

the rule is that individuals should be able to perform more than 3 but no more than 12 repetitions (3 to 12 RM) for adequate strength gains. For example, if a person is training with a resistance of 55 kg and cannot lift it more than 12 times, the training stimulus (weight) is adequate for development of strength.

Once the person can lift the resistance more than 12 times, the resistance should be increased by 2.5 to 5 kg and the person again should build up to 12 repetitions. This is referred to as **progressive resistance training**.

Research on strength indicates that the closer a person trains to the 1 RM, the greater are the strength gains. A disadvantage of working constantly at or near the 1 RM is that it increases the risk for injury.

Highly trained athletes seeking maximum strength development often use 1 to 6 repetitions maximum. Working around 10 repetitions maximum seems to produce the best results in terms of muscular hypertrophy (information on dietary guidelines to optimize muscle strength and hypertrophy is provided under the section "Healthy Weight Gain" in Chapter 5, page 137). Eccentric contractions are also more effective in producing muscle hypertrophy but result in greater muscle soreness.[12] If training is conducted with more than 12 repetitions, primarily muscular endurance will be developed.

Body builders tend to work with moderate resistance levels (60 to 85 percent of the 1 RM) and perform 8 to 20 repetitions to near fatigue. A foremost objective of body building is to increase muscle size. Moderate resistance promotes blood flow to the muscles, "pumping up the muscles" (also known as "the pump") and making them look much larger than they do in a resting state.

From a health-fitness point of view, 8 to 12 repetitions maximum are recommended for adequate development. We live in a dynamic world in which both muscular strength and endurance are required to lead an enjoyable life. Therefore, working near a 10-repetition threshold seems to improve overall performance most effectively.

Sets

In strength training, a **set** is the number of repetitions performed for a given exercise. For example, a person lifting 55 kg eight times has performed one set of 8 repetitions (1 $\times$ 8 $\times$ 55).

When you work with 8 to 12 repetitions maximum, the recommendation is three sets per exercise. Because of the characteristics of muscle fibre, the number of sets that can be done is limited. As the number of sets increases, so does the amount of muscle fatigue and subsequent recovery time. Therefore, strength gains may be lessened by performing too many sets.

A recommended program for beginners in their first year of training is one or two light warm-up sets per exercise using about 50 percent of the 1 RM (no warm-up sets are necessary for subsequent exercises that use the same muscle group) followed by three heavy sets. At least one of these three sets should be performed to exhaustion or near exhaustion (up to the maximum number of repetitions selected). Maintaining a resistance and effort that will exhaust a muscle in 8 to 12 repetitions in at least one of these three heavy sets is critical to achieve optimal progress. Because of the lower resistances used in body building, four to eight sets can be done for each exercise.

To avoid muscle soreness and stiffness, new participants ought to build up gradually to the three sets of maximal repetitions. This can be done by performing only one set of each exercise with a lighter resistance on the first day, two sets of each exercise on the second day—the first light and the second with the regular resistance—and three sets on the third day—one light and two heavy. After that, a person should be able to do all three heavy sets.

The time necessary to recover between sets depends mainly on the resistance used during each set. In strength training, the energy to lift heavy weights is derived primarily from the ATP-CP or phosphagen system (see Chapter 3, "Energy (ATP) Production," pages 78–79). Ten seconds of maximal exercise nearly depletes the CP stores in the exercised muscle(s). These stores are replenished in about three minutes of recovery.

Based on this principle, a rest period of about three minutes between sets is necessary for people who are trying to maximize their strength gains. Individuals training for health-fitness purposes might allow two minutes of rest between sets. Body builders should rest no more than one minute to maximize the "pumping" effect. The exercise program will be more time-effective by alternating two or three exercises that require different muscle groups, called **circuit training**. In this way, an individual will not have to wait two to three minutes before proceeding to a new set on a different exercise. For example, the bench press, leg extension, and abdominal curl-up exercises may be combined so the person can go almost directly from one set to the next.

Men and women alike should observe the guidelines given previously. Many women, however, do not follow these guidelines. They erroneously believe that training with low resistances and many repetitions is best to enhance body composition and maximize energy expenditure. Unless a person is seeking to increase muscular endurance for a specific sport-related activity, the use of low resistances and high repetitions is not recommended to achieve optimal strength-fitness goals and maximize long-term energy expenditure (also see "Exercise: The Key to Weight Management" in Chapter 5, pages 134–137).

Frequency

Strength training should be done either through a total body workout two to three times a week, or more frequently if using a split-body routine (upper body one day, lower body the next). After a maximum strength workout, the muscles should be rested for about two to three days to allow adequate recovery. If not completely recovered in two to three days, the person most likely is overtraining and therefore not reaping the full benefits of the program. In that case, the person should do fewer sets of exercises than in the previous workout. A summary of strength training guidelines for health-fitness purposes is provided in Figure 7.5.

To achieve significant strength gains, a minimum of eight weeks of consecutive training is necessary. After an individual has achieved a recommended strength level, from a health-fitness standpoint, one training session per week will be sufficient to maintain the new strength level. Highly trained athletes will need to train two times per week to maintain their strength level.

Frequency of strength training for body builders varies from person to person. Because they use moderate resistance, daily or even two-a-day workouts are common. The frequency depends on the amount of resistance, number of sets performed per session, and the person's ability to recover from the previous exercise bout (see Table 7.4). The latter often is dictated by level of conditioning.

Resistance Amount of weight that is lifted.

Progressive resistance training A gradual increase of resistance over a period of time.

Set A fixed number of repetitions; one set of bench presses might be 10 repetitions.

Circuit training Alternating exercises by performing them in a sequence of three to six or more.

FIGURE 7.5 Strength-training guidelines

Mode: 8 to 10 dynamic strength-training exercises involving the body's major muscle groups

Resistance: Enough resistance to perform 8 to 12 repetitions to near-fatigue (10 to 15 repetitions for older and more frail individuals)

Sets: A minimum of 1 set

Frequency: At least two times per week

Based on "The Recommended Quantity and Quality of Exercise for Developing and Maintaining Cardiorespiratory and Muscular Fitness, and Flexibility in Healthy Adults," *Medicine and Science in Sports and Exercise* 30 (1998): 975–991.

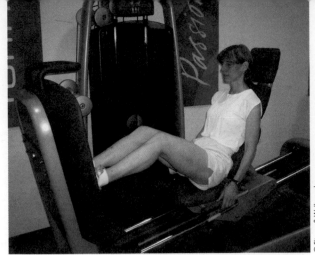

From a health fitness standpoint, one strength-training session per week is sufficient to maintain strength.

TABLE 7.4 Guidelines for Various Strength-Training Programs

Strength-Training Program	Resistance	Sets	Rest Between Sets*	Frequency (workouts per week)**
Health fitness	8–12 reps max	3	2 min	2–3
Maximal strength	1–6 reps max	3–6	3 min	2–3
Muscular endurance	10–30 reps	3–6	2 min	3–6
Body building	8–20 reps near max	3–8	0–1 min	4–12

* Recovery between sets can be decreased by alternating exercises that use different muscle groups.

** Weekly training sessions can be increased by using a split-body routine.

Training Volume

Volume refers to the sum of all the repetitions performed multiplied by the resistances used during a strength-training session.[13] Volume is frequently used to quantify the amount of work performed in a given training session—in the example under "Sets" on page 210, the volume of a single set was calculated to be 440. The volume of training done in a strength-training session can be modified by changing the total number of exercises performed—either by changing the number of sets done per exercise or the number of repetitions performed per set. High initial training volumes and low intensities are used for muscle hypertrophy, whereas low volumes and high intensities are used to increase strength and power.

Altering training volume and intensity is known as **periodization**, a training approach frequently used by athletes to achieve peak fitness and prevent **overtraining**. Periodization means cycling of one's training objectives (hypertrophy, strength, and endurance), with each phase of the program lasting anywhere from 2 to 12 weeks. To prevent overtraining during periodization, the volume should not increase by more than 5 percent from one phase to the next.

Periodization is also used by fitness participants who want to achieve higher levels of fitness. A more thorough discussion on periodization is provided in Chapter 9 (pages 287–288).

Plyometrics

Strength, speed, and explosiveness are all crucial for success in athletics. All three of these factors are enhanced with a progressive resistance training program, but greater increases in speed and explosiveness are thought possible with **plyometric exercise**. The objective is to generate the greatest amount of force in the shortest amount of time. A sound strength base is necessary before attempting plyometric exercises.

Plyometric training is popular in sports that require powerful movements, such as basketball, volleyball, sprinting, jumping, and gymnastics. A typical plyometric exercise involves jumping off and back onto a box, attempting to rebound as quickly as possible on each jump. Box heights are increased progressively from about 30 to 55 cm.

The bounding action attempts to take advantage of the stretch-recoil and stretch reflex characteristics of muscle. The rapid stretch applied to the muscle during contact with the ground is thought to augment muscle contraction, leading to more explosiveness. Plyometrics can be used, too, for strengthening upper body muscles. An example is doing push-ups so the extension of the arms is forceful enough to drive the hands (and body) completely off the floor during each repetition.

A drawback of plyometric training is its higher risk for injuries compared to conventional modes of progressive resistance training. For instance, the potential for injury in rebound exercise escalates with the increase in box height or the number of repetitions.

Strength Gains

A common question by many strength-training participants is: How quickly can strength gains be observed? Strength-training studies have revealed that most of the strength gains are seen in the first eight weeks of training. The amount of improvement, however, is related to previous training status. Increases of 40 percent are seen in individuals with no previous strength-training experience, 16 percent in previously strength-trained people, and 10 percent in advanced individuals.[14] Adhering to a periodized strength-training program will yield further improvements (see Chapter 9, pages 287–288).

Strength-Training Exercises With and Without Weights

The two strength-training programs introduced on pages 221–234 provide a complete body workout. The major muscles of the human body referred to in the exercises are pointed out in Figure 7.6, page 218.

Only a minimum of equipment is required for the first program, Strength-Training Exercises without Weights (Exercises 1 through 14). This program can be conducted in your own home. Your body weight is used as the primary resistance for most exercises. A few exercises call for a friend's help or some basic implements from around your house to provide greater resistance.

Strength-Training Exercises with Weights (Exercises 15 through 35) require machines (shown in the accompanying photographs). These exercises can be conducted on either fixed-resistance or variable-resistance equipment. Many of these exercises can also be performed with free weights. The first twelve exercises (15 to 26) are recommended to get a complete workout. You can do these exercises as circuit training. If time is a factor, as a minimum, perform the first eight (15 through 22) exercises. Exercises 27 to 35 are supplemental or can be used to replace some of the basic twelve (for instance, substitute Exercise 27 or 28 for 15; 29 for 16; 30 for 19; 31 for 20; 32 for 23; 33 or 34 for 25).

Core Strength Training

The trunk (spine) and pelvis are referred to as the "core" of the body. Core muscles include the abdominal muscles (rectus, transversus, and internal and external obliques), hip muscles (front and back), and spinal muscles (lower and upper back muscles). These muscle groups are responsible for maintaining the stability of the spine and pelvis.

Many of the major muscle groups of the legs, shoulder, and arms attach to the core. A strong core allows a person to perform activities of daily living with greater ease, improve sports performance through a more effective energy transfer from large to small body parts, and decrease the incidence of low-back pain.

Interest in **core strength training** programs has increased recently. A major objective of core training is to exercise the abdominal and lower back muscles in unison. Furthermore, individuals should spend as much time training the back muscles as they do the abdominal muscles. Besides enhancing stability, core training improves dynamic balance, which is often required during physical activity and sports participation.

Key core-training exercises include the abdominal crunch and bent-leg curl-up, reverse crunch, pelvic tilt, lateral bridge, prone bridge, leg press, seated back, lat pull-down, back extension, supine bridge, and pelvic clock (Exercises 4, 11, 12, 13, 14, 16, 21, 23, and 35 in this chapter and Exercises 26 and 27 in Chapter 8, respectively).

When core training is used in athletic conditioning programs, athletes attempt to mimic the dynamic

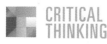

CRITICAL THINKING

Your roommate started a strength-training program last year and has seen good results. He is now strength-training on a nearly daily basis and taking performance-enhancing supplements hoping to accelerate results. What are your feelings about his program? What would you say (and not say) to him?

Volume (in strength training) The sum of all the repetitions performed multiplied by the resistances used during a strength-training session.

Periodization A training approach that divides the season into cycles using a systematic variation in intensity and volume of training to enhance fitness and performance.

Overtraining An emotional, behavioural, and physical condition marked by increased fatigue, decreased performance, persistent muscle soreness, mood disturbances, and feelings of "staleness" or "burnout" as a result of excessive physical training.

Plyometric exercise Explosive jump training, incorporating speed and strength training to enhance explosiveness.

Core strength training A training program designed to strengthen the abdominal, hip, and spinal muscles (the core of the body).

skills they use in their sport. To do so, they use special equipment such as balance boards, stability balls, and foam pads. The use of this equipment allows the athletes to train the core while seeking balance and stability in a sport-specific manner.[15]

Pilates Exercise System

Pilates exercises have become increasingly popular in recent years. Previously, Pilates training was used primarily by dancers, but now this exercise modality is embraced by a large number of fitness participants, rehab patients, models, actors, and even professional athletes. Pilates studios, university and college courses, and classes at health clubs are available nationwide.

The Pilates training system was originally developed in the 1920s by German physical therapist Joseph Pilates. The exercises are designed to help strengthen the body's core by developing pelvic stability and abdominal control—coupled with focused breathing patterns.

Pilates exercises are performed either on a mat (floor) or specialized equipment to help increase strength and flexibility of deep postural muscles. The intent is to improve muscle tone and length (a limber body), instead of increasing muscle size (hypertrophy).

Pilates mat classes focus on body stability and correct body mechanics. The exercises are performed in a slow, controlled, and precise manner. Properly performed, these exercises require intense concentration. Initial Pilates training should be conducted under the supervision of certified instructors with extensive Pilates teaching experience.

Fitness goals of Pilates programs include better flexibility, muscle tone, posture, spinal support, body balance, low-back health, sports performance, and mind–body awareness. Individuals with loose or unstable joints benefit from Pilates because the exercises are designed to enhance joint stability. The Pilates program is also used to help lose weight, increase lean tissue, and manage stress. Although Pilates programs are quite popular, research is required to corroborate the benefits attributed to this training system.

Exercise Guidelines

As you prepare to design your strength training program, keep the following guidelines in mind:

1. Select exercises that will involve all major muscle groups: chest, shoulders, back, legs, arms, hip, and trunk.
2. Select exercises that will strengthen the core. Use controlled movements and start with light

to moderate resistances (athletes may later use explosive movements with heavier resistances).

3. Never lift weights alone. Always have someone work out with you in case you need a spotter or help with an injury. When you use free weights, one to two spotters are recommended for certain exercises (for example, bench press, squats, overhead press).
4. Warm up properly prior to lifting weights by performing a light- to moderate-intensity aerobic activity (five to seven minutes) and some gentle stretches for a few minutes.
5. Use proper lifting technique for each exercise. Correct lifting technique will involve only those muscles and joints intended for a specific exercise. Involving other muscles and joints to "cheat" during the exercise to complete a repetition or to be able to lift a greater resistance decreases the long-term effectiveness of the exercise and can lead to injury (such as arching the back during the push-up, squat, or bench press exercises).

    Proper lifting technique also implies performing the exercises in a controlled manner and throughout the entire range of motion. Avoid fast and jerky movements and do not throw the entire body into the lifting motion. Do not arch the back when lifting a weight.

6. Maintain proper body balance while lifting. Proper balance involves good posture, a stable body position, and correct seat and arm/leg settings on exercise machines. Loss of balance places undue strain on smaller muscles and leads to injuries because of the heavy resistances suddenly placed on them.

    In the early stages of a program, first-time lifters often struggle with bar control and balance when using free weights. This problem is quickly overcome with practice following a few training sessions.

7. Exercise larger muscle groups (such as those in the chest, back, and legs) before exercising smaller muscle groups (arms, abdominals, ankles, neck). For example, the bench press exercise works the chest, shoulders, and back of the upper arms (triceps), whereas the triceps extension works the back of the upper arms only.
8. Exercise opposing muscle groups for a balanced workout. When you work the chest (bench press), also work the back (rowing torso). If you work the biceps (arm curl), also work the triceps (triceps extension).
9. Breathe naturally. Inhale during the eccentric phase (bringing the weight down) and exhale during the concentric phase (lifting or pushing

the weight up). Practise proper breathing with lighter weights when you are learning a new exercise.

10. Avoid holding your breath while straining to lift a weight. Holding your breath greatly increases the pressure inside the chest and abdominal cavity, making it practically impossible for the blood in the veins to return to the heart. Although rare, a sudden high intrathoracic pressure may lead to dizziness, a blackout, a stroke, a heart attack, or a hernia.

11. Based on the program selected, allow adequate recovery time between sets of exercises (see Table 7.4, page 212).

12. Discontinue training if you experience unusual discomfort or pain. High tension loads used in strength training can exacerbate potential injuries. Discomfort and pain are signals to stop and determine what's wrong. Be sure to properly evaluate your condition before you continue training.

13. Use common sense on days when you feel fatigued or when you are performing sets to complete fatigue. Excessive fatigue affects lifting technique, body balance, muscles involved, and range of motion—all of which increase the risk for injury. A spotter is recommended when sets are performed to complete fatigue. The spotter's help through the most difficult part of the repetition will relieve undue stress on muscles, ligaments, and tendons—and help ensure you perform the exercise correctly.

14. Stretch out for a few minutes at the end of each strength-training workout to help your muscles return to their normal resting length and to minimize muscle soreness and risk for injury.

Setting Up Your Own Strength-Training Program

The same pre-exercise guidelines outlined for cardiorespiratory endurance training apply to strength training (see Physical Activity Readiness Questionnaire (PAR-Q) on page 23). If you have any concerns about your present health status or ability to participate safely in strength training, consult a physician before you start. Strength training is not advised for people with advanced heart disease.

Before you proceed to write your strength-training program, you should determine your

stage of change for this fitness component in Lab 7B. Next, if you are prepared to do so, and depending on the facilities available, you can choose one of the training programs outlined in this chapter (use Lab 7B). Once you begin your strength-training program, you may use the form provided in Figure 7.7 (pages 219–220) to keep a record of your training sessions.

The resistance and the number of repetitions you use with your program should be based on whether you want to increase muscular strength or muscular endurance as follows:

■ For strength gains, do up to 12 repetitions maximum, and, for muscular endurance, more than 12. For most people, three training sessions per week on nonconsecutive days is an ideal arrangement for proper development.

■ For both strength and endurance gains, the recommendation is three sets of about 12 repetitions maximum for each exercise. In doing this, you will obtain good strength gains and yet be close to the endurance threshold.

■ If you are training for reasons other than health fitness, review Table 7.4, page 212, for a summary of the guidelines.

Perhaps the only exercise that calls for more than 12 repetitions is the abdominal group of exercises. The abdominal muscles are considered primarily antigravity or postural muscles. Hence, a little more endurance may be required. When doing abdominal work, most people perform about 20 repetitions.

If time is a concern in completing a strength training exercise program, the American College of Sports Medicine[16] recommends as a minimum (a) one set of 8 to 12 repetitions performed to near fatigue, and (b) 8 to 10 exercises involving the major muscle groups of the body, conducted twice a week. The recommendation is based on research showing that this training generates 70 to 80 percent of the improvements reported in other programs using three sets of about 10 RM.

Pilates A training program that uses exercises designed to help strengthen the body's core by developing pelvic stability and abdominal control; exercises are coupled with focused breathing patterns.

ASSESS YOUR KNOWLEDGE

1. The ability of a muscle to exert submaximal force repeatedly over time is known as:
   a. muscular strength.
   b. plyometric training.
   c. muscular endurance.
   d. isokinetic training.
   e. isometric training.

2. Each additional 0.45 kilogram of muscle tissue increases resting metabolism by:
   a. 10 Calories.
   b. 17 Calories.
   c. 23 Calories.
   d. 35 Calories.
   e. 50 Calories.

3. The Hand Grip Strength Test is an example of
   a. an isometric test.
   b. an isotonic test.
   c. a dynamic test.
   d. an isokinetic test.
   e. a plyometric test.

4. A 70 percentile rank places an individual in the _____ fitness category.
   a. excellent
   b. good
   c. average
   d. fair
   e. poor

5. During an eccentric muscle contraction
   a. the muscle shortens as it overcomes the resistance.
   b. there is little or no movement during the contraction.
   c. a joint has to move through the entire range of motion.
   d. the muscle lengthens as it contracts.
   e. the speed is kept constant throughout the range of motion.

6. The training concept stating that the demands placed on a system must be increased systematically and progressively over time to cause physiological adaptation is referred to as
   a. the overload principle.
   b. positive-resistance training.
   c. specificity of training.
   d. variable-resistance training.
   e. progressive resistance.

7. A set in strength training implies
   a. the starting position for an exercise.
   b. the recovery time required between exercises.
   c. a given number of repetitions.
   d. the starting resistance used in an exercise.
   e. the sequence in which exercises are performed.

8. For health-fitness, a person should perform between
   a. 1 and 6 reps max.
   b. 4 and 10 reps max.
   c. 8 and 12 reps max.
   d. 8 and 20 reps max.
   e. 10 and 30 reps max.

9. Plyometric training is frequently used to help with performance in
   a. gymnastics.
   b. basketball.
   c. volleyball.
   d. sprinting.
   e. all of these sports.

10. The posterior deltoid, rhomboids, and trapezius muscles can be developed with the following exercise:
    a. bench press
    b. lat pull-down
    c. rotary torso
    d. squat
    e. rowing torso

Correct answers can be found at the back of the book.

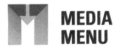

MEDIA MENU

INTERNET CONNECTIONS

■ Canadian Society for Exercise Physiology (CSEP). This is a voluntary organization composed of professionals interested and involved in the scientific study of exercise physiology, exercise biochemistry, fitness, and health.
  http://www.csep.ca

■ National Strength and Conditioning Association (NSCA). NSCA is a worldwide authority on strength and conditioning. It supports and disseminates research-based knowledge and its practical applications to improve athletic performance and fitness.
  http://www.nsca-lift.org/

■ Muscle and Fitness. This comprehensive site features information on intermediate and advanced training techniques, with photographs and informative articles on the use of dietary supplements as well as the importance of mind-body activities to enhance your workout.
  http://www.muscleandfitness.com

■ Strength Training Muscle Map & Explanation. This site provides an anatomical map of the body's muscles. Click on the muscle for exercises designed to specifically strengthen that particular muscle, complete with a video and safety information.
  http://www.global-fitness.com/strength/s_muscle map.html

■ Strengthcoach.com. This comprehensive site features articles on a variety of strength-training topics. The virtual weight room features written descriptions of muscles used and proper movements as well as a video demonstration illustrating proper workout techniques that will improve muscle strength of abdominals, back, biceps, chest, and legs, plus information about plyometrics and speed development.

http://www.strengthcoach.com

Notes

1. C. Castaneda, et al., "A Randomized Controlled Trial of Resistance Exercise Training to Improve Glycemic Control in Older Adults with Type 2 Diabetes," *Diabetes Care* 25 (2202): 2335–2341.

2. W. W. Campbell, M. C. Crim, V. R. Young, and W. J. Evans, "Increased Energy Requirements and Changes in Body Composition with Resistance Training in Older Adults," *American Journal of Clinical Nutrition* 60 (1994): 167–175.

3. W. J. Evans, "Exercise, Nutrition and Aging," *Journal of Nutrition* 122 (1992): 796–801.

4. Campbell et al., "Increased Energy Requirements and Changes in Body Composition with Resistance Training in Older Adults."

5. P. E. Allsen, *Strength Training: Beginners, Body Builders and Athletes* (Dubuque, IA: Kendall/Hunt, 2003).

6. Canadian Centre for Ethics in Sport, "Doping Free Sport: International Doping Control." Retrieved January 22, 2008 from: http://www.cces.ca/forms/index.cfm?dsp=template&act=view3&template_id=142&lang-e.

7. Canadian Body Building Federation, "CBBF Positive Drug Test Appeals," June 3, 2007. Retrieved January 23, 2008, from www.cbbf.ca/info_full.asp?id=23.

8. American College of Sports Medicine, "Progression Models in Resistance Training for Healthy Adults," *Medicine and Science in Sports and Exercise* 34 (2002): 364–380.

9. J. K. Kraemer and N. A. Ratamess, "Fundamentals of Resistance Training: Progression and Exercise Prescription," *Medicine and Science in Sports and Exercise* 36 (2004): 674–688.

10. S. P. Messier, and M. Dill, "Alterations in Strength and Maximal Oxygen Uptake Consequent to Nautilus Circuit Weight Training," *Research Quarterly for Exercise and Sport* 56 (1985): 345–351.

    T. V. Pipes, "Variable Resistance Versus Constant Resistance Strength Training in Adult Males," *European Journal of Applied Physiology* 39 (1978): 27–35.

11. W. W. K. Hoeger, D. R. Hopkins, S. L. Barette, and D. F. Hale, "Relationship Between Repetitions and Selected Percentages of One Repetition Maximum: A Comparison Between Untrained and Trained Males and Females," *Journal of Applied Sport Science Research* 4, no. 2 (1990): 47–51.

12. B. M. Hather, P. A. Tesch, P. Buchanan, and G. A. Dudley, "Influence of Eccentric Actions on Skeletal Muscle Adaptations to Resistance Training," *Acta Physiologica Scandinavica* 143 (1991): 177–185.

    C. B. Ebbeling and P. M. Clarkson, "Exercise-Induced Muscle Damage and Adaptation," *Sports Medicine* 7 (1989): 207–234.

13. American College of Sports Medicine, "Progression Models in Resistance Training for Healthy Adults."

14. American College of Sports Medicine, "Progression Models in Resistance Training for Healthy Adults."

15. Gatorade Sports Science Institute, "Core Strength Training," *Sports Science Exchange Roundtable* 13, no. 1 (2002): 1–4; J. Compton, S. Scott, and M. Tyler, *Ball Bearings* (Victoria, BC: Trafford Publishing, 2003). See also www.BallBearings.org.

16. "The Recommended Quantity and Quality of Exercise for Developing and Maintaining Cardiorespiratory and Muscular Fitness and Flexibility in Healthy Adults," *Medicine and Science in Sports and Exercise* 30 (1998): 975–991.

Suggested Readings

American College of Sports Medicine. "Progression Models in Resistance Training for Healthy Adults." *Medicine and Science in Sports and Exercise* 34 (2002): 364–380.

Hesson, J. L. *Weight Training for Life*. Belmont, CA: Wadsworth/Thomson Learning, 2005.

Heyward, V. H. *Advanced Fitness Assessment and Exercise Prescription*. Champaign, IL: Human Kinetic Press, 2002.

Hoeger, W. W. K., and S. A. Hoeger. *Lifetime Physical Fitness and Wellness: A Personalized Program*. Belmont, CA: Wadsworth/Thomson Learning, 2005.

Kell, R. T., G. Bell, and A. Quinney. "Musculoskeletal Fitness, Health Outcomes and Quality of Life." *Sports Medicine*, 31(2001): 863–873.

Kraemer, J. K., and N. A. Ratamess. "Fundamentals of Resistance Training: Progression and Exercise Prescription." *Medicine and Science in Sports and Exercise* 36 (2004): 674–688.

Liemohn, W. and G. Pariser. "Core Strength: Implications for Fitness and Low Back Pain." *ACSM's Health and Fitness Journal* 6, no. 5 (2002): 10–16.

Mannie, K. "Barbells Versus Machines: Balancing a Weighty Issue." *Coach and Athletic Director* 67 (1998): 6–7.

Payne N., N. Gledhill, P.T. Katzmarzyk, V. Jamnik and S. Ferguson. "Health Implication of Musculoskeletal Fitness." *Canadian Journal of Applied Physiology*, 25 (2000): 114–126.

Volek, J. "Influence of Nutrition on Responses to Resistance Training" *Medicine and Science in Sports and Exercise* 36 (2004): 689–696.

Warburton, D. E., N. Gledhill, and A. Quinney. "The Effects of Changes in Musculoskeletal Fitness on Health." *Canadian Journal of Applied Physiology*, 26 (2001): 161–216.

Wescott, W. L., and T. R. Baechle. *Strength Training for Seniors*. Champaign, IL: Human Kinetic Press, 1999.

FIGURE 7.6 Major muscles of the human body

THE MUSCULAR SYSTEM

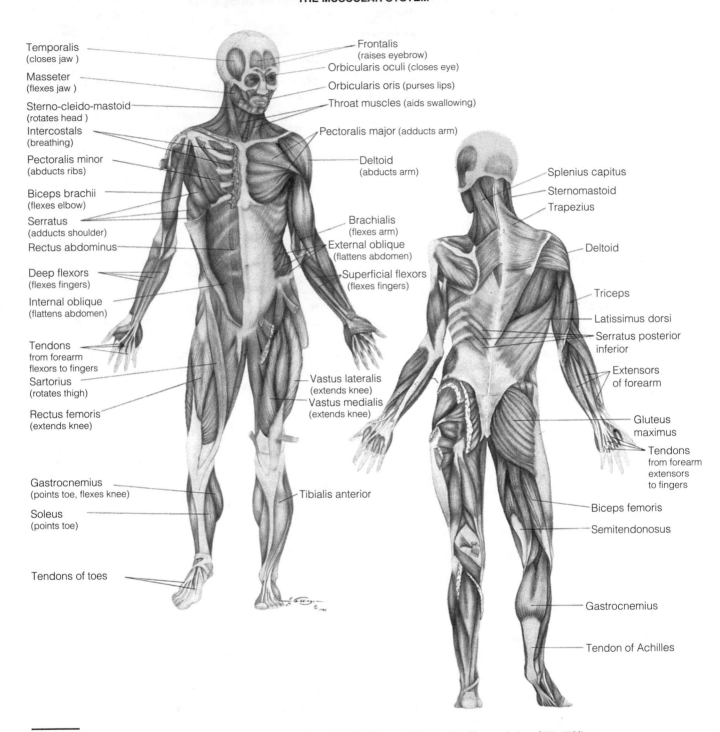

Temporalis
(closes jaw)

Masseter
(flexes jaw)

Sterno-cleido-mastoid
(rotates head)

Intercostals
(breathing)

Pectoralis minor
(abducts ribs)

Biceps brachii
(flexes elbow)

Serratus
(adducts shoulder)

Rectus abdominus

Deep flexors
(flexes fingers)

Internal oblique
(flattens abdomen)

Tendons
from forearm
flexors to fingers

Sartorius
(rotates thigh)

Rectus femoris
(extends knee)

Gastrocnemius
(points toe, flexes knee)

Soleus
(points toe)

Tendons of toes

Frontalis
(raises eyebrow)

Orbicularis oculi (closes eye)

Orbicularis oris (purses lips)

Throat muscles (aids swallowing)

Pectoralis major (adducts arm)

Deltoid
(abducts arm)

Brachialis
(flexes arm)

External oblique
(flattens abdomen)

Superficial flexors
(flexes fingers)

Vastus lateralis
(extends knee)

Vastus medialis
(extends knee)

Tibialis anterior

Splenius capitus

Sternomastoid

Trapezius

Deltoid

Triceps

Latissimus dorsi

Serratus posterior
inferior

Extensors
of forearm

Gluteus
maximus

Tendons
from forearm
extensors
to fingers

Biceps femoris

Semitendonosus

Gastrocnemius

Tendon of Achilles

From *Prehospital Emergency Care and Crisis Intervention* by Brent Q. Hafen and Keith J. Karren, 1983. Reprinted by permission of F.D. Giddings.

FIGURE 7.7 Strength training record form

Name

Date												
Exercise	St/Reps/Res*	St/Reps/Res*	St/Reps/Res*	St/Reps/Res*	St/Reps/Res*	St/Reps/Res*	St/Reps/Res*	St/Reps/Res*	St/Reps/Res*	St/Reps/Res*	St/Reps/Res*	St/Reps/Res*

(continued)

*Sets, Repetitions, and Resistance (e.g., 1/6/55 = 1 set of 6 repetitions with 55 kg)

PRINCIPLES & LABS

FIGURE 7.7 Strength training record form

Name _____

Date											
Exercise	St/Reps/Res*	St/Reps/Res*	St/Reps/Res*	St/Reps/Res*	St/Reps/Res*	St/Reps/Res*	St/Reps/Res*	St/Reps/Res*	St/Reps/Res*	St/Reps/Res*	St/Reps/Res*

*Sets, Repetitions, and Resistance (e.g., 1/6/55 = 1 set of 6 repetitions with 55 kg)

Strength-Training Exercises without Weights

Exercise 1
Step-Up

Action Step up and down using a box or chair approximately 30 to 38 cm high (a). Conduct one set using the same leg each time you go up, and then conduct a second set using the other leg. You also could alternate legs on each step-up cycle. You may increase the resistance by holding an object in your arms (b). Hold the object close to the body to avoid increased strain in the lower back.

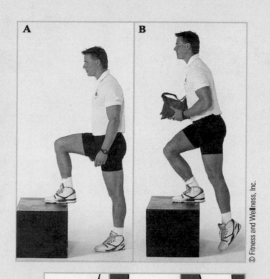

Muscles Developed
Gluteal muscles, quadriceps, gastrocnemius, and soleus

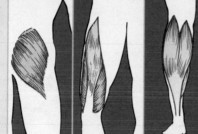

Back   Front   Back

Exercise 2
Rowing Torso

Action Raise your arms laterally (abduction) to a horizontal position and bend your elbows to 90°. Have a partner apply enough pressure on your elbows to gradually force your arms forward (horizontal flexion) while you try to resist the pressure. Next, reverse the action, horizontally forcing the arms backward as your partner applies sufficient forward pressure to create resistance.

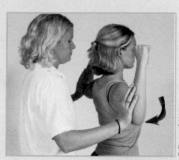

Muscles Developed
Posterior deltoid, rhomboids, and trapezius

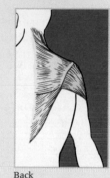

Back

Exercise 3
Push-Up

Action Maintaining your body as straight as possible (a), flex the elbows, lowering the body until you almost touch the floor (b), then raise yourself back up to the starting position. If you are unable to perform the push-up as indicated, decrease the resistance by supporting the lower body with the knees rather than the feet (c) or using an incline plane and supporting your hands at a higher point than the floor (d). If you wish to increase the resistance, have someone else add resistance to your shoulders as you are coming back up (e).

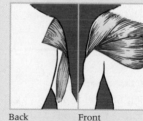

Back   Front   Front

Muscles Developed
Triceps, deltoid, pectoralis major, abdominals, and erector spinae

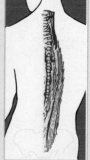

Back

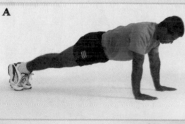

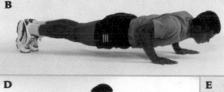

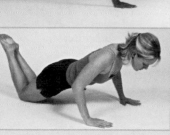

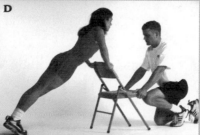

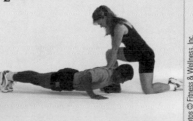

Exercise 4
Abdominal Crunch and Bent-Leg Curl-Up

Action   Start with your head and shoulders off the floor, arms crossed on your chest, and knees slightly bent (a). The greater the flexion of the knee, the more difficult the curl-up. Now curl up to about 30° (abdominal crunch—illustration b) or curl up all the way (abdominal curl-up—illustration c), then return to the starting position without letting the head or shoulders touch the floor or allowing the hips to come off the floor. If you allow the hips to raise off the floor and the head and shoulders to touch the floor, you most likely will "swing up" on the next crunch or curl-up, which minimizes the work of the abdominal muscles. If you cannot curl up with the arms on the chest, place the hands by the side of the hips or even help yourself up by holding on to your thighs (d and e). Do not perform the sit-up exercise with your legs completely extended, because this will strain the lower back. For additional resistance during the abdominal crunch, have a partner add slight resistance to your shoulders as you "crunch up" (f).

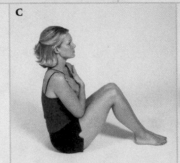
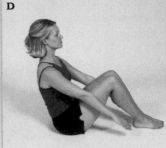
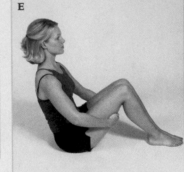
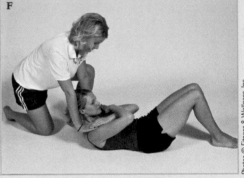
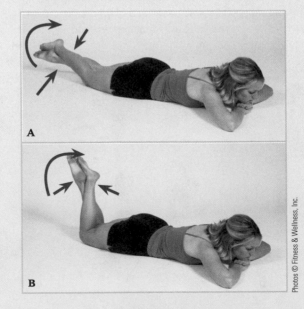

Muscles Developed
Abdominal muscles and hip flexors

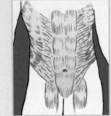

Front

Note: The abdominal curl-up exercise should be used only by individuals of at least average fitness without a history of lower back problems. New participants and those with a history of lower back problems should use the abdominal crunch exercise in its place.

Photos © Fitness & Wellness, Inc.

Exercise 5
Leg Curl

Action   Lie on the floor face down. Cross the right ankle over the left heel (a). Apply resistance with your right foot while you bring the left foot up to 90° at the knee joint (b). Apply enough resistance so the left foot can only be brought up slowly. Repeat the exercise, crossing the left ankle over the right heel.

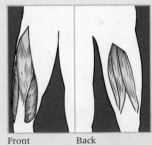

Front   Back

Muscles Developed
Hamstrings (and quadriceps)

Photos © Fitness & Wellness, Inc.

Exercise 6
Modified Dip

Action   Using a gymnasium bleacher or box and with the help of a partner, sit in front of the box with your back against it and reach back and press up. Dip down at least to a 90° angle at the elbow joint and then return to the initial position.

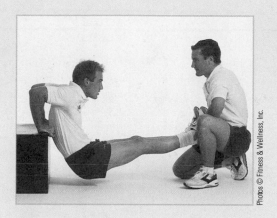

Photos © Fitness & Wellness, Inc.

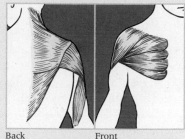

Back   Front

Muscles Developed   Triceps, deltoid, and pectoralis major

Exercise 7
Pull-Up

Action   Suspend yourself from a bar with a pronated (thumbs-in) grip (a). Pull your body up until your chin is above the bar (b), then lower yourself slowly to the starting position. If you are unable to perform the pull-up as described, have a partner hold your feet to help you push off and facilitate the movement upward (c and d).

Muscles Developed
Biceps, brachioradialis, brachialis, trapezius, and latissimus dorsi

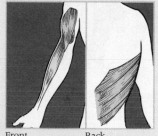

Front   Back

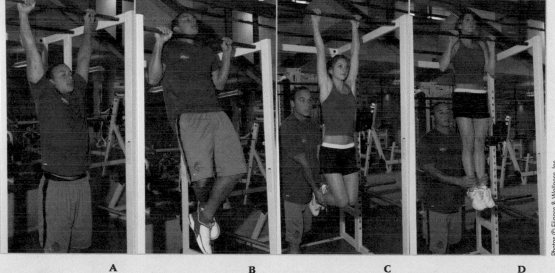

Photos © Fitness & Wellness, Inc.

A   B   C   D

MUSCULAR STRENGTH AND ENDURANCE

Exercise 8
Arm Curl

Action   Using a palms-up grip, start with the arm completely extended and, with the aid of a sandbag or bucket filled (as needed) with sand or rocks (a), curl up as far as possible (b), then return to the initial position. Repeat the exercise with the other arm.

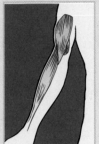

Front

Muscles Developed
Biceps, brachioradialis, and brachialis

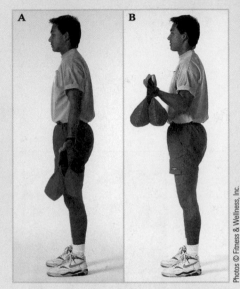

Exercise 9
Heel Raise

Action   From a standing position with feet flat on the floor (a), raise and lower your body weight by moving at the ankle joint only (b). For added resistance, have someone else hold your shoulders down as you perform the exercise.

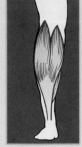

Back

Muscles Developed
Gastrocnemius and soleus

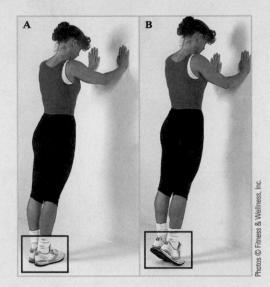

Exercise 10
Leg Abduction and Adduction

Action   Both participants sit on the floor. The person on the left places the feet on the inside of the other person's feet. Simultaneously, the person on the left presses the legs laterally (to the outside—abduction), while the person on the right presses the legs medially (adduction). Hold the contraction for 5 to 10 seconds. Repeat the exercise at all three angles, and then reverse the pressing sequence: The person on the left places the feet on the outside and presses inward, while the person on the right presses outward.

Muscles Developed   Hip abductors (rectus femoris, sartori, gluteus medius and minimus) and adductors (pectineus, gracilis, adductor magnus, adductor longus, and adductor brevis)

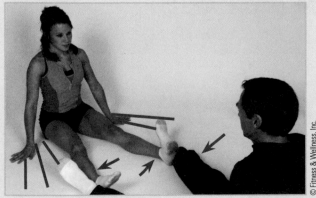

Exercise 11
Reverse Crunch

Action   Lie on your back with arms to the sides and knees and hips flexed at about 90° (a). Now attempt to raise the pelvis off the floor by lifting vertically from the knees and lower legs (b). This is a challenging exercise that may be difficult for beginners to perform.

Muscles Developed
Abdominals

Front

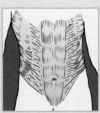

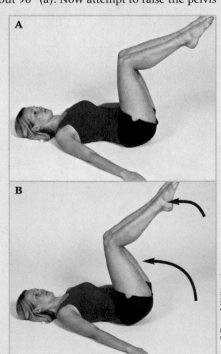

Exercise 12
Pelvic Tilt

Action   Lie flat on the floor with the knees bent at about a 90° angle (a). Tilt the pelvis by tightening the abdominal muscles, flattening your back against the floor, and raising the lower gluteal area ever so slightly off the floor (b). Hold the final position for several seconds.

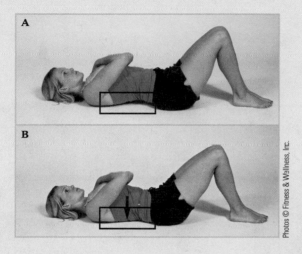

A

B

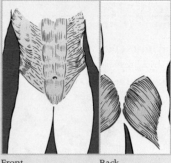

Front   Back

Areas Stretched
Low back muscles and ligaments

Areas Strengthened
Abdominal and gluteal muscles

Photos © Fitness & Wellness, Inc.

Exercise 13
Lateral Bridge

Action   Lie on your side with legs bent (a: easier version) or straight (b: harder version) and support the upper body with your arm. Straighten out your body by raising the hip off the floor and hold the position for several seconds. Repeat the exercise with the other side of the body.

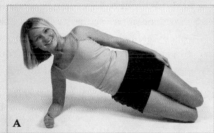

A

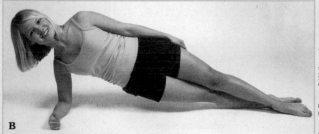

B

Photos © Fitness & Wellness, Inc.

Muscles Developed
Abdominals (obliques and transversus abdominus) and quadratus lumborum (lower back)

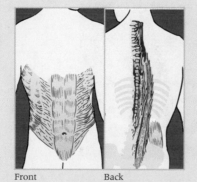

Front   Back

Exercise 14
Prone Bridge

Action   Starting in a prone position on a floor mat, balance yourself on the tips of your toes and elbows while attempting to maintain a straight body from head to toes (do not arch the lower back). You can increase the difficulty of this exercise by placing your hands in front of you and straightening out the arms (elbows off the floor).

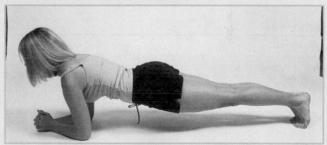

© Fitness & Wellness, Inc.

Muscles Developed
Anterior and posterior muscle groups of the trunk and pelvis

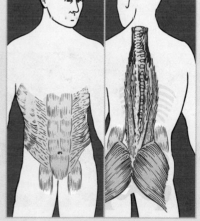

Front   Back

Strength-Training Exercises with Weights

Exercise 15
Bench (Chest) Press

Machine From a seated position, grasp the bar handles (a) and press forward until the arms are completely extended (b), then return to the original position. Do not arch the back during this exercise.

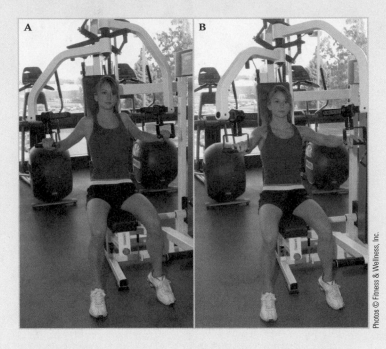

Photos © Fitness & Wellness, Inc.

Muscles Developed Pectoralis major, triceps, and deltoid

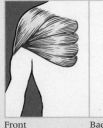

Front   Back

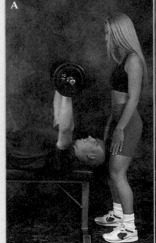
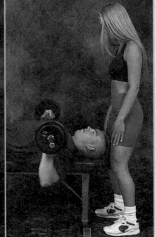

© Eric Risberg

Free Weights Lie on the bench with arms extended and have one or two spotters help you place the barbell directly over your shoulders (a). Lower the weight to your chest (b) and then push it back up until you achieve full extension of the arms. Do not arch the back during this exercise.

Exercise 16
Leg Press

Action From a sitting position with the knees flexed at about 90° and both feet on the footrest (a), extend the legs fully (b), then return slowly to the starting position.

Muscles Developed Quadriceps and gluteal muscles

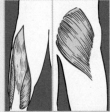

Front   Back

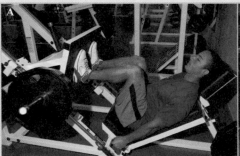
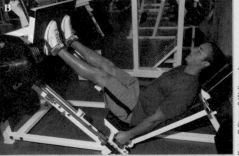

Photos © Fitness & Wellness, Inc.

Exercise 17
Abdominal Crunch

Action Sit in an upright position. Grasp the handles over your shoulders and crunch forward. Return slowly to the original position.

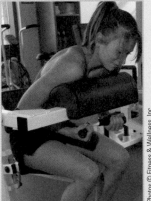

Photos © Fitness & Wellness, Inc.

Muscles Developed Abdominals

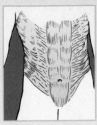

Front

Exercise 18
Rowing Torso

Action   Sit in the machine and grasp the handles in front of you, (a). Press back as far as possible, drawing the shoulder blades together (b). Return to the original position.

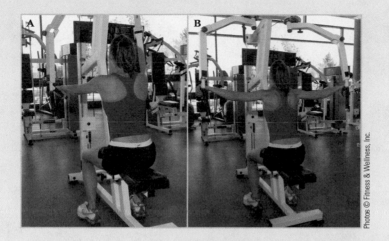

Photos © Fitness & Wellness, Inc.

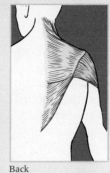

Back

Muscles Developed
Posterior deltoid, rhomboids, and trapezius

Bent-Over Lateral Raise

Action   Bend over with your back straight and knees bent at about 5 to 10° (a). Hold one dumbbell in each hand. Raise the dumbbells laterally to about shoulder level (b) and then slowly return them to the starting position.

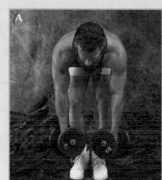
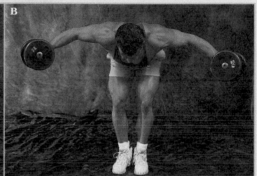

© Eric Risberg

Exercise 19
Arm Curl

Machine   Using a supinated (palms-up) grip, start with the arms almost completely extended (a). Curl up as far as possible (b), then return to the starting position.

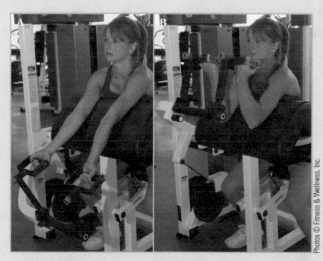

Photos © Fitness & Wellness, Inc.

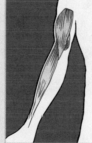

Front

Muscles Developed
Biceps, brachioradialis, and brachialis

Free Weights   Standing upright, hold a barbell in front of you at about shoulder width with arms extended and the hands in a thumbs-out position (supinated grip) (a). Raise the barbell to your shoulders (b) and slowly return it to the starting position.

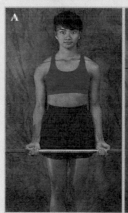
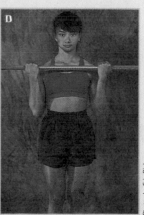

Photos by Eric Risberg

Exercise 20
Leg Curl

Action Lie with the face down on the bench, legs straight, and place the back of the feet under the padded bar (a). Curl up to at least 90° (b), and return to the original position.

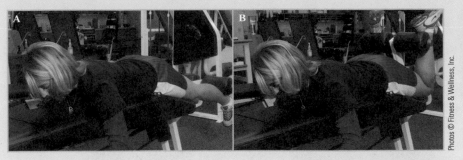

Photos © Fitness & Wellness, Inc.

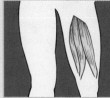

Back

Muscles Developed
Hamstrings

Exercise 21
Seated Back

Action Sit in the machine with your trunk flexed and the upper back against the shoulder pad. Place the feet under the padded bar and hold on with your hands to the bars on the sides (a). Start the exercise by pressing backward, simultaneously extending the trunk and hip joints (b). Slowly return to the original position.

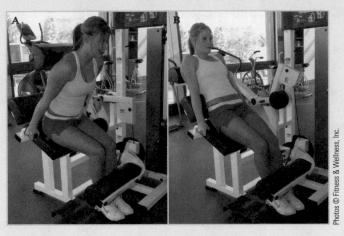

Photos © Fitness & Wellness, Inc.

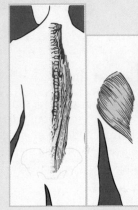

Back   Back

Muscles Developed
Erector spinae and gluteus maximus

Exercise 22
Calf Press

Machine Start with your feet flat on the plate (a), then extend the ankles by pressing on the plate with the balls of your feet (b).

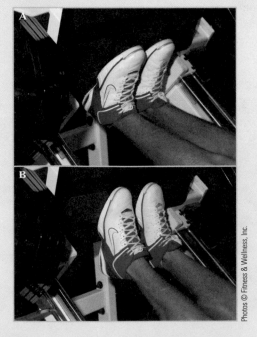

Photos © Fitness & Wellness, Inc.

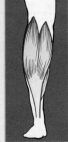

Back

Muscles Developed
Gastrocnemius, soleus

Free Weights In a standing position, place a barbell across the shoulders and upper back. Grip the bar away from the shoulders as far out as needed (a). Place the balls of your feet over a weight plate or a small board so that your heels are lower than the front of your feet. Raise your heels off the floor as far as possible (b) and then slowly return them to the starting position.

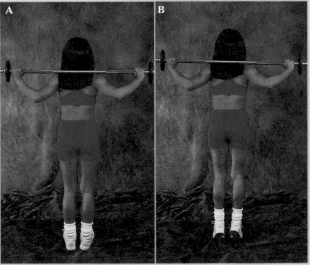

© Eric Risberg

Exercise 23
Lat Pull-Down

Action Starting from a sitting position, hold the exercise bar with a wide grip (a). Pull the bar down in front of you until it reaches the base of the neck (b), then return to the starting position.

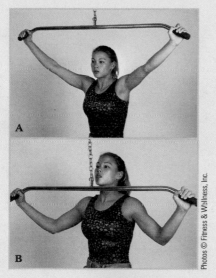

A

B

Photos © Fitness & Wellness, Inc.

Muscles Developed Latissimus dorsi, pectoralis major, and biceps

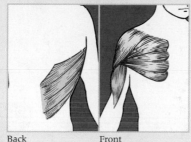

Back   Front

Exercise 24
Rotary Torso

Machine Sit upright in the machine and place the elbows behind the padded bars. Rotate the torso as far as possible to one side and then return slowly to the starting position. Repeat the exercise to the opposite side.

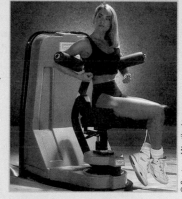

© Courtesy of Nautilus Inc.

Free Weights Stand with your feet slightly apart. Place a barbell across your shoulders and upper back, holding on to the sides of the barbell. Now gently, and in a controlled manner, twist your torso to one side as far as possible and then do so in the opposite direction.

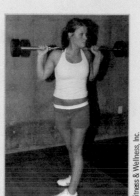

© Fitness & Wellness, Inc.

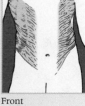

Front

Muscles Developed Internal and external obliques (abdominal muscles)

Exercise 25
Triceps Extension

Machine Sit in an upright position and grasp the bar behind the shoulders (a). Fully extend the arms (b) and then return to the original position.

Muscles Developed Triceps

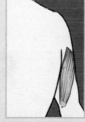

Back

Free Weights In a standing position, hold a barbell with both hands overhead and with the arms in full extension (a). Slowly lower the barbell behind your head (b) and then return it to the starting position.

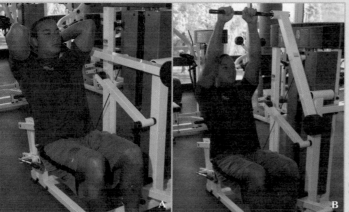

A   B

Photos © Fitness & Wellness, Inc.

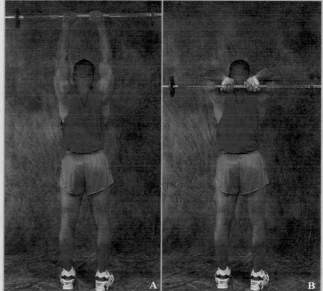

A   B

© Eric Fisberg

Exercise 26
Leg Extension

Action Sit in an upright position with the feet under the padded bar and grasp the handles at the sides (a). Extend the legs until they are completely straight (b), then return to the starting position.

Muscles Developed
Quadriceps

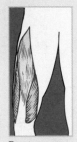

Front

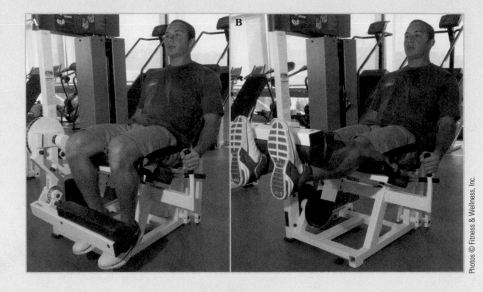

Photos © Fitness & Wellness, Inc.

Exercise 27
Shoulder Press

Machine Sit in an upright position and grasp the bar wider than shoulder width (a). Press the bar all the way up until the arms are fully extended (b), then return to the initial position.

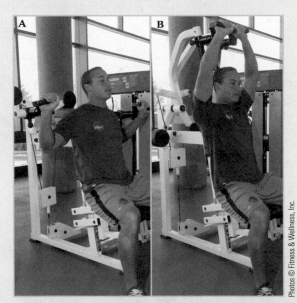

Photos © Fitness & Wellness, Inc.

Muscles Developed
Triceps, deltoid, and pectoralis major

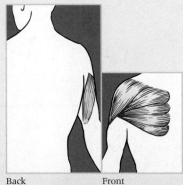

Back   Front

Free Weights Place a barbell on your shoulders in front of the body (a) and press the weight overhead until complete extension of the arms is achieved (b). Then return the weight to the original position. Be sure not to arch the back or lean back during this exercise.

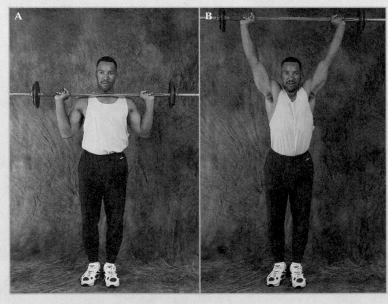

© Eric Risberg

Exercise 28
Chest Press

Action Start with the arms up to the side, and grasp the handle bars with the arms straight (a). Press the movement arms forward until they are completely in front of you (b). Slowly return to the starting position.

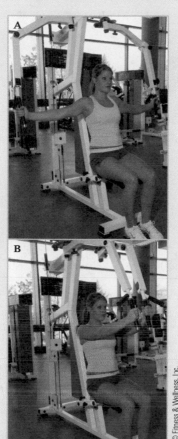

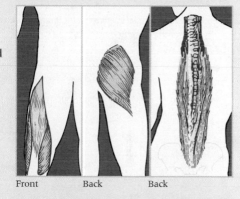

Front

Muscles Developed
Pectoralis major and deltoid

Photos © Fitness & Wellness, Inc.

Bent-Arm Flyes
Action Lie down on your back on a bench and hold a dumbbell in each hand directly overhead (a). Keeping your elbows slightly bent, lower the weights laterally to a horizontal position (b) and then bring them back up to the starting position.

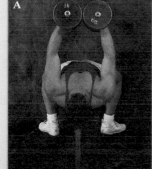

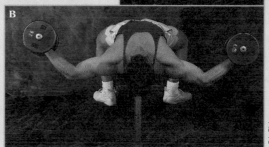

© Eric Risberg

Exercise 29
Squat

Machine Place the shoulders under the pads and grasp the bars by the sides of the shoulders (A). Completely extend the legs (B), then return to the original position.

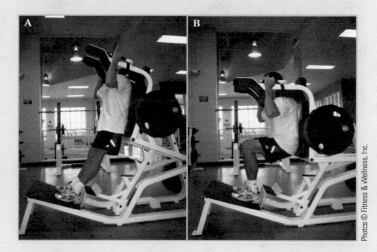

Photos © Fitness & Wellness, Inc.

Muscles Developed
Quadriceps, gluteus maximus, erector spinae

Front   Back   Back

Free Weights From a standing position, and with a spotter to each side, support a barbell over your shoulders and upper back (a). Keeping your head up and back straight, bend at the knees and the hips until you achieve an approximate 120° angle at the knees (b). Then return to the starting position. *Do not perform this exercise alone.* If no spotters are available, use a squat rack to ensure that you will not get trapped under a heavy weight.

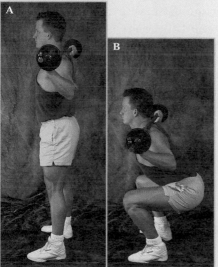

© Eric Risberg

Exercise 30
Upright Rowing

Machine Start with the arms extended and grip the handles with the palms down (a). Pull all the way up to the chin (b), then return to the starting position.

Free Weights Hold a barbell in front of you, with the arms fully extended and hands in a thumbs-in (pronated) grip less than shoulder-width apart (a). Pull the barbell up until it reaches shoulder level (b) and then slowly return it to the starting position.

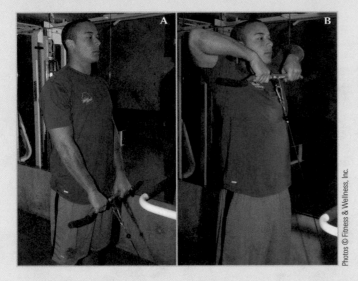

Photos © Fitness & Wellness, Inc.

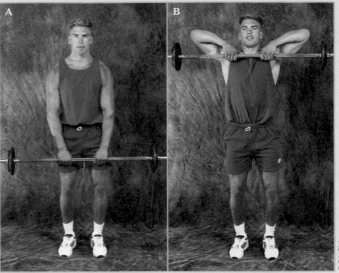

© Eric Risberg

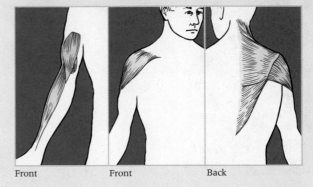

Front   Front   Back

Muscles Developed
Biceps, brachioradialis, brachialis, deltoid, and trapezius

Exercise 31
Seated Leg Curl

Action Sit in the unit and place the strap over the upper thighs. With legs extended, place the back of the feet over the padded rollers (a). Flex the knees until you reach a 90° to 100° angle (b). Slowly return to the starting position.

Muscles Developed
Hamstrings

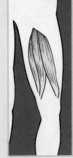

Back

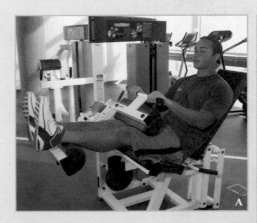

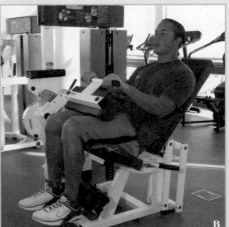

Photos © Fitness & Wellness, Inc.

Exercise 32
Bent-Arm Pullover

Machine Sit back into the chair and grasp the bar behind your head (a). Pull the bar over your head all the way down to your abdomen (b) and slowly return to the original position.

Free Weights Lie on your back on an exercise bench with the head over the edge of the bench. Hold a barbell over your chest with the hands less than shoulder-width apart (a). Keeping the elbows shoulder-width apart, lower the weight over your head until your shoulders are completely extended (b). Slowly return the weight to the starting position.

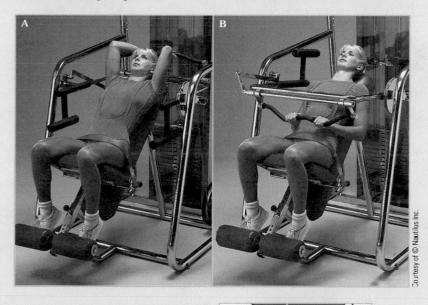

Courtesy of © Nautilus Inc.

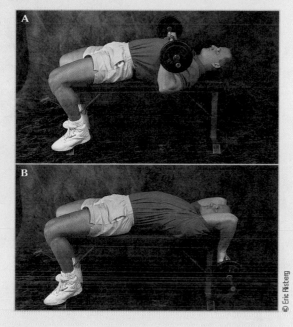

© Eric Risberg

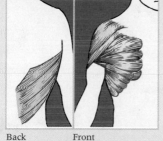

Back   Front

Muscles Developed
Latissimus dorsi, pectoral muscles, deltoid, and serratus anterior

Exercise 33
Triceps Extension

Action Using a palms-down grip, grasp the bar slightly closer than shoulder-width and start with the elbows almost completely bent (a). Extend the arms fully (b), then return to starting position.

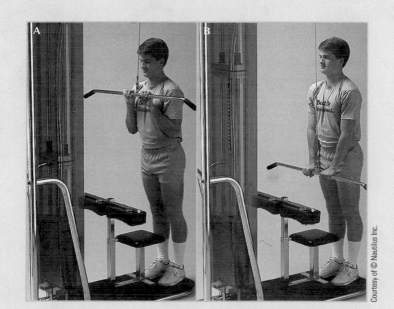

Courtesy of © Nautilus Inc.

Back

Muscles Developed
Triceps

Exercise 34
Dip

Action   Start with the elbows flexed (a), then extend the arms fully (b), and return slowly to the initial position.

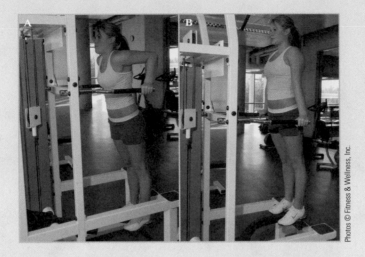

Photos © Fitness & Wellness, Inc.

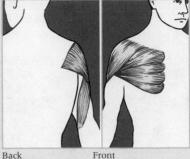

Back   Front

Muscles Developed
Triceps, deltoid, and pectoralis major

Exercise 35
Back Extension

Action   Place your feet under the ankle rollers and the hips over the padded seat. Start with the trunk in a flexed position and the arms crossed over the chest (a). Slowly extend the trunk to a horizontal position (b), hold the extension for two to five seconds, then slowly flex (lower) the trunk to the original position.

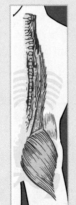

Muscles Developed
Erector spinae, gluteus maximus, and quadratus lumborum (lower back)

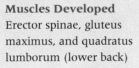

Back

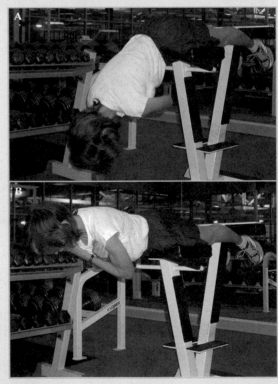

Photos © Fitness & Wellness, Inc.

Chapter 8

Muscular Flexibility

© Polka Dot Images/Jupiter Images

Objectives

- Explain the importance of muscular flexibility to adequate fitness and preventive health care.
- Identify the factors that affect muscular flexibility.
- Explain the health fitness benefits of stretching.
- Become familiar with a battery of tests to assess overall body flexibility (Trunk Forward Flexion Test, Total Body Rotation Test, Shoulder Rotation Test).
- Be able to interpret flexibility test results according to health-fitness and physical-fitness standards.
- Learn the principles that govern muscular flexibility development.
- List some exercises that may cause injury.
- Become familiar with a program for preventing and rehabilitating low-back pain.

Most fitness participants underestimate and overlook the contribution of good muscular flexibility to overall fitness and preventive health care. **Flexibility** refers to the achievable range of motion at a joint or group of joints without causing injury. Most people who exercise don't take the time to stretch, and many of those who do stretch don't stretch properly. When joints are not regularly moved through their normal range of motion, muscles and ligaments shorten in time, and flexibility decreases.

Some muscular/skeletal problems and injuries are related to a lack of flexibility. In daily life, we often have to make rapid or strenuous movements we are not accustomed to making. Abruptly forcing a tight muscle beyond its achievable range of motion may lead to injury.

A decline in flexibility can cause poor posture and subsequent aches and pains that lead to limited and painful joint movement. Inordinate tightness is uncomfortable and debilitating. According to the Arthritis Society, almost 20 million Canadians will suffer from at least one episode of back pain during their lifetime, and 1 in 50 Canadians will be disabled by it.[1] And, in the United States, approximately 80 percent of all low-back problems stem from improper alignment of the vertebral column and pelvic girdle, a direct result of inflexible and weak muscles. This backache syndrome costs billions of dollars each year in lost productivity, health care, and workers' compensation.

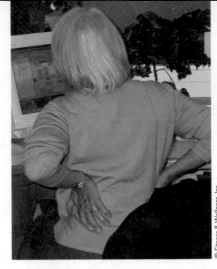

Excessive sitting and lack of physical activity lead to chronic back pain.

© Fitness & Wellness, Inc.

Benefits of Good Flexibility

Improving and maintaining good range of motion in the joints enhances the quality of life. Good flexibility promotes healthy muscles and joints. Improving elasticity of muscles and connective tissue around joints enables greater freedom of movement and the individual's ability to participate in many types of sports and recreational activities. Adequate flexibility also makes activities of daily living such as turning, lifting, and bending much easier to perform. A person must take care, however, not to overstretch joints. Too much flexibility leads to unstable and loose joints, which may increase injury rate, including joint dislocation and **subluxation**.

Taking part in a regular **stretching** program increases circulation to the muscle(s) being stretched, prevents low-back and other spinal column problems, improves and maintains good postural alignment, promotes proper and graceful body movement, improves personal appearance and self-image, and helps to develop and maintain motor skills throughout life.

Flexibility exercises have been prescribed successfully to treat **dysmenorrhea**[2] (painful menstruation), general neuromuscular tension (stress), and knots (trigger points) in muscles and fascia. Regular stretching helps decrease the aches and pains caused by psychological stress and contributes to a decrease in anxiety, blood pressure, and breathing rate.[3] Stretching also helps relieve muscle cramps encountered at rest or during participation in exercise.

Mild stretching exercises, in conjunction with calisthenics, are helpful in warm-up routines to prepare for more vigorous aerobic or strength-training exercises, and in cool-down routines following exercise to facilitate the return to a normal resting state. Fatigued muscles tend to contract to a shorter-than-average resting length, and stretching exercises help fatigued muscles reestablish their normal resting length.

Flexibility in Older Adults

Similar to muscular strength, good range of motion is critical in older life (see discussion in Chapter 9). Because of decreased flexibility, older adults lose mobility and may be unable to perform simple daily tasks such as bending forward or turning. Many older adults cannot turn their head or rotate their trunk to look over their shoulder but, rather, must step around 90° to 180° to see behind them. Adequate flexibility is also important for driving. Individuals who lose range of motion with age are unable to look over their shoulder to switch lanes or to parallel-park, increasing the risk for automobile accidents.

Physical activity and exercise can be hampered severely by lack of good range of motion. Because of the pain during activity, older people who have tight hip flexors (muscles) cannot jog or walk very far. A vicious circle ensues, because the condition usually worsens with further inactivity. Lack of flexibility also may be a cause of falls and subsequent injury in older adults. A simple stretching program can alleviate or prevent this problem and help people return to an exercise program.

Factors Affecting Flexibility

Total range of motion around a joint is highly specific and varies from one joint to another (hip, trunk, shoulder), as well as from one individual to the next. Muscular flexibility relates primarily to genetic factors and to physical activity. Joint structure (shape of the bones), joint cartilage, ligaments, tendons, muscles, skin, tissue injury, and adipose tissue (fat)—all influence range of motion about a joint. Body temperature, age, and gender also affect flexibility.

The range of motion about a given joint depends mostly on the structure of that joint. Greater range of motion, however, can be attained through plastic and elastic elongation. **Plastic elongation** is the permanent lengthening of soft tissue. Even though joint capsules, ligaments, and tendons are basically nonelastic, they can undergo plastic elongation. This permanent lengthening, accompanied by increased range of motion, is best attained through slow-sustained stretching exercises.

Elastic elongation is the temporary lengthening of soft tissue. Muscle tissue has elastic properties and responds to stretching exercises by undergoing elastic or temporary lengthening. Elastic elongation increases extensibility, or ability to stretch the muscles.

Changes in muscle temperature can increase or decrease flexibility by as much as 20 percent. Individuals who warm up properly have better flexibility than people who do not. Cool temperatures have the opposite effect, impeding range of motion. Because of the effects of temperature on muscular flexibility, many people prefer to do their stretching exercises after the aerobic phase of their workout. Aerobic activities raise body temperature, facilitating plastic elongation.

Another factor that influences flexibility is the amount of adipose (fat) tissue in and around joints and muscle tissue. Excess adipose tissue will increase resistance to movement, and the added bulk also hampers joint mobility because of the contact between body surfaces.

On the average, women have better flexibility than men do, and they seem to retain this advantage throughout life. Aging does decrease the extensibility of soft tissue, though, resulting in less flexibility in both sexes.

The most significant contributor to lower flexibility is sedentary living. With less physical activity, muscles lose their elasticity, and tendons and ligaments tighten and shorten. Inactivity also tends to be accompanied by an increase in adipose tissue, which further decreases the range of motion around a joint. Finally, injury to muscle tissue and tight skin from excessive scar tissue have negative effects on range of motion.

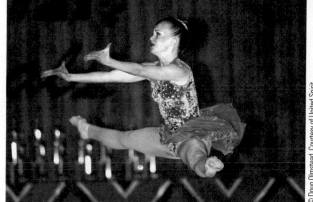

Adequate flexibility helps to develop and maintain sports skill throughout life.

Assessment of Flexibility

Many flexibility tests developed over the years were specific to certain sports or not practical for the general population. Their application in health and fitness programs was limited. For example, the Front-to-Rear Splits Test and the Bridge-Up Test had applications in sports such as gymnastics and several track-and-field events, but they did not represent actions that most people encounter in daily life.

Because of the lack of practical flexibility tests, most health and fitness centres rely strictly on the Trunk Forward Flexion (Sit-and-Reach) Test as an indicator of overall flexibility. This test measures flexibility of the hamstring muscles (back of the thigh) and, to a lesser extent, the lower back muscles.

Flexibility is joint-specific. This means that a lot of flexibility in one joint does not necessarily indicate that other joints are just as flexible. Therefore, the Total Body Rotation Test and the Shoulder Rotation Test—indicators of ability to perform everyday movements such as reaching, bending, and turning—are included to determine your flexibility profile.

The Trunk Forward Flexion Test has been modified from the traditional test to take length of arms and legs into consideration in determining the score (see Figure 8.1). In the original Trunk Forward Flexion Test, the 38 cm mark of the metre stick used to measure flexibility was always set at the edge of the box where the feet are placed. This does not take into consideration an individual with long arms and/or short legs or one with short arms and/or long legs.[4] All other factors being equal, an individual with longer arms or shorter legs, or both, receives a better rating because of the structural advantage.

Flexibility Refers to the achievable range of motion at a joint or group of joints without causing injury.

Subluxation Partial dislocation of a joint.

Stretching Moving the joints beyond the accustomed range of motion.

Dysmenorrhea Painful menstruation.

Plastic elongation Permanent lengthening of soft tissue.

Elastic elongation Temporary lengthening of soft tissue.

FIGURE 8.1 Procedure for the Trunk Forward Flexion (Sit-and-Reach) Test

To perform this test you will need a Sit-and-Reach Box available from a number of sources.* You may also place a metre stick on top of a box approximately 30 cm high.

1. Warm up properly before your first trial.
2. Remove your shoes for the test. Place your feet flat against the box.
3. Sit in an upright position.
4. Keep your feet flat against the box. Keep your legs straight. Do not have your legs held in place.
5. Extend your hands, with your palms facing downward.
6. Reach as far forward as possible. Don't jerk or bounce.
7. Hold this position for two seconds.
8. You may lower your head as you stretch forward.
9. This test should be done with a slow, controlled reach.
10. Repeat this test three times.
11. Measure the distance you reach to the nearest centimetre.
12. Average your scores for your final score.

* The Acuflex Flexibility Tester for the Sit and Reach Test can be obtained from Jansen Medical at 1-888-896-4050 or ordered online at http://www.jansenmedical.net/Acuflex-I-Modified-Flexibility-Sit-and-Reach-Test-Box-pr-2380.html.

TABLE 8.1 Percentile Ranks for the Trunk Forward Flexion (Sit-and-Reach) Test

15–19 Years of Age

Gender	Male	Female
Excellent	≥39	≥43
Very good	34–38	38–42
Good	29–33	34–37
Fair	24–28	29–33
Needs improvement	≤23	≤28

40–49 Years of Age

Gender	Male	Female
Excellent	≥35	≥38
Very good	29–34	34–37
Good	24–28	30–33
Fair	18–23	25–29
Needs improvement	≤17	≤24

20–29 Years of Age

Gender	Male	Female
Excellent	≥40	≥41
Very good	34–39	37–40
Good	30–33	33–36
Fair	25–29	28–32
Needs improvement	≤24	≤27

50–59 Years of Age

Gender	Male	Female
Excellent	>35	≥39
Very good	28–34	33–38
Good	24–27	30–32
Fair	16–23	25–29
Needs improvement	≤15	≤24

30–39 Years of Age

Gender	Male	Female
Excellent	≥38	≥41
Very good	33–37	36–40
Good	28–32	32–35
Fair	23–27	27–31
Needs improvement	≤22	≤26

60–69 Years of Age

Gender	Male	Female
Excellent	≥33	≥35
Very good	25–32	31–34
Good	20–24	27–30
Fair	15–19	23–26
Needs improvement	≤14	≤23

Source: *Canadian Physical Activity Fitness & Lifestyle Approach: CSEP-Health & Fitness Program's Health-Related Appraisal & Counselling Strategy*, Third Edition, © 2003. Reprinted with permission from the Canadian Society for Exercise Physiology.

FIGURE 8.2 Procedure for the Total Body Rotation Test

An Acuflex II* Total Body Rotation Flexibility Tester or a measuring scale with a sliding panel is needed to administer this test. The Acuflex II or scale is placed on the wall at shoulder height and should be adjustable to accommodate individual differences in height. If you need to build your own scale, use two measuring tapes and glue them above and below the sliding panel centred at the 38 cm mark. Each tape should be at least 76 cm long. If no sliding panel is available, simply tape the measuring tapes onto a wall oriented in opposite directions as shown below. A line also must be drawn on the floor and centred with the 38 cm mark.

1. Warm up properly before beginning this test.
2. Stand with one side toward the wall, an arm's length away from the wall, with the feet straight ahead, slightly separated, and the toes touching the centre line drawn on the floor. Hold out the arm away from the wall horizontally from the body, making a fist with the hand. The Acuflex II measuring scale or tapes should be shoulder height at this time.
3. Rotate the trunk, the extended arm going backward (always maintaining a horizontal plane) and making contact with the panel, gradually sliding it forward as far as possible. If no panel is available, slide the fist alongside the tapes as far as possible. Hold the final position at least two seconds. Position the hand with the little finger side forward during the entire sliding movement. **Proper hand position is crucial. Many people attempt to open the hand, or push with extended fingers, or slide the panel with the knuckles—none of which is acceptable.** During the test the knees can be bent slightly, but **the feet cannot be moved or rotated**—they must point forward. The body must be kept as straight (vertical) as possible.
4. Conduct the test on either the right or the left side of the body. Perform two trials on the selected side. Record the farthest point reached, measured to the nearest centimetre and held for at least two seconds. Use the average of the two trials as the final test score. Refer to Tables 8.2 and 8.4 to determine the percentile rank and flexibility fitness category for this test.

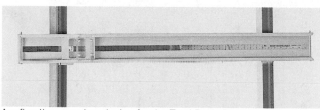

Acuflex II measuring device for the Total Body Rotation Test.

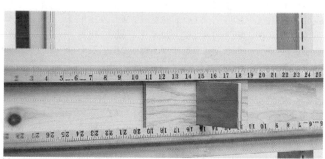

Homemade measuring device for the Total Body Rotation Test.

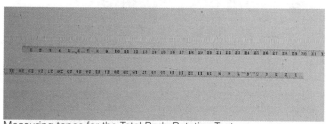

Measuring tapes for the Total Body Rotation Test.

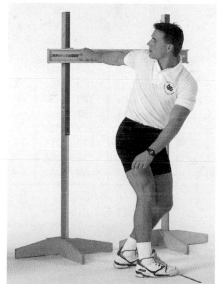

Total Body Rotation Test.

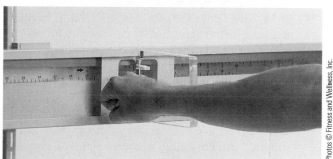

Proper hand position for the Total Body Rotation Test.

Photos © Fitness and Wellness, Inc.

---

* The Acuflex II Flexibility Tester for Total Body Rotation Test can be obtained from Jansen Medical at 1-888-896-4050 or ordered online at http://www.jansenmedical.net/Acuflex-II-Trunk-Rotation-Test-pr-2381.html.

TABLE 8.2 Percentile Ranks for the Total Body Rotation Test

	Percentile Rank	Left Rotation								Right Rotation							
		≤18		19–35		36–49		≥50		≤18		19–35		36–49		≥50	
		in.	cm	in.	cm	in.	cm	in.	cm	in.	cm	in.	cm	in.	cm	in.	cm
Men	99	29.1	73.9	28.0	71.1	26.6	67.6	21.0	53.3	28.2	71.6	27.8	70.6	25.2	64.0	22.2	56.4
	95	26.6	67.6	24.8	63.0	24.5	62.2	20.0	50.8	25.5	64.8	25.6	65.0	23.8	60.5	20.7	52.6
	90	25.0	63.5	23.6	59.9	23.0	58.4	17.7	45.0	24.3	61.7	24.1	61.2	22.5	57.1	19.3	49.0
	80	22.0	55.9	22.0	55.9	21.2	53.8	15.5	39.4	22.7	57.7	22.3	56.6	21.0	53.3	16.3	41.4
	70	20.9	53.1	20.3	51.6	20.4	51.8	14.7	37.3	21.3	54.1	20.7	52.6	18.7	47.5	15.7	39.9
	60	19.9	50.5	19.3	49.0	18.7	47.5	13.9	35.3	19.8	50.3	19.0	48.3	17.3	43.9	14.7	37.3
	50	18.6	47.2	18.0	45.7	16.7	42.4	12.7	32.3	19.0	48.3	17.2	43.7	16.3	41.4	12.3	31.2
	40	17.0	43.2	16.8	42.7	15.3	38.9	11.7	29.7	17.3	43.9	16.3	41.4	14.7	37.3	11.5	29.2
	30	14.9	37.8	15.0	38.1	14.8	37.6	10.3	26.2	15.1	38.4	15.0	38.1	13.3	33.8	10.7	27.2
	20	13.8	35.1	13.3	33.8	13.7	34.8	9.5	24.1	12.9	32.8	13.3	33.8	11.2	28.4	8.7	22.1
	10	10.8	27.4	10.5	26.7	10.8	27.4	4.3	10.9	10.8	27.4	11.3	28.7	8.0	20.3	2.7	6.9
	05	8.5	21.6	8.9	22.6	8.8	22.4	0.3	0.8	8.1	20.6	8.3	21.1	5.5	14.0	0.3	0.8
	01	3.4	8.6	1.7	4.3	5.1	13.0	0.0	0.0	6.6	16.8	2.9	7.4	2.0	5.1	0.0	0.0
Women	99	29.3	74.4	28.6	72.6	27.1	68.8	23.0	58.4	29.6	75.2	29.4	74.7	27.1	68.8	21.7	55.1
	95	26.8	68.1	24.8	63.0	25.3	64.3	21.4	54.4	27.6	70.1	25.3	64.3	25.9	65.8	19.7	50.0
	90	25.5	64.8	23.0	58.4	23.4	59.4	20.5	52.1	25.8	65.5	23.0	58.4	21.3	54.1	19.0	48.3
	80	23.8	60.5	21.5	54.6	20.2	51.3	19.1	48.5	23.7	60.2	20.8	52.8	19.6	49.8	17.9	45.5
	70	21.8	55.4	20.5	52.1	18.6	47.2	17.3	43.9	22.0	55.9	19.3	49.0	17.3	43.9	16.8	42.7
	60	20.5	52.1	19.3	49.0	17.7	45.0	16.0	40.6	20.8	52.8	18.0	45.7	16.5	41.9	15.6	39.6
	50	19.5	49.5	18.0	45.7	16.4	41.7	14.8	37.6	19.5	49.5	17.3	43.9	14.6	37.1	14.0	35.6
	40	18.5	47.0	17.2	43.7	14.8	37.6	13.7	34.8	18.3	46.5	16.0	40.6	13.1	33.3	12.8	32.5
	30	17.1	43.4	15.7	39.9	13.6	34.5	10.0	25.4	16.3	41.4	15.2	38.6	11.7	29.7	8.5	21.6
	20	16.0	40.6	15.2	38.6	11.6	29.5	6.3	16.0	14.5	36.8	14.0	35.6	9.8	24.9	3.9	9.9
	10	12.8	32.5	13.6	34.5	8.5	21.6	3.0	7.6	12.4	31.5	11.1	28.2	6.1	15.5	2.2	5.6
	05	11.1	28.2	7.3	18.5	6.8	17.3	0.7	1.8	10.2	25.9	8.8	22.4	4.0	10.2	1.1	2.8
	01	8.9	22.6	5.3	13.5	4.3	10.9	0.0	0.0	8.9	22.6	3.2	8.1	2.8	7.1	0.0	0.0

▓ High physical fitness standard   ░ Health fitness standard

The procedures and norms for the flexibility tests are described in Figures 8.1 through 8.3 and Tables 8.1 through 8.3. The flexibility test results in these three tables are provided in both inches (in.) and centimetres (cm). Be sure to use the proper column to read your percentile score based on your test results. For the flexibility profile, you should take all three tests. You will be able to assess your flexibility profile in Lab 8A. Because of the specificity of flexibility, pinpointing an "ideal" level of flexibility is difficult. Nevertheless, flexibility is important to health and independent living, so assessment will give an indication of level of flexibility.

Interpreting Flexibility Test Results

After obtaining your scores and fitness ratings for each test, you can determine the fitness category for each flexibility test using the guidelines given in Table 8.4. You also should look up the number of points assigned for each fitness category in this table. The overall flexibility fitness category is obtained by totalling the number of points from all three tests and using the ratings given in Table 8.5.

Evaluating Body Posture

Posture tests are used to detect deviations from normal body alignment and prescribe corrective exercises or procedures to improve alignment. These analyses are best conducted early in life, because certain postural deviations are more difficult to correct in older people. If deviations are allowed to go uncorrected, they usually become more serious as the person grows older. Consequently, corrective exercises or other medical procedures should be used to stop or slow postural degeneration.

A leading cause of chronic low-back problems is faulty posture together with weak and inelastic muscles. Thus, evaluation is crucial to prevent and rehabilitate low-back pain. The results of these tests can be used to prescribe corrective exercises.

FIGURE 8.3 Procedure for the Shoulder Rotation Test

This test can be done using the Acuflex III* Flexibility Tester, which consists of a shoulder caliper and a measuring device for shoulder rotation. If this equipment is unavailable, you can construct your own device quite easily. The caliper can be built with three regular metre sticks. Nail and glue two of the metre sticks at one end at a 90° angle, and use the third one as the sliding end of the caliper. Construct the rotation device by placing a 150 cm measuring tape on an aluminum or wood stick, starting at about 15 or 20 cm from the end of the stick.

1. Warm up before the test.
2. Using the shoulder caliper, measure the biacromial width to the nearest 0.5 cm (use the top scale on the Acuflex III). Measure biacromial width between the lateral edges of the acromion processes of the shoulders.
3. Place the Acuflex III or homemade device behind the back and use a reverse grip (thumbs out) to hold on to the device. Place the index finger of the right hand next to the zero point of the scale or tape (lower scale on the Acuflex III) and hold it firmly in place throughout the test. Place the left hand on the other end of the measuring device wherever comfortable.

4. Standing straight up and extending both arms to full length, with elbows locked, slowly bring the measuring device over the head until it reaches about forehead level. For subsequent trials, depending on the resistance encountered when rotating the shoulders, move the left grip 1 cm at a time, and repeat the task until you no longer can rotate the shoulders without undue strain or starting to bend the elbows. Always keep the right-hand grip against the zero point of the scale. Measure the last successful trial to the nearest centimetre. Take this measurement at the inner edge of the left hand on the side of the little finger.

5. Determine the final score for this test by subtracting the biacromial width from the best score (shortest distance) between both hands on the rotation test. For example, if the best score is 90 cm and the biacromial width is 40 cm, the final score is 50 cm (90 − 40 = 50). Using Tables 8.3 and 8.4, determine the percentile rank and flexibility fitness category for this test.

*The Acuflex III Flexibility Tester for the Shoulder Rotation Test can be obtained from Jansen Medical at 1-888-896-4050 or ordered online at http://www.jansenmedical.net/Acuflex-III-Shoulder-Rotation-Test-pr-2382.html.

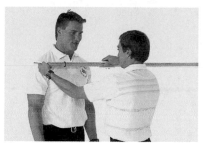

Measuring biacromial width.

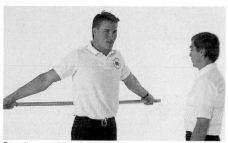

Starting position for the shoulder rotation test (note the reverse grip used for this test).

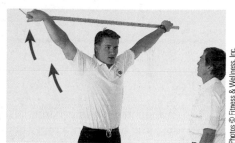

Shoulder rotation test.

Photos © Fitness & Wellness, Inc.

TABLE 8.3 Percentile Ranks for the Shoulder Rotation Test

	Age Category—Men								Age Category—Women							
Percentile Rank	≤18		19–35		36–49		≥50		Percentile Rank	≤18		19–35		36–49		≥50	
	in.	cm	in.	cm	in.	cm	in.	cm		in.	cm	in.	cm	in.	cm	in.	cm
99	2.2	5.6	−1.0	−2.5	18.1	46.0	21.5	54.6	99	2.6	6.6	−2.4	−6.1	11.5	29.2	13.1	33.3
95	15.2	38.6	10.4	26.4	20.4	51.8	27.0	68.6	95	8.0	20.3	6.2	15.7	15.4	39.1	16.5	41.9
90	18.5	47.0	15.5	39.4	20.8	52.8	27.9	70.9	90	10.7	27.2	9.7	24.6	16.8	42.7	20.9	53.1
80	20.7	52.6	18.4	46.7	23.3	59.2	28.5	72.4	80	14.5	36.8	14.5	36.8	19.2	48.8	22.5	57.1
70	23.0	58.4	20.5	52.1	24.7	62.7	29.4	74.7	70	16.1	40.9	17.2	43.7	21.5	54.6	24.3	61.7
60	24.2	61.5	22.9	58.2	26.6	67.6	29.9	75.9	60	19.2	48.8	18.7	47.5	23.1	58.7	25.1	63.8
50	25.4	64.5	24.4	62.0	28.0	71.1	30.5	77.5	50	21.0	53.3	20.0	50.8	23.5	59.7	26.2	66.5
40	26.3	66.8	25.7	65.3	30.0	76.2	31.0	78.7	40	22.2	56.4	21.4	54.4	24.4	62.0	28.1	71.4
30	28.2	71.6	27.3	69.3	31.9	81.0	31.7	80.5	30	23.2	58.9	24.0	61.0	25.9	65.8	29.9	75.9
20	30.0	76.2	30.1	76.5	33.3	84.6	33.1	84.1	20	25.0	63.5	25.9	65.8	29.8	75.7	31.5	80.0
10	33.5	85.1	31.8	80.8	36.1	91.7	37.2	94.5	10	27.2	69.1	29.1	73.9	31.1	79.0	33.1	84.1
05	34.7	88.1	33.5	85.1	37.8	96.0	38.7	98.3	05	28.0	71.1	31.3	79.5	33.4	84.8	34.1	86.6
01	40.8	103.6	42.6	108.2	43.0	109.2	44.1	112.0	01	32.5	82.5	37.1	94.2	34.9	88.6	35.4	89.9

■ High physical fitness standard   ▢ Health fitness standard

TABLE 8.4 Flexibility Fitness Categories According to Percentile Ranks

Percentile Rank	Fitness Category	Points
≥90	Excellent	5
70–80	Good	4
50–60	Average	3
30–40	Fair	2
≤20	Poor	1

TABLE 8.5 Overall Flexibility Fitness Categories

Total Points	Flexibility Category
≥13	Excellent
10–12	Good
7–9	Average
4–6	Fair
≤3	Poor

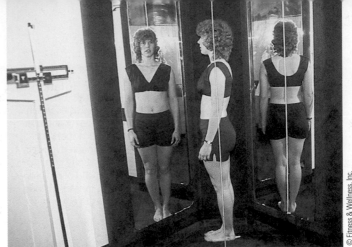

Photographic technique used for posture evaluation.

© Fitness & Wellness, Inc.

TABLE 8.6 Posture Evaluation Standards

Total Points	Category
≥45	Excellent
40–44	Good
30–39	Average
20–29	Fair
≤19	Poor

Adequate body mechanics also help alleviate chronic low-back pain. Proper body mechanics means using correct positions in all the activities of daily life, including sleeping, sitting, standing, walking, driving, working, and exercising. Because of the high incidence of low-back pain, illustrations of proper body mechanics and a series of corrective and preventive exercises are shown in Figure 8.7 on pages 253–254.

Most people are unaware of how faulty their posture is until they see themselves in a photograph. This can be quite a shock and is often enough to motivate them to institute change.

Besides engaging in the recommended exercises to elicit changes in postural alignment, individuals need to be continually aware of the corrections they are trying to make. As their posture improves, people frequently become motivated to change other aspects, such as improving muscular strength and flexibility and decreasing body fat.

Proper body alignment has been difficult to evaluate because most experts still don't know exactly what constitutes good posture. To objectively analyze a person's posture, an observer either must be adequately trained or must have some guidelines to identify abnormalities and assign ratings according to the amount of deviation from "normal" posture.

A posture rating chart, such as that in Lab 8B, provides simple guidelines for evaluating posture. Assuming that the drawings in the left column illustrate proper alignment and the drawings in the right column are extreme deviations from normal, an observer is able to rate each body segment on a scale from 1 to 5.

Postural analysis can be done with more precision with the aid of a plumb line, two mirrors, and a Polaroid camera. The mirrors are placed at an 80 to 85 percent angle, and the plumb line is centred in front of the mirrors. Another line is drawn down the centre of the mirror on the right. The person should stand with the left side to the plumb line. The plumb line is used as a reference to divide the body into front and back halves (try to centre the line with the hip joint and the shoulder). The line on the back (right) mirror should divide the body into right and left halves. A picture then is taken (like the photo above) that can be compared to the rating chart given in Lab 8B.

The photographic procedure allows for a better comparison of the different body segment alignments and a more objective analysis. If no mirrors and camera are available, the participant should stand with his or her side to the line, then repeat with the back to the line, while the evaluator does the assessment.

A final posture score is determined according to the sum of the ratings obtained for each body segment. Table 8.6 contains the various categories as determined by the final posture score.

Principles of Muscular Flexibility Prescription

Even though genetics play a crucial role in body flexibility, the range of joint mobility can be increased and maintained through a regular stretching program. Because range of motion is highly specific to each body part (ankle, trunk, shoulder), a comprehensive stretching program should include all body parts and follow the basic guidelines for flexibility development.

The overload and specificity of training principles (discussed in conjunction with strength development in Chapter 7) also apply to the development of muscular flexibility. To increase the total range of motion of a joint, the specific muscles surrounding that joint have to be stretched progressively beyond their accustomed length. The principles of mode, intensity, repetitions, and frequency of exercise can also be applied to flexibility programs.

Mode of Training

Three modes of stretching exercises can increase flexibility:

1. Ballistic stretching.
2. Slow-sustained stretching.
3. Proprioceptive neuromuscular facilitation (PNF) stretching.

Although research has indicated that all three types of stretching are effective in improving flexibility, each technique has certain advantages.

BALLISTIC STRETCHING

Ballistic (or **dynamic**) **stretching** exercises are done with jerky, rapid, and bouncy movements that provide the necessary force to lengthen the muscles. This type of stretching helps to develop flexibility, but the ballistic actions may cause muscle soreness and injury from small tears to the soft tissue.

Precautions must be taken not to overstretch ligaments, because they will undergo plastic or permanent elongation. If the stretching force cannot be controlled—as often occurs in fast, jerky movements—ligaments can easily be overstretched. This, in turn, leads to excessively loose joints, increasing the risk for injuries. Slow, gentle, and **controlled ballistic stretching** (instead of jerky, rapid, and bouncy movements), however, is effective in developing flexibility, and most individuals can perform it safely.

SLOW-SUSTAINED STRETCHING

With the **slow-sustained stretching** technique, muscles are lengthened gradually through a joint's complete range of motion and the final position is held for a few seconds. A slow-sustained stretch causes the muscles to relax and thereby achieve greater length. This type of stretch causes little pain and has a low risk for injury. Slow-sustained stretching exercises are the most frequently used and recommended in flexibility-development programs.

PROPRIOCEPTIVE NEUROMUSCULAR FACILITATION (PNF)

Proprioceptive neuromuscular facilitation (PNF) stretching is based on a "contract-and-relax" method and requires the assistance of another person. The procedure is as follows:

1. The person assisting with the exercise provides initial force by pushing slowly in the direction of the desired stretch. This first stretch does not cover the entire range of motion.
2. The person being stretched then applies force in the opposite direction of the stretch, against the assistant, who tries to hold the initial degree of stretch as close as possible. This results in an isometric contraction at the angle of the stretch.
3. After four or five seconds of isometric contraction, the person being stretched relaxes the target muscle completely. The assistant then increases the degree of stretch slowly to a greater angle.
4. The isometric contraction is repeated for another four or five seconds, after which the muscle is relaxed again. The assistant then can increase the degree of stretch, slowly, one more time.

Steps 1 through 4 are repeated two to five times, until the exerciser feels mild discomfort. On the last trial, the final stretched position should be held for several seconds.

Theoretically, with the PNF technique, the isometric contraction helps relax the muscle being stretched, which results in lengthening the muscle. Some fitness leaders believe PNF is more effective than slow-sustained stretching. Another benefit of PNF is an increase in strength of the muscle(s) being stretched. Research has shown approximately 17 and 35 percent increases in absolute strength and muscular endurance, respectively, in the hamstring muscle group after 12 weeks of PNF stretching.[5] The

---

Ballistic (dynamic) stretching Exercises done with jerky, rapid, bouncy movements, or slow, short, and sustained movements.

Controlled ballistic stretching Exercises done with slow, short, and sustained movements.

Slow-sustained stretching Exercises in which the muscles are lengthened gradually through a joint's complete range of motion.

Proprioceptive neuromuscular facilitation (PNF) Mode of stretching that uses reflexes and neuromuscular principles to relax the muscles that are being stretched.

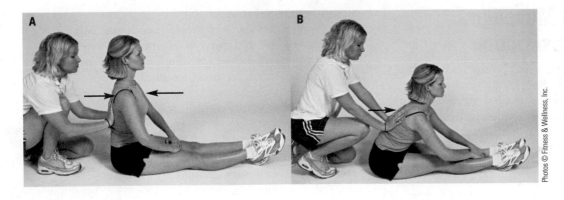

Proprioceptive neuromuscular facilitation (PNF) stretching technique: (A) isometric phase, (B) stretching phase.

results were consistent in both men and women and are attributed to the isometric contractions performed during PNF. Disadvantages of PNF are (1) more pain, (2) the need for a second person to assist, and (3) the need for more time to conduct each session.

Intensity

The **intensity**, or degree of stretch, when doing flexibility exercises should be only to a point of mild discomfort. Pain does not have to be part of the stretching routine. Excessive pain is an indication that the load is too high and may cause injury.

All stretching should be done to slightly below the pain threshold. As participants reach this point, they should try to relax the muscle being stretched as much as possible. After completing the stretch, the body part is brought back gradually to the starting point.

CRITICAL THINKING

Carefully consider the relevance of stretching exercises to your personal fitness program. How much importance do you place on these exercises? Have some conditions improved through your stretching program, or have certain specific exercises contributed to your health and well-being?

Repetitions

The time required for an exercise session for flexibility development is based on the number of **repetitions** and the length of time each repetition is held in the final stretched position. As a general recommendation, each exercise should be done four or five times, holding the final position each time for 10 to 30 seconds.

As flexibility increases, a person can gradually increase the time each repetition is held, to a maximum of one minute. Individuals who are susceptible to flexibility injuries should limit each stretch to 20 seconds. Pilates exercises are recommended for these individuals, as they increase joint stability (also see Chapter 7, page 214).

FIGURE 8.4 Guidelines for flexibility development

Mode:	Static or dynamic (slow ballistic or proprioceptive neuromuscular facilitation) stretching to include every major joint of the body
Intensity:	Stretch to the point of mild discomfort
Repetitions:	Repeat each exercise at least 4 times and hold the final stretched position for 10 to 30 seconds
Frequency:	2–3 days per week

Based on American College of Sports Medicine, "Position Stand: The Recommended Quantity and Quality of Exercise for Developing and Maintaining Cardiorespiratory and Muscular Fitness, and Flexibility in Healthy Adults," *Medical Science Sports Exercise* 30 (1998): 975–991.

Frequency of Exercise

Flexibility exercises should be conducted five or six times a week in the early stages of the program. After six to eight weeks of almost daily stretching, flexibility can be maintained with only two or three sessions per week, doing about three repetitions of 10 to 30 seconds each. Figure 8.4 summarizes the flexibility development guidelines.

When to Stretch?

Many people do not differentiate a warm-up from stretching. Warming up means starting a workout slowly with walking, cycling, or slow jogging, followed by gentle stretching (not through the entire range of motion). Stretching implies movement of joints through their full range of motion and holding the final degree of stretch according to recommended guidelines.

A warm-up that progressively increases muscle temperature and mimics movement that will occur during training enhances performance. For some activities, gentle stretching is recommended in conjunction with warm-up routines. Before steady activities (walking, jogging, cycling), a warm-up of three to five minutes is recommended. Up to 10 minutes is the recommendation before stop-and-go activities (racquet sports, basketball, soccer) and athletic participation in general (football, gymnastics). Activities that require abrupt changes in direction are more likely to cause muscle strains if they are performed without proper warm-up that includes mild stretching.

Sports-specific/pre-exercise stretching can improve performance in sports that require greater-than-average range of motion, such as gymnastics, dance, swimming, and figure skating. Some evidence, however, suggests that intense stretching during warm-up can lead to a temporary short-term (up to 60 minutes) decrease in strength. Thus extensive stretching conducted prior to participation in athletic events that rely on strength and power for peak performance is not recommended.[6]

With regard to preventing injuries, the best time to stretch is controversial. In limited studies on athletic populations, the evidence is unclear as to whether stretching before or after exercise is more beneficial in preventing injury. Additional research is necessary to clarify this issue.

In general, a good time to stretch is after aerobic workouts. Higher body temperature in itself helps to increase the joint range of motion. Muscles also are fatigued following exercise, and a fatigued muscle tends to shorten, which can lead to soreness and spasms. Stretching exercises help fatigued muscles reestablish their normal resting length and prevent unnecessary pain.

Flexibility Exercises

To improve body flexibility, each major muscle group should be subjected to at least one stretching exercise. A complete set of exercises for developing muscular flexibility is presented on pages 257–260.

You may not be able to hold a final stretched position with some of these exercises (such as lateral head tilts and arm circles), but you still should perform the exercise through the joint's full range of motion. Depending on the number and length of repetitions, a complete workout will last between 15 and 30 minutes.

Contraindicated Exercises

Most strength and flexibility exercises are relatively safe to perform, but even safe exercises can be hazardous if they are performed incorrectly. Some exercises may be safe to perform occasionally but, when executed repeatedly, may cause trauma and

injury. Preexisting muscle or joint conditions (old sprains or injuries) can further increase the risk of harm during certain exercises. As you develop your exercise program, you are encouraged to follow the exercise descriptions and guidelines given in this book.

A few exercises, however, are not recommended because of the potential high risk for injury. These exercises are sometimes performed in videotaped workouts and some fitness classes. **Contraindicated exercises** may cause harm because of the excessive strain placed on muscles and joints, in particular the spine, lower back, knees, neck, or shoulders.

Illustrations of contraindicated exercises are presented in Figure 8.5. Safe alternative exercises are listed below each contraindicated exercise and are illustrated in the exercises for strength (pages 221–234) and flexibility (pages 257–260). In isolated instances, a qualified physical therapist may select one or a few of the contraindicated exercises to treat a specific injury or disability in a carefully supervised setting. You might also see some of these exercises being taught in specialized fitness sessions such as Pilates and Yoga classes. Unless you are specifically instructed to use one of these exercises, it is best that you select safe exercises from this book.

Preventing and Rehabilitating Low-Back Pain

Few people make it through life without having low-back pain at some point. An estimated 60 to 80 percent of the population has been afflicted by back pain or injury.

Back pain is considered chronic if it persists longer than three months. It has been determined that backache syndrome is preventable about 80 percent of the time, and is caused by (a) physical inactivity, (b) poor postural habits and body mechanics, (c) excessive body weight, and/or (d) psychological stress. Data also indicate that back injuries are more common among smokers.

More than 95 percent of all back pain is related to muscle or tendon injury, and only 1 to 5 percent is related to intervertebral disk damage.[7] Usually, back pain is the result of repeated micro-injuries that occur over an extended time (sometimes years) until a certain movement, activity, or excessive overload causes a significant injury to the tissues.[8]

Intensity (for flexibility exercises) Degree of stretch when doing flexibility exercises.

Repetitions Number of times a given resistance is performed.

Contraindicated exercises Exercises that are not recommended because they may cause injury to a person.

FIGURE 8.5 Contraindicated exercises

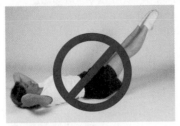

Double-Leg Lift

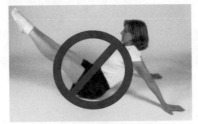

Upright Double-Leg Lifts

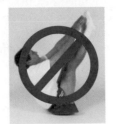

V-Sits

All three of these exercises cause excessive strain on the spine and may harm disks.

Alternatives: Strength Exercises 4 and 17, pages 222 and 226

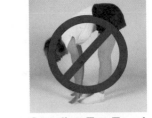

Standing Toe Touch

Excessive strain on the knee and lower back.

Alternative: Flexibility Exercise 12, page 258

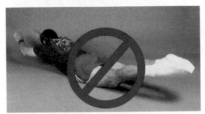

Swan Stretch

Excessive strain on the spine; may harm intervertebral disks.

Alternative: Flexibility Exercise 20, page 259

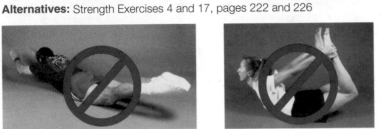

Cradle

Excessive strain on the spine, knees, and shoulders.

Alternatives: Flexibility Exercises 20, 8, and 6, pages 259, 258, and 257

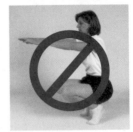

Full Squat

Excessive strain on the knees.

Alternatives: Flexibility Exercise 8, page 258; Strength Exercises 1, 16, 27, pages 221, 226, and 230

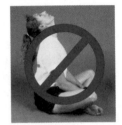

Head Rolls

May injure neck disks.

Alternative: Flexibility Exercise 1, page 257

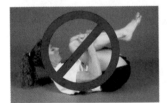

Knee to Chest

(with hands over the shin) Excessive strain on the knee.

Alternative: Flexibility Exercises 15 and 16, page 259

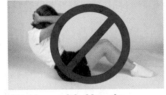

Sit-Ups with Hands Behind the Head

Excessive strain on the neck.

Alternatives: Strength Exercises 4 and 17, pages 222 and 226

Yoga Plow

Excessive strain on the spine, neck, and shoulders.

Alternatives: Flexibility Exercises 12, 15, 16, 17, and 19, pages 258–259

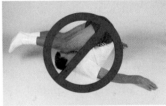
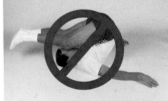

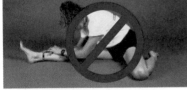

Hurdler Stretch

Excessive strain on the bent knee.

Alternatives: Flexibility Exercises 8 and 12, page 258

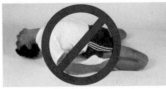

The Hero

Excessive strain on the knees.

Alternatives: Flexibility Exercises 8 and 14, pages 258 and 259

Windmill

Excessive strain on the spine and knees.

Alternatives: Flexibility Exercises 12 and 21, pages 258 and 260

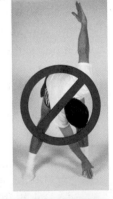

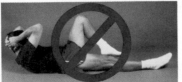

Straight-Leg Sit-Ups

Alternating Bent-Leg Sit-Ups

These exercises strain the lower back.

Alternatives: Strength Exercises 4 and 17, pages 222 and 226

Donkey Kicks

Excessive strain on the back, shoulders, and neck.

Alternatives: Flexibility Exercises 20, 14, and 1, pages 259 and 257

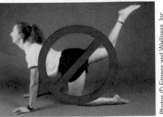

Photos © Fitness and Wellness, Inc.

FIGURE 8.6 Incorrect (left) and correct (right) pelvic alignment

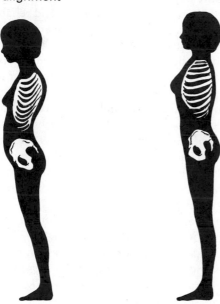

People tend to think of back pain as a problem with the skeleton. In fact, the spine's curvature, alignment, and movement are controlled by surrounding muscles. Lack of physical activity is the most common reason for chronic low-back pain. In particular, a major contributor to back pain is excessive sitting, which causes back muscles to shorten, stiffen, and become weaker.

Deterioration or weakening of the abdominal and gluteal muscles, along with tightening of the lower back (erector spinae) muscles, brings about an unnatural forward tilt of the pelvis (Figure 8.6). This tilt puts extra pressure on the spinal vertebrae, causing pain in the lower back. Accumulation of fat around the midsection of the body contributes to the forward tilt of the pelvis, which further aggravates the condition.

Low-back pain frequently is associated with faulty posture and improper body mechanics, or body positions in all of life's daily activities, including sleeping, sitting, standing, walking, driving, working, and exercising. Incorrect posture and poor mechanics, such as prolonged static postures, repetitive bending and pushing, twisting a loaded spine, and prolonged sitting with little movement (more than an hour) increase strain on the lower back and many other bones, joints, muscles, and ligaments. Figure 8.7 provides a summary of proper body mechanics that promote back health.

In the majority of back injuries, pain is present only with movement and physical activity. If the pain is severe and persists even at rest, the first step

is to consult a physician, who can rule out any disc damage and may prescribe proper bed rest using several pillows under the knees for leg support (see Figure 8.7). This position helps release muscle spasms by stretching the muscles involved. In addition, a physician may prescribe a muscle relaxant or anti-inflammatory medication (or both) and some type of physical therapy.

In most cases of low-back pain, even with severe pain, people feel better within days or weeks without treatment from health care professionals.[9] To relieve symptoms, you may use over-the-counter pain relievers and hot or cold packs. You should also stay active to avoid further weakening of the back muscles. Low-impact activities such as walking, swimming, water aerobics, and cycling are recommended. Once you are pain-free in the resting state, you need to start correcting the muscular imbalance by stretching the tight muscles and strengthening the weak ones. Stretching exercises always are performed first.

If there is no indication of disease or injury (such as leg numbness or pain), a herniated disk, or fractures, spinal manipulation by a chiropractor or other health care professional can provide pain relief. Spinal manipulation as a treatment modality for low-back pain has been endorsed by the Canadian Chiropractic Association (www.ccachiro.org). The guidelines suggest that spinal manipulation may help to alleviate discomfort and pain during the first few weeks of an acute episode of low-back pain. Generally, benefits are seen in fewer than 10 treatments. People who have had chronic pain for more

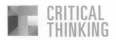

CRITICAL THINKING

Consider your own low-back health. Have you ever experienced episodes of low-back pain? If so, how long did it take you to recover, and what helped you recover from this condition?

than six months should avoid spinal manipulation until they have been thoroughly examined by a physician.

Back pain can be reduced greatly through aerobic exercise, muscular flexibility exercise, and muscular strength and endurance training that includes specific exercises to strengthen the spine-stabilizing muscles. Exercise requires effort by the patient, and it may create discomfort initially, but exercise promotes circulation, healing, muscle size, and muscle strength and endurance. Many patients abstain from aggressive physical therapy because they are unwilling to commit the time required for the program.

Aerobic exercise is beneficial because it helps decrease body fat and psychological stress. During an episode of back pain, however, people often avoid activity and cope by getting more rest. Rest is recommended if the pain is associated with a herniated disc, but if your physician rules out a serious problem, exercise is a better choice of treatment. Exercise helps restore physical function, and individuals who start and maintain an aerobic exercise program have back pain less frequently. Individuals who exercise are also less likely to require surgery or other invasive treatments.

With regard to flexibility, regular stretching exercises that help the hip and trunk go through a functional range of motion, as opposed to increasing the range of motion, are recommended. That is, for proper back care, stretching exercises should not be performed to the extreme range of motion. Individuals with a greater spinal range of motion also have a higher incidence of back injury. Spinal stability, instead of mobility, is desirable for back health.[10]

A strengthening program for a healthy back should be conducted around the endurance threshold—10 to 12 repetitions to near fatigue. Muscular endurance of the muscles that support the spine is more important than absolute strength because these muscles perform their work during the course of an entire day.

Several exercises for preventing and rehabilitating the backache syndrome are given on pages 259–260. These exercises can be done twice or more daily when a person has back pain. Under normal circumstances, doing these exercises three or four times a week is enough to prevent the syndrome. Using some of the additional core exercises listed in Chapter 7 (pages 221–226) will further enhance your low-back management program. Data have shown that back pain recurs more often in people who rely solely on medication, compared with people who use both medication and exercise therapy to recover.[11]

Lab 8C allows you to develop your own flexibility and low-back conditioning programs. The recommendation calls for isometric contractions of 2 to 20 seconds during each repetition for some of the exercises listed for back health (see Lab 8C) to further increase spinal stability and muscular strength endurance. The length of the hold depends on your current fitness level and the difficulty of each exercise. For most exercises, you may start with a 2- to 10-second hold. Over the course of several weeks, you can increase the length of the hold from 10 to 30 seconds.

Psychological stress may also lead to back pain.[12] Excessive stress causes muscles to contract. In the case of the lower back, frequent tightening of the muscles can throw the back out of alignment and constrict blood vessels that supply oxygen and nutrients to the back. Chronic stress also increases the release of hormones that have been linked to muscle and tendon injuries. Furthermore, people under stress tend to forget proper body mechanics, placing themselves at unnecessary risk for injury. If you are undergoing excessive stress and back pain at the same time, proper stress management (see Chapter 10) should be a part of your comprehensive back-care program.

FIGURE 8.7 Your back and how to care for it

Whatever the cause of low-back pain, part of its treatment is the correction of faulty posture. But good posture is not simply a matter of "standing tall." It refers to correct use of the body at all times. In fact, for the body to function in the best of health it must be so used that no strain is put upon the muscles, joints, bones, and ligaments. To prevent low-back pain, avoiding strain must become a way of life, practised while lying, sitting, standing, walking, working, and exercising. When body position is correct, internal organs have enough room to function normally and blood circulates more freely.

With the help of this guide, you can begin to correct the positions and movements that bring on or aggravate backache. Particular attention should be paid to the positions recommended for resting, since it is possible to strain the muscles of the back and neck even while lying in bed. By learning to live with good posture, under all circumstances, you will gradually develop the proper carriage and stronger muscles needed to protect and support your hard-working back.

Source: Schering Corporation

How to Stay on Your Feet Without Tiring Your Back

To prevent strain and pain in everyday activities, it is restful to change from one task to another before fatigue sets in. People doing housework can lie down between chores; others should check body position frequently, drawing in the abdomen, flattening the back, bending the knees slightly.

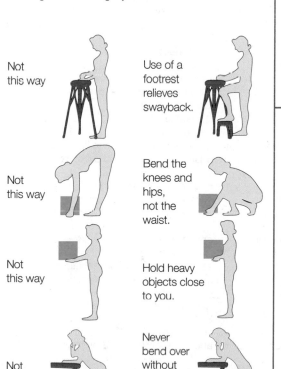

Not this way

Use of a footrest relieves swayback.

Not this way

Bend the knees and hips, not the waist.

Not this way

Hold heavy objects close to you.

Not this way

Never bend over without bending the knees.

Check Your Carriage Here

In correct, fully erect posture, a line dropped from the ear will go through the tip of the shoulder, middle of hip, back of kneecap, and front of anklebone.

Incorrect
Lower back is arched or hollow.

Incorrect
Upper back is stooped, lower back is arched, abdomen sags.

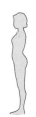
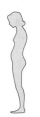

Incorrect
Note how, in strained position, pelvis tilts forward, chin is out, and ribs are down, crowding internal organs.

Correct
In correct position, chin is in, head up, back flattened, pelvis held straight.

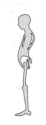
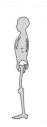

To find the correct standing position: Stand one foot away from wall. Now sit against wall, bending knees slightly. Tighten abdominal and buttock muscles. This will tilt the pelvis back and flatten the lower spine. Holding this position, inch up the wall to standing position, by straightening the legs. Now walk around the room, maintaining the same posture. Place back against wall again to see if you have held it.

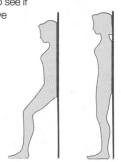

How to Sit Correctly

A back's best friend is a straight, hard chair. If you can't get the chair you prefer, learn to sit properly on whatever chair you get. *To correct sitting position from forward slump:* Throw head well back, then bend it forward to pull in the chin. This will straighten the back. Now tighten abdominal muscles to raise the chest. Check position frequently.

Use of footrest relieves swayback. Aim is to have knees higher than hips.

Correct way to sit while driving, close to pedals. Use seat belt or hard backrest, available commercially.

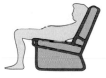

TV slump leads to "dowager's hump," strains neck and shoulders.

If chair is too high, swayback is increased.

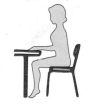

Keep neck and back in as straight a line as possible with the spine. Bend forward from hips.

Driver's seat too far from pedals emphasizes curve in lower back.

Strained reading position. Forward thrusting strains muscles of neck and head.

(continued)

FIGURE 8.7 (Continued)

How to Put Your Back to Bed

For proper bed posture, a firm mattress is essential. Bedboards, sold commercially, or devised at home, may be used with soft mattresses. Bedboards, preferably, should be made of 2 cm plywood. Faulty sleeping positions intensify swayback and result not only in backache but in numbness, tingling, and pain in arms and legs.

Incorrect:

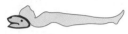

Lying flat on back makes swayback worse.

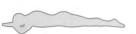

Use of high pillow strains neck, arms, shoulders.

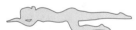

Sleeping face down exaggerates swayback, strains neck and shoulders.

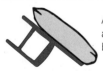

Bending one hip and knee does not relieve swayback.

Correct:

Lying on side with knees bent effectively flattens the back. Flat pillow may be used to support neck, especially when shoulders are broad.

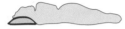

Sleeping on back is restful and correct when knees are properly supported.

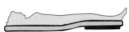

Raise the foot of the mattress 20 cm to discourage sleeping on the abdomen.

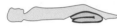

Proper arrangement of pillows for resting or reading in bed.

A straight-back chair used behind a pillow makes a serviceable backrest.

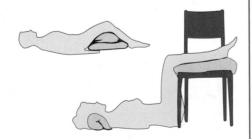

When Doing Nothing, Do it Right

- Rest is the first rule for the tired, painful back. The above positions relieve pain by taking all pressure and weight off the back and legs.
- Note pillows under knees to relieve strain on spine.
- For complete relief and relaxing effect, these positions should be maintained from 5 to 25 minutes.

Exercise Without Getting Out of Bed

Exercises to be performed while lying in bed are aimed not so much at strengthening muscles as at teaching correct positioning. But muscles used correctly become stronger and in time are able to support the body with the least amount of effort.

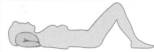

Do all exercises in this position. Legs should not be straightened.

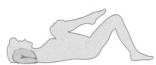

Bring knee up to chest. Lower slowly but do not straighten leg. Relax. Repeat with each leg 10 times.

Exercise Without Attracting Attention

Use these inconspicuous exercises whenever you have a spare moment during the day, both to relax tension and improve the tone of important muscle groups.

1. Rotate shoulders, forward and backward.
2. Turn head slowly side to side.
3. Watch an imaginary plane take off, just below the right shoulder. Stretch neck, follow it slowly as it moves up, around and down, disappearing below the other shoulder. Repeat, starting on left side.
4. Slowly, slowly, touch left ear to left shoulder, right ear to right shoulder. Raise both shoulders to touch ears, drop them as far down as possible.
5. At any pause in the day—waiting for an elevator to arrive, for a specific traffic light to change—pull in abdominal muscles, tighten, hold it for the count of eight without breathing. Relax slowly. Increase the count gradually after the first week, practise breathing normally with the abdomen flat and contracted. Do this sitting, standing, and walking.

Bring both knees slowly up to chest (place your hands on the lower thigh behind the knees). Tighten muscles of abdomen, press back flat against bed. Hold knees to chest 20 seconds, then lower slowly. Relax. Repeat five times. This exercise gently stretches the shortened muscles of the lower back, while strengthening abdominal muscles.

Rules to Live By—From Now On

1. Never bend from the waist only; bend the hips and knees.
2. Never lift a heavy object higher than your waist.
3. Always turn and face the object you wish to lift.
4. Avoid carrying unbalanced loads; hold heavy objects close to your body.
5. Never carry anything heavier than you can manage with ease.
6. Never lift or move heavy furniture. Wait for someone to do it who knows the principles of leverage.
7. Avoid sudden movements, sudden "overloading" of muscles. Learn to move deliberately, swinging the legs from the hips.
8. Learn to keep the head in line with the spine, when standing, sitting, lying in bed.
9. Put soft chairs and deep couches on your "don't sit" list. During prolonged sitting, cross your legs to rest your back.
10. Your doctor is the only one who can determine when low-back pain is due to faulty posture and he is the best judge of when you may do general exercises for physical fitness. When you do, omit any exercise that arches or overstrains the lower back: backward bends, or forward bends, touching the toes with the knees straight.
11. Wear shoes with moderate heels, all about the same height. Avoid changing from high to low heels.
12. Put a footrail under the desk and a footrest under the crib.
13. Diaper the baby sitting next to him or her on the bed.
14. Don't stoop and stretch to hang the wash; raise the clothesbasket and lower the washline.
15. Beg or buy a rocking chair. Rocking rests the back by changing the muscle groups used.
16. Train yourself vigorously to use your abdominal muscles to flatten your lower abdomen. In time, this muscle contraction will become habitual, making you the envied possessor of a youthful body profile!
17. Don't strain to open windows or doors.
18. For good posture, concentrate on strengthening "nature's corset"—the abdominal and buttock muscles. The pelvic roll exercise is especially recommended to correct the postural relation between the pelvis and the spine.

Source: Schering Corporation

ASSESS YOUR KNOWLEDGE

1. Muscular flexibility is defined as
   a. the capacity of joints and muscles to work in a synchronized manner.
   b. the ability of a joint to move freely through its full range of motion.
   c. the capability of muscles to stretch beyond their normal resting length without injury to the muscles.
   d. the capacity of muscles to return to their proper length following the application of a stretching force.
   e. the limitations placed on muscles as the joints move through their normal planes.

2. Good flexibility
   a. promotes healthy muscles and joints.
   b. decreases the risk of injury.
   c. improves posture.
   d. decreases the risk of chronic back pain.
   e. All are correct choices.

3. Plastic elongation is a term used in reference to
   a. permanent lengthening of soft tissue.
   b. increased flexibility achieved through dynamic stretching.
   c. temporary elongation of muscles.
   d. the ability of a muscle to achieve a complete degree of stretch.
   e. lengthening of a muscle against resistance.

4. The most significant contributors to loss of flexibility are
   a. sedentary living and lack of physical activity.
   b. weight and power training.
   c. age and injury.
   d. muscular strength and endurance.
   e. excessive body fat and low lean tissue.

5. Which of the following is *not* a mode of stretching?
   a. proprioceptive neuromuscular facilitation
   b. elastic elongation
   c. ballistic stretching
   d. slow-sustained stretching
   e. All are modes of stretching.

6. PNF can help increase
   a. muscular strength.
   b. muscular flexibility.
   c. muscular endurance.
   d. range of motion.
   e. All are correct choices.

7. When performing stretching exercises, the degree of stretch should be
   a. through the entire arc of movement.
   b. to about 80 percent of capacity.
   c. to the point of mild discomfort.
   d. applied until the muscle(s) start shaking.
   e. progressively increased until the desired stretch is attained.

8. When stretching, the final stretch should be held for
   a. 1 to 10 seconds.
   b. 10 to 30 seconds.
   c. 30 to 90 seconds.
   d. 1 to 3 minutes.
   e. as long as the person is able to sustain the stretch.

9. Low-back pain is primarily associated with
   a. physical inactivity.
   b. faulty posture.
   c. excessive body weight.
   d. improper body mechanics.
   e. All are correct choices.

10. The following exercise helps stretch the lower back and hamstring muscles:
    a. adductor stretch
    b. trunk forward flexion stretch
    c. back extension stretch
    d. single-knee-to-chest stretch
    e. quad stretch

Correct answers can be found at the back of the book.

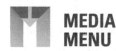

MEDIA MENU

INTERNET CONNECTIONS

■ Healthy Ontario. This site provides viewers with a number of watch-and-learn videos, including one on stretching. Related links include information on yoga, tai chi, and general stretching techniques and exercises.

http://www.healthyontario.com/MultimediaVideo2.aspx

■ Stretching and Flexibility: Everything You Never Wanted to Know. This very comprehensive and academic site describes the physiology of muscles, types of flexibility, types of stretching, and factors limiting flexibility. It includes how to stretch and specific exercises, as well as references.

http://www.cmcrossroads.com/bradapp/docs/rec/stretching/

■ Yoga and other stretching exercises. This site features information on the techniques of yoga, Pilates, and other forms of stretching exercises.

http://www.yoga.com

■ Stretching to Increase Flexibility. In addition to a comprehensive description of the health benefits of regular stretching, this site features a series of exercises tailored to one of three levels of fitness levels based on the frequency that you perform stretching exercises.

http://k2.kirtland.cc.mi.us/~balbachl/flex.htm

Notes

1. The Arthritis Society. Chronic Back Injury. Quick Facts. 21 Dec 2007. Retrieved 25 Jan 2008 from http://www.arthritis.ca/types%20of%20arthritis/chronic back/quick%20facts/default.asp?s=1.

2. American College of Obstetricians and Gynecologists, *Guidelines for Exercise During Pregnancy*, 1994.

3. "Stretch Yourself Younger," *Consumer Reports on Health* 11 (August 1999): 6–7.

4. W. W. K. Hoeger and D. R. Hopkins, "A Comparison Between the Sit and Reach and the Modified Sit and Reach in the Measurement of Flexibility in Women," *Research Quarterly for Exercise and Sport* 63 (1992): 191–195.

   W. W. K. Hoeger, D. R. Hopkins, S. Button, and T. A. Palmer, "Comparing the Sit and Reach with the Modified Sit and Reach in Measuring Flexibility in Adolescents," *Pediatric Exercise Science* 2 (1990): 156–162.

   D. R. Hopkins and W. W. K. Hoeger, "A Comparison of the Sit and Reach and the Modified Sit and Reach in the Measurement of Flexibility for Males," *Journal of Applied Sports Science Research* 6 (1992): 7–10.

5. J. Kokkonen and S. Lauritzen, "Isotonic Strength and Endurance Gains Through PNF Stretching," *Medicine and Science in Sports and Exercise* 27 (1995): S22, 127.

6. S. B. Thacker, J. Gilchrist, D. F. Stroup, and C. D. Kimsey. Jr., "The Impact of Stretching on Sports Injury Risk: A Systematic Review of the Literature," *Medicine and Science in Sports and Exercise* 36 (2004): 371–378.

7. D. B. J. Andersson, L. J. Fine, and B. A. Silverstein, "Musculoskeletal Disorders," Occupational Health: Recognizing and Preventing Work-Related Disease, edited by B. S. Levy and D. H. Wegman (Boston: Little, Brown and Company, 1995).

8. M. R. Bracko, "Can We Prevent Back Injuries?" *ACSM's Health & Fitness Journal* 8, no. 4 (2004): 5–11.

9. R. Deyo, "Chiropractic Care for Back Pain: The Physician's Perspective," *HealthNews* 4 (September 10, 1998).

10. Bracko, "Can We Prevent Back Injuries?"

11. J. A. Hides, G. A. Jull, and C. A. Richardson, "Long-Term Effects of Specific Stabilizing Exercises for First-Episode Low Back Pain," *Spine* 26 (2001): E243–248.

12. A. Brownstein, "Chronic Back Pain Can Be Beaten," *Bottom Line/Health* 13 (October 1999): 3–4.

Suggested Readings

Alter, M. J. *The Science of Stretching*. Champaign, IL: Human Kinetic Press, 1996.

Alter, M. J. *Sports Stretch*. Champaign, IL: Human Kinetics, 2004.

Anderson, B. *Stretching*. Bolinas, CA: Shelter Publications, 1999.

Bracko, M. R. "Can We Prevent Back Injuries?" *ACSM's Health & Fitness Journal* 8, no. 4 (2004): 5–11.

Canadian Centre for Occupational Health and Safety. OSH Answers. Ergonomics. Back Injury Prevention. http://www.ccohs.ca/oshanswers/ergonomics/inj_prev.html

Hoeger, W. W. K. *The Assessment of Muscular Flexibility: Test Protocols and National Flexibility Norms for the Modified Sit-and-Reach Test, Total Body Rotation Test, and Shoulder Rotation Test*. Rockton, IL: Figure Finder Collection Novel Products, Inc., 2004.

Liemohn, W. and G. Pariser. "Core Strength: Implications for Fitness and Low Back Pain." *ACSM's Health and Fitness Journal* 6, no. 5 (2002): 10–16.

McAtee, R. E. and J. Charland. *Facilitated Stretching*. Champaign, IL: Human Kinetics, 1999.

Schultz, S. E, and Kopec, J. A. Impact of chronic conditions. Health Reports 2003; 14 (4): 41–53. [Statistics Canada, Catalogue 82-003].

WorkSafe BC. Safety at Work. Back at Work. Watch your back: back health in the workplace. http://www2.work safebc.com/Topics/Ergonomics/BackAtWork.asp?Report ID=33765

Flexibility Exercises

Exercise 1
Lateral Head Tilt

Action Slowly and gently tilt the head laterally. Repeat several times to each side.

Areas Stretched
Neck flexors and extensors; ligaments of the cervical spine

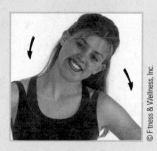

Exercise 2
Arm Circles

Action Gently circle your arms all the way around. Conduct the exercise in both directions.

Areas Stretched
Shoulder muscles and ligaments

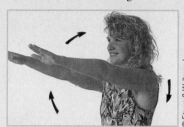

Exercise 3
Side Stretch

Action Stand straight up, feet separated to shoulder-width, and place your hands on your waist. Now move the upper body to one side and hold the final stretch for a few seconds. Repeat on the other side.

Areas Stretched
Muscles and ligaments in the pelvic region

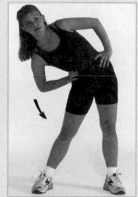

Exercise 4
Body Rotation

Action Place your arms slightly away from your body and rotate the trunk as far as possible, holding the final position for several seconds. Conduct the exercise for both the right and left sides of the body. You also can perform this exercise by standing about 60 cm away from the wall (back toward the wall) and then rotating the trunk, placing the hands against the wall.

Areas Stretched
Hip, abdominal, chest, back, neck, and shoulder muscles; hip and spinal ligaments

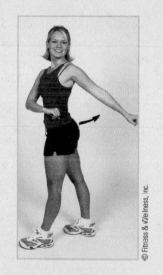

Exercise 5
Chest Stretch

Action Place your hands on the shoulders of your partner, who will in turn push you down by your shoulders. Hold the final position for a few seconds.

Areas Stretched
Chest (pectoral) muscles and shoulder ligaments

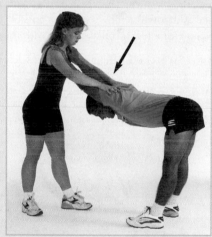

Exercise 6
Shoulder Hyperextension Stretch

Action Have a partner grasp your arms from behind by the wrists and slowly push them upward. Hold the final position for a few seconds.

Areas Stretched
Deltoid and pectoral muscles; ligaments of the shoulder joint

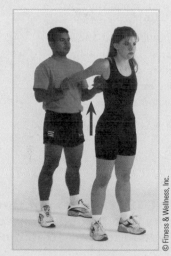

Exercise 7
Shoulder Rotation Stretch

Action With the aid of surgical tubing or an aluminum or wood stick, place the tubing or stick behind your back and grasp the two ends using a reverse (thumbs-out) grip. Slowly bring the tubing or stick over your head, keeping the elbows straight. Repeat several times (bring the hands closer together for additional stretch).

Areas Stretched
Deltoid, latissimus dorsi, and pectoral muscles; shoulder ligaments

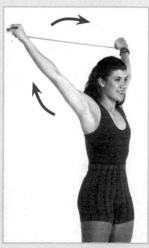

Exercise 8
Quad Stretch

Action   Lie on your side and move one foot back by flexing the knee. Grasp the front of the ankle and pull the ankle toward the gluteal region. Hold for several seconds. Repeat with the other leg.

Areas Stretched   Quadriceps muscle, hip flexors; knee and ankle ligaments

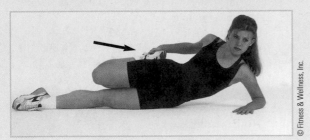

Exercise 10
Adductor Stretch

Action   Stand with your feet about twice shoulder-width apart and place your hands slightly above the knees. Flex one knee and slowly go down as far as possible, holding the final position for a few seconds. Repeat with the other leg.

Areas Stretched   Hip adductor muscles

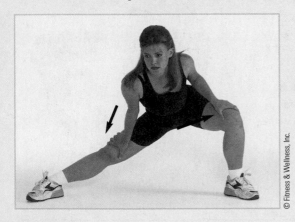

Exercise 12
Sit-and-Reach Stretch

Action   Sit on the floor with legs together and gradually reach forward as far as possible. Hold the final position for a few seconds. This exercise also may be performed with the legs separated, reaching to each side as well as to the middle.

Areas Stretched Hamstrings and lower back muscles; lumbar spine ligaments

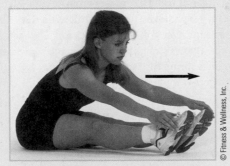

Exercise 9
Heel Cord Stretch

Action   Stand against the wall or at the edge of a step and stretch the heel downward, alternating legs. Hold the stretched position for a few seconds.

Areas Stretched Heel cord (Achilles tendon), gastrocnemius and soleus muscles

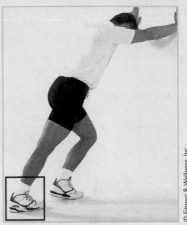

Exercise 11
Sitting Adductor Stretch

Action   Sit on the floor and bring your feet in close to you, allowing the soles of the feet to touch each other. Now place your forearms (or elbows) on the inner part of the thighs and push the legs downward, holding the final stretch for several seconds.

Areas Stretched Hip adductor muscles

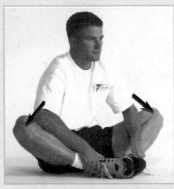

Exercise 13
Triceps Stretch

Action   Place the right hand behind your neck. Grasp the right arm above the elbow with the left hand. Gently pull the elbow backward. Repeat the exercise with the opposite arm.

Areas Stretched Back of upper arm (triceps muscle); shoulder joint

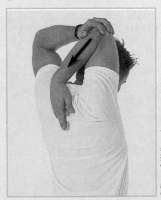

> **NOTE: Exercises 14 through 21 and 23 are also flexibility exercises and can be added to your stretching program.**

Exercises for the Prevention and Rehabilitation of Low-Back Pain

Exercise 14
Hip Flexors Stretch

Action Kneel down on an exercise mat or a soft surface, or place a towel under your knees. Raise the left knee off the floor and place the left foot about 90 cm in front of you. Place your left hand over your left knee and the right hand over the back of the right hip. Keeping the lower back flat, slowly move forward and downward as you apply gentle pressure over the right hip. Repeat the exercise with the opposite leg forward.

Areas Stretched Flexor muscles in front of the hip joint

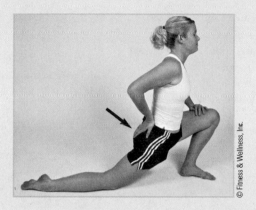

Exercise 15
Single-Knee-to-Chest Stretch

Action Lie down flat on the floor. Bend one leg at approximately 100° and gradually pull the opposite leg toward your chest. Hold the final stretch for a few seconds. Switch legs and repeat the exercise.

Areas Stretched Lower back and hamstring muscles; lumbar spine ligaments

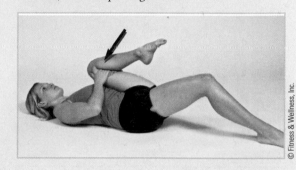

Exercise 16
Double-Knee-to-Chest Stretch

Action Lie flat on the floor and then curl up slowly into a fetal position. Hold for a few seconds.

Areas Stretched Upper and lower back and hamstring muscles; spinal ligaments

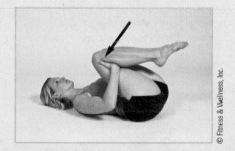

Exercise 17
Upper- and Lower-Back Stretch

Action Sit on the floor and bring your feet in close to you, allowing the soles of the feet to touch each other. Holding on to your feet, bring your head and upper chest gently toward your feet.

Areas Stretched Upper and lower back muscles and ligaments

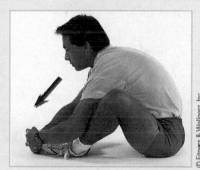

Exercise 18
Sit-and-Reach Stretch

(see Exercise 12, in this chapter, on page 258)

Exercise 19
Gluteal Stretch

Action Sit on the floor, bend your right leg, and place your right ankle slightly above the left knee. Grasp the left thigh with both hands and gently pull the leg toward your chest. Repeat the exercise with the opposite leg.

Areas Stretched Buttock area (gluteal muscles)

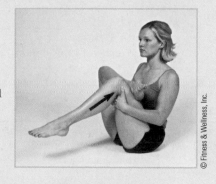

Exercise 20
Back Extension Stretch

Action Lie face down on the floor with the elbows by the chest, forearms on the floor, and the hands beneath the chin. Gently raise the trunk by extending the elbows until you reach an approximate 90° angle at the elbow joint. Be sure the forearms remain in contact with the floor at all times. DO NOT extend the back beyond this point. Hyperextension of the lower back may lead to or aggravate an existing back problem. Hold the stretched position for about 10 seconds.

Areas Stretched Abdominal region

Additional Benefits Restore lower back

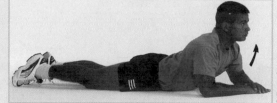

Exercise 21
Trunk Rotation and Lower Back Stretch

Action   Sit on the floor and bend the right leg, placing the right foot on the outside of the left knee. Place the left elbow on the right knee and push against it. At the same time, try to rotate the trunk to the right (clockwise). Hold the final position for a few seconds. Repeat the exercise with the other side.

Areas Stretched
Lateral side of the hip and thigh; trunk and lower back

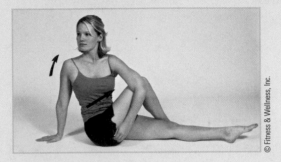

Exercise 22
Pelvic Tilt

(see Exercise 12 in Chapter 7, page 225)

Note:
This is perhaps the most important exercise for the care of the lower back. It should be included as a part of your daily exercise routine and should be performed several times throughout the day when pain in the lower back is present as a result of muscle imbalance.

Exercise 23
The Cat

Action   Kneel on the floor and place your hands in front of you (on the floor) about shoulder-width apart. Relax your trunk and lower back (a). Now arch the spine and pull in your abdomen as far as you can and hold this position for a few seconds (b). Repeat the exercise 4–5 times.

Areas Stretched
Low back muscles and ligaments

Areas Strengthened
Abdominal and gluteal muscles

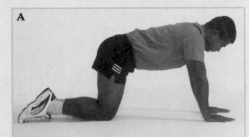

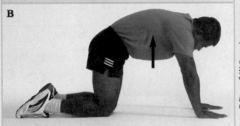

Exercise 24
Abdominal Crunch or Abdominal Curl-Up

(see Exercise 4 in Chapter 7, page 222)

It is important that you do not stabilize your feet when performing either of these exercises, because doing so decreases the work of the abdominal muscles. Also, remember not to "swing up" but, rather, to curl up as you perform these exercises.

Exercise 25
Reverse Crunch

(see Exercise 11 in Chapter 7, page 224)

Exercise 26
Supine Bridge

Action   Lie face up on the floor with the knees bent at about 120°. Do a pelvic tilt (Exercise 12, page 225) and maintain the pelvic tilt while you raise the hips off the floor until the upper body and upper legs are in a straight line. Hold this position for several seconds.

Areas Strengthened
Gluteal and abdominal flexor muscles

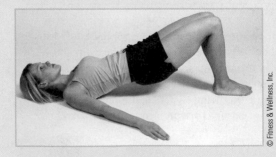

Exercise 27
Pelvic Clock

Action   Lie face up on the floor with the knees bent at about 120°. Fully extend the hips as in the supine bridge (Exercise 26). Now progressively rotate the hips in a clockwise manner (2 o'clock, 4 o'clock, 6 o'clock, 8 o'clock, 10 o'clock, and 12 o'clock), holding each position in an isometric contraction for about 1 second. Repeat the exercise counterclockwise.

Areas Strengthened
Gluteal, abdominal, and hip flexor muscles

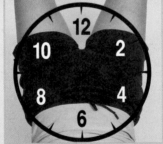

Exercise 28
Lateral Bridge
(see Exercise 13 in Chapter 7, page 225)

Exercise 29
Prone Bridge
(see Exercise 14 in Chapter 7, page 225)

Exercise 30
Leg Press
(see Exercise 16 in Chapter 7, page 226)

Exercise 31
Seated Back
(see Exercise 21 in Chapter 7, page 228)

Exercise 32
Lat Pull-Down
(see Exercise 23 in Chapter 7, page 229)

Exercise 33
Back Extension
(see Exercise 35 in Chapter 7, page 234)

Lab 8A

MUSCULAR FLEXIBILITY ASSESSMENT

Name: _____ Date: _____ Grade: _____

Instructor: _____ Course: _____ Section: _____

Necessary Lab Equipment

Acuflex I, Acuflex II, and Acuflex III Flexibility Testers* or homemade flexibility testing equipment as described in Figures 8.1, 8.2, and 8.3.

Objective

To assess muscular flexibility and the respective fitness categories.

Lab Preparation

The procedures for the flexibility tests* administered in this lab are explained in this chapter (Figures 8.1, 8.2, and 8.3, pages 242–245. It is important that you warm up properly before you perform any of these tests. Do gentle stretching exercises specific to the tests that will be administered. Wear loose exercise clothing for this lab.

I. Modified Sit-and-Reach Test (page 242)

Trials: 1. _____ cm   2. _____ cm

Average score: _____ cm   Percentile rank: _____   Points: _____

(Table 8.4, page 246)

Fitness category: _____

II. Total Body Rotation Test (pages 243–244)

Right Side   Left Side   (circle one)

Trials: 1. _____ cm   2. _____ cm

Average score: _____ cm   Percentile rank: _____   Points: _____

(Table 8.4, page 246)

Fitness category: _____

III. Shoulder Rotation Test (page 245)

Biacromial width: _____ cm   Rotation score: _____ cm

Final score = Rotation score − biacromial width

Final score = _____ − _____ = _____ cm   Percentile rank: _____

Fitness category: _____   Points: _____

(Table 8.4, page 246)

---

* The Acuflex I, II, and III Flexibility Testers can be obtained from Jansen Medical at 1-888-896-4050 or ordered online at http://www.jansenmedical.net.

IV. Overall Flexibility Rating

Test	Points
Modified sit-and-reach:	
Total body rotation (right, left — circle one):	
Shoulder rotation:	
	Total Points:
Overall flexibility category (see Table 8.5, page 246):	

V. Flexibility Goals

1. Indicate the flexibility category that you would like to achieve by the end of the term:

2. Describe your feelings about your current body flexibility and any potential implications that your current flexibility levels may have on your health and wellness. Also, briefly state how you plan to achieve your flexibility objective by the end of the term.

Lab 8B

POSTURE EVALUATION

Name: _____   Date: _____   Grade: _____

Instructor: _____   Course: _____   Section: _____

Necessary Lab Equipment

A plumb line, two large mirrors set at about an 85° angle, and a Polaroid camera (the mirrors and the camera are optional—see "Evaluating Body Posture" (pages 244 and 246).

Objective

To determine current body alignment.

Lab Preparation

To conduct the posture analysis, men should wear shorts only and women, shorts and a tank top. Shoes should also be removed for this test.

Lab Assignment

The class should be divided in groups of four students each. The group should carefully study the posture form given in this lab, then proceed to fill out the form for each member according to the instructions given under "Evaluating Body Posture" (pages 244 and 246). If no mirrors and camera are available, three members of the group are to rate the fourth person's posture while he/she first stands with the side of the body and then with the back to the plumb line. A final score is obtained by totalling the points given for each body segment and looking up the posture rating according to the total score found in the table provided below.

Results

Total points: _____

Category: _____

Posture Evaluation Standards	
Total Points	**Category**
≥45	Excellent
40–44	Good
30–39	Average
20–29	Fair
≤19	Poor

Posture Improvement

Indicate how you feel about your posture, identify areas to correct, and specify the steps you can take to make those improvements.

_____

_____

_____

_____

_____

_____

_____

_____

_____

	Good — 5	Fair — 3	Poor — 1	Score
HEAD Left Right	head erect, gravity passes directly through centre	head twisted or turned to one side slightly	head twisted or turned to one side markedly	
SHOULDERS Left Right	shoulders level horizontally	one shoulder slightly higher	one shoulder markedly higher	
SPINE Left Right	spine straight	spine slightly curved	spine markedly curved laterally	
HIPS Left Right	hips level horizontally	one hip slightly higher	one hip markedly higher	
KNEES and ANKLES	feet pointed straight ahead, legs vertical	feet pointed out, legs deviating outward at the knee	feet pointed out markedly, legs deviate markedly	
NECK and UPPER BACK	neck erect, head in line with shoulders, rounded upper back	neck slightly forward, chin out, slightly more rounded upper back	neck markedly forward, chin markedly out, markedly rounded upper back	
TRUNK	trunk erect	trunk inclined to rear slightly	trunk inclined to rear markedly	
ABDOMEN	abdomen flat	abdomen protruding	abdomen protruding and sagging	
LOWER BACK	lower back normally curved	lower back slightly hollow	lower back markedly hollow	
LEGS	legs straight	knees slightly hyper-extended	knees markedly hyper-extended	
			Total Score	

Adapted from *The New York Physical Fitness Test: A Manual for Teachers of Physical Education,* New York State Education Department (Division of HPER), 1958. Used with permission.

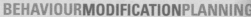

Lab 8C

FLEXIBILITY DEVELOPMENT AND LOW-BACK CONDITIONING PROGRAMS

Name: _____   Date: _____   Grade: _____

Instructor: _____   Course: _____   Section: _____

Necessary Lab Equipment

Minor implements such as a chair, a table, an elastic band (surgical tubing or a wood or aluminum stick), and a stool or steps.

Objective

To develop a flexibility exercise program and a conditioning program for the prevention and rehabilitation of low-back pain.

Lab Preparation

Wear exercise clothing and prepare to participate in a sample stretching exercise session. All of the flexibility and low-back conditioning exercises are illustrated on pages 257–260.

I. Stage of Change for Flexibility Training

Using Figure 2.4 (page 41) and Table 2.3 (page 41), identify your current stage of change for participation in a muscular stretching program: _____

II. Instruction

Perform all the recommended flexibility exercises given on pages 257–258. Use a combination of slow-sustained and proprioceptive neuromuscular facilitation stretching techniques. Indicate the technique(s) used for each exercise and, where applicable, the number of repetitions performed and the length of time that the final degree of stretch was held.

Stretching Exercises

Exercise	Stretching Technique	Repetitions	Length of Final Stretch
Lateral head tilt			NA*
Arm circles			NA
Side stretch			
Body rotation			
Chest stretch			
Shoulder hyperextension stretch			
Shoulder rotation stretch			NA
Quad stretch			
Heel cord stretch			
Adductor stretch			
Sitting adductor stretch			
Trunk forward flexion stretch			
Triceps stretch			

*Not Applicable

Stretching Schedule (Indicate days, time, and place where you will stretch):

Flexibility-training days: M ☐ T ☐ W ☐ Th ☐ F ☐ Sa ☐ Su ☐ Time of day: ☐ Place: ☐

Low-Back Conditioning Program

Perform all the recommended exercises for the prevention and rehabilitation of low-back pain given on pages 259–260. Indicate the number of repetitions performed for each exercise.

Flexibility Exercises	Repetitions	Strength/Endurance Exercises	Repetitions	Seconds Held
Hip flexors stretch		Pelvic tilt		
Single-knee-to-chest stretch		The cat		
Double-knee-to-chest stretch		Abdominal crunch or abdominal curl-up		
Upper- and lower-back stretch		Reverse crunch		
Trunk forward flexion stretch		Supine bridge		
Gluteal stretch		Pelvic clock		
Back extension stretch		Lateral bridge		
Trunk rotation and lower back stretch		Prone bridge		
		Leg press		
		Seated back		
		Lat pull-down		
		Back extension		

Proper Body Mechanics

Perform the following tasks using the proper body mechanics given in Figure 8.7 (pages 253–254). Check off each item as you perform the task:

☐ Standing (carriage) position   ☐ Resting position for tired and painful back

☐ Sitting position   ☐ Lifting an object

☐ Bed posture

"Rules to Live By — From Now On"

Read the 18 "Rules to Live By—From Now On" given in Figure 8.7 (pages 253–254) and indicate below those rules that you need to work on to improve posture and body mechanics and prevent low-back pain.

_____

_____

_____

_____

_____

_____

_____

_____

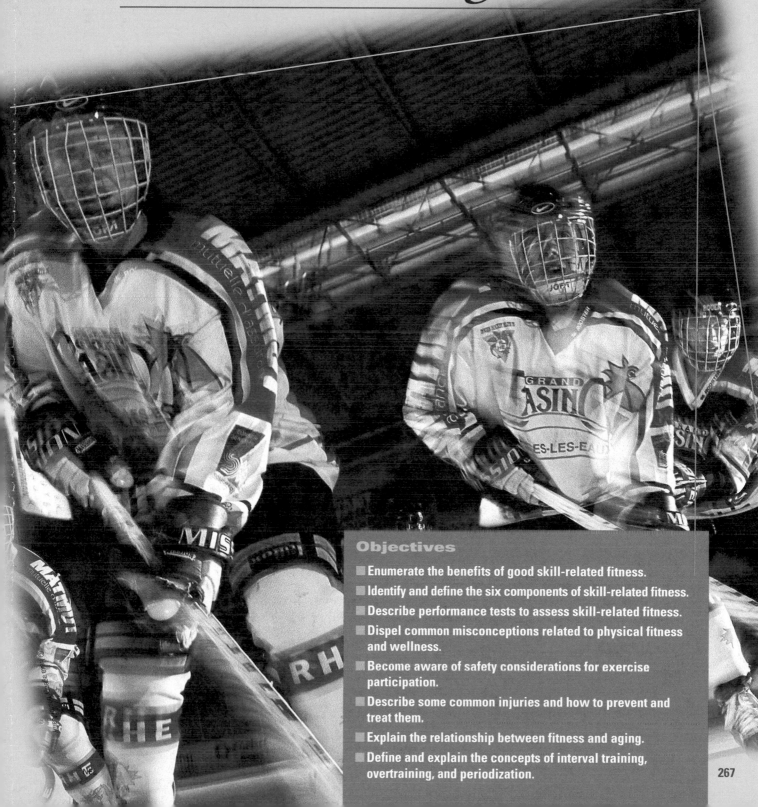

Chapter 9

Skill Fitness
and Fitness Programming

Objectives

- Enumerate the benefits of good skill-related fitness.
- Identify and define the six components of skill-related fitness.
- Describe performance tests to assess skill-related fitness.
- Dispel common misconceptions related to physical fitness and wellness.
- Become aware of safety considerations for exercise participation.
- Describe some common injuries and how to prevent and treat them.
- Explain the relationship between fitness and aging.
- Define and explain the concepts of interval training, overtraining, and periodization.

Skill-related fitness is important for successful motor performance in athletic events and in lifetime sports and activities such as basketball, racquetball, golf, hiking, soccer, and water skiing. Good skill-related fitness also enhances overall quality of life by helping people cope more effectively in emergency situations.

Outstanding gymnasts, for example, must achieve good skill-related fitness in all six components. A significant amount of *agility* is necessary to perform a double back somersault with a full twist—a skill during which the athlete must simultaneously rotate around one axis and twist around a different one. They must have good *balance*. Static balance is essential for maintaining a handstand or a scale. Dynamic balance is needed to perform many of the gymnastics routines (such as those on the balance beam, parallel bars, and pommel horse). *Coordination* is important to successfully integrate multiple skills, each with its own degree of difficulty, into one routine. *Power* and *speed* are needed to propel the body into the air, such as when tumbling or vaulting. Quick *reaction* time is necessary to determine when to end rotation upon a visual clue, such as spotting the floor on a dismount.

The principle of specificity of training applies to skill-related components just as it does to health-related fitness components. The development of agility, balance, coordination, and reaction time is highly task-specific. That is, to develop a certain task or skill, the individual must practise that same task many times. There seems to be very little crossover learning effect.

For instance, properly practising a handstand (balance) will lead eventually to performing the skill successfully, but complete mastery of this skill does not ensure that the person will have immediate success when attempting to perform other static-balance positions in gymnastics. In contrast, power and speed may improve with a specific strength-training program or frequent repetition of the specific task to be improved, or both.

The rate of learning in skill-related fitness varies from person to person, mainly because these components seem to be determined to a large extent by genetics. Individuals with good skill-related fitness tend to do better and learn faster when performing a wide variety of skills, but few individuals enjoy complete success in all skill-related components. Although skill-related fitness can be enhanced with practice, improvements in reaction time and speed are limited and seem to be related to genetic endowment.

Benefits of Skill-Related Fitness

Although we do not know how much skill-related fitness is desirable, everyone should attempt to develop and maintain a better-than-average level.

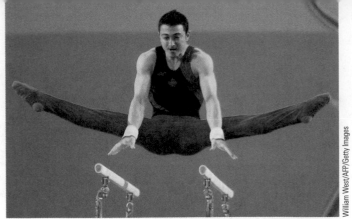
Successful gymnasts demonstrate high levels of skill fitness.

As pointed out earlier, this type of fitness is crucial for athletes, and it also enables fitness participants to lead a better and happier life. Improving skill-related fitness affords an individual more enjoyment and success in lifetime sports (for example, tennis, racquetball, basketball) and also can help a person cope more effectively in emergency situations. Some of the benefits are as follows.

1. Good reaction time, balance, coordination, and/or agility can help you avoid a fall or break a fall and thereby minimize injury.
2. The ability to generate maximum force in a short time (power) may be crucial to ameliorate injury or even preserve life if you ever have to lift a heavy object that has fallen on another person or even on yourself.
3. In our society, where the average lifespan continues to expand, maintaining speed can be especially important for elderly people. Many of these individuals and, for that matter, many unfit or overweight young people no longer have the speed they need to cross an intersection safely before the light changes or run for help if someone else needs assistance.

Regular participation in a health-related fitness program can heighten performance of skill-related components. For example, significantly overweight people do not have good agility or speed. Because participating in aerobic and strength-training programs helps take off body fat, an overweight individual who loses weight through such an exercise program can improve agility and speed. A sound flexibility program decreases resistance to motion about body joints, which may increase agility, balance, and overall coordination. Improvements in strength definitely help develop power. People who have good

CRITICAL THINKING

If you are interested in health fitness, should you participate in skill-fitness activities? Explain the pros and cons of participating in skill-fitness activities. Should you participate in skill-fitness activities to get fit, or should you get fit to participate in skill-fitness activities?

skill-related fitness usually participate in lifetime sports and games, which in turn helps develop and/or maintain health-related fitness.

Performance Tests for Skill-Related Fitness

The performance tests described below will assist you in assessing a number of components of skill-related fitness. Although this is not a comprehensive review of skill-related fitness, basic tests for agility, balance, and power are included in this chapter.

For students interested in obtaining full testing instruments for other skill-related and motor-performance tests such as coordination, reaction time, and speed, consult Ronald F. Kirby's 1991 *Kirby's Guide to Fitness and Motor Performance Tests.*

Agility

Agility is the ability to quickly and efficiently change body position and direction. Agility is important in sports such as basketball, soccer, and racquetball, in which the participant must change direction rapidly and also maintain proper body control.

SEMO AGILITY TEST[1]

Objective

To measure general body agility

Procedure

The free-throw area of a basketball court or any other smooth area 12 feet (4 m) by 19 feet (6 m) with adequate running space around it can be used for this test. Four plastic cones or similar objects are needed, with one placed at each corner of the free-throw lane, as shown in Figure 9.1.

Start on the outside of the free-throw lane at point A, with your back to the free-throw line. When

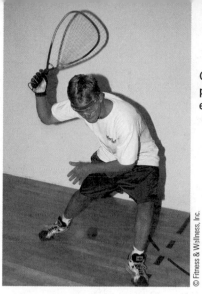

Good racquetball players have excellent agility.

© Fitness & Wellness, Inc.

FIGURE 9.1 Graphic depiction of the SEMO test for agility

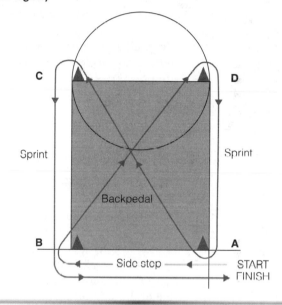

given the "go" command, side-step from A to B (do not make cross-oversteps), backpedal from B to D, sprint forward from D to A, again backpedal from A to C, sprint forward from C to B, and side-step from B to the finish line at A.

During the test, always go outside each corner cone. A stopwatch is started at the "go" command and stopped when you cross the finish line. Take a practice trial, and then use the best of two trials as the final test score. Record the time to the nearest tenth of a second. (See Lab 9A to record your results.)

TABLE 9.1 Norms in Seconds for SEMO Agility Test, College Students[a]

Performance Level	Score	
	Men	**Women**
Advanced	10.72 and below	12.19 and below
Advanced intermediate	11.49–10.73	12.99–12.20
Intermediate	13.02–11.50	13.90–13.00
Advanced beginner	13.79–13.03	14.49–13.91
Beginner	13.80 and above	14.50 and above

[a]Scores for men were obtained by Dr. Ronald Kirby, Southeast Missouri State University, Cape Girardeau, MO., 1971. Scores for women were from a small group of subjects from Corpus Christi State University, Corpus Christi TX, 1976.

Source: Table 13.4, p. 230 from PRACTICAL MEASUREMENTS FOR EVALUATION IN PHYSICAL EDUCATION by Barry L. Johnson and Jack K. Nelson. Copyright © 1986 by Macmillan Publishing Company. Reprinted by permission of Pearson Education, Inc

Skill-related fitness Fitness components important for success in skillful activities and athletic events; encompasses agility, balance, coordination, power, reaction time, and speed.

Agility Ability to change body position and direction quickly and efficiently.

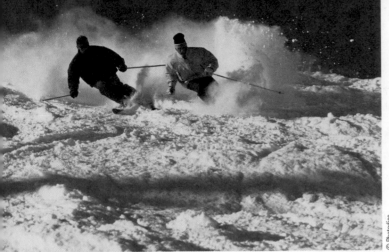

Alpine skiing requires good balance.

© Photodisc

TABLE 9.2 Norms in Seconds for Stork Stand, College Students[a]

Performance Level	Men	Women
Advanced	51 and above	28 and above
Advanced intermediate	37–50	23–27
Intermediate	15–36	8–22
Advanced beginner	5–14	3–7
Beginner	0–4	0–2

[a]Based on the scores of 50 men and 50 women at Corpus Christi (Texas) State University, 1976.

Source: Table 14.1, p. 238 from PRACTICAL MEASUREMENTS FOR EVALUATION IN PHYSICAL EDUCATION by Barry L. Johnson and Jack K. Nelson. Copyright © 1986 by Macmillan Publishing Company. Reprinted by permission of Pearson Education, Inc.

Balance

The ability to maintain the body in proper equilibrium, **balance**, is vital in activities such as gymnastics, diving, ice skating, skiing, and even football and wrestling, in which the athlete attempts to upset the opponent's equilibrium.

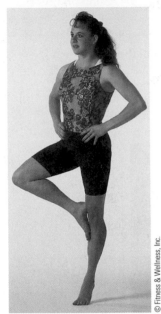

One-Foot Stand Test for balance.

© Fitness & Wellness, Inc.

STORK STAND TEST

Objective

To measure the static balance of the participant.

Procedure

A flat, smooth floor, not carpeted, is used for this test. Remove your shoes and socks and stand on your preferred or dominant foot, placing the other foot on the inside of the supporting knee, and the hands on the sides of the hips. When the "go" command is given, raise your heel off the floor and balance yourself as long as possible without moving the ball of the foot from its initial position. Balance time is recorded to the nearest whole second. Three trials are given; the score is the time of the longest balance.

The test is terminated when any of the following conditions occur:

1. The supporting foot moves (shuffles).
2. The raised heel touches the floor.
3. The hands are moved from the hips.

(See Lab 9A to record your results.)

Power

Power is defined as the ability to produce maximum force in the shortest time. The two components of power are speed and force (strength). An effective combination of these two components allows a person to produce explosive movements such as in jumping, putting the shot, and spiking, throwing, or hitting a ball.

Power is necessary to perform many activities of daily living that require strength and speed, such as climbing stairs, lifting objects, preventing falls, or hurrying to catch a bus. Power is also beneficial in sports such as soccer, tennis, softball, golf, volleyball, and basketball.

VERTICAL JUMP

Objective

To measure power of the leg extensor muscles.

Procedure

Administrator: This test requires a measuring tape that can be attached to a wall at a height appropriate for the participant being tested. Chalk dust or a piece of chalk can be used to record the height of the jump. A weigh scale is also needed.

Participant:

1. Take a standing position facing sideways to the wall on which the measuring tape has been attached.
2. Standing erect, with feet flat on the floor, reach as high as possible on the tape with the arm and fingers fully extended and the palm toward the wall. This is recorded as the ***Stand and Reach Height*** to the nearest 0.5 cm.
3. Next, move a safe distance away from the wall (with your hand on your hip, your elbow should barely reach the wall).
4. No run up, step up, or pre-jump is permitted.
5. Bring your arm downward and backward while bending your knees to a balanced semi-squat position.
6. Jump as high as possible, touching the measuring tape at the peak height of the jump with your arm and fingers fully extended.
7. Three trials are allowed.
8. Record the ***Peak Height*** after each trial.

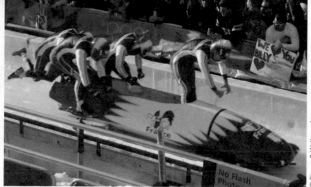
Fast starts in bob sleigh require exceptional leg power.

9. Rest periods of 10 to 15 seconds are allowed between trials.
10. Subtract the **Stand and Reach Height** from the **Peak Height** of the best of the three trials. This is the vertical **Jump Height** used in the equation to determine leg power.
11. Insert your Body Mass (kg) and vertical **Jump Height** measures as recorded into the Sayers equation. This equation determines **Peak Leg Power** in Watts (W):

Peak Leg Power (W) = [60.7 $\times$ jump height (cm)] + 45.3 $\times$ body mass (kg) – 2055.

12. Refer to Table 9.3 to determine your Health Benefit Rating for leg power from the Healthy Musculoskeletal Fitness Norms from the manual *Canadian Physical Activity, Fitness and Lifestyle Approach*, 3rd edition.

Source: *The Canadian Physical Activity, Fitness & Lifestyle Approach: CSEP-Health & Fitness Program's Health-Related Appraisal and Counselling Strategy*, Third edition, © 2003, p. 7–44. Used with permission from the Canadian Society for Exercise Physiology.

Reaction Time

Reaction time is defined as the time required to initiate a response to a given stimulus. Good reaction time is important for starts in track and swimming, when playing tennis at the net, and in sports such as Ping Pong, boxing, and karate.

METRE STICK TEST
(preferred hand)

Objective
To measure hand reaction time in response to a visual stimulus

Procedure
Administrator: For this test you will need a regular metre stick with a shaded "concentration zone" marked on the first 5 cm of the stick. Administer the test with the participant sitting in a chair adjacent to a table and the preferred forearm and hand resting on the table.

Participant: Hold the tips of the thumb and fingers in a "ready-to-pinch" position, about 2 cm apart and 8 cm beyond the edge of the table, with the upper edges of the thumb and index finger parallel to the floor. With the person administering the test holding the metre stick near the upper end and the zero point of the stick even with the upper edge of your thumb and index finger (the administrator may steady the middle of the stick with the other hand), look at the "concentration zone" and react by catching the stick when it is dropped. Do not look at the administrator's hand or move your hand up or down while trying to catch the stick.

Twelve trials make up the test, each preceded by the preparatory command "ready." The administrator makes a random 1- to 3-second count between the "ready" command and each drop of the stick. Each trial is scored to the nearest

Balance Ability to maintain the body in proper equilibrium.

Power The ability to produce maximum force in the shortest time.

Reaction time The time required to initiate a response to a given stimulus.

TABLE 9.3 Health Benefit Rating for Leg Power—Vertical Jump Test

Category	Age (yr) 15–19	Age (yr) 20–29	Age (yr) 30–39	Age (yr) 40–49	Age (yr) 50–59	Age (yr) 60–69
Excellent	≥56	≥58	≥52	≥43	≥41	≥33
Very Good	51–55	54–57	46–51	36–42	34–40	29–32
Good	46–50	48–53	40–45	32–35	28–33	25–28
Fair	42–45	42–47	31–39	26–31	18–27	18–24
Needs Improvement	≤41	≤41	≤30	≤25	≤17	≤17

The Canadian Physical Activity, Fitness & Lifestyle Approach: CSEP-Health & Fitness Program's Health-Related Appraisal and Counselling Strategy, 3rd edition, © 2003, p. 7–47. Used with permission from the Canadian Society for Exercise Physiology.

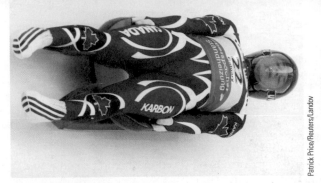

Luge athletes exhibit excellent reaction time and coordination.

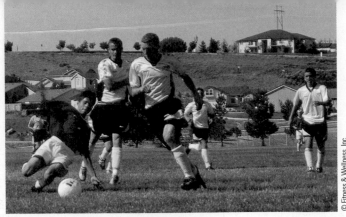

Speed is essential in the sport of soccer.

TABLE 9.4 Skill-Fitness Categories

Percentile Rank	Fitness Category
≥81	Excellent
61–80	Good
41–60	Average
21–40	Fair
≤20	Poor

centimetre, read just above the upper edge of the thumb. Three practice trials are given before the actual test to be sure the person understands the procedure. The three lowest and the three highest scores are discarded, and the average of the middle six is used as the final test score. The testing area should be as free from distractions as possible.

Speed

Speed is the ability to rapidly propel the body or a part of the body from one point to another. Examples of activities that require good speed for success are soccer, basketball, sprints in track, and stealing a base in baseball. In everyday life, speed can be important in a wide variety of emergency situations.

50-METRE DASH[3]

Objective

To measure speed

Procedure

Two participants take their positions behind the starting line. The starter raises one arm and asks, "Are you ready?" and then gives the command "go" while swinging the raised arm downward as a signal for the timer (or timers) at the finish line to start the stopwatch (or stopwatches).

The score is the time that elapses between the starting signal and the moment the participant crosses the finish line, recorded to the nearest tenth of a second.

Interpreting Test Results

Look up your score for each test in Table 9.1 to 9.3, then use Table 9.4 to see your level of fitness in that skill.

Specific Exercise Considerations

In addition to the exercise-related issues already discussed in this book, many other concerns require clarification or are somewhat controversial. Let's examine some of these issues.

1. Does aerobic exercise make a person immune to heart and blood vessel disease?

Although aerobically fit individuals as a whole have a lower incidence of cardiovascular disease, a regular aerobic exercise program by itself does not offer an absolute guarantee against cardiovascular disease. Overall management of the risk factors is the best way to minimize the risk for cardiovascular disease. Many factors, including a genetic predisposition, can increase the person's risk. In any case, experts believe that a regular aerobic exercise program will delay the onset of cardiovascular problems and also will improve the chances of surviving a heart attack.

Even moderate increases in aerobic fitness significantly lower the incidence of premature deaths from cardiovascular diseases. Data from the research study on death rates by physical fitness groups (illustrated in Chapter 1) indicate that the decrease in cardiovascular mortality is greatest between the unfit and the moderately fit groups. A further decrease in cardiovascular mortality is observed between the moderately fit and the highly fit groups, although the difference is not as pronounced as that between the unfit and the moderately fit groups.

2. How much aerobic exercise is required to decrease the risk for cardiovascular disease?

Even though research has not yet indicated the exact amount of aerobic exercise required to lower the risk for cardiovascular disease, some general recommendations have been set forth. In their study, Dr. Ralph Paffenbarger and his co-researchers showed that expending 2,000 Calories per week as a result of physical activity yielded the lowest risk for cardiovascular disease among a group of almost 17,000 Harvard alumni.[4] The expenditure of 2,000 Calories per week represents about 300 Calories per daily exercise session.

3. Do people get a "physical high" during aerobic exercise?

During vigorous exercise, **endorphins** are released from the pituitary gland in the brain. Endorphins can create feelings of euphoria and natural well-being. Higher levels of endorphins often result from aerobic endurance activities and may remain elevated for as long as 30 to 60 minutes following exercise. Many experts believe these higher levels explain the physical high that some people get during and after prolonged exercise.

Endorphin levels have also been shown to increase during pregnancy and childbirth. Endorphins act as painkillers. The higher levels could explain a woman's greater tolerance for the pain and discomfort of natural childbirth and her pleasant feelings shortly after the baby's birth. Several reports have indicated that well-conditioned women have shorter and easier labour. These women may attain higher endorphin levels during delivery, making childbirth less traumatic than it is for untrained women.

4. Can people with asthma exercise?

Asthma, a condition that causes difficulty in breathing, is characterized by coughing, wheezing, and shortness of breath induced by narrowing of the airway passages because of contraction (bronchospasm) of the airway muscles, swelling of the mucous membrane, and excessive secretion of mucus. In a few people, asthma can be triggered by exercise itself, particularly in cool and dry environments. This type of condition is referred to as *exercise-induced asthma* (EIA).

People with asthma need to obtain proper medication from a physician prior to initiating an exercise program. A regular program is best, because random exercise bouts are more likely to trigger asthma attacks. In the initial stages of exercise, an intermittent program (with frequent rest periods during the exercise session) is recommended. Gradual warm-up and cool-down are also essential to reduce the risk of an acute attack. Furthermore, exercising in warm and humid conditions (such as swimming) is better because it helps to moisten the airways and thus minimizes the asthmatic response. For land-based activities (such as walking or aerobics), drinking water before, during, and after exercise helps to keep the

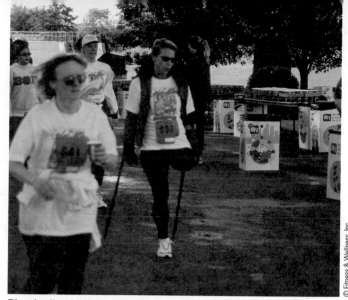

Physically challenged people can participate in and derive health and fitness benefits from a high-intensity exercise program.

airways moist, decreasing the risk of an attack. During the winter months, wearing an exercise mask is recommended to increase warmth and humidity of inhaled air. People with asthma should not exercise alone and should always carry their medication with them during workouts.

5. What types of activities are recommended for people with arthritis?

Individuals who have arthritis should participate in a combined stretching, aerobic, and strength-training program. Mild stretching should be performed prior to aerobic exercise to relax tight muscles. A regular flexibility program following aerobic exercise is encouraged to help maintain good joint mobility. During the aerobic portion of the exercise program, people with arthritis should avoid high-impact activities, because they may cause greater trauma to arthritic joints. Low-impact activities such as swimming, water aerobics, or cycling are recommended. A complete strength-training program is also recommended, with special emphasis on exercises that will help support the affected joint(s). As with any other program, individuals with arthritis should start with low intensity or resistance and build up gradually to a higher fitness level.

6. What precautions should diabetics take with respect to exercise?

According to the Canadian Diabetes Association, more than 2 million Canadians have diabetes and the number will probably rise to 3 million by

Speed The ability to propel the body or a part of the body rapidly from one point to another.

Endorphins Morphine-like substances released from the pituitary gland (in the brain) during prolonged aerobic exercise; thought to induce feelings of euphoria and natural well-being.

the end of the decade. The increasing number of people developing diabetes is largely a result of an aging population and increasing obesity rates. There are two types of diabetes:

- type 1, or insulin-dependent diabetes (IDDM)
- type 2, or non–insulin-dependent diabetes (NIDDM).

In type 1, found primarily in young people, the pancreas produces little or no insulin. With type 2, the pancreas may not produce enough insulin or the cells become insulin-resistant, thereby keeping glucose from entering the cell. Type 2 accounts for more than 90 percent of all diabetes cases, and it occurs mainly in overweight people. (A more thorough discussion of the types of diabetes is given in Chapter 11.)

If you have diabetes, consult your physician before you start exercising. You may not be able to start until the diabetes is under control. Never exercise alone, and always wear a bracelet that identifies your condition. If you take insulin, the amount and timing of each dose may have to be regulated with your physician. If you inject insulin, do so over a muscle that won't be exercised, then wait an hour before exercising. For type 1 diabetics, it is recommended that you ingest 15 to 30 grams of carbohydrates during each 30 minutes of intense exercise and follow it with a carbohydrate snack after exercise.

Both types of diabetes improve with exercise, although the results are more notable in patients with type 2 diabetes. Exercise usually lowers blood sugar and helps the body use food more effectively. The degree to which blood glucose level can be controlled in overweight type 2 diabetics seems to be directly related to how long and how hard a person exercises. Normal or near-normal blood glucose levels can be achieved through a proper exercise program.

As with any fitness program, the exercise must be done regularly to be effective against diabetes. The benefits of a single exercise bout on blood glucose are highest between 12 and 24 hours following exercise. These benefits are completely lost within 72 hours after exercise. Thus, regular participation is crucial to derive ongoing benefits. With regard to fitness, all diabetic patients can achieve higher fitness levels, including reductions in weight, blood pressure, and total cholesterol and triglycerides.

According to the Canadian Diabetes Association, patients with type 2 diabetes should adhere to the following guidelines to make their exercise program safe and derive the most benefit:[5]

- Expend a minimum of 1,000 calories per week through your exercise program.
- Exercise at a low-to-moderate intensity (40 to 70 percent of HRR). Start your program with 10 to 15 minutes per session, on at least three nonconsecutive days, but preferably exercise five days per week. Gradually increase the time you exercise to 30 minutes until you achieve your goal of at least 1,000 calories weekly. Diabetic individuals with a weight problem should build up daily physical activity to 60 minutes per session.
- Choose an activity that you enjoy doing and stay with it. As you select your activity, be aware of your condition. For example, if you have lost sensation in your feet, swimming or stationary cycling is better than walking or jogging to minimize the risk for injury.
- Check blood glucose levels before and after exercise. If you are on insulin or diabetes medication, monitor blood glucose regularly and check it at least twice within 30 minutes of starting exercise.
- Schedule your exercise one to three hours after a meal, and avoid exercise when your insulin is peaking.
- Be ready to treat low blood glucose with a source of fast-acting carbohydrate, such as juice, raisins, or other source recommended by your doctor.
- Discontinue exercise immediately if you feel that a reaction is about to occur. Check your blood glucose level and treat the condition as needed.
- When you exercise outdoors, always do so with someone who knows what to do in a diabetes-related emergency.

In addition, strength training twice per week, using 8 to 10 exercises with a minimum of one set of 10 to 15 repetitions to near fatigue, is recommended for individuals with diabetes. A complete description of strength-training programs is provided in Chapter 7.

7. Is exercise safe during pregnancy?

Exercise is beneficial during pregnancy. According to guidelines approved by the Society of Obstetricians and Gynaecologists of Canada (SOGC) and the Canadian Society for Exercise Physiology (CSEP), all women without contraindications should be encouraged to participate in aerobic and strength-conditioning exercises as part of a healthy lifestyle during their pregnancy.[6] In addition, a PAR-medX for pregnancy that provides guidelines for health screening prior to exercising has been developed by CSEP. Pregnant women, however, should consult with their physicians to ensure that there are no contraindications to exercise during pregnancy (see Table 9.5).

As a general rule, healthy pregnant women can also accumulate 30 minutes of moderate-intensity physical activity on most, if not all, days of the week. Physical activity strengthens the body and helps prepare for the challenges of labour and childbirth.

The average labour and delivery lasts 10 to 12 hours. In most cases, labour and delivery are highly intense, with repeated muscular contractions interspersed with short rest periods. Proper

TABLE 9.5 Considerations for Exercise During Pregnancy

- If a woman has not been active prior to pregnancy, it is recommended that an exercise routine be started in the second trimester.
- If an increase in training is desired, a woman should wait until the second trimester.
- Third-trimester exercise should be more conservative and adaptations to the exercises should be made to accommodate body changes.
- Stretching should not be vigorous.
- Be sure to hydrate with a glass of fluid before and after exercising.
- Stop exercise and seek medical advice if you experience any of the following symptoms.
    - Unusual pain or discomfort is felt, especially in the chest or abdominal area.
    - Cramping, primarily in the pelvic or lower back areas
    - Muscle weakness, excessive fatigue, or shortness of breath
    - Abnormally high heart rate or a pounding (palpitations) heart rate
    - Decreased fetal movement
    - Insufficient weight gain
    - Amniotic fluid leakage
    - Nausea, dizziness, or headaches
    - Persistent uterine contractions
    - Vaginal bleeding or rupture of the membranes
    - Swelling of ankles, calves, hands, or face

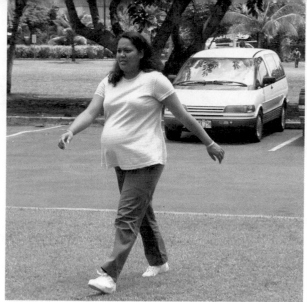

Mild-to-moderate intensity exercise is recommended throughout pregnancy.

conditioning will better prepare the body for childbirth. Moderate exercise during pregnancy also helps to prevent back pain and excessive weight gain, and it speeds up recovery following childbirth.

The most common recommendations for exercise during pregnancy for healthy pregnant women with no additional risk factors are as follows:

- Do not start a new or more rigorous exercise program without proper medical clearance.
- Accumulate 30 minutes of moderate-intensity physical activities on most days of the week.
- Instead of using heart rate to monitor intensity, exercise at an intensity level between "fairly light" and "somewhat hard," using the Rate of Perceived Exertion (RPE) scale in Chapter 6 (see page 176).
- Gradually switch from weight-bearing and high-impact activities such as jogging and aerobics, to nonweight-bearing/lower-impact activities such as walking, stationary cycling, swimming, and water aerobics. The latter activities minimize the risk of injury and may allow exercise to continue throughout pregnancy.
- Avoid exercising at an altitude above 1,800 m; and scuba diving which may compromise availability of oxygen to the fetus.

- Women who are accustomed to strenuous exercise may continue in the early stages of pregnancy but should gradually decrease the amount, intensity, and exercise mode as pregnancy advances (most healthy pregnant women, however, slow down during the first few weeks of pregnancy until morning sickness and fatigue subside).
- Pay attention to the body's signals of discomfort and distress, and never exercise to exhaustion. When fatigued, slow down or take a day off. Do not stop exercising altogether unless you experience any of the contraindications for exercise listed in Table 9.5.
- To prevent fetal injury, avoid activities that involve potential contact, loss of balance, or cause even mild trauma to the abdomen. Examples of these activities are basketball, soccer, volleyball, alpine or water skiing, ice skating, road cycling, horseback riding, and motorcycle riding.
- Do not exercise for weight-loss purposes during pregnancy.
- Get proper nourishment (pregnancy requires between 150 and 300 extra Calories per day), and eat a small snack or drink some juice 20 to 30 minutes prior to exercise.
- Prevent dehydration by drinking 250 mL of fluids 20 to 30 minutes before exercise, and drink 250 mL of liquid every 15 to 20 minutes during exercise.
- During the first three months in particular, do not exercise in the heat. Wear clothing that allows for proper dissipation of heat. A body temperature above 39.2°C can harm the fetus.
- After the first trimester, avoid exercises that require lying on the back. This position can block blood flow to the uterus and the baby.
- Perform stretching exercises gently because hormonal changes during pregnancy increase the

SKILL FITNESS AND FITNESS PROGRAMMING

laxity of muscles and connective tissue. Although these changes facilitate delivery, they also make women more susceptible to injuries during exercise.

8. Does exercise help relieve dysmenorrhea?

Even though exercise has not been shown to either cure or aggravate **dysmenorrhea**, it has been shown to relieve menstrual cramps because it improves circulation to the uterus. Less severe menstrual cramps also could be related to higher levels of endorphins produced during prolonged physical activity, which may counteract pain. Particularly, stretching exercises of the muscles in the pelvic region seem to reduce and prevent painful menstruation that is not the result of disease.[7]

9. Does participation in exercise hinder menstruation?

In some instances, highly trained athletes develop **amenorrhea** during training and competition. This condition is seen most often in extremely lean women who also engage in sports that require strenuous physical effort over a sustained time. It is by no means irreversible. At present, we do not know whether the condition is caused by physical or emotional stress related to high-intensity training, excessively low body fat, or other factors.

Although, on the average, women have a lower physical capacity during menstruation, medical surveys at the Olympic games have shown that women have broken Olympic and world records at all stages of the menstrual cycle. Menstruation should not keep a woman from exercising, and it will not necessarily have a negative impact on performance.

10. Does exercise offset the detrimental effects of cigarette smoking?

Physical exercise often motivates a person to stop smoking, but it does not offset any ill effects of smoking. Smoking greatly decreases the ability of the blood to transport oxygen to working muscles.

Oxygen is carried in the circulatory system by hemoglobin, the iron-containing pigment of the red blood cells. Carbon monoxide, a byproduct of cigarette smoke, has 210 to 250 times greater affinity for hemoglobin over oxygen. Consequently, carbon monoxide combines much faster with hemoglobin, decreasing the oxygen-carrying capacity of the blood.

Chronic smoking also increases airway resistance, requiring the respiratory muscles to work much harder and consume more oxygen just to ventilate a given amount of air. If a person quits smoking, exercise does help increase the functional capacity of the pulmonary system.

A regular exercise program seems to be a powerful incentive to quit smoking. A random survey of 1,250 runners conducted at a 10 km race in Atlanta, Georgia, provided impressive results. The survey indicated that, of the men and women who smoked

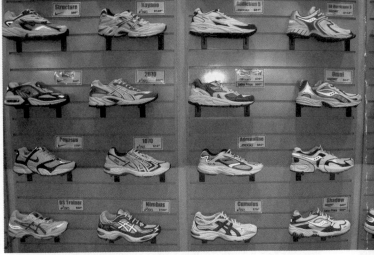

Activity-specific shoes are recommended to prevent lower-extremity injuries.

cigarettes when they started running, 81 percent and 75 percent, respectively, had quit before the date of the race.

11. How long should a person wait after a meal before exercising strenuously?

The length of time to wait before exercising after a meal depends on the amount of food eaten. On the average, after a regular meal, you should wait about two hours before participating in strenuous physical activity. A walk or some other light physical activity is fine following a meal, though. If anything, it helps burn extra calories and may help the body metabolize fats more efficiently.

12. What type of clothing should I wear when I exercise?

The type of clothing you wear during exercise is important. In general, clothing should fit comfortably and allow free movement of the various body parts. Select clothing according to air temperature, humidity, and exercise intensity. Avoid nylon and rubberized materials and tight clothes that interfere with the cooling mechanism of the human body or obstruct normal blood flow. Choose fabrics made of polypropylene, Capilene, Thermax, or any synthetic that draws (wicks) moisture away from the skin, enhancing evaporation and cooling of the body. It's also important to consider your exercise intensity, because the harder you exercise, the more heat your body produces.

When exercising in the heat, avoid the hottest time of the day—between 11:00 A.M. and 5:00 P.M. Surfaces such as asphalt, concrete, and artificial turf absorb heat, which then radiates to the body. Therefore, these surfaces are not recommended. (Also see the discussion about heat and humidity in Question 14, pages 277–278.)

Only a minimal amount of clothing is necessary during exercise in the heat, to allow for maximal evaporation. Clothing should be lightweight, light-coloured, loose-fitting, airy, and absorbent. Examples of commercially available products that can be

FIGURE 9.2 What to look for in a good pair of shoes

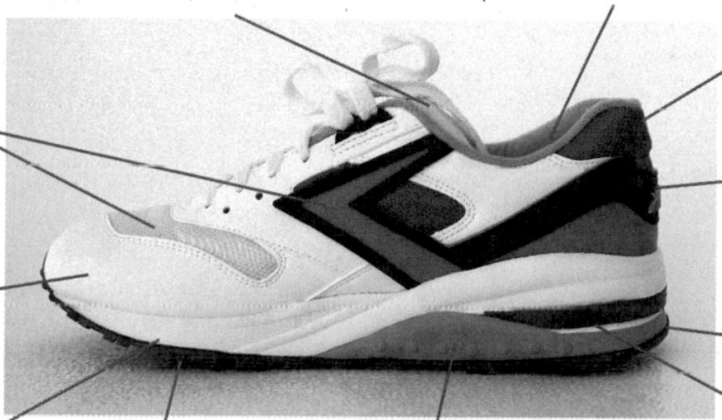

Choosing the Right Shoe

Tongue
Should be well-padded to prevent irritation of the top of the foot.

Collar
About 0.5 cm rim of soft material to protect the heel cord.

Upper
Leather, nylon mesh, or other breathable materials are best for ventilation.

Achilles Pad
Not too high to prevent irritation to the tendon or blistering of the skin.

Firm Heel Counter
Durable plastic cup placed in the heel of the shoe to help stability.

Toe Box
Allow enough space for the toes to fit comfortably.

Flared Heel
Added for support

© Fitness & Wellness, Inc.

External Stabilizer
Supports the heel counter and offers extra stability.

Flexibility under forefoot.

Outsole
Solid or carbon rubber outsoles are best for running, walking, and cross-training traction.

Midsole
Principal shock-absorbing feature of the shoe. Usually becomes worn out after 800 to 950 km of use. Multi-density EVA or polyurethane midsoles offer best support and durability.

used during exercise in the heat are Asic's Perma Plus, Cool-max, and Nike's Dri-F.I.T. Double-layer acrylic socks are more absorbent than cotton and help to prevent blistering and chafing of the feet. A straw-type hat can be worn to protect the eyes and head from the sun. (Clothing for exercise in the cold is discussed in Question 16, page 279–280.)

A good pair of shoes is vital to prevent injuries to lower limbs. Shoes manufactured specifically for your choice of activity are a must (see Figure 9.2). When selecting proper footwear, you should consider body type, tendency toward pronation (rotating foot outward) or supination (rotating foot inward), and exercise surfaces. Shoes should have good stability, motion control, and comfortable fit. Purchase shoes in the middle of the day when your feet have expanded and might be one-half size larger. For increased breathability, choose shoes with nylon or mesh uppers. Generally, salespeople at reputable athletic shoe stores are knowledgeable and can help you select a good shoe that fits your needs. After 500 to 800 km or six months, examine your shoes and obtain a new pair if they are worn out. Old shoes are frequently responsible for injuries to the lower limbs.

13. What time of the day is best for exercise?

You can do intense exercise almost any time of the day, with the exception of about two hours following a heavy meal or the mid-day and early afternoon hours on hot, humid days. Moderate exercise seems to be beneficial shortly after a meal, because exercise enhances the **thermogenic response**. A walk shortly after a meal burns more calories than a walk several hours after a meal.

Many people enjoy exercising early in the morning because it gives them a boost to start the day. People who exercise in the morning also seem to stick with it more than others, because the chances of putting off the exercise session for other reasons are minimized. Some prefer the lunch hour for weight-control reasons. By exercising at noon, they do not eat as big a lunch, which helps keep down the daily caloric intake. Highly stressed people seem to like the evening hours because of the relaxing effects of exercise.

14. Why is exercising in hot and humid conditions unsafe?

When a person exercises, only 30 to 40 percent of the energy the body produces is used for

Dysmenorrhea Painful menstruation.

Amenorrhea Cessation of regular menstrual flow.

Thermogenic response Amount of energy required to digest food.

SYMPTOMS OF HEAT ILLNESS

If any of these symptoms occur, stop physical activity, get out of the sun, and start drinking fluids.

- Decreased perspiration
- Cramping
- Weakness
- Flushed skin
- Throbbing head
- Nausea/vomiting
- Diarrhea
- Numbness in the extremities
- Blurred vision
- Unsteadiness
- Disorientation
- Incoherency

mechanical work or movement. The rest of the energy (60 to 70 percent) is converted into heat. If this heat cannot be dissipated properly because the weather is too hot or the relative humidity is too high, body temperature increases and, in extreme cases, it can result in death.

The specific heat of body tissue (the heat required to raise the temperature of the body by 1 degree C) is 0.84 calories per kilogram of body weight (0.84 kcal/kg). This indicates that if no body heat is dissipated, a 70 kg person has to burn only 59 Calories (kcals) (70 × 0.84) to increase total body temperature by 1 degree C. If this person were to conduct an exercise session requiring 300 Calories (e.g., running about 5 km) without any heat dissipation, the inner body temperature would increase by 5.3° C, which is the equivalent of going from 37° C to 42.3° C.

This example illustrates clearly the need for caution when exercising in hot or humid weather. If the relative humidity is too high, body heat cannot be lost through evaporation because the atmosphere already is saturated with water vapour. In one instance, a football casualty occurred when the temperature was only 18° C—but the relative humidity was 100 percent. People must be cautious when air temperature is above 32° C and the relative humidity is above 60 percent.

The American College of Sports Medicine recommends avoiding strenuous physical activity when the readings of a wet-bulb globe thermometer exceed 28.8° C. With this type of thermometer, the wet bulb is cooled by evaporation, and on dry days it shows a lower temperature than the regular (dry) thermometer. On humid days, the cooling effect is less because of less evaporation; hence, the difference between the wet and dry readings is not as great.

Following are descriptions of, and first-aid measures for, the three major signs of heat illness:

- **Heat cramps**. Symptoms include cramps, spasms, and muscle twitching in the legs, arms, and abdomen. To relieve heat cramps, stop exercising, get out of the heat, massage the painful area, stretch slowly, and drink plenty of fluids (water, fruit drinks, or electrolyte beverages).

- **Heat exhaustion**. Symptoms include fainting; dizziness; profuse sweating; cold, clammy skin; weakness; headache; and a rapid, weak pulse. If you incur any of these symptoms, stop and find a cool place to rest. If conscious, drink cool water. Do not give water to an unconscious person. Loosen or remove clothing, and rub your body with a cool, wet towel or apply ice packs. Place yourself in a supine position with the legs elevated 20 to 30 cm. If you are not fully recovered in 30 minutes, seek immediate medical attention.

- **Heat stroke**. Symptoms include serious disorientation; warm, dry skin; no sweating; rapid, full pulse; vomiting; diarrhea; unconsciousness; and high body temperature. As the body temperature climbs, unexplained anxiety sets in. When the body temperature reaches 40° C to 40.5° C, the individual may feel a cold sensation in the trunk of the body, goosebumps, nausea, throbbing in the temples, and numbness in the extremities. Most people become incoherent after this stage. When body temperature reaches 40.5° C to 41° C, disorientation, loss of fine-motor control, and muscular weakness set in. If the temperature exceeds 41° C, serious neurologic injury and death may be imminent.

Heat stroke requires immediate emergency medical attention. Request help and get out of the sun and into a cool, humidity-controlled environment. While you are waiting to be taken to the hospital emergency room, you should be placed in a semi-seated position and your body should be sprayed with cool water and rubbed with cool towels. If possible, cold packs should be placed in areas that receive an abundant blood supply, such as the head, neck, armpits, and groin. Fluids should not be given if you are unconscious. In any case of heat-related illness, if the person refuses water, vomits, or starts to lose consciousness, call for an ambulance immediately. Proper initial treatment of heat stroke is critical.

15. What should a person do to replace fluids lost during prolonged aerobic exercise?

The main objective of fluid replacement during prolonged aerobic exercise is to maintain the blood volume so circulation and sweating can continue at normal levels. Adequate water replacement is the most important factor in preventing heat disorders. Drinking about 200 to 250 mL of cool water every 15 to 20 minutes during exercise is ideal to prevent dehydration. Cold fluids seem to be absorbed more rapidly from the stomach.

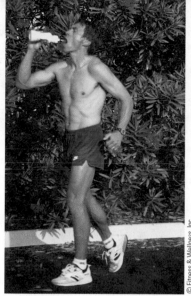
Fluid and carbohydrate replacement are essential when exercising in the heat or for a prolonged period.

© Fitness & Wellness, Inc.

Other relevant points are the following:

■ Drinking commercially prepared sports drinks is recommended when exercise will be strenuous and carried out for more than an hour. For exercise lasting less than an hour, water is just as effective in replacing lost fluid. The sports drinks you select may be based on your personal preference. Try different drinks at 6 to 8 percent glucose concentration to see which drink you tolerate best and suits your tastes as well.

■ Commercial fluid-replacement solutions (such as Powerade and Gatorade) contain about 6 to 8 percent glucose, which seems to be optimal for fluid absorption and performance. Sugar does not become available to the muscles until about 30 minutes after a glucose solution is consumed.

■ Drinks high in fructose or with a glucose concentration above 8 percent are not recommended because they slow down water absorption when exercising in the heat.

■ Most soft drinks (both cola, and non-cola) contain between 10 and 12 percent glucose, which is too high for proper rehydration during exercise in the heat.

16. What precautions must a person take when exercising in the cold?

When exercising in the cold, the two factors to consider are frostbite and **hypothermia**. In contrast to hot and humid conditions, cold weather usually does not threaten health because clothing can be selected for heat conservation, and exercise itself increases the production of body heat.

Most people actually overdress for exercise in the cold. Because exercise increases body temperature, a moderate workout on a cold day makes a person feel that the temperature is about 10° C warmer than it actually is. Overdressing for exercise can make the clothes damp from excessive perspiration. The risk for hypothermia increases when a

person is wet or after exercise stops—when the person is not moving around sufficiently to increase (or maintain) body heat.

Initial warning signs of hypothermia include shivering, loss of coordination, and difficulty speaking. With a continued drop in body temperature, shivering stops, the muscles weaken and stiffen, and the person has feelings of elation or intoxication and eventually loses consciousness. To prevent hypothermia, use common sense, dress properly, and be aware of environmental conditions.

The popular belief that exercising in cold temperatures (0° C and lower) freezes the lungs is false, because the air is warmed properly in the air passages before it reaches the lungs. Cold is not what poses a threat; wind velocity is what increases the chill factor most.

For example, exercising at a temperature of −4° C with adequate clothing is not too cold to exercise, but if the wind is blowing at 40 km/h, the chill factor lowers the actual temperature to −10° C. This effect is even worse if a person is wet and exhausted. When the weather is windy, the individual should exercise (jog or cycle) against the wind on the way out and with the wind upon returning.

Even though the lungs are under no risk when you exercise in the cold, your face, head, hands, and feet should be protected, because they are subject to frostbite. Watch for signs of frostbite—numbness and discoloration. In cold temperatures, as much as half of the body's heat can be lost through an unprotected head and neck. A wool or synthetic cap, hood, or hat will help to hold in body heat. Mittens are better than gloves, because they keep the fingers together so the surface area from which to lose heat is less. Inner linings of synthetic material to wick moisture away from the skin are recommended. Avoid cotton next to the skin, because once cotton gets wet—whether from perspiration, rain, or snow—it loses its insulating properties.

Wearing several layers of lightweight clothing is preferable to wearing one single, thick layer because warm air is trapped between layers of clothes, enabling greater heat conservation. As body temperature increases, you can remove layers as necessary.

The first layer of clothes should wick moisture away from the skin. Polypropylene, Capilene, and

Heat cramps Muscle spasms caused by heat-induced changes in electrolyte balance in muscle cells.

Heat exhaustion Heat-related fatigue.

Heat stroke Emergency situation resulting from the body being subjected to high atmospheric temperatures.

Hypothermia A breakdown in the body's ability to generate heat; a drop in body temperature below 35° C.

Thermax are recommended materials. Next, a layer of wool, dacron, or polyester fleece insulates well even when wet. Lycra tights or sweatpants help protect the legs. The outer layer should be waterproof, wind-resistant, and breathable. A synthetic material such as Gortex is best, so moisture can still escape from the body. A ski mask or face mask helps protect the face. In extremely cold conditions, exposed skin, such as the nose, cheeks, and around the eyes, can be insulated with petroleum jelly.

For lengthy or long-distance workouts (cross-country skiing or long runs), take a small backpack to carry the clothing that is removed. You also can carry extra warm and dry clothes in case you stop exercising away from shelter. If you remain outdoors following exercise, added clothing and continuous body movement are essential to maintain body temperature and avoid hypothermia.

17. Should I exercise when I have a cold or the flu?

The most important consideration in deciding to exercise when you have a cold or flu is to use common sense and pay attention to your symptoms. Typically, you may continue to exercise if your symptoms are limited to a runny nose, sneezing, or a scratchy throat, but if your symptoms include fever, muscle ache, vomiting, diarrhea, or a hacking cough, you should avoid exercise. Following an illness, be sure to ease back gradually into your program. Do not attempt to return at the same intensity and duration that you were used to prior to your illness.

Exercise-Related Injuries

To enjoy and maintain physical fitness, preventing injury during a conditioning program is essential. Exercise-related injuries, nonetheless, are common in individuals who participate in exercise programs. Surveys indicate that more than half of all new participants incur injuries during the first six months after beginning the conditioning program.

Causes of Injuries

The four most common causes of injuries are:

1. High-impact activities
2. Rapid conditioning programs (doing too much too quickly)
3. Improper shoes or training surfaces
4. Anatomical predisposition (body propensity)

By far the most common causes of injuries are high-impact activities and a significant increase in quantity, intensity, and duration of activities. The body requires time to adapt to more intense activities. Most of these injuries can be prevented through a more gradual and correct conditioning (low-impact) program.

Proper shoes for specific activities are essential. Shoes should be replaced when they show a lot of wear and tear. Softer training surfaces, such as grass and dirt, produce less trauma than asphalt and concrete.

Because few people have perfect body alignment, injuries associated with overtraining may occur eventually. In case of injury, proper treatment can avert a lengthy recovery process. A summary of common exercise-related injuries and how to manage them follows.

Acute Sports Injuries

The best treatment always has been prevention. If an activity causes unusual discomfort or chronic irritation, you need to treat the cause by decreasing the intensity, switching activities, substituting equipment, or upgrading clothing (such as buying proper-fitting shoes).

In cases of acute injury, the standard treatment is protection, rest, cold application, compression or splinting (or both), and elevation of the affected body part. This is commonly referred to as "**PRICE**":

P = protection
R = rest
I = ice (cold) application
C = compression
E = elevation

An injury or possible injury should be protected against further problems. An injured person often wants to return to his or her activities as soon as possible. However, if he or she returns too soon, additional damage or complications can occur. Immobilizing, splinting, or limiting further activity (no weight bearing) can protect against further injury.

Cold should be applied three to five times a day for 15 minutes at a time during the first 24 to 36 hours, by submerging the injured area in cold water, using an ice bag, or applying ice massage to the affected part. An elastic bandage or wrap can be used for compression. Elevating the body part decreases blood flow (and therefore swelling) in that body part.

The purpose of these treatment modalities is to minimize swelling in the area, and thus hasten recovery time. After the first 36 to 48 hours, heat can be used if the injury shows no further swelling or inflammation. If you have doubts as to the nature or seriousness of the injury (such as suspected fracture), you should seek a medical evaluation.

Obvious deformities (exhibited by fractures, dislocations, or partial dislocations, as examples) call for splinting, cold application with an ice bag, and medical attention. Do not try to reset any of these conditions by yourself, because you could further damage muscles, ligaments, and nerves. Treatment of these injuries always should be in the

TABLE 9.6 Reference Guide for Exercise-Related Problems

Injury	Signs/Symptoms	Treatment*
Bruise (contusion)	Pain, swelling, discoloration	Cold application, compression, rest
Dislocation / Fracture	Pain, swelling, deformity	Splinting, cold application, seek medical attention
Heat cramp	Cramps, spasms, and muscle twitching in the legs, arms, and abdomen	Stop activity, get out of the heat, stretch, massage the painful area, drink plenty of fluids
Heat exhaustion	Fainting, profuse sweating, cold/clammy skin, weak/rapid pulse, weakness, headache	Stop activity, rest in a cool place, loosen clothing, rub body with cool/wet towel, drink plenty of fluids, stay out of heat for 2–3 days
Heat stroke	Hot/dry skin, no sweating, serious disorientation, rapid/full pulse, vomiting, diarrhea, unconsciousness, high body temperature	**Seek immediate medical attention**, request help and get out of the sun, bathe in cold water/spray with cold water/ rub body with cold towels, drink plenty of cold fluids
Joint sprain	Pain, tenderness, swelling, loss of use, discoloration	Cold application, compression, elevation, rest, heat after 36 to 48 hours (if no further swelling)
Muscle cramp	Pain, spasm	Stretch muscle(s), use mild exercises for involved area
Muscle soreness and stiffness	Tenderness, pain	Mild stretching, low-intensity exercise, warm bath
Muscle strain	Pain, tenderness, swelling, loss of use	Cold application, compression, elevation, rest, heat after 36 to 48 hours (if no further swelling)
Shin splints	Pain, tenderness	Cold application prior to and following any physical activity, rest, heat (if no activity is carried out)
Side stitch	Pain on the side of the abdomen below the rib cage	Decrease level of physical activity or stop altogether, gradually increase level of fitness
Tendinitis	Pain, tenderness, loss of use	Rest, cold application, heat after 48 hours

* Cold should be applied three to four times a day for 15 minutes. Heat can be applied three times a day for 15 to 20 minutes.

hands of specialized medical personnel. A quick reference guide for the signs or symptoms and treatment of exercise-related problems is provided in Table 9.6.

Muscle Soreness and Stiffness

Individuals who begin an exercise program or participate after a long layoff from exercise often develop muscle soreness and stiffness. The acute soreness that sets in the first few hours after exercise is thought to be related to a lack of blood (oxygen) flow and general fatigue of the exercised muscles.

Delayed muscle soreness that appears several hours after exercise (usually about 12 hours later) and lasts two to four days may be related to actual tiny tears in muscle tissue, muscle spasms that increase fluid retention (stimulating the pain nerve endings), and overstretching or tearing of connective tissue in and around muscles and joints.

Mild stretching before and adequate stretching after exercise help to prevent soreness and stiffness. Gradually progressing into an exercise program is important, too. A person should not attempt to do too much too quickly. To relieve pain, mild stretching, low-intensity exercise to stimulate blood flow, and a warm bath might help.

Exercise Intolerance

When starting an exercise program, participants should stay within the safe limits. The best method to determine whether you are exercising too strenuously is to check your heart rate and make sure it does not exceed the limits of your target zone. Exercising above this target zone may not be safe for unconditioned or high-risk individuals. You do not have to exercise beyond your target zone to gain the desired cardiorespiratory benefits.

PRICE An acronym used to describe the standard treatment procedure for acute sports injuries: *Protecting, Rest, Ice* (cold application), *Compression,* and *Elevation.*

Several physical signs will tell you when you are exceeding your functional limitations—that is, experiencing **exercise intolerance**. Signs of intolerance include rapid or irregular heart rate, difficult breathing, nausea, vomiting, lightheadedness, headache, dizziness, unusually flushed or pale skin, extreme weakness, lack of energy, shakiness, sore muscles, cramps, and tightness in the chest. Learn to listen to your body. If you notice any of these symptoms, seek medical attention before continuing your exercise program.

Recovery heart rate is another indicator of overexertion. To a certain extent, recovery heart rate is related to fitness level. The higher your cardiorespiratory fitness level, the faster your heart rate will decrease following exercise. As a rule, heart rate should be below 120 beats per minute 5 minutes into recovery. If your heart rate is above 120, you most likely have overexerted yourself or possibly could have some other cardiac abnormality. If you lower the intensity or duration of exercise, or both, and you still have a fast heart rate 5 minutes into recovery, you should consult your physician.

Side Stitch

Side stitch can develop in the early stages of participation in exercise. It occurs primarily in unconditioned beginners and in trained individuals when they exercise at higher intensities than usual. As one's physical condition improves, this condition tends to disappear unless training is intensified.

The exact cause is unknown. Some experts suggest that it could relate to a lack of blood flow to the respiratory muscles during strenuous physical exertion. Some people encounter side stitch during downhill running. If you experience side stitch during exercise, slow down. If it persists, stop altogether. Lying down on your back and gently bringing both knees to the chest and holding that position for 30 to 60 seconds also helps.

Some people get side stitch if they eat or drink juice shortly before exercise. Drinking only water one to two hours prior to exercise sometimes prevents side stitch. Other individuals have problems with commercially available sports drinks during high-intensity exercise. Unless carbohydrate replacement is crucial to complete an event (such as a marathon or a triathlon), drink cool water for fluid replacement or try a different carbohydrate solution.

Shin Splints

Shin splints, one of the most common injuries to the lower limbs, usually results from one or more of the following: (a) lack of proper and gradual conditioning, (b) doing physical activities on hard surfaces (wooden floors, hard tracks, cement, or asphalt), (c) fallen arches, (d) chronic overuse, (e) muscle fatigue, (f) faulty posture, (g) improper shoes, or (h) participating in weight-bearing activities when excessively overweight.

To manage shin splints:

1. Remove or reduce the cause (exercise on softer surfaces, wear better shoes or arch supports, or completely stop exercise until the shin splints heal);
2. Do stretching exercises before and after physical activity;
3. Use ice massage for 10 to 20 minutes before and after exercise;
4. Apply active heat (whirlpool and hot baths) for 15 minutes, two to three times a day; or
5. Use supportive taping during physical activity (a qualified athletic trainer can teach you the proper taping technique).

Muscle Cramps

Muscle cramps are caused by the body's depletion of essential electrolytes or a breakdown in the coordination between opposing muscle groups. If you have a muscle cramp, you should first attempt to stretch the muscles involved. In the case of the calf muscle, for example, pull your toes up toward the knees. After stretching the muscle, rub it down gently, and, finally, do some mild exercises requiring the use of that muscle.

In pregnant and lactating women, muscle cramps often are related to a lack of calcium. If women get cramps during these times, calcium supplements usually relieve the problem. Tight clothing also can cause cramps by decreasing blood flow to active muscle tissue.

Leisure-Time Physical Activity

Recognizing that individuals have notable differences, the average person in developed countries has about 3.5 hours of "free" or leisure time daily. In our current automated society, most of this time is spent in sedentary living. People would be better off doing some physical activities based on personal interests. Motivational factors include health, aesthetics, weight control, competition and challenge, fun, social interaction, mental arousal, relaxation, and stress management.

Frequently, leisure-time physical activity does not include exercise performed during a regular exercise program. It consists of activities such as walking, hiking, gardening, yardwork, occupational work and chores, and moderate sports such as tennis, table tennis, badminton, golf, or croquet.

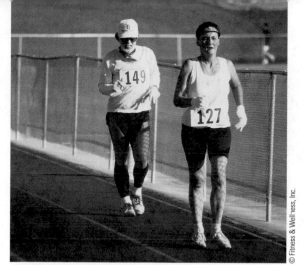

Older adults who exercise enjoy better health, increase their quality of life, and live longer than physically inactive adults.

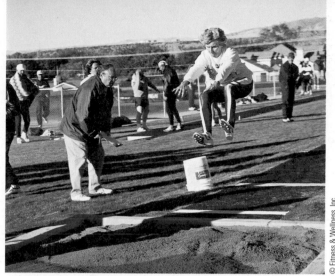

A high level of physical fitness can be maintained throughout the life span.

Every small increase in daily physical activity contributes to better health and wellness. Small increases in physical activity have a large impact in decreasing early risks for disease and premature death. Therefore, a new, concerted effort must be made to spend leisure time in activities that will promote the expenditure of energy, provide a break from daily tasks, and contribute to health-related fitness.

Exercise and Aging

For the first time in North American history, the elderly constitute the fastest-growing segment of the population. The 2001 Canadian Census showed seniors (individuals 65 years old and over) accounted for 13 percent of the Canadian population. This figure will likely reach 15 percent by 2011. For many years the median age in Canada was between 20 and 30 years old, but by 2011 the median age is expected to be over 40 years old.

The main objective of fitness programs for older adults should be to help them improve their functional status and contribute to healthy aging. This implies the ability to maintain independent living status and to avoid disability. Older adults are encouraged to participate in programs that will help develop cardiorespiratory endurance, muscular strength and endurance, muscular flexibility, agility, balance, and motor coordination.

Physical Training in Older Adults

Regular participation in physical activity provides both physical and psychological benefits to older adults.[8] Cardiorespiratory endurance training helps to increase functional capacity, decrease the risk for disease, improve health status, and increase life expectancy. Strength training decreases the rate at which strength and muscle mass are lost. Among the psychological benefits are preserved cognitive function, reduced symptoms and behaviours related to depression, and improved self-confidence and self-esteem.

The trainability of older men and women alike and the effectiveness of physical activity in enhancing health have been demonstrated in prior

TABLE 9.7 Effects of Physical Activity and Inactivity on Older Men

	Exercisers	Non-exercisers
Age (yrs)	68.0	69.8
Weight (kg)	72.8	84.7
Resting heart rate (bpm)	55.8	66.0
Maximal heart rate (bpm)	157.0	146.0
Heart rate reserve* (bpm)	101.2	80.0
Blood pressure (mm Hg)	120/78	150/90
Maximal oxygen uptake (mL/kg/min)	38.6	20.3

*Heart rate reserve = maximal heart rate − resting heart rate.

Data from F. W. Kash, J. L. Boyer, S. P. Van Camp, L. S. Verity, and J. P. Wallace, "The Effect of Physical Activity on Aerobic Power in Older Men (A Longitudinal Study)," *The Physician and Sports Medicine* 18, no. 4 (1990): 73–83.

CRITICAL THINKING

You have been exercising regularly and you are enjoying many exercise-related benefits. Other friends and members of your family, however, do not exercise and think that something is wrong with you because of your love for physical activity. How do you respond so that they will be supportive and maybe even start an exercise program of their own?

Exercise intolerance Inability to function during exercise because of excessive fatigue or extreme feelings of discomfort.

Side stitch A sharp pain in the side of the abdomen.

Shin splints Injury to the lower leg characterized by pain and irritation in the shin region of the leg.

research. Older adults who increase their physical activity experience significant changes in cardio-respiratory endurance, strength, and flexibility. The extent of the changes depends on their initial fitness level and the types of activities they select for their training (walking, cycling, strength training, and so on).

Improvements in maximal oxygen uptake in older adults are similar to those of younger people, although older people seem to require a longer training period to achieve these changes. Declines in maximal oxygen uptake average about 1 percent per year between age 25 and 75.[9] A slower rate of decline is seen in people who maintain a lifetime aerobic exercise program.

Results of research on the effects of aging on the cardiorespiratory system of male exercisers versus non-exercisers showed that the maximal oxygen uptake of regular exercisers was almost twice that of the non-exercisers (see Table 9.7).[10] The study revealed a decline in maximal oxygen uptake between ages 50 and 68 of only 13 percent in the active group, compared to 41 percent in the inactive group. These changes indicate that about one-third of the loss in maximal oxygen uptake results from aging and two-thirds of the loss comes from inactivity. Blood pressure, heart rate, and body weight also were remarkably better in the exercising group. Furthermore, aerobic training seems to decrease high blood pressure in the older patients at the same rate as in young hypertensive people.[11]

Muscle strength declines by 10 to 20 percent between ages 20 and 50, but between ages 50 and 70, it drops by another 25 to 30 percent. Through strength training, frail adults in their 80s or 90s can double or triple their strength in just a few months. The amount of muscle hypertrophy achieved, how-ever, decreases with age. Strength gains close to 200 percent have been found in previously inactive adults over age 90.[12] In fact, research has shown that regular strength training improves balance, gait, speed, **functional independence**, morale, depres-sion symptoms, and energy intake.[13] (The health-related components of strength and flexibility fitness are addressed in Chapters 7 and 8, respectively.)

Although muscle flexibility drops by about 5 percent per decade of life, 10 minutes of stretching every other day can prevent most of this loss as a person ages.[14] Improved flexibility also enhances mobility skills.[15] The latter promotes independence because it helps older adults successfully perform activities of daily living.

With regard to body composition, inactive adults continue to gain body fat after age 60 despite their tendency toward lower body weight. The increase in body fat is most likely related to a decrease in basal metabolic rate and physical activity

along with increased caloric intake above that required to maintain daily energy requirements.[16]

Older adults who wish to initiate or continue an exercise program are strongly encouraged to have a complete medical exam, including a stress electrocardiogram test (see Chapter 11). Recom-mended activities for older adults include calis-thenics, walking, jogging, swimming, cycling, and water aerobics.

Older people should avoid isometric and very high intensity weight-training exercises (see Chap-ter 7). Activities that require all-out effort or require participants to hold their breath tend to lessen blood flow to the heart, cause a significant increase in blood pressure, and increase the load placed on the heart. Older adults should participate in activities that require continuous and rhythmic muscular activity (about 40 to 60 percent of HRR). These activities do not cause large increases in blood pressure or overload the heart.

Preparing for Participation in Sports*

To enhance your participation in sports, keep in mind that in most cases it is better to get fit before playing sports instead of playing sports to get fit. A good pre-season training program will help make the season more enjoyable and prevent exercise-related injuries.

Properly conditioned individuals can safely participate in sports and enjoy the activities to their fullest with few or no limitations. Unfortunately, sport injuries are often the result of poor fitness and a lack of sport-specific conditioning. Many injuries occur when fatigue sets in following overexertion by unconditioned individuals.

Base Fitness Conditioning

Pre-activity screening that includes a health history (see page 23) and/or a medical evaluation appropri-ate to your sport selection is recommended. Once cleared for exercise, start by building a base of general athletic fitness that includes the four health-related fitness components: cardiorespiratory fitness, muscular strength and endurance, flexibility, and rec-ommended body composition. The base fitness condi-tioning program should last a minimum of six weeks.

As explained in Chapter 6, for cardiorespiratory fitness select an activity that you enjoy (such as walk-ing, jogging, cycling, step aerobics, cross-country

---

* Adapted from W. W. K. Hoeger and J. R. Moore, "Preparing for Outdoor Winter Sports," *ACSM Fit Society Page*, Fall 2002 (www.acsm.org).

skiing, stair climbing, endurance games) and train three to five times per week at a minimum of 20 minutes of continuous activity per session. Exercise in the moderate- to high-intensity zones for adequate conditioning. You should feel as though you are training "somewhat hard" to "hard" at these intensity levels.

Strength (resistance) training helps maintain and increase muscular strength and endurance. Following the guidelines provided in Chapter 7, select 8 to 10 exercises that involve the major muscle groups of the body and train two or three times per week on nonconsecutive days. Select a resistance (weight) that allows you to do 8 to 12 repetitions to near fatigue. That is, the resistance will be heavy enough so that when you perform a set of an exercise, you will not be able to do more than 12 repetitions at that weight. Begin your program slowly and perform between one and three sets of each exercise. Recommended exercises include the bench press, lat pulldown, leg press, leg curl, triceps extension, arm curl, rowing torso, heel raise, abdominal crunch, and back extension.

Flexibility is important in sports participation to enhance the range of motion in the joints. Using the guidelines from Chapter 8, schedule flexibility training two or three days per week. Perform each stretching exercise four times, and hold each stretch for 10 to 30 seconds. Examples of stretching exercises include the side body stretch, body rotation, chest stretch, shoulder stretch, trunk forward flexion stretch, adductor stretch, quad stretch, heel cord stretch, and knee-to-chest stretch.

With regard to body composition, excess body fat hinders sports performance and increases the risk for injuries. Depending on the nature of the activity, fitness goals for body composition range from 12 percent to 20 percent body fat for men and 17 percent to 25 percent for most women.

Sport-Specific Conditioning

Once the general fitness base is achieved, continue with the program but make adjustments to add sport-specific training. This training should match the sport's requirements for aerobic/anaerobic capabilities, muscular strength and endurance, and range of motion.

During the sport-specific training, about half of your aerobic/anaerobic training should involve the same muscles used during your sport. Ideally, allocate four weeks of sport-specific training before you start participating in the sport. Then continue the sport-specific training on a more limited basis throughout the season. Depending on the nature of the sport (aerobic versus anaerobic—discussed next), once the season starts, sports participation itself can take the place of some or all of your aerobic workouts.

The next step is to look at the demands of the sport. For example, soccer, bicycle racing, cross-country skiing, and snowshoeing are aerobic activities, whereas basketball, racquetball, alpine skiing, snowboarding, and ice hockey are stop-and-go sports that require a combination of aerobic and anaerobic activity. Consequently, aerobic training may be appropriate for cross-country skiing, but it will do little to prepare your muscles for the high-intensity requirements of combined aerobic and anaerobic sports.

Interval training, performed twice per week, is added to the program at this time. The intervals consist of a 1:3 work-to-rest ratio. This means you'll work at a fairly high intensity for, say, 15 seconds, and then spend 45 seconds on low-intensity recovery. Be sure to keep moving during the recovery phase. Perform four or five intervals at first, then gradually progress to 10 intervals. As your fitness improves, progressively lengthen the high-intensity proportion of the intervals to 1 minute and use a 1:2 work-to-rest ratio—wherein you work at high intensity for 1 minute and then at low intensity for 2 minutes.

For aerobic sports, interval training once a week also improves performance. These intervals, however, can be done on a 3-minute to 3-minute work-to-rest ratio. A 5- to 10-minute work interval followed by 1 to 2 minutes of recovery can also be done, but the intensity of these longer intervals should not be as high, and only three to five intervals are recommended. Your interval-training workouts are not performed in addition to the regular aerobic workouts but, instead, take the place of one of these workouts.

Consider sport-specific strength requirements as well. Look at the primary muscles used in your sport, and make sure your choice of exercises works those muscles. Try to perform your strength training through a range of motion similar to that used in your sport. Aerobic/anaerobic sports require greater strength; during the season, three sets of 8 to 12 repetitions to near fatigue are recommended two or three times per week. For aerobic endurance sports, the recommendation is a minimum of one set of 8 to 12 repetitions to near fatigue performed once or twice per week during the season.

For some winter sports, such as alpine skiing and snowboarding, gravity supplies most of the

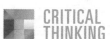

CRITICAL THINKING

Sports participation is a good predictor of adherence to exercise later in life. What experiences have you had with youth sports? Were these experiences positive, and what effect do they have on your current physical activity patterns?

Functional independence Ability to carry out activities of daily living without assistance from other individuals.

Interval training A training program where high-intensity speed intervals are followed by short recovery intervals.

propulsion and the body acts more as a shock absorber. Muscles in the hips, knees, and trunk are used to control the forces on the body and equipment. Multi-joint exercises, such as the leg press, squats, and lunges, are suggested for these activities.

Before the season starts, make sure your equipment is in proper working condition. For example, alpine skiers' bindings should be cleaned and adjusted properly so they will release as needed. This is one of the most important things you can do to help prevent knee injuries. A good pair of bindings may be all that stands between you and knee surgery.

The first few times you participate in the sport of your choice, go easy, practise technique, and do not continue once fatigued. Gradually increase the length and intensity of your workouts. Consider taking a lesson to have someone watch your technique and help correct flaws early in the season. Even Olympic athletes have coaches watching them. Proper conditioning allows for a more enjoyable and healthier season.

Overtraining

Rest is important in any fitness conditioning program. Although the term **overtraining** is most frequently associated with athletic performance, it applies just as well to fitness participants. We all know that hard work improves fitness and performance. Hard training without adequate recovery, however, breaks down the body and leads to loss of fitness.

Physiological improvements in fitness and conditioning programs occur during the rest periods following training. As a rule, a hard day of training must be followed by a rest day or a day of light training. Equally, a few weeks of increased training

COMMON SIGNS AND SYMPTOMS OF OVERTRAINING

- Decreased fitness
- Decreased sports performance
- Increased fatigue
- Loss of concentration
- Staleness and burnout
- Loss of competitive drive
- Increased resting and exercise heart rate
- Decreased appetite
- Loss of body weight
- Altered sleep patterns
- Decreased sex drive
- Generalized body aches and pains
- Increased susceptibility to illness and injury
- Mood disturbances
- Depression

volume are to be followed by a few days of light recovery work. During these recovery periods, body systems strengthen and compensate for the training load, leading to a higher level of fitness. If proper recovery is not built into the training routine, overtraining occurs. Decreased performance, staleness, and injury are frequently seen with overtraining. Thus, to obtain optimal results, training regimens are altered during different phases of the year.

Periodization

Periodization is a training approach that uses a systematic variation in intensity and volume to enhance fitness and performance. This model was designed on the premise that the body becomes stronger as a result of training, but if similar workouts are constantly repeated, the body tires and enters a state of staleness and fatigue.

Periodization is used most frequently for athletic conditioning. Because peak fitness cannot be maintained during an entire season, most athletes seeking peak performance use a periodized training approach. Studies have documented that greater improvements in fitness are achieved by using a variety of training loads. Using the same program and attempting to increase volume and intensity over a prolonged time will be manifested in overtraining.

The periodization training system involves three cycles:

1. macrocycles
2. mesocycles
3. microcycles

These cycles vary in length depending on the requirements of the sport. Typically, the overall training period (season or year) is referred to as a macrocycle. For athletes who need to peak twice a year, such as cross-country and track runners, two macrocycles can be developed within the year.

Macrocycles are divided into smaller weekly or monthly training phases known as mesocycles. A typical season, for example, is divided into the following mesocycles: base fitness conditioning (off-season), pre-season or sport-specific conditioning, competition, peak performance, and transition (active recovery from sport-specific training and competition). In turn, mesocycles are divided into smaller weekly or daily microcycles. During microcycles, training follows the general objective of the mesocycle, but the workouts are altered to avoid boredom and fatigue.

The concept behind periodizing can be used in both aerobic and anaerobic sports. In the case of a long-distance runner, for instance, training can start with a general strength-conditioning program and cardiorespiratory endurance cross-training (jogging,

TABLE 9.8 Periodization Program for Strength

	One Macrocycle			
	Mesocycle 1*	Mesocycle 2*	Mesocycle 3*	Mesocycle 4*
	Hypertrophy	**Strength & Hypertrophy**	**Strength & Power**	**Peak Performance**
Sets per exercise	3–5	3–5	3–5	1–3
Repetitions	8–12	6–9	1–5	1–3
Intensity (resistance)	Low	Moderate	High	Very High
Volume	High	Moderate	Low	Very Low
Weeks (microcycles)	6–8	4–6	3–5	1–2

*Each mesocycle is followed by several days of light training.

cycling, swimming) during the off-season. In pre-season, the volume of strength training is decreased and the total weekly running distance, at moderate intensities, is progressively increased. During the competitive season, the athlete maintains a limited strength-training program but now increases the intensity of the runs while decreasing the total weekly distance. During the peaking phase, volume (kilometres) of training is reduced even further while the intensity is maintained at a high level. At the end of the season, a short transition period of two to four weeks, involving low- to moderate-intensity activities other than running and lifting weights, is recommended.

Periodization is frequently used for muscular strength development, progressively cycling through the various components (hypertrophy, strength, and power) of strength training. A sample sequence—one macrocycle—of periodized training is provided in Table 9.8. The program starts with high volume and low intensity. During subsequent mesocycles (divided among the objectives of hypertrophy, strength, and power), the volume is decreased and the intensity (resistance) increases. Following each mesocycle, up to seven days of very light training are recommended. This brief resting period allows the body to fully recuperate, preventing overtraining and risk for injury. Other models of periodization exist, but the previous example is the most commonly used training model.

Altering or cycling workouts has become popular in recent years among fitness participants. Research indicates that periodization is not limited to athletes but has been used successfully by fitness enthusiasts who are preparing for a special event such a 10 km run, a triathlon, a bike race, or who are simply aiming for higher fitness. Altering training is also recommended for people who progressed nicely in the initial weeks of a program but now feel "stale" and "stagnant." Studies indicate that even among general fitness participants, systematically altering volume and intensity of training is most effective for progression in long-term fitness. Because training phases continually change during a macrocycle, periodization breaks staleness and the monotony of repeated workouts.

For the non-athlete, a periodization program does not have to account for every detail of the sport. You can periodize workouts by altering mesocycles every two to eight weeks. You can use different exercises, change the number of sets and repetitions, vary the speed of the repetitions, alter recovery time between sets, and even cross-train.

Periodization is not for everyone. People who are starting an exercise program, who enjoy a set routine, or who are satisfied with their fitness routine and fitness level do not need to periodize. For new participants, the goal is to start and adhere to exercise long enough to adopt the exercise behaviour.

Personal Fitness Programming: An Example

Now that you understand the principles of fitness assessment and exercise prescription given in Chapters 6 through 8 and this chapter, you can review this program to cross-check and improve the design of your own fitness program.

Mary is 20 years old. She participated in organized sports on and off throughout high school.

Overtraining An emotional, behavioural, and physical condition marked by increased fatigue, decreased performance, persistent muscle soreness, mood disturbances, and feelings of "staleness" or "burnout" as a result of excessive physical training.

Volume (of training) The total amount of training performed in a given work period (day, week, month, or season).

Periodization A training approach that divides the season into three cycles (macrocycles, mesocycles, and microcycles) using a systematic variation in intensity and volume of training to enhance fitness and performance.

During the last two years, however, she has only minimally participated in physical activity. She was not taught the principles for exercise prescription and has not participated in regular exercise to improve and maintain the various health-related components of fitness.

Mary became interested in fitness and contemplated signing up for a fitness and wellness course. As she was preparing her class schedule for the semester, she noted a "Lifetime Fitness and Wellness" course. In registering for the course, Mary anticipated some type of structured aerobic exercise. She knew that good fitness was important to health and weight management, but she didn't quite know how to plan and implement a program.

Once the new course started, she and her classmates received the "Stages of Change Questionnaire." Mary learned that she was in the Contemplation stage for cardiorespiratory endurance, the Precontemplation stage for muscular strength and endurance, the Maintenance stage for flexibility, and the Preparation stage for body composition (see Transtheoretical Model in Chapter 2, pages 34–36). Various fitness assessments determined that her cardiorespiratory endurance level was fair, her muscular strength and endurance was poor, her flexibility was good, and her percent body fat was 25 percent (Moderate classification).

CRITICAL THINKING

In your own experience with personal fitness programs throughout the years, what factors have motivated you and helped you the most to stay with the program? What factors have kept you from being physically active and what can you do to change these factors?

Cardiorespiratory Endurance

At the beginning of the semester, the instructor informed the students that the course required self-monitored participation in activities outside the regularly scheduled class hours. Thus, Mary entered the Preparation stage for cardiorespiratory endurance. She knew she would be starting exercise in the next couple of weeks.

While in this Preparation stage, Mary chose three processes of change to help her implement her program (see Table 2.1, page 37). She thought she could adopt an aerobic exercise program (Positive Outlook process of change) and set a realistic goal to reach the "Good" category for cardiorespiratory endurance by the end of the semester (Goal Setting). By staying in this course, she committed to go through with exercise (Commitment). She prepared a 12-week Personalized Cardiorespiratory Exercise Prescription (see Figure 9.3), wrote down her goal, signed the prescription (now a contract), and shared the program with her instructor and roommates.

As her exercise modalities, Mary selected walking/jogging and aerobics. Initially she walked/jogged twice a week and did aerobics once a week. By the 10th week of the program, she was jogging three times per week and participating in aerobics twice a week. She also selected Self-monitoring, Self-reevaluation, and Countering as techniques of change (see Table 2.2, page 40). Using the exercise log in Figure 6.10 (pages 184–185), she monitored her exercise program (see Figure 9.4). At the end of six weeks, she scheduled a follow-up cardiorespiratory assessment test (Self-reevaluation process of change), and she's replaced her evening television hour with aerobic training (Countering).

Mary also decided to increase her daily physical activity. She chose to walk 10 minutes to and from school, take the stairs instead of elevators whenever possible, and add 5-minute walks every hour during study time. On Saturdays, she cleaned her apartment and went to a school-sponsored dance at night. On Sundays, she opted to walk to and from church and took a 30-minute leisurely walk after the dinner meal. Mary now was fully in the Action stage of change for cardiorespiratory endurance.

Muscular Strength and Endurance

After Mary had started her fitness and wellness course, she wasn't yet convinced that she wanted to strength-train. Still, she contemplated strength training because a small part of her grade depended on it. When she read the information on the importance of lean body mass in regulating basal metabolic rate and weight maintenance (the Consciousness-raising process of change), she thought that perhaps it would be good to add strength training to her program. She was also contemplating the long-term consequences of loss of lean body mass, its effect on her personal appearance, and the potential for decreased independence and quality of life (Emotional Arousal process of change).

Mary visited with her course instructor for additional guidance. Following this meeting, Mary committed herself to strength-train. While yet in the Preparation stage, she outlined a 10-week periodized training program (see Figure 9.5) and opted to aim for the "Good" strength category by the end of the program.

Because this was the first time Mary had lifted weights, the course instructor introduced Mary to two other students who were already lifting (Helping Relationships process of change). She also monitored her program with the form provided in Figure 7.7 on pages 219–220. Mary promised herself a movie and dinner out if she completed the first 5 weeks of strength training, and a new blouse if she made it through 10 weeks (Rewards process and technique for change).

FIGURE 9.3 Sample computerized cardiorespiratory exercise prescription

Personalized Cardiorespiratory Exercise Prescription
Fitness & Wellness Series

Mary Johnson   September 1, 2008
Maximal heart rate: 200 bpm   Resting heart rate: 76 bpm
Present cardiorespiratory fitness level: Fair   Age: 20

The following is your personal program for cardiorespiratory fitness development and maintenance. If you have been exercising regularly and you are in the average or good category, you may start at week five. If you are in the excellent category, you can start at week ten.

Week	Time (min.)	Frequency (per week)	Training Intensity (beats per minute)	Pulse (10 sec. count)
1	15	3	126 - 138	21 - 23 beats
2	15	4	126 - 138	21 - 23 beats
3	20	4	126 - 138	21 - 23 beats
4	20	5	126 - 138	21 - 23 beats
5	20	4	138 - 150	23 - 25 beats
6	20	5	138 - 150	23 - 25 beats
7	30	4	138 - 150	23 - 25 beats
8	30	5	138 - 150	23 - 25 beats
9	30	4	150 - 181	25 - 30 beats
10	30	5	150 - 181	25 - 30 beats
11	30-40	5	150 - 181	25 - 30 beats
12	30-40	5-6	150 - 181	25 - 30 beats

You may participate in any combination of activities which are aerobic and continuous in nature such as walking, jogging, swimming, cross country skiing, aerobelt exercise, rope skipping, cycling, aerobic dancing, racquetball, stair climbing, stationary running or cycling, etc. As long as the heart rate reaches the desired rate, and it stays at that level for the period of time indicated, the cardiorespiratory system will improve.

Following the twelve week program, in order to maintain your fitness level, you should exercise between 150 and 181 bpm for about 30 minutes, a minimum of three times per week on non-consecutive days. When you exercise, allow about 5 minutes for a gradual warm-up period and another 5 for gradual cool-down. Also, when you check your exercise heart rate, only count your pulse for 10 seconds (start counting with 0) and then refer to the above 10 second pulse count. You may also multiply by 6 to obtain your rate in beats per minute.

Good cardiorespiratory fitness will greatly contribute toward the enhancement and maintenance of good health. It is especially important in the prevention of cardiovascular disease. We encourage you to be persistent in your exercise program and to participate regularly.

Training days: ✓ M ✓ T ___ W ___ Th ✓ F ✓ S ___ S   Training time: *7:00 am*

Signature: *Mary Johnson*   Goal: *Good*   Date: *9-01-08*

FIGURE 9.4 Sample computerized exercise record

Exercise Log
Fitness & Wellness Series

Mary Johnson

Date	Exercise	Body Weight (kg)	Heart Rate (bpm)	Duration (min)	Distance (km)	Calories Burned
09/01/2008	Walking (7km/hr)	63.5	138	15	1.75	95
09/03/2008	Aerobics/Moderate	63.5	144	20		182
09/05/2008	Walking (7km/hr)	64	138	15	1.75	95
09/06/2008	Dance/Moderate	64	100	60		254
09/07/2008	Walking (7km/hr)	63.5	132	30	3.50	189
09/08/2008	Jogging (7min/km)	63.5	138	15	2.00	147
09/10/2008	Aerobics/Moderate	63.5	138	20		182
09/11/2008	Jogging (7min/km)	63	138	15	2.00	146
09/12/2008	Jogging (7min/km)	63	134	15	2.00	146
09/13/2008	Dance/Moderate	63.5	96	75		315
09/14/2008	Walking (7km/hr)	63	126	30	4.00	188
09/15/2008	Jogging (7min/km)	63	134	20	3.50	195
09/16/2008	Strength Training	62.5	96	30		207
09/17/2008	Step-Aerobics	63	138	30		292
09/18/2008	Jogging (7min/km)	62.5	138	20	3.50	193
09/19/2008	Jogging (7min/km)	62.5	138	20	3.50	193
	Strength Training	62.5	96	30		207
09/20/2008	Dance/Moderate	62.5	90	30		124
09/21/2008	Walking (7km/hr)	62.5	126	30	4.00	186
09/22/2008	Jogging (7min/km)	62	136	20	3.50	192
09/23/2008	Step-Aerobics	62.5	138	30		290
	Strength Training	62.5	96	40		276
09/24/2008	Jogging (5.5min/km)	62.5	144	20	4.00	248
09/25/2008	Step-Aerobics	62	136	20		192
09/26/2008	Strength Training	62	92	40		274
	Jogging (5.5min/km)	62	140	20	4.00	247
09/27/2008	Dance/Moderate	61.5	94	90		367
09/28/2008	Walking (7km/hr)	61.5	120	30	4.00	184
Totals				13 hr 50 min	47.00	5806
Average per exercise session		63	124	30	1.88	207
Number of exercise sessions:	28					
Average per day exercised				33		232
Number of days exercised:	25					

Distance summary

Total km run:	22.5
Total km walked:	17.5

FIGURE 9.5 Sample starting muscular strength and endurance periodization program

	Learning Lifting Technique	Muscular Strength	Muscular Endurance	Muscular Strength
Sets per exercise	1–2	2	2	3
Repetitions	10	12	18–20	8–12 (RM)
Intensity (resistance)	Very low	Moderate	Low	High
Volume	Low	Moderate	Moderate	High
Sessions per week	2	2	2	3
Weeks	2	3	2	3

Selected exercises: Bench press, leg press, leg curl, lat pull-down, rowing torso, rotary torso, seated back, and abdominal crunch.

Training days: ☐M ☑T ☐W ☐Th ☐F ☑S ☐S   Training time: **3:00 pm**

Signature: _Mary Johnson_   Goal: _Good_   Date: _9-10-08_

Muscular Flexibility

Good flexibility was not a problem for Mary because she regularly stretched 15 to 30 minutes while watching the evening news on television. She had developed this habit the last two years of high school to maintain flexibility as a member of the dance-drill team (Environment Control process of change—as a team member she needed good flexibility).

Because Mary had been stretching regularly for more than three years, she was in the Maintenance stage for flexibility. The flexibility fitness tests revealed that she had good flexibility. These results allowed her to pursue her stretching program because she thought she would be excellent for this fitness component (Self-evaluation process of change).

To gain greater improvements in flexibility, Mary chose slow-sustained stretching and proprioceptive neuromuscular facilitation (PNF). She would need help to carry out the PNF technique. She spoke to one of her lifting classmates, and together they decided to allocate 20 minutes at the end of strength training to stretching (Helping Relationships process of change) and they chose the sequence of exercises presented in Lab 8C, pages 265–266 (Consciousness-raising and Goal Setting).

Body Composition

One of the motivational factors to enroll in a fitness course was Mary's desire to learn how to better manage her weight. She had gained a couple of kilograms since entering college. To prevent further weight gain, she thought it was time to learn sound principles for weight management (Behaviour Analysis process of change). She was in the Preparation stage of change because she was planning to start a diet and exercise program but wasn't sure how to get it done. All Mary needed was a little Consciousness-raising to get her into the Action stage.

With the knowledge she had now gained, Mary planned her program. At 25 percent body fat and 63.5 kg, she decided to aim for 23 percent body fat so she would be in the "Good" category for body composition (Goal Setting). This meant she would have to lose 1.8 kg (see Lab 4B, page 118).

Being moderately active, Mary's daily estimated energy requirement was about 1,890 Calories. Mary also figured out that she was expending an additional 450 Calories per day through her newly adopted exercise program and increased level of daily physical activity. Thus, her total daily energy intake would be around 2,340 Calories (1,890 + 450).

To lose weight, Mary could decrease her caloric intake by 700 Calories per day (body weight × 5— see Lab 5A, page 149), yielding a target daily intake of 1,640 Calories. By decreasing the intake by 700 daily Calories daily, Mary should achieve her target weight in about 20 days (1.8 kg of fat × 3,500 Calories per kilogram of fat ÷ 700 fewer Calories per day = 20 days).

Mary picked the 1,500 Calorie diet and allowed herself one additional serving of fruit and two servings of vegetables to meet her estimated 1,640 daily Calorie needs.

The processes of change that will help Mary in the Action stage for weight management are Goal Setting, Countering (exercising instead of watching television), Monitoring, Environment Control, and Rewards. To monitor her daily caloric intake, Mary uses the 1,500-Calorie diet plan in Lab 5B. To further exert control over her environment, she gave away all of her junk food. She determined that she would not eat out while on the diet, and she bought only low-to-moderate fat/complex carbohydrate foods during the three weeks. As her reward, she achieved her target body weight of 62 kg.

You Can Do It

Once the proper exercise, nutrition, and behaviour modification guidelines are understood, implementing a fitness lifestyle program is not as difficult as people think. With adequate preparation and a personal behavioural analysis, you are now ready to design, implement, evaluate, and adhere to a lifetime fitness program that can enhance your functional capacity and zest for life.

According to the concepts provided thus far in this book, three case studies are given in Lab 9B for you to evaluate how well you have learned and are able to apply the principles of exercise prescription. You also have an opportunity to update your current stage of change and fitness category for each health-related component of physical fitness.

 ASSESS YOUR KNOWLEDGE

1. Which of the following is *not* a skill-related fitness component?
   a. agility
   b. speed
   c. power
   d. strength
   e. balance

2. The ability to quickly and efficiently change body position and direction is known as
   a. agility.
   b. coordination.
   c. speed.
   d. reaction time.
   e. mobility.

3. The two components of power are
   a. strength and endurance.
   b. speed and force.
   c. speed and endurance.
   d. strength and force.
   e. strength and speed.
   f. endurance and force.

4. Diabetics should
   a. not exercise alone.
   b. wear a bracelet that identifies their condition.
   c. exercise at a low-to-moderate intensity.
   d. check blood glucose levels before and after exercise.
   e. All four guidelines above.

5. Exercise intensity during pregnancy should be decreased by about _____ percent from the pre-pregnancy program.
   a. 5
   b. 10
   c. 20
   d. 25
   e. 50

6. During exercise in the heat, drinking about a 250 mL of cool water every _____ minutes seems to be ideal to prevent dehydration.
   a. 5
   b. 15 to 20
   c. 30
   d. 30 to 45
   e. 60

7. One of the most common causes of activity-related injuries is
   a. high-impact activities.
   b. low level of fitness.
   c. exercising without stretching.
   d. improper warm-up.
   e. All choices result in about an equal number of injuries.

8. Improvements in maximal oxygen uptake in older adults (as compared to younger adults) as a result of cardiorespiratory endurance training are
   a. lower.
   b. higher.
   c. difficult to determine.
   d. nonexistent.
   e. similar.

9. To participate in sports, it is recommended that you have
   a. base fitness and sport-specific conditioning.
   b. at least a "Good" rating on skill fitness.
   c. good to excellent agility.
   d. basic speed.
   e. All of the above are recommended.

10. Periodization is a training approach that
    a. uses a systematic variation in intensity and volume.
    b. enhances fitness and performance.
    c. is commonly used by athletes.
    d. helps to prevent staleness and overtraining.
    e. All are correct choices.

Correct answers can be found at the back of the book.

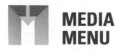

MEDIA MENU

INTERNET CONNECTIONS

■ Canadian Fitness and Lifestyle Research Institute (CFLRI). This site provides research, monitors trends, and makes recommendations to increase Canadians' levels of physical activity and improve their health.

http://www.cflri.ca/eng/index.php

■ Canadian Fitness Matters. This is a web-based consumer's shopping guide to the fitness industry in Canada. The site contains an online directory of more than 10,000 fitness-related facilities.

www.canadianfitnessmatters.ca

■ Canadian Centre for Activity and Aging (CCAA). CCAA is an organization affiliated with a university, a research institute, and a hospital and specializes in research and outreach related to physiological aspects of aging.

www.uwo.ca/actage

■ Canadian Society for Exercise Physiology (CSEP). This voluntary organization is involved in the scientific study of exercise physiology, exercise biochemistry, fitness, and health.

http://www.csep.ca

■ Fitness Jumpsite. This site features information on nutrition, weight management, fitness equipment, and healthy lifestyles. A comprehensive search engine is also available.

http://www.primusweb.com/fitnesspartner

■ Fitness online. This site features information on fitness goals and programs, fitness adventures, injury prevention, nutrition, and mental fitness.

http://www.fitnessonline.com/

Notes

1. R. F. Kirby, "A Simple Test of Agility," *Coach and Athlete*, June 1971: 30–31.

2. American Alliance for Health, Physical Education, Recreation and Dance (AAHPERD). *Youth Fitness: Test Manual.* Reston, VA: AAHPERD, 1976.

3. AAHPERD, *Youth Fitness.*

4. R. S. Paffenbarger, Jr., R. T. Hyde, A. L. Wing, and C. H. Steinmetz, "A Natural History of Athleticism and Cardiovascular Health," *Journal of the American Medical Association* 252 (1984): 491–495.

5. Canadian Diabetes Association, "Physical Activity and Type 2 Diabetes." Retrieved January 22, 2008, from www.diabetes.ca/Section_About/firststep.asp.

6. Joint SOGC/CSEP Clinical Practice Guideline. Exercise in Pregnancy and the Postpartum Period. No 129, June 2003.

7. American College of Obstetricians and Gynecologists, "Exercise During Pregnancy and the Postpartum Period" (ACOG Committee Opinion No. 267), *International Journal of Gynecology and Obstetrics* 77 (2002): 79–81.

8. American College of Sports Medicine, "Position Stand: Exercise and Physical Activity for Older Adults," *Medicine and Science in Sports and Exercise* 30 (1998): 992–1008.

9. R. J. Shephard, "Exercise and Aging: Extending Independence in Older Adult," *Geriatrics* 48 (1993): 61–64.

10. F. W. Kash, J. L. Boyer, S. P. Van Camp, L. S. Verity, and J. P. Wallace, "The Effect of Physical Activity on Aerobic Power in Older Men (A Longitudinal Study)," *Physician and Sports Medicine* 18, no. 4 (1990): 73–83.

11. J. Hagberg, S. Blair, A. Ehsani, N. Gordon, N. Kaplan, C. Tipton, and E. Zambraski, "Position Stand: Physical Activity, Physical Fitness, and Hypertension," *Medicine and Science in Sports and Exercise* 25 (1993): i–x.

12. W. S. Evans, "Exercise, Nutrition and Aging," *Journal of Nutrition* 122 (1992): 796–801.

13. E. J. Marcinick, J. Potts, G. Schlabach, S. Will, P. Dawson, and B. F. Hurley, "Effects of Strength Training on Lactate Threshold and Endurance Performance," *Medicine and Science in Sports and Exercise* 23 (1991): 739–743.

14. The Editors, "Exercise for the Ages," *Consumer Reports on Health* (Yonkers, NY: July, 1996).

15. J. M. Walker, D. Sue, N. Miles-Elkousy, G. Ford, and H. Trevelyan, "Active Mobility of the Extremities in Older Subjects," *Physical Therapy* 64 (1994): 919–923.

16. S. B. Roberts, et al., "What are the Dietary Needs of Adults?" *International Journal of Obesity* 16 (1992): 969–976.

Suggested Readings

American College of Obstetricians and Gynecologists. "Exercise During Pregnancy and the Postpartum Period (ACOG Committee Opinion No. 267). *International Journal of Gynecology and Obstetrics* 77 (2002): 79–81.

Coleman, E. *Eating for Endurance*. Palo Alto, CA: Bull Publishing, 2003.

Katzmarzyk, P. T., C. L. Craig, and L. Gauvin. "A Diposity, Physical Fitness and Incident Diabetes: The Physical Activity Longitudinal Study." *Diabetologia* 50 (2007): 538–544.

Mason, C., S. E. Brien, C. L. Craig, L. Gauvin and P. T. Katzmarzyk. "Musculoskeletal Fitness and Weight Gain in Canada." *Medicine and Science in Sports and Exercise* 39 (2007): 38–43.

Pfeiffer, R. P., and B. C. Mangus. *Concepts of Athletic Training.* Boston: Jones and Bartlett, 2005.

Prentice, W., and D. D. Arnheim. *Arnheim's Principles of Athletic Training.* Boston: McGraw–Hill, 2003.

Unruh, N., S. Unruh, and E. Scantling. "Heat Can Kill: Guidelines to Prevent Heat Illness in Athletics and Physical Education." *Journal of Physical Education, Recreation & Dance* 73 no. 6 (2002): 36–38.

Lab 9A

ASSESSMENT OF SKILL-RELATED COMPONENTS OF FITNESS

Name: _____   Date: _____

Instructor: _____   Course: _____   Section: _____

Necessary Lab Equipment

Agility: Free-throw area of a basketball court (or any area 4 × 6 metres with sufficient running space around it), four plastic cones, and a stopwatch.

Balance: Any flat, smooth floor (not carpeted) and a stopwatch.

Power: A flat smooth surface, a wall, and a measuring tape.

Objective

To assess the fitness level for each skill-related fitness component.

Lab Preparation

Wear exercise clothing, including running shoes for the agility and power tests. Do not exercise strenuously several hours prior to this lab.

Instructions

Perform all three tests for the fitness-related components as outlined in Chapter 9. Report the results below and answer the questions given at the end of this lab.

Skill-Related Fitness:	Test Results

1. Agility   SEMO Agility Test

Trial: 1. ⬜⬜ . ⬜   2. ⬜⬜ . ⬜

See Table 9.1, Norms in Seconds for SEMO Agility Test, College Students page 269 to compare your results.

2. Balance   Stork Stand Test

Trial: 1. ⬜ . ⬜   2. ⬜ . ⬜   3. ⬜ . ⬜

See Table 9.2 Norms in Seconds for Stork Stand, College Students page 270 to compare your results.

3. Power   Vertical Jump Test

Stand and Reach Height (cm): ⬜⬜⬜

Peak Height: Trial: 1. ⬜⬜⬜   2. ⬜⬜⬜   3 ⬜⬜⬜

Jump Height: Peak Height (best Trial) ⬜⬜ − Stand and Reach Height ⬜⬜ = ⬜⬜

Peak Leg Power in Watts (W): ⬜⬜⬜

Calculate as follows using Sayers Equation:

Peak Leg Power (W) = [60.7 − jump height (cm)] × 45.3 × body mass (kg) − 2055.

Peak Leg Power (W) = [60.7 × ⬜⬜⬜ (jump height)] + 45.3 × ⬜⬜⬜ body mass (kg) − 2055

= ⬜⬜⬜ Watts

= ⬜⬜⬜ Rating

See Table 9.3—Health Benefit Rating for Leg Power—Vertical Jump Test (page 271) to compare your results.

Refer to the Table below to compare your results for Log Power is Watts.

Table 9A.1 Norms and Health Benefit Zones for Leg Power in Watts—for Males

Category	Age (yr) 15–19	Age (yr) 20–29	Age (yr) 30–39	Age (yr) 40–49	Age (yr) 50–59	Age (yr) 60–69
Excellent	≥4644	≥5094	≥4860	≥4320	≥4019	≥3764
Very Good	4185–4643	4640–5093	4389–4859	3700–4319	3567–4018	3291–3763
Good	3858–4184	4297–4639	3967–4388	3242–3699	2937–3566	2843–3290
Fair	3323–3857	3775–4296	3485–3966	2708–3241	2512-2936	2383–2842
Needs Improvement	≤3322	≤3774	≤3484	≤2707	≤2511	≤2382

Table 9A.2 Norms and Health Benefit Zones for Leg Power in Watts—for Females

Category	Age (yr) 15–19	Age (yr) 20–29	Age (yr) 30–39	Age (yr) 40–49	Age (yr) 50–59	Age (yr) 60–69
Excellent	≥3167	≥3250	≥3193	≥2675	≥2559	≥2475
Very Good	2795–3166	2804–3249	2550–3192	2288–2674	2161–2558	1718–2474
Good	2399–2794	2478–2803	2335–2549	2101–2287	1701–2160	1317–1717
Fair	2156–2398	2271–2477	2147–2334	1688–2100	1386–1700	1198–1316
Needs Improvement	≤2155	≤2270	≤2146	≤1687	≤1385	≤1197

Interpretation of Test Results

1. What conclusions can you draw from your test results?

_____

_____

_____

_____

_____

2. Briefly state how you could improve your test results and what activities you could engage in to obtain the desired results.

_____

_____

_____

_____

_____

3. Did you ever participate in organized sports, or have you found success in a particular game or sport? ☐ Yes ☐ No

3a. If your answer is yes, list the sports, games, or events in which you enjoy(ed) success.

_____

_____

3b. Is there a relationship between your answers to question 3a and your test results in this lab?

_____

_____

_____

Lab 9B

HEALTH-RELATED FITNESS CASE STUDIES

Name: _____   Date: _____   Grade: _____

Instructor: _____   Course: _____   Section: _____

Necessary Lab Equipment
None.

Objective
To provide an opportunity to apply exercise prescriptions concepts and to determine progress in your personal fitness goals.

I. Indicate the procedure that you would follow to clear a 66-year-old woman who wishes to initiate an exercise program. Be specific in your recommendations.

_____

_____

_____

_____

_____

_____

_____

_____

II. Design a periodized strength-training program for a 22-year-old sprint athlete who wishes to reach peak performance in 18 weeks. Include in your program the exercises (lifts), sets, and number of repetitions maximum that are to be used with each mesocycle (use additional paper as necessary).

III. Using the information that you have thus far learned in this course, design a 16-week exercise prescription for a previously inactive 60-year-old male with a resting heart rate of 76 beats per minute. Other than some minor knee problems, the individual has been cleared for cardiorespiratory exercise by a physician. Use a weekly progressive approach as outlined in Lab 6D (pages 195–196) and Figure 9.3 (page 289) that includes intensity, duration, frequency, and mode(s) of exercise.

IV. Indicate your stage of change and fitness category for the health-related components of fitness.

Fitness Component	Initial Rating		Current Rating	
	Stage of Change	Fitness Category	Stage of Change	Fitness Category
Cardiorespiratory endurance				
Muscular strength and endurance				
Muscular flexibility				
Body composition				

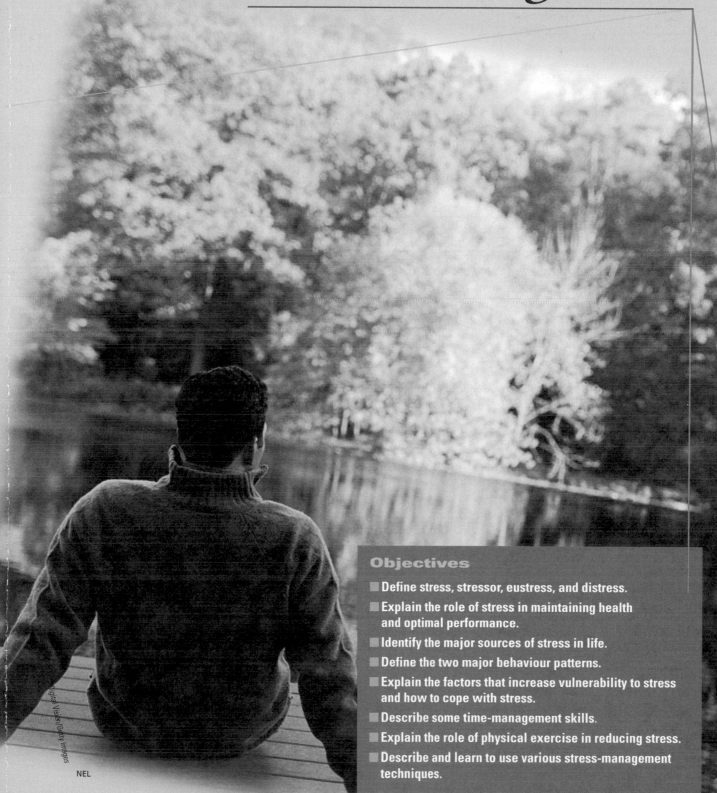

Chapter 10

Stress Management

Objectives

- Define stress, stressor, eustress, and distress.
- Explain the role of stress in maintaining health and optimal performance.
- Identify the major sources of stress in life.
- Define the two major behaviour patterns.
- Explain the factors that increase vulnerability to stress and how to cope with stress.
- Describe some time-management skills.
- Explain the role of physical exercise in reducing stress.
- Describe and learn to use various stress-management techniques.

Living in today's world is nearly impossible without encountering **stress**. In an unpredictable world that changes with every new day, most people find that stress has become the norm rather than the exception. Further, stress undermines our ability to stay well.[1] The cost of work time lost to stress in Canada is $12 billion, and 47 percent of employed Canadians reported "a great deal of stress at work." Not surprisingly, more Canadians are feeling "severe stress," which manifests itself in many ways. Many medical and stress researchers believe that "stress should carry a health warning" as well.[2]

The good news is that stress can be self-controlled. Too often, people have accepted stress as a normal part of daily life and, even though everyone has to deal with it, few seem to understand it or know how to cope effectively. It is difficult to live fully without "runs, hits, and errors." Actually, stress should not be avoided entirely. A certain amount of stress is necessary for optimum health, performance, and well-being.

Just what is stress? Dr. Hans Selye, a Hungarian physicist who worked at McGill University and was one of the foremost authorities on stress, defined it as "the nonspecific response of the human organism to any demand that is placed upon it."[3] "Nonspecific" indicates that the body reacts in a similar fashion regardless of the nature of the event. In simpler terms, stress is the body's mental, emotional, and physiological response to any situation that is new, threatening, frightening, or exciting.

The body's response to stress has been the same ever since humans were first put on the earth. Stress prepares the organism to react to the stress-causing event, also called the **stressor**. The problem, though, is the way in which we react to stress. Many people thrive under stress; others, under similar circumstances, are unable to handle it. An individual's reaction to a stress-causing agent determines whether that stress is positive or negative.

Dr. Selye defined the ways in which we react to stress as either eustress or distress. In both cases, the nonspecific response is almost the same. In the case of **eustress**, on the one hand, health and performance continue to improve even as stress increases. On the other hand, **distress** refers to the unpleasant or harmful stress under which health and performance begin to deteriorate. The relationship between stress and performance is illustrated in Figure 10.1.

Stress is a fact of modern life, and every person does need an optimal level of stress that is most

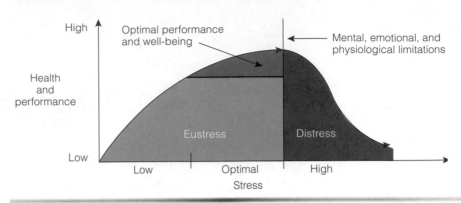

FIGURE 10.1 Relationship between stress and health and performance

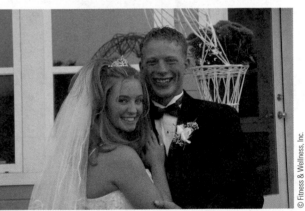

Vandalism causes distress or negative stress.

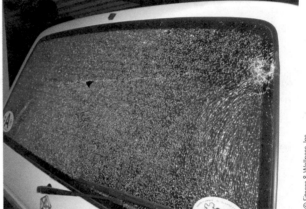

Marriage is an example of positive stress, also known as eustress.

conducive to adequate health and performance. When stress levels reach mental, emotional, and physiological limits, however, stress becomes distress and the person no longer functions effectively.

Chronic distress raises the risk for many health disorders—including coronary heart disease, hypertension, eating disorders, ulcers, diabetes, asthma, depression, migraine headaches, sleep disorders, and chronic fatigue—and may even play a role in

FIGURE 10.2 General adaptation syndrome: The body's response to stress

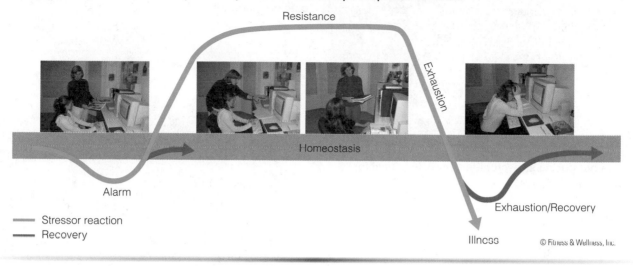

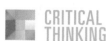

CRITICAL THINKING

Can you identify sources of eustress and distress in your personal life during this past year? Explain your emotional and physical response to each stressor and how the two differ.

the development of certain types of cancers.[4] Recognizing this and overcoming the problem quickly and efficiently are crucial in maintaining emotional and physiological stability.

Adapting to Stress

The body continually strives to maintain a constant internal environment. This state of physiological balance, known as **homeostasis**, allows the body to function as effectively as possible. When a stressor triggers a nonspecific response, homeostasis is disrupted. This reaction to stressors is best explained by Dr. Hans Selye, as the **general adaptation syndrome (GAS)**, composed of three stages—alarm reaction, resistance, and exhaustion/recovery.

Alarm Reaction

The alarm reaction is the immediate response to a stressor (whether positive or negative). During the alarm reaction, the body evokes an instant physiological reaction that mobilizes internal systems and processes to minimize the threat to homeostasis (see also "Coping with Stress" on pages 309–310). If the stressor subsides, the body recovers and returns to homeostasis.

Resistance

If the stressor persists, the body calls upon its limited reserves to build up its resistance as it strives to

maintain homeostasis. For a short while, the body copes effectively and meets the challenge of the stressor until it can be overcome (see Figure 10.2).

Exhaustion/Recovery

If stress becomes chronic and intolerable, the body spends its limited reserves and loses its ability to cope. It enters the exhaustion/recovery stage. During this stage the body functions at a diminished capacity while it recovers from stress. In due time, following an "adequate" recovery period (which varies greatly), the body recuperates and is able to return to homeostasis. If chronic stress persists during the exhaustion stage, however, the immune function is compromised, which can damage body systems and lead to disease.

An example of the stress response through the general adaptation syndrome can be illustrated in a test performance. As you prepare to take an exam,

---

Stress The mental, emotional, and physiological response of the body to any situation that is new, threatening, frightening, or exciting.

Stressor Stress-causing event.

Eustress Positive stress: Health and performance continue to improve, even as stress increases.

Distress Negative stress: Unpleasant or harmful stress under which health and performance begin to deteriorate.

Homeostasis A natural state of equilibrium; the body attempts to maintain this equilibrium by constantly reacting to external forces that attempt to disrupt this fine balance.

General adaptation syndrome (GAS) A theoretical model that explains the body's adaptation to sustained stress which includes three stages: Alarm reaction, resistance, and exhaustion/recovery.

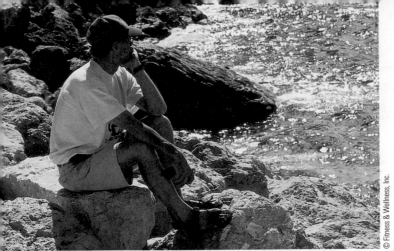

Taking time out during stressful life events is critical for good health and wellness.

you experience an initial alarm reaction. If you understand the material, study for the exam, and do well (eustress), the body recovers and stress is dissipated. If, however, you are not adequately prepared and fail the exam, you trigger the resistance stage. You are now concerned about your grade, and you remain in the resistance stage until the next exam. If you prepare and do well, the body recovers. But if you fail once again and can no longer bring up your grade, exhaustion sets in and physical and emotional breakdowns may occur. Exhaustion may be further aggravated if you are struggling in other courses as well.

The exhaustion stage is often manifested by athletes and the most ardent fitness participants. Staleness is usually a manifestation of overtraining. Peak performance can be sustained for only about two to three weeks at a time. Any attempts to continue intense training after peaking leads to exhaustion, diminished fitness, and the mental and physical problems associated with overtraining (see Chapter 9, pages 286–287). Thus, athletes and some fitness participants also need an active recovery phase after attaining peak fitness.

Sources of Stress

Several instruments have been developed to assess sources of stress in life. The most practical of these is the **Life Experiences Survey**, presented in Lab 10A, in which you identify the life changes within the last 12 months that may have an impact on your physical and psychological well-being.

The Life Experiences Survey is divided into two sections. Section 1, to be completed by all respondents, contains a list of 47 life events plus three blank spaces for other events experienced but not listed in the survey. Section 2 contains an additional 10 questions designed for students only (students should fill out both sections). Common stressors in the lives of university and college students are depicted in Figure 10.3.

FIGURE 10.3 Stressors in the lives of university and college students

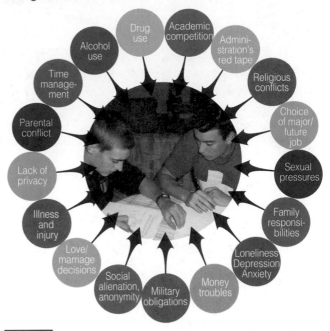

Adapted from W.W.K. Hoeger, L.W. Turner, and B.Q. Hafen. *Wellness: Guidelines for a Healthy Lifestyle.* Wadsworth/Thomson Learning, 2002.

The survey requires the testee to rate the extent to which his or her life events had a positive or negative impact on his or her life at the time these events occurred. The ratings are on a 7-point scale. A rating of –3 indicates an extremely undesirable impact. A rating of zero (0) suggests neither a positive nor a negative impact, called **neustress**. A rating of +3 indicates an extremely desirable impact.

After the person evaluates his or her life events, the negative and the positive points are totalled separately. Both scores are expressed as positive numbers (for example, positive ratings of 2, 1, 3, and 3 = 9 points positive score; negative ratings of −3, −2, −2, −1, and −2 = 10 points negative score). A final "total life change" score can be obtained by adding the positive score and the negative score together as positive numbers (total life change score: 9 + 10 = 19 points).

Because negative and positive changes alike can produce nonspecific responses, the total life change score is a good indicator of total life stress. Most research in this area, however, suggests that the negative change score is a better predictor of

CRITICAL THINKING

Technological advances provide many benefits to our lives. What positive and negative effects do these advances have upon your daily living activities, and what impact are they having on your stress level?

- Make a contract with yourself to slow down and take it easy. Put it in writing. Post it in a conspicuous spot, then stick to the terms you set up. Be specific. Abstracts ("I'm going to be less uptight") don't work.
- Work on only one or two things at a time. Wait until you change one habit before you tackle the next one.
- Eat more slowly and eat only when you are relaxed and sitting down.
- If you smoke, quit.
- Cut down on your caffeine intake, because it increases the tendency to become irritated and agitated.
- Take regular breaks throughout the day, even as brief as 5 or 10 minutes, when you totally change what you're doing. Get up, stretch, get a drink of cool water, walk around for a few minutes.
- Work on fighting your impatience. If you're standing in line at the grocery store, study the interesting things people have in their carts instead of getting upset.
- Work on controlling hostility. Keep a written log. When do you flare up? What causes it? How do you feel at the time? What preceded it? Look for patterns and figure out what sets you off. Then do something about it. Either avoid the situations that cause you hostility or practise reacting to them in different ways.
- Plan some activities just for the fun of it. Load a picnic basket in the car and drive to the country with a friend. After a stressful physics class, stop at a theatre and see a good comedy.
- Choose a role model, someone you know and admire who does not have a Type A personality. Observe the person carefully, then try out some techniques the person demonstrates.
- Simplify your life so you can learn to relax a little bit. Figure out which activities or commitments you can eliminate right now, then get rid of them.
- If morning is a problem time for you and you get too hurried, set your alarm clock half an hour earlier.
- Take time out during even the most hectic day to do something truly relaxing. Because you won't be used to it, you may have to work at it at first. Begin by listing things you'd really enjoy that would calm you. Include some things that take only a few minutes: Watch a sunset, lie out on the lawn at night and look at the stars, call an old friend and catch up on news, take a nap, sauté a pan of mushrooms and savour them slowly.
- If you're under a deadline, take short breaks. Stop and talk to someone for 5 minutes, take a short walk, or lie down with a cool cloth over your eyes for 10 minutes.
- Pay attention to what your own body clock is saying. You've probably noticed that every 90 minutes or so, you lose the ability to concentrate, get a little sleepy, and have a tendency to daydream. Instead of fighting the urge, put down your work and let your mind wander for a few minutes. Use the time to imagine and let your creativity run wild.
- Learn to treasure unplanned surprises: a friend dropping by unannounced, a hummingbird outside your window, a child's tightly clutched bouquet of wildflowers.
- Savour your relationships. Think about the people in your life. Relax with them and give yourself to them. Give up trying to control others and resist the urge to end relationships that don't always go as you'd like them to.

From W. W. K. Hoeger, L. W. Turner, and B. Q. Hafen, *Wellness: Guidelines for a Healthy Lifestyle* (3rd ed.) (Belmont, CA: Wadsworth/Thomson Learning, 2002).

---

potential physical and psychological illness than the total change score. More research is necessary to establish the role of total change and the role of the ratio of positive to negative stress.

Behaviour Patterns

Common life events are not the only source of stress in life. All too often, individuals bring on stress as a result of their behaviour patterns. The two main behaviour patterns, Type A and Type B, are based on several observable characteristics.

Several attempts have been made to develop an objective scale to identify Type A individuals properly,

but these questionnaires are not as valid and reliable as researchers would like them to be. Consequently, the main assessment tool to determine behavioural type is still the **structured interview**, during which a person is asked to reply to several questions that describe Type A and Type B behaviour patterns.

Life Experiences Survey A questionnaire used to assess sources of stress in life.

Neustress Neutral stress; stress that is neither harmful nor helpful.

Structured interview Assessment tool used to determine behavioural patterns that define Type A and B personalities.

The interviewer notes the responses to the questions as well as the individual's mental, emotional, and physical behaviours as he or she replies to each question.

Based on the answers and the associated behaviours, the interviewer rates the person along a continuum ranging from Type A to Type B. Along this continuum, behavioural patterns are classified into five categories: A-1, A-2, X (a mix of Type A and Type B), B-3, and B-4. The Type A-1 exhibits all of the Type A characteristics, and the B-4 shows a relative absence of Type A behaviours. The Type A-2 does not exhibit a complete Type A pattern, and the Type B-3 exhibits only a few Type A characteristics.

Type A behaviour characterizes a primarily hard-driving, overambitious, aggressive, at times hostile and overly competitive person. Type A individuals often set their own goals, are self-motivated, try to accomplish many tasks at the same time, are excessively achievement-oriented, and have a high degree of time urgency.

In contrast, **Type B** behaviour is characteristic of calm, casual, relaxed, easygoing individuals. Type B people take one thing at a time, do not feel pressured or hurried, and seldom set their own deadlines.

Over the years, experts have indicated that individuals classified as Type A are under too much stress and have a significantly higher incidence of coronary heart disease. Based on these findings, Type A individuals have been counselled to lower their stress level by modifying their Type A behaviours.

Many of the Type A characteristics are learned behaviours. Consequently, if people can identify the sources of stress and make changes in their behavioural responses, they can move along the continuum and respond more like Type B's. The debate, however, has centred on which Type A behaviours should be changed, because not all of them are undesirable.

Even though personality questionnaires are not as valid and reliable as the structured interview in identifying Type A individuals, Drs. Meyer Friedman and Ray Rosenman, two San Francisco scientists, constructed a Type A personality assessment form, adapted from the structured interview method, to give people a general idea of Type A behavioural patterns. This assessment form is found in Lab 10A. You can use it to understand your own behavioural patterns better. If you obtain a high rating, you probably are Type A.

We also know that many individuals perform well under pressure. They typically are classified as Type A but do not demonstrate any of the detrimental effects of stress. Drs. Robert and Marilyn Kriegel came up with the term and concept of Type C to characterize people with these behaviours.[5]

Type C individuals are just as highly stressed as Type A's but do not seem to be at higher risk for

BEHAVIOUR MODIFICATION PLANNING

TIPS TO MANAGE ANGER

■ Commit to change and gain control over the behaviour.
■ Remind yourself that chronic anger leads to illness and disease and may eventually kill you.
■ Recognize when feelings of anger are developing and ask yourself the following questions:
 ■ Is the matter really that important?
 ■ Is the anger justified?
 ■ Can I change the situation without getting angry?
 ■ Is it worth risking my health over it?
 ■ How will I feel about the situation in a few hours?
■ Tell yourself, "Stop, my health is worth it" every time you start to feel anger.
■ Prepare for a positive response: Ask for an explanation or clarification of the situation, walk away and evaluate the situation, exercise, or use appropriate stress management techniques (breathing, meditation, imagery) before you become angry and hostile.
■ Manage anger at once; do not let it build up.
■ Never attack anyone verbally or physically.
■ Keep a journal and ponder the situations that cause you to be angry.
■ Seek professional help if you are unable to overcome anger by yourself: You are worth it.

disease than Type B's. The keys to successful Type C performance are *commitment, confidence,* and *control.* Type C people are highly committed to what they are doing, have a great deal of confidence in their ability to do their work, and are in constant control of their actions. In addition, they enjoy their work and maintain themselves in top physical condition to be able to meet the mental and physical demands of their work.

Type A behaviour by itself is no longer viewed as a major risk factor for coronary heart disease, but Type A individuals who commonly express anger and hostility are at higher risk. Therefore, many behavioural modification counsellors now work on changing the latter behaviours to prevent disease. The questionnaire provided at the end of Lab 10A can help you determine whether you have a hostile personality.

Anger increases heart rate and blood pressure and leads to constriction of blood vessels. Over time, these changes are thought to cause damage to the arteries and eventually lead to a heart attack. Several studies indicate that chronically angry people have up to a threefold increased risk for CHD and are seven times more likely to suffer a fatal heart attack by age 50.

Many experts also believe that emotional stress is far more likely than physical stress to trigger a

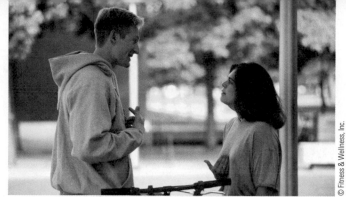
Anger and hostility can increase the risk for disease.

heart attack. People who are impatient and readily annoyed when they have to wait for someone or something—an employee, a traffic light, a table in a restaurant—are especially vulnerable.

Research is also focusing on individuals who have anxiety, depression, and feelings of helplessness when they encounter setbacks and failures in life. People who lose control of their lives or who give up on their dreams in life, knowing that they could and should be doing better, probably are more likely to have heart attacks than hard-driving people who enjoy their work.

Vulnerability to Stress

Researchers have identified a number of factors that can affect the way in which people handle stress. How people deal with these factors can actually increase or decrease vulnerability to stress. The questionnaire provided in Lab 10B lists these factors so you can determine your vulnerability rating. Many of the items on this questionnaire are related to health, social support, self-worth, and nurturance (sense of being needed). All of these factors are crucial to a person's physical, social, mental, and emotional well-being and are essential to cope effectively with stressful life events. The more integrated people are in society, the less vulnerable they are to stress and illness.

Positive correlations have been found between social support and health outcomes. People can draw upon social support to weather crises. Knowing that someone else cares, that people are there to lean on, that support is out there, is valuable for survival (or growth) in times of need.

The health benefits of physical fitness have already been discussed extensively. The questionnaire in Lab 10B will help you identify specific areas in which you can make improvements to help you cope more efficiently.

As you complete Lab 10B, you will notice that many of the items describe situations and behaviours that are within your own control. To make yourself less vulnerable to stress, you will want to improve the behaviours that make you more

vulnerable to stress. You should start by modifying the behaviours that are easiest to change before undertaking some of the most difficult ones.

Time Management

According to Benjamin Franklin, "Time is the stuff life is made of." The present hurry-up style of Canadian life is not conducive to wellness. The hassles involved in getting through a routine day often lead to stress-related illnesses. People who do not manage their time properly will quickly experience chronic stress, fatigue, despair, discouragement, and illness.

Surveys indicate that many people think time moves too fast for them, and more than half of those surveyed think they have to get everything done. The younger the respondents, the more they struggle with lack of time. Almost half wish they had more time for exercise and recreation, hobbies, and family.

Healthy and successful people are good time managers, able to maintain a pace of life within their comfort zone. In a survey of 1954 Harvard graduates from the school of business, only 27 percent had reached the goals they established in college. Every one had rated himself a superior time manager, and only 8 percent of the remaining graduates perceived themselves as superior time managers. The successful graduates attributed their success to smart work, not necessarily hard work.

Five Steps to Time Management

Trying to achieve one or more goals in a limited time can create a tremendous amount of stress. Many people don't seem to have enough hours in the day to accomplish their tasks. The greatest demands on our time, nonetheless, frequently are self-imposed. We try to do too much, too fast, too soon.

Some time killers, such as eating, sleeping, and recreation, are necessary for health and wellness, but in excess they'll lead to stress in life. You can follow five basic steps to make better use of your time (also see Lab 10C):

Type A Behaviour pattern characteristic of a hard-driving, overambitious, aggressive, at times hostile, and overly competitive person.

Type B Behaviour pattern characteristic of a calm, casual, relaxed, and easy-going individual.

Type C Behaviour pattern of individuals who are just as highly stressed as the Type A but do not seem to be at higher risk for disease than the Type B.

BEHAVIOUR MODIFICATION PLANNING

COMMON TIME KILLERS

- Watching television
- Listening to radio/music
- Sleeping
- Eating
- Daydreaming
- Shopping
- Socializing/parties
- Recreation
- Talking on the telephone
- Worrying
- Procrastinating
- Drop-in visitors
- Confusion (unclear goals)
- Indecision (what to do next)
- Interruptions
- Perfectionism (every detail must be done)

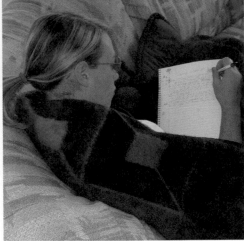

Planning and prioritizing activities will simplify your days.

1. Find the time killers. Many people do not know how they spend each part of the day. Keep a four- to seven-day log and record your activities at half-hour intervals. Record the activities as you go through your typical day so you will remember all of them. At the end of each day, decide when you wasted time. You may be shocked by the amount of time you spent on the phone, on the Internet, sleeping (more than eight hours per night), or watching television.

2. Set long-range and short-range goals. Setting goals requires some in-depth thinking and helps put your life and daily tasks in perspective: What do I want out of life? Where do I want to be 10 years from now? Next year? Next week? Tomorrow? You can use Lab 10C to list these goals.

3. Identify your immediate goals and prioritize them for today and this week (Use Lab 10C—make as many copies as necessary). Each day sit down and determine what you need to accomplish that day and that week. Rank your "today" and "this week" tasks in four categories: (a) top-priority, (b) medium-priority, (c) low-priority, and (d) trash.

    Top-priority tasks are the most important. If you were to reap most of your productivity from 30 percent of your activities, which would they be? Medium-priority activities are those that must be done but can wait a day or two. Low-priority activities are those to be done only upon completing all top- and middle-priority activities. Trash activities are not worth your time (for example, cruising the hallways, channel-surfing).

4. Use a daily planner to help you organize and simplify your day. In this way, you can access your priority list, appointments, notes, references, names, places, phone numbers, and addresses conveniently from your coat pocket or purse.

Many people think that planning daily and weekly activities is a waste of time. A few minutes to schedule your time each day, however, may pay off in hours saved.

As you plan your day, be realistic and find your comfort zone. Determine the best way to organize your day. Which is the most productive time for work? study? errands? Are you a morning person, or are you getting most of your work done when people are quitting for the day? Pick your best hours for top-priority activities. Be sure to schedule enough time for exercise and relaxation. Recreation is not necessarily wasted time. You need to take care of your physical and emotional well-being. Otherwise your life will be seriously imbalanced.

5. Conduct nightly audits. Take 10 minutes each night to figure out how well you accomplished your goals that day. Successful time managers evaluate themselves daily. This simple task will help you see the entire picture. Cross off the goals you accomplished, and carry over to the next day those you did not get done. You also may realize that some goals can be moved down to low-priority or be trashed.

Time-Management Skills

In addition to the five major steps, the following can help you make better use of your time:

- *Delegate.* If possible, delegate activities that someone else can do for you. Having another person type your paper while you prepare for an exam might be well worth the expense and your time.

- *Say "no."* Learn to say no to activities that keep you from getting your top priorities done. You can do only so much in a single day. Nobody has enough time to do everything he or she would like to get done. Don't overload either. Many people are afraid to say no because they feel guilty if they do. Think ahead, and consider the consequences. Are you doing this to please others? What will it do to your well-being? Can you handle one more task? At some point, you have to balance your activities and look at life and time realistically.

■ *Protect against boredom*. Doing nothing can be a source of stress. People need to feel that they are contributing and that they are productive members of society. It is also good for self-esteem and self-worth. Set realistic goals and work toward them each day.

■ *Plan ahead for disruptions*. Even a careful plan of action can be disrupted. An unexpected phone call or visitor can ruin your schedule. Planning your response ahead will help you deal with these saboteurs.

■ *Get it done*. Select only one task at a time, concentrate on it, and see it through. Many people do a little here, do a little there, then do something else. In the end, nothing gets done. An exception to working on just one task at a time occurs when you are doing a difficult task. Rather than "killing yourself," interchange with another activity that is not as hard.

■ *Eliminate distractions*. If you have trouble adhering to a set plan, remove distractions and trash activities from your eyesight. Television, radio, magazines, open doors, or studying in a park might distract you and become time killers.

■ *Set aside "overtimes."* Regularly schedule as overtime the time you didn't think you would need to complete unfinished projects. Most people underschedule rather than overschedule time. The result is (usually late-night) burnout! If you schedule overtimes and get your tasks done, enjoy some leisure time, get ahead on another project, or work on some of your trash activities.

■ *Plan time for you*. Set aside special time for yourself daily. Life is not meant to be all work. Use your time to walk, read, or listen to your favourite music.

■ *Reward yourself*. As with any other healthy behaviour, positive change or a job well done deserves a reward. We often overlook the value of rewards, even if they are self-given. People practise behaviours that are rewarded and discontinue those that are not.

One more activity that you should perform weekly is to go through the list of strategies in Lab 10C to determine if you are becoming a good time manager. Provide a yes or no answer to each statement. If you are able to answer yes to most questions, congratulations. You are becoming a good time manager.

BEHAVIOUR MODIFICATION PLANNING

COMMON SYMPTOMS OF STRESS

- Headaches
- Muscular aches (mainly in neck, shoulders, and back)
- Grinding teeth
- Nervous tick, finger tapping, toe tapping
- Increased sweating
- Increase in or loss of appetite
- Insomnia
- Nightmares
- Fatigue
- Dry mouth
- Stuttering
- High blood pressure
- Tightness or pain in the chest
- Impotence
- Hives
- Dizziness
- Depression
- Irritation
- Anger
- Hostility
- Fear, panic, anxiety
- Stomach pain, flutters
- Nausea
- Cold, clammy hands
- Poor concentration
- Pacing
- Restlessness
- Rapid heart rate
- Low-grade infection
- Loss of sex drive
- Rash or acne

Coping with Stress

The ways in which people perceive and cope with stress seem to be more important in the development of disease than the amount and type of stress itself. If individuals perceive stress as a definite problem in their lives or if it interferes with their optimal level of health and performance, they can call upon several excellent stress-management techniques to help them cope more effectively.

First, of course, the person must recognize that a problem exists. Many people either do not want to believe they are under too much stress or they fail to recognize some of the typical symptoms of distress. Noting some of the stress-related symptoms (see "Common Symptoms of Stress") will help a person respond more objectively and initiate an adequate coping response.

When people have stress-related symptoms, they should first try to identify and remove the stressor or stress-causing agent. This is not as simple as it may seem, because in some situations eliminating the stressor is not possible, or a person may not even know the exact causal agent. If the cause is unknown, keeping a log of the time and days when the symptoms occur, as well as the events preceding and following the onset of symptoms, may be helpful.

In many instances, the stressor cannot be removed. Examples of these situations are the death of a close family member, the first year on the job, an intolerable boss, or a change in work responsibility. Nevertheless, stress can be managed through relaxation techniques.

The body responds to stress by activating the **fight-or-flight** mechanism, which prepares a person to take action by stimulating the body's vital defence systems. This stimulation originates in the hypothalamus and the pituitary gland in the brain. The hypothalamus activates the sympathetic nervous system, and the pituitary activates the release of catecholamines (hormones) from the adrenal glands.

These hormonal changes increase heart rate, blood pressure, blood flow to active muscles and the brain, glucose levels, oxygen consumption, and strength—all necessary for the body to fight or flee. For the body to relax, one of these actions must take place. If the person is unable to take action, however, the muscles tense up and tighten (see Figure 10.4). This increased tension and tightening can be dissipated effectively through some coping techniques, described in the following pages.

Physical Activity

The benefits of physical activity in reducing the physiological and psychological responses to stress are well-established.[6] Exercise is one of the simplest tools to control stress. The value of exercise in reducing stress is related to several factors, the main one being a decrease in muscular tension. For example, a person can be distressed because he or she has had a miserable eight hours of work with an intolerable boss, or you have had a difficult day at school, you are behind in your reading, and you are worried about preparing for examinations that are coming up soon. To make matters worse, it is late and, on the way home, the car in front is going much slower than the speed limit. The fight-or-flight mechanism—already activated during the stressful day—begins again: catecholamines rise, heart rate and blood pressure shoot up, breathing quickens and deepens, muscles tense up, and all systems say "go." No action can be initiated or stress dissipated, though, because the person cannot just hit the boss or the car in front or eliminate your school troubles.

A real remedy would be to take action by "hitting" the swimming pool, the tennis ball, the weights, or the jogging trail. Engaging in physical activity reduces the muscular tension and metabolizes the increased catecholamines (which were triggered by the fight-or-flight mechanism and brought about the physiological changes). Although exercise does not solve problems at work or at school, or take care of slow drivers, it certainly can help a person cope with stress and can prevent stress from becoming a chronic problem.

Some studies suggest that students who are making a transition from high school to college or university are faced with a number of barriers with regard to participating in physical activity. These barriers include lack of time, lack of facilities, and lack of encouragement by others.[7] However, other studies on college and university student life show that participation in regular physical activity does help to alleviate stress and is an effective strategy for improving moods.[8]

Many people can relate to exercise as a means of managing stress by remembering how good they felt the last time they concluded a strenuous exercise session after a long, difficult day. A fatigued muscle is a relaxed muscle. For this reason, people often say that the best part of exercise is the shower afterward.

Research has also shown that physical exercise requiring continuous and rhythmic muscular activity, such as aerobic exercise, stimulates alpha-wave activity in the brain. These are the same wave patterns seen commonly during meditation and relaxation.

Further, during vigorous aerobic exercise lasting 30 minutes or longer, morphine-like substances called **endorphins** are thought to be released from the pituitary gland in the brain. These substances

FIGURE 10.4 Physiological response to stress: fight-or-flight mechanism

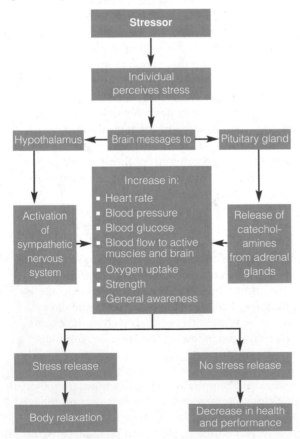

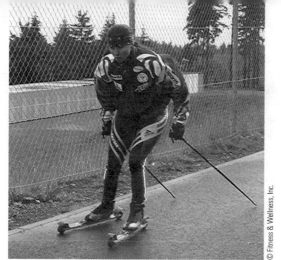
Physical activity: an excellent tool to control stress.

act as painkillers and also seem to induce the soothing, calming effect often associated with aerobic exercise.

Another way by which exercise helps lower stress is to deliberately divert stress to various body systems. Dr. Selye explains in his book *Stress without Distress* that, when one specific task becomes difficult, a change in activity can be as good as or better than rest itself.[9] For example, if a person is having trouble with a task and does not seem to be getting anywhere, jogging or swimming for a while is better than sitting around and getting frustrated. In this way, the mental strain is diverted to the working muscles and one system helps the other to relax.

Other psychologists indicate that when muscular tension is removed from the emotional strain, the emotional strain disappears. In many cases, the change of activity suddenly clears the mind and helps put the pieces together.

Researchers have found that physical exercise gives people a psychological boost because exercise does all the following:

■ Lessens feelings of anxiety, depression, frustration, aggression, anger, and hostility.
■ Alleviates insomnia.
■ Provides an opportunity to meet social needs and develop new friendships.
■ Allows the person to share common interests and problems.
■ Develops discipline.
■ Provides the opportunity to do something enjoyable and constructive that will lead to better health and total well-being.

Beyond the short-term benefits of exercise in lessening stress, a regular aerobic exercise program actually strengthens the cardiovascular system itself. Because the cardiovascular system seems to be affected seriously by stress, a stronger system should be able to cope more effectively. For instance, good

cardiorespiratory endurance has been shown to lower the resting heart rate and blood pressure. Because both heart rate and blood pressure rise in stressful situations, initiating the stress response at a lower baseline will counteract some of the negative effects of stress. Cardiorespiratory-fit individuals can cope more effectively and are less affected by the stresses of daily living.

Relaxation Techniques

Although benefits are reaped immediately after engaging in any of the several relaxation techniques, several months of regular practice may be necessary for total mastery. The relaxation exercises that follow should not be considered cure-alls. If these exercises do not prove to be effective, more specialized textbooks and professional help are called for. (Some symptoms may not be caused by stress but instead may be related to a medical disorder.)

BIOFEEDBACK

Clinical application of **biofeedback** has been used to treat various medical disorders for many years. Besides its successful application in managing stress, it is commonly used to treat medical disorders such as essential hypertension, asthma, disturbances in heart rhythm and rate, cardiac neurosis, eczematous dermatitis, fecal incontinence, insomnia, and stuttering. Biofeedback as a treatment modality has been defined as a technique in which a person learns to influence physiological responses that are not typically under voluntary control or responses that normally are regulated but regulation has broken down as a result of injury, trauma, or illness.

In simpler terms, biofeedback is the interaction with the interior self. This interaction allows a person to learn the relationship between the mind and the biological response. The person actually can "feel" how thought processes influence biological responses (such as heart rate, blood pressure, body temperature, and muscle tension) and how biological responses in turn influence the thought process.

Fight or flight Physiological response of the body to stress that prepares the individual to take action by stimulating the body's vital defence systems.

Endorphins Morphine-like substances released from the pituitary gland in the brain during prolonged aerobic exercise. They are thought to induce feelings of euphoria and natural well-being.

Biofeedback A stress-management technique in which a person learns to influence physiological responses that are not typically under voluntary control or responses that typically are regulated but for which regulation has broken down as a result of injury, trauma, or illness.

As an illustration of this process, consider the association between a strange noise in the middle of a dark, quiet night and the heart rate response. At first the heart rate shoots up because of the stress the unknown noise induces. The individual may even feel the heart palpitating in the chest and, while still uncertain about the noise, attempts to avoid panic to prevent an even faster heart rate. Upon realizing that all is well, the person can take control and influence the heart rate to come down. The mind, now calm, is able to exert almost complete control over the biological response.

Complex electronic instruments are required to conduct biofeedback. The process itself entails a three-stage, closed-loop feedback system:

1. A biological response to a stressor is detected and amplified.
2. The response is processed.
3. Results of the response are fed back to the individual immediately.

The person uses this new input and attempts to change the physiological response voluntarily. This attempt, in turn, is detected, amplified, and processed. The results then are fed back to the person. The process continues with the intent of teaching the person to reliably influence the physiological response for the better (see Figure 10.5). The most common methods used to measure physiological responses are monitoring the heart rate, finger temperature, and blood pressure; electromyograms; and electroencephalograms. The goal of biofeedback training is to transfer the experiences learned in the laboratory to everyday living.

Although biofeedback has significant applications in treating various medical disorders, including stress, it requires adequately trained personnel and, in many cases, costly equipment. Therefore, several alternative methods that yield similar results are frequently substituted for biofeedback. For example, research has shown that exercise and progressive muscle relaxation, used successfully in stress management, seem to be just as effective as biofeedback in treating essential hypertension.

PROGRESSIVE MUSCLE RELAXATION

Progressive muscle relaxation, developed by Dr. Edmund Jacobsen in the 1930s, enables individuals to relearn the sensation of deep relaxation. The technique involves progressively contracting and relaxing muscle groups throughout the body. Because chronic stress leads to high levels of muscular tension, acute awareness of how progressively tightening and relaxing the muscles feels can release the tension in the muscles and teach the body to relax at will.

Feeling the tension during the exercises also helps the person to be more alert to signs of distress, because this tension is similar to that experienced in stressful situations. In everyday life, these feelings then can cue the person to do relaxation exercises.

Relaxation exercises should be done in a quiet, warm, well-ventilated room. The recommended exercises and the duration of the routine vary from one person to the next. Most important is that the individual pay attention to the sensation that he or she feels each time the muscles are tensed and relaxed.

The exercises should encompass all muscle groups of the body. Following is an example of a sequence of progressive muscle relaxation exercises. The instructions for these exercises can be read to the person, memorized, or tape-recorded. At least 20 minutes should be set aside to complete the entire sequence. Doing the exercises any faster will defeat their purpose. Ideally, the sequence should be done twice a day.

The individual performing the exercises stretches out comfortably on the floor, face up, with a pillow under the knees, and assumes a passive attitude, allowing the body to relax as much as possible. Each muscle group is to be contracted in sequence, taking care to avoid any strain. Muscles should be tightened to only about 70 percent of the total possible tension to avoid cramping or injury to the muscle itself.

To produce the relaxation effects, the person must pay attention to the sensation of tensing up and relaxing. The person holds each contraction about five seconds and then allows the muscles to go totally limp. The person should take enough time to contract and relax each muscle group before going on to the next.

An example of a complete progressive muscle relaxation sequence is as follows:

1. Point your feet, curling the toes downward. Study the tension in the arches and the top of the feet. Hold, continue to note the tension, then relax. Repeat once.

FIGURE 10.5 Biofeedback mechanism

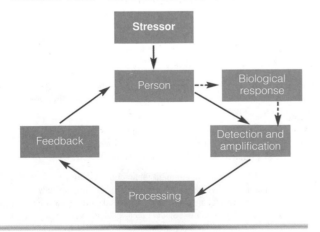

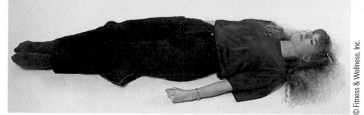

Practising progressive muscle relaxation on a regular basis helps reduce stress.

2. Flex the feet upward toward the face and note the tension in your feet and calves. Hold and relax. Repeat once.

3. Push your heels down against the floor as if burying them in the sand. Hold and note the tension at the back of the thigh. Relax. Repeat once.

4. Contract the right thigh by straightening the leg, gently raising the leg off the floor. Hold and study the tension. Relax. Repeat with the left leg. Hold and relax. Repeat each leg.

5. Tense the buttocks by raising your hips ever so slightly off the floor. Hold and note the tension. Relax. Repeat once.

6. Contract the abdominal muscles. Hold them tight and note the tension. Relax. Repeat once.

7. Suck in your stomach. Try to make it reach your spine. Flatten your lower back to the floor. Hold and feel the tension in the stomach and lower back. Relax. Repeat once.

8. Take a deep breath and hold it, then exhale. Repeat. Note your breathing becoming slower and more relaxed.

9. Place your arms at the sides of your body and clench both fists. Hold, study the tension, and relax. Repeat.

10. Flex the elbow by bringing both hands to the shoulders. Hold tight and study the tension in the biceps. Relax. Repeat.

11. Place your arms flat on the floor, palms up, and push the forearms hard against the floor. Note the tension on the triceps. Hold, and relax. Repeat.

12. Shrug your shoulders, raising them as high as possible. Hold and note the tension. Relax. Repeat.

13. Gently push your head backward. Note the tension in the back of the neck. Hold, and relax. Repeat.

14. Gently bring the head against the chest, push forward, hold, and note the tension in the neck. Relax. Repeat.

15. Press your tongue toward the roof of your mouth. Hold, study the tension, and relax. Repeat.

16. Press your teeth together. Hold, and study the tension. Relax. Repeat.

17. Close your eyes tightly. Hold them closed and note the tension. Relax, leaving your eyes closed. Do this one more time.

BEHAVIOUR MODIFICATION PLANNING

CHARACTERISTICS OF GOOD STRESS MANAGERS

Good stress managers
- are physically active, eat a healthy diet, and get adequate rest every day.
- believe they have control over events in their life (have an internal locus of control, see pages 33–34).
- understand their own feelings and accept their limitations.
- recognize, anticipate, monitor, and regulate stressors within their capabilities.
- control emotional and physical responses when distressed.
- use appropriate stress management techniques when confronted with stressors.
- recognize warning signs and symptoms of excessive stress.
- schedule daily time to unwind, relax, and evaluate the day's activities.
- control stress when called upon to perform.
- enjoy life despite occasional disappointments and frustrations.
- look success and failure squarely in the face and keep moving along a predetermined course.
- move ahead with optimism and energy and do not spend time and talent worrying about failure.
- learn from previous mistakes and use them as building blocks to prevent similar setbacks in the future.
- give of themselves freely to others.
- have a deep meaning in life.

18. Wrinkle your forehead and note the tension. Hold and relax. Repeat.

When time is a factor during the daily routine and an individual is not able to go through the entire sequence, he or she may do only the exercises specific to the area that feels most tense. Performing a partial sequence is better than not doing the exercises at all. Completing the entire sequence, of course, yields the best results.

BREATHING TECHNIQUES FOR RELAXATION

Breathing exercises also can be an antidote to stress. These exercises have been used for centuries in Asia and India to improve mental, physical, and emotional stamina. In breathing exercises, the person concentrates on "breathing away" the tension and inhaling a large amount of air with each breath. Breathing exercises can be learned in only a few minutes and require considerably less time than the progressive muscle relaxation exercises.

Progressive muscle relaxation A stress management technique that involves progressive contraction and relaxation of muscle groups throughout the body.

Breathing exercises A stress management technique wherein the individual concentrates on "breathing away" the tension and inhaling fresh air to the entire body.

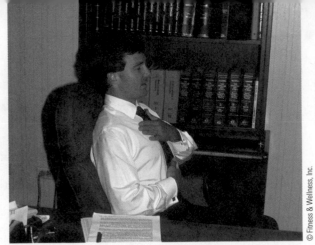
Breathing exercises help dissipate stress.

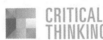

CRITICAL THINKING

List the three most common stressors you face as a post secondary student. What techniques have you used to manage these situations, and in what way have they helped you cope?

As with any other relaxation technique, these exercises should be done in a quiet, pleasant, well-ventilated room. Any of the three examples of breathing exercises presented here will help relieve tension induced by stress.

1. *Deep breathing*. Lie with your back flat against the floor, and place a pillow under your knees. Separate the feet slightly, with the toes pointing outward. (The exercise also may be done while sitting up in a chair or standing straight up.) Place one hand on your abdomen and the other hand on your chest.

   Slowly breathe in and out so the hand on your abdomen rises when you inhale and falls as you exhale. The hand on the chest should not move much at all. Repeat the exercise about 10 times. Next, scan your body for tension and compare your present tension with the tension you felt at the beginning of the exercise. Repeat the entire process once or twice.

2. *Sighing*. Using the abdominal breathing technique, breathe in through your nose to a specific count (e.g., 4, 5, or 6). Now exhale through pursed lips to double the intake count (e.g., 8, 10, or 12). Repeat the exercise 8 to 10 times whenever you feel tense.

3. *Complete natural breathing*. Sit in an upright position, or stand straight up. Breathing through your nose, gradually fill your lungs from the bottom up. Hold your breath for several seconds. Now exhale slowly, allowing your chest and abdomen to relax completely. Repeat the exercise 8 to 10 times.

Visual Imagery

Visual or mental **imagery** has been used as a healing technique for centuries in various cultures around the world. In Western medicine, the practice of imagery is relatively new and not widely accepted among health-care professionals. Research is now being done to study the effects of imagery on the treatment of conditions such as cancer, hypertension, asthma, chronic pain, and obesity.

Visual imagery involves the creation of relaxing visual images and scenes in times of stress to elicit body and mind relaxation. Imagery works by off-setting the stressor with the visualization of relaxing scenes such as a sunny beach, a beautiful meadow, a quiet mountaintop, or some other peaceful setting. Imagery can also be used in conjunction with breathing exercises, meditation, or yoga.

As with other stress management techniques, imagery should be performed in a quiet and comfortable environment. You can either sit or lie down for the exercise. If you lie down, use a soft surface and place a pillow under your knees. Be sure that your clothes are loose and that you are as comfortable as you can be.

To start the exercise, close your eyes and take a few breaths using one of the breathing techniques previously described. You can then proceed to visualize one of your favourite scenes in nature. You may place yourself right into the scene and visualize yourself moving about and experiencing nature to its fullest. Enjoy the people, the animals, the colours, the sounds, the smells, and even the temperature in your scene. After 10 to 20 minutes of visualization, open your eyes and compare the tension in your body and mind at this point with how you felt prior to the exercise. You can repeat this exercise as often as you deem necessary when you are feeling tension or stress.

You may not always be able to find a quiet, comfortable setting in which to sit or lie down for 10 to 20 minutes. If you think imagery works for you, however, you can perform this technique while standing or sitting in an active setting. If you are able, close your eyes and disregard your surroundings for a moment and visualize one of your favourite scenes. Once you feel you have regained some control over the stressor, open your eyes and continue with your assigned tasks.

Autogenic Training

Autogenic training is a form of self-suggestion in which people place themselves in an autohypnotic state by repeating and concentrating on feelings of heaviness and warmth in the extremities. This technique was developed by Johannes Schultz, a German psychiatrist, who noted that hypnotized individuals developed sensations of warmth and heaviness in the limbs and torso. The sensation of warmth is

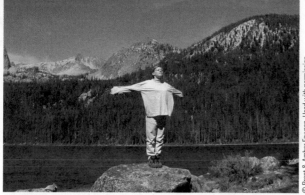

Visual imagery of beautiful and relaxing scenes helps attenuate the stress response.

caused by dilation of blood vessels, which increases blood flow to the limbs. Muscular relaxation produces the feeling of heaviness.

In this technique, the person lies down or sits in a comfortable position, eyes closed, and concentrates progressively on six fundamental stages and says (or thinks) the following:

1. Heaviness
   My right (left) arm is heavy.
   Both arms are heavy.
   My right (left) leg is heavy.
   Both legs are heavy.
   My arms and legs are heavy.
2. Warmth
   My right (left) arm is warm.
   Both arms are warm.
   My right (left) leg is warm.
   Both legs are warm.
   My arms and legs are warm.
3. Heart
   My heartbeat is calm and regular. (Repeat four or five times.)
4. Respiration
   My body breathes itself. (Repeat four or five times.)
5. Abdomen
   My abdomen is warm. (Repeat four or five times.)
6. Forehead
   My forehead is cool. (Repeat four or five times.)

The autogenic training technique is more difficult to master than any of those mentioned previously. The person should not move too fast through the entire exercise, because this actually may interfere with learning and relaxation. Each stage must be mastered before proceeding to the next.

Meditation

Meditation is a mental exercise that can bring about psychological and physical benefits. Regular meditation has been shown to decrease blood pressure, stress, anger, anxiety, fear, negative feelings, chronic pain, and increase activity in the brain's left frontal region—an area associated with positive emotions.[10] The objective of meditation is to gain control over one's attention by clearing the mind and blocking out the stressor(s) responsible for the higher tension.

This technique can be learned rather quickly, but first-time users often drop out before reaping benefits because they feel intimidated, confused, bored, or frustrated. In such cases, a group setting is best to get started. Many colleges, community programs, health clubs, and hospitals offer classes.

Initially, the person who is learning to meditate should choose a room that is comfortable, quiet, and free of all disturbances (including telephones). After learning the technique, the person will be able to meditate just about anywhere. A time block of approximately 10 to 15 minutes is adequate to start, but as you become more comfortable with meditation, you can lengthen the time to 30 minutes or longer. To use meditation effectively, it is best to meditate daily, as only once or twice a week may not provide noticeable benefits.

Of the several forms of meditation, the following routine is recommended to get started.

1. Sit in a chair in an upright position with the hands resting either in your lap or on the arms of the chair. Close your eyes and focus on your breathing. Allow your body to relax as much as possible. Do not try to consciously relax, because trying means work. Rather, assume a passive attitude and concentrate on your breathing.
2. Allow the body to breathe regularly, at its own rhythm, and repeat in your mind the word "one" every time you inhale, and the word "two" every time you exhale. Paying attention to these two words keeps distressing thoughts from entering into your mind.
3. Continue to breathe in this way for about 15 minutes. Because the objective of meditation is

Imagery Mental visualization of relaxing images and scenes to induce body relaxation in times of stress or as an aid in the treatment of certain medical conditions such as cancer, hypertension, asthma, chronic pain, and obesity.

Autogenic training A stress management technique using a form of self-suggestion, wherein an individual is able to place himself or herself in an autohypnotic state by repeating and concentrating on feelings of heaviness and warmth in the extremities.

Meditation A stress management technique used to gain control over one's attention by clearing the mind and blocking out the stressor(s) responsible for the increased tension.

to bring about a hypometabolic state leading to body relaxation, do not use an alarm clock to remind you that the 15 minutes have expired. The alarm will only trigger your stress response again, defeating the purpose of the exercise. Opening your eyes once in a while to keep track of the time is fine, but do not rush or anticipate the end of the session. This time has been set aside for meditation, and you need to relax, take your time, and enjoy the exercise.

Yoga exercises help induce the relaxation response.

Yoga

Yoga is an excellent stress-coping technique. It is a school of thought in the Hindu religion that seeks to help the individual attain a higher level of spirituality and peace of mind. Although its philosophical roots can be considered spiritual, yoga is based on principles of self-care.

Yoga practitioners adhere to a specific code of ethics and a system of mental and physical exercises that promote control of the mind and the body. In Western countries, many people are familiar mainly with the exercise portion of yoga. This system of exercises (postures or asanas) can be used as a relaxation technique for stress management. The exercises include a combination of postures, diaphragmatic breathing, muscle relaxation, and meditation that help buffer the biological effects of stress.

Western interest in yoga exercises gradually developed over the last century, particularly since the 1970s. The practice of yoga exercises helps align the musculoskeletal system and increases muscular flexibility, muscular strength and endurance, and balance.[11] People pursue yoga exercises to help dispel stress by raising self-esteem, clearing the mind, slowing respiration, promoting neuromuscular relaxation, and increasing body awareness. In addition, the exercises help relieve back pain and control involuntary body functions like heart rate, blood pressure, oxygen consumption, and metabolic rate. Yoga is also used in many hospital-based programs for cardiac patients to help manage stress and decrease blood pressure.

In addition, yoga exercises have been used to help treat chemical dependency, insomnia, and prevent injury. New research on patients with coronary heart disease who practised yoga (among other lifestyle changes) has shown that it slows down or even reverses atherosclerosis. These patients were compared with others who did not use yoga as one of the lifestyle changes.[12]

There are many different styles of yoga, and more than 60 styles are presently taught in North America. Classes vary according to their emphasis. Some styles of yoga are athletic, and others are passive in nature.

The most popular variety in the Western world is hatha yoga, which incorporates a series of static-stretching postures, performed in specific sequences ("asanas") that help induce the relaxation response. The postures are held for several seconds while participants concentrate on breathing patterns, meditation, and body awareness.

Most yoga classes are now variations of **hatha yoga**, and many of the typical stretches used in flexibility exercises today have been adapted from hatha yoga. Examples include:

1. *integral yoga* and *viny yoga*, which focus on gentle/static stretches
2. *iyengar yoga*, which promotes muscular strength and endurance
3. *yogalates*, incorporating Pilates exercises to increase muscular strength
4. *power yoga* or *yogarobics*, a high-energy form that links many postures together in a dance-like routine to promote cardiorespiratory fitness

As with flexibility exercises, the stretches in hatha yoga should not be performed to the point of discomfort. Instructors should not push participants beyond their physical limitations. Similar to other stress-management techniques, yoga exercises are best performed in a quiet place for about 15 to 60 minutes per session. Many yoga participants like to perform the exercises daily.

To appreciate yoga exercises, a person has to experience them. This section, nonetheless, serves only as an introduction. Although yoga exercises can be practised with the instruction of a book or video, most participants take classes. Many of the postures are difficult and complex, and few individuals can master the entire sequence in the first few weeks.

Individuals who are interested in yoga exercises should initially pursue it under qualified instruction. Many universities offer yoga courses, and you can also check the phone book for a listing of yoga instructors or classes. Yoga courses are offered at many health clubs and recreation centres. Because instructors and yoga styles vary, you may want to sit in on a class before enrolling. The most important thing is to look for an instructor whose views on wellness parallel your own. There are no national certification standards for instructors. If you are new to yoga, you are encouraged to compare a couple of instructors before you select a class.

Which Technique Is Best?

Each person reacts to stress differently. Therefore, the best coping strategy depends mostly on the individual. Which technique is used does not really matter, as long as it works. An individual may want to experiment with several or all of them to find out which works best. A combination of two or more is best for many people.

All the coping strategies discussed here help to block out stressors and promote mental and physical relaxation by diverting attention to a different,

nonthreatening action. Some of the techniques are easier to learn and may take less time per session. As a part of your class experience, you may participate in a stress-management session (see Lab 10D). Regardless of which technique you select, the time spent doing stress-management exercises (several times a day, as needed) is well worth the effort when stress becomes a significant problem in life.

People need to learn to relax and take time out for themselves. Stress is not what makes people ill; it's the way they react to the stress-causing agent. Individuals who learn to be diligent and start taking control of themselves find that they can enjoy a better, happier, and healthier life.

Yoga A school of thought in the Hindu religion that seeks to help the individual attain a higher level of spirituality and peace of mind.

Hatha yoga A form of yoga that incorporates specific sequences of static-stretching postures to help induce the relaxation response.

 ASSESS YOUR KNOWLEDGE

1. Positive stress is also referred to as
   a. eustress.
   b. poststress.
   c. functional stress.
   d. distress.
   e. physiostress.

2. Which of the following is not a stage of the general adaptation syndrome?
   a. alarm reaction
   b. resistance
   c. compliance
   d. exhaustion/recovery
   e. All are stages of the general adaptation syndrome.

3. The behaviour pattern of highly stressed individuals who do not seem to be at higher risk for disease is known as Type
   a. A.
   b. B.
   c. C.
   d. X.
   e. Z.

4. Effective time managers
   a. delegate.
   b. learn to say "no."
   c. protect from boredom.
   d. set aside "overtimes."
   e. All of the above.

5. Hormonal changes that occur during a stress response
   a. decrease heart rate.
   b. sap the body's strength.
   c. diminish blood flow to the muscles.
   d. induce relaxation.
   e. increase blood pressure.

6. Exercise decreases stress levels by
   a. deliberately diverting stress to various body systems.
   b. metabolizing excess catecholamines.
   c. diminishing muscular tension.
   d. stimulating alpha-wave activity in the brain.
   e. All of the above.

7. Biofeedback is
   a. the interaction with the interior self.
   b. the biological response to stress.
   c. the nonspecific response to a stress-causing agent.
   d. used to identify biological factors that cause stress.
   e. most readily achieved while in a state of self-hypnosis.

8. The technique whereby a person breathes in through the nose to a specific count and then exhales through pursed lips to double the intake count is known as
   a. sighing.
   b. deep breathing.
   c. meditation.
   d. autonomic ventilation.
   e. release management.

9. During autogenic training, a person
   a. contracts each muscle to about 70 percent of capacity.
   b. concentrates on feelings of warmth and heaviness.
   c. visualizes relaxing scenes to induce body relaxation.
   d. learns to reliably influence physiological responses.
   e. notes the positive and negative impact of frequent stressors on various body systems.

10. Yoga exercises have been used successfully to
    a. stimulate ventilation.
    b. increase metabolism during stress.
    c. slow down atherosclerosis.
    d. decrease body awareness.
    e. Accomplish all of the above.

Correct answers can be found at the back of the book.

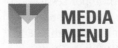

MEDIA MENU

■ Stress: Effects on Health. This site discusses symptoms of poor coping and mental health problems. The Canadian Heart & Stroke Foundation also provides a stress index quiz that can be taken online.

   http://ww2.heartandstroke.ca/Page.asp?PageID= 1613&ContentID=10337&ContentTypeID=1

■ Stress: Who Has Time For It? A visually appealing site that describes the symptoms of stress and how to manage your daily stress.

   http://www.familydoctor.org/handouts/278.html

■ Workplace Stress. This site, sponsored by the American Institute of Stress, provides research-based practical information on occupational stress and its effect on health.

   http://www.stress.org/job.htm

Notes

1. R. Booth et al., "The State of the Science: The Best Evidence for the Involvement of Thoughts and Feelings in Physical Health," *Advances in Mind–Body Medicine* 17, no. 1 (2001): 2.

2. K. Senior, "Should Stress Carry a Health Warning? *Lancet* 357 (2001): 126.

3. H. Selye, *Stress without Distress* (New York: Signet, 1974).

4. E. Gullete et al., "Effects of Mental Stress on Myocardial Ischemia during Daily Life," *Journal of the American Medical Association* 277 (1997): 1521–1525.

   C. A. Lengacher et al., "Psychoneuroimmunology and Immune System Link for Stress, Depression, Health Behaviors, and Breast Cancer," *Alternative Health Practitioner* 4 (1998): 95–108.

5. R. J. Kriegel and M. H. Kriegel, *The C Zone: Peak Performance Under Stress* (Garden City, NY: Anchor Press/ Doubleday, 1985).

6. Lengacher, "Psychoneuroimmunology and Immune System Link for Stress, Depression, Health Behaviors and Breast Cancer."

   J. Moses et al., "The Effects of Exercise Training on Mental Well-Being in the Normal Population: A Controlled Trial," *Journal of Psychosomatic Research* 33 (1989): 47–61.

C. Shang, "Emerging Paradigms in Mind-Body Medicine," *Journal of Complementary and Alternative Medicine* 7 (2001): 83–91.

7. L. Grubbs and J. Carter. "The Relationship of Perceived Benefits and Barriers to Reported Exercise Behavior in College Undergraduates," *Family and Community Health* 25 (2002): 76–84.

   J. Buckworth, "Exercise Adherence in College Students: Issues and Preliminary Results," Quest 53 (2001): 335–345.

8. Y. Iwasaki. "Roles of Leisure in Coping with Stress among University Students: A Repeated Assessment Field Study," *Anxiety, Stress and Coping* 16 (2003): 31–57.

9. Booth et al., "The State of Science."

10. S. Bodian, "Meditate Your Way to Much Better Health," *Bottom Line/Health* 18 (June 2004): 11–13.

11. D. Mueller, "Yoga Therapy," *ACSM's Health & Fitness Journal* 6 (2002): 18–24.

12. S. C. Manchanda et al., "Retardation of Coronary Atherosclerosis with Yoga Lifestyle Intervention," *Journal of the Association of Physicians of India* 48 (2000): 687–694.

Suggested Readings

Girdano, D. A., D. E. Dusek, and G. S. Everly. *Controlling Stress and Tension*. San Francisco: Benjamin Cummings, 2005.

Greenberg, J. S. *Comprehensive Stress Management*. New York: McGraw-Hill/Primis Custom Publishing, 2002.

Schafer, W. *Stress Management for Wellness*. Belmont, CA: Wadsworth/Thomson Learning, 2000.

Schwartz, M. S., and F. Andrasik. *Biofeedback: A Practitioner's Guide*. New York: Guilford Press, 2004.

Selye, H. *The Stress of Life*. New York: McGraw–Hill, 1978.

Smith, J. S. *Stress Management: A Comprehensive Handbook of Techniques and Strategies*. New York: Springer, 2002.

Lab 10A

LIFE EXPERIENCES SURVEY AND TYPE A PERSONALITY ASSESSMENT

Name: _____   Date: _____   Grade: _____

Instructor: _____   Course: _____   Section: _____

Necessary Lab Equipment

None required.

Objective

To determine stressful life experiences within the last 12 months that may affect your physical and psychological well-being and your Type A personality rating.

I. Life Experiences Survey

Introduction

The Life Experiences Survey contains a list of events that sometimes bring about change in the lives of those who experience them and that necessitate social readjustment. Please check events that you have experienced in the past 12 months. Be sure all checkmarks are directly across from the items to which they correspond (check only those that apply). For each item checked, please indicate the type and extent of impact the event had on your life at the time the event occurred. A rating of −3 would indicate an extremely negative impact. A rating of 0 suggests no impact either positive or negative. A rating of +3 would indicate an extremely positive impact.

Section 1

1. Marriage	−3	−2	−1	0	+1	+2	+3
2. Detention in jail or comparable institution	−3	−2	−1	0	+1	+2	+3
3. Death of spouse	−3	−2	−1	0	+1	+2	+3
4. Major change in sleeping habits (much more or much less sleep)	−3	−2	−1	0	+1	+2	+3
5. Death of close family member:							
a. mother	−3	−2	−1	0	+1	+2	+3
b. father	−3	−2	−1	0	+1	+2	+3
c. brother	−3	−2	−1	0	+1	+2	+3
d. sister	−3	−2	−1	0	+1	+2	+3
e. grandmother	−3	−2	−1	0	+1	+2	+3
f. grandfather	−3	−2	−1	0	+1	+2	+3
g. other (specify)	−3	−2	−1	0	+1	+2	+3
6. Major change in eating habits (much more or much less food intake)	−3	−2	−1	0	+1	+2	+3
7. Foreclosure on mortgage or loan	−3	−2	−1	0	+1	+2	+3
8. Death of close friend	−3	−2	−1	0	+1	+2	+3
9. Outstanding personal achievement	−3	−2	−1	0	+1	+2	+3
10. Minor law violations (traffic tickets, disturbing the peace, etc.)	−3	−2	−1	0	+1	+2	+3
11. Male: Wife/girlfriend's pregnancy	−3	−2	−1	0	+1	+2	+3
12. Female: Pregnancy	−3	−2	−1	0	+1	+2	+3
13. Changed work situation (different work responsibility, major change in working conditions or working hours, etc.)	−3	−2	−1	0	+1	+2	+3
14. New job	−3	−2	−1	0	+1	+2	+3

Continued

Adapted from Sarason, I.G., et al., "Assessing the Impact of Life Changes: Development of the Life Experiences Survey," *Journal of Consulting and Clinical Psychology* 46 (1978), pp. 932–946. Copyright © 1978 by the American Psychological Association. Adapted with permission. No further reproduction or distribution is permitted without written permission from the American Psychological Association.

15. Serious illness or injury of close family member:

a. father	−3	−2	−1	0	+1	+2	+3
b. mother	−3	−2	−1	0	+1	+2	+3
c. sister	−3	−2	−1	0	+1	+2	+3
d. brother	−3	−2	−1	0	+1	+2	+3
e. grandfather	−3	−2	−1	0	+1	+2	+3
f. grandmother	−3	−2	−1	0	+1	+2	+3
g. spouse	−3	−2	−1	0	+1	+2	+3
h. other (specify)	−3	−2	−1	0	+1	+2	+3
16. Sexual difficulties	−3	−2	−1	0	+1	+2	+3
17. Trouble with employer (in danger of losing job or of being suspended or demoted, etc.)	−3	−2	−1	0	+1	+2	+3
18. Trouble with in-laws	−3	−2	−1	0	+1	+2	+3
19. Major change in financial status (a lot better off or a lot worse off)	−3	−2	−1	0	+1	+2	+3
20. Major change in closeness of family members (increased or decreased closeness)	−3	−2	−1	0	+1	+2	+3
21. Gaining a new family member (through birth, adoption, family member moving in, etc.)	−3	−2	−1	0	+1	+2	+3
22. Change of residence	−3	−2	−1	0	+1	+2	+3
23. Marital separation from mate (due to conflict)	−3	−2	−1	0	+1	+2	+3
24. Major change in church activities (increased or decreased attendance)	−3	−2	−1	0	+1	+2	+3
25. Marital reconciliation with mate	−3	−2	−1	0	+1	+2	+3
26. Major change in number of arguments with spouse (a lot more or a lot fewer arguments)	−3	−2	−1	0	+1	+2	+3
27. Married male: Change in wife's work outside the home (beginning work, ceasing work, changing to a new job, etc.)	−3	−2	−1	0	+1	+2	+3
28. Married female: Change in husband's work (loss of job, beginning new job, retirement, etc.)	−3	−2	−1	0	+1	+2	+3
29. Major change in usual type and/or amount of recreation	−3	−2	−1	0	+1	+2	+3
30. Borrowing more than $10,000 (buying home, business, etc.)	−3	−2	−1	0	+1	+2	+3
31. Borrowing less than $10,000 (buying car or TV, getting school loan, etc.)	−3	−2	−1	0	+1	+2	+3
32. Being fired from job	−3	−2	−1	0	+1	+2	+3
33. Male: Wife/girlfriend having abortion	−3	−2	−1	0	+1	+2	+3
34. Female: Having abortion	−3	−2	−1	0	+1	+2	+3
35. Major personal illness or injury	−3	−2	−1	0	+1	+2	+3
36. Major change in social activities (participation in parties, movies, visiting, etc.)	−3	−2	−1	0	+1	+2	+3
37. Major change in living conditions of family (building new home or remodelling, deterioration of home or neighbourhood, etc.)	−3	−2	−1	0	+1	+2	+3
38. Divorce	−3	−2	−1	0	+1	+2	+3
39. Serious injury or illness of close friend	−3	−2	−1	0	+1	+2	+3
40. Retirement from work	−3	−2	−1	0	+1	+2	+3
41. Son or daughter leaving home (because of marriage, college, etc.)	−3	−2	−1	0	+1	+2	+3
42. End of formal schooling	−3	−2	−1	0	+1	+2	+3
43. Separation from spouse (because of work, travel, etc.)	−3	−2	−1	0	+1	+2	+3
44. Engagement	−3	−2	−1	0	+1	+2	+3

45. Breaking up with boyfriend/girlfriend	-3	-2	-1	0	+1	+2	+3
46. Leaving home for the first time	-3	-2	-1	0	+1	+2	+3
47. Reconciliation with boyfriend/girlfriend	-3	-2	-1	0	+1	+2	+3
48. Others____	-3	-2	-1	0	+1	+2	+3
49. ____	-3	-2	-1	0	+1	+2	+3
50. ____	-3	-2	-1	0	+1	+2	+3

Section 2

51. Beginning a new school experience at a higher academic level (college, university, graduate school, professional school, etc.)	-3	-2	-1	0	+1	+2	+3
52. Changing to a new school at the same academic level (undergraduate, graduate, etc.)	-3	-2	-1	0	+1	+2	+3
53. Academic probation	-3	-2	-1	0	+1	+2	+3
54. Being dismissed from dormitory or other residence	-3	-2	-1	0	+1	+2	+3
55. Failing an important exam	-3	-2	-1	0	+1	+2	+3
56. Changing a major	-3	-2	-1	0	+1	+2	+3
57. Failing a course	-3	-2	-1	0	+1	+2	+3
58. Dropping a course	-3	-2	-1	0	+1	+2	+3
59. Joining a fraternity/sorority	-3	-2	-1	0	+1	+2	+3
60. Financial problems concerning school (in danger of not having sufficient money to continue)	-3	-2	-1	0	+1	+2	+3

How to Score

After determining the life events that have taken place, sum the negative and the positive points separately (e.g., positive ratings: 3, 2, 1, 2 = 8 points positive score; negative ratings: -1, -3, -1, -3, -2, -3 = 13 negative points score). A final "total life change" score is obtained by adding the positive and negative scores together as positive numbers (e.g., total life change score: 8 + 13 = 21 points). The various stress ratings for the Life Experiences Survey are given below. Your negative score is the best indicator of stress (distress or negative stress) in your life.

Score Interpretation*

Stress Category	Negative Score		Total Score	
	Men	Women	Men	Women
Poor	≥13	≥15	≥27	≥27
Fair	7–12	8–14	17–26	18–26
Average	6	7	16	17
Good	1–5	1–6	5–15	6–16
Excellent	0	0	1–4	1–5

Life Experiences Survey Results

	Points	Stress Category
Negative score:		
Positive score:		
Total life change score:		

*Adapted from Sarason, I.G., et al., "Assessing the Impact of Life Changes: Development of the Life Experiences Survey," *Journal of Consulting and Clinical Psychology* 46 (1978), pp. 932–946. Copyright © 1978 by the American Psychological Association. Adapted with permission. No further reproduction or distribution is permitted without written permission from the American Psychological Association.

II. Type A Behaviour

Instructions

Please answer "yes" or "no" for each of the items listed below. For questions 7, 15, and 16, give yourself one point for each "yes" answer. For the rest of the questions, give yourself one point for each "no" answer.

Yes   No

1. Do you feel your job carries heavy responsibility?

2. Would you describe yourself as a hard-driving, ambitious type of person?

3. Do you usually try to get things done as quickly as possible?

4. Would family members and close friends describe you as hard-driving and ambitious?

5. Have people close to you ever asked you to slow down in your work?

6. Do you think you drive harder to accomplish things than most of your associates do?

7. When you play games with people your own age, do you play just for the fun of it?

8. If there's competition in your job, do you enjoy this?

9. When you are driving and there is a car in your lane going much too slowly for you, do you mutter and complain? Would anyone riding with you know you are annoyed?

10. If you make an appointment with someone, are you there on time in almost all cases?

11. If you are kept waiting, do you resent it?

12. If you see someone doing a job rather slowly and you know you could do it faster and better yourself, does it make you restless to watch him or her?

13. Would you be tempted to step in and do it yourself?

14. Do you eat rapidly? Walk rapidly?

15. After you've finished eating, do you like to sit around the table and chat?

16. When you go out to a restaurant and find eight or ten people waiting ahead of you for a table, will you wait?

17. Do you really resent having to wait in line at the bank or post office?

18. Do you always feel anxious to get going and finish whatever you have to do?

19. Do you have the feeling that time is passing too rapidly for you to accomplish all the things you'd like to get done in one day?

20. Do you often feel a sense of time urgency or time pressure?

21. Do you hurry in doing most things?

Form revised from *The Structured Interview from the Forum on Type A Behaviour*, National Heart/Lung/Blood Institute, Ray M. Rosenman, MD, 1981. This form is reprinted from R. W. Patton et. al., *Implementing Health/Fitness Programs* (Champaign, IL: Human Kinetics Publisher, 1986). Adapted by permission of the authors.

How to Score

Results   **Points**

Questions 7, 15, 16: [   ]   (1 point for each "yes" answer)

All other questions: [   ]   (1 point for each "no" answer)

Total score: [   ]

Your level of Type A: [   ]

Score Interpretation

Rating	Points
High	0–7
Medium	8–13
Low	14–21

III. Hostile Personality Assessment

Hostility could harm your heart. Experts now conclude that feelings of hostility increase your risk of heart disease. Dr. Redford Williams, of Duke University Medical Center, designed a questionnaire to help you determine whether you have a hostile personality. Circle the answer that most closely fits how you would respond to the given situation:

1. **A teenager drives by my yard blasting the car stereo:**
   A. I begin to understand why teenagers can't hear.
   B. I can feel my blood pressure starting to rise.

2. **A boyfriend/girlfriend calls at the last minute "too tired to go out tonight." I'm stuck with two $15 tickets:**
   A. I find someone else to go with.
   B. I tell my friend how inconsiderate he/she is.

3. **Waiting in the express checkout line at the supermarket where a sign says "No More Than 10 Items Please":**
   A. I pick up a magazine and pass the time.
   B. I glance to see if anyone has more than 10 items.

4. **Most homeless people in large cities:**
   A. Are down and out because they lack ambition.
   B. Are victims of illness or some other misfortune.

5. **At times when I've been very angry with someone:**
   A. I was able to stop short of hitting him/her.
   B. I have, on occasion, hit or shoved him/her.

6. **When I am stuck in a traffic jam:**
   A. I am usually not particularly upset.
   B. I quickly start to feel irritated and annoyed.

7. **When there's a really important job to be done:**
   A. I prefer to do it myself.
   B. I am apt to call on my friends to help.

8. **The cars ahead of me start to slow and stop as they approach a curve:**
   A. I assume there is a construction site ahead.
   B. I assume someone ahead had a fender-bender.

9. **An elevator stops too long above where I'm waiting:**
   A. I soon start to feel irritated and annoyed.
   B. I start planning the rest of my day.

10. **When a friend or co-worker disagrees with me:**
    A. I try to explain my position more clearly.
    B. I am apt to get into an argument with him or her.

11. **At times when I was really angry in the past:**
    A. I have never thrown things or slammed a door.
    B. I've sometimes thrown things or slammed a door.

12. **Someone bumps into me in a store:**
    A. I pass it off as an accident.
    B. I feel irritated at their clumsiness.

13. **When my spouse (significant other) is fixing a meal:**
    A. I keep an eye out to make sure nothing burns.
    B. I talk about my day or read the paper.

14. **Someone is hogging the conversation at a party:**
    A. I look for an opportunity to put him/her down.
    B. I soon move to another group.

15. **In most arguments:**
    A. I am the angrier one.
    B. The other person is angrier than I am.

How to Score

Score one point for each of these answers: 1. B, 2. B, 3. B, 4. A, 5. B, 6. B, 7. A, 8. B, 9. A, 10. B, 11. B, 12. B, 13. A, 14. A, 15. A. If you scored 4 or more points you may be hostile. Questions 1, 6, 9, 12, and 15 reflect anger. Questions 2, 5, 10, 11, 14, reflect aggression. Questions 3, 4, 7, 8, 13 reflect cynicism. If you scored 2 points in any category, you should work on that area of your personality.

Hostility score ☐   Anger score ☐   Aggression score ☐   Cynicism score ☐

From *Anger Kills: 17 Strategies* by Redford B. Williams and Virginia Williams, copyright © 1993 by Redford B. Williams, M.D. and Virginia Williams, Ph.D. Used by permission of Crown Publishers, a division of Random House, Inc.

IV. In your own words, summarize the results of all three assessment tools and express your feelings about how stress and your personality affect you in daily life.

_____
_____
_____
_____
_____
_____
_____
_____
_____
_____
_____
_____
_____
_____
_____
_____
_____
_____
_____
_____
_____
_____
_____
_____
_____
_____
_____

Lab 10B

STRESS VULNERABILITY QUESTIONNAIRE

Name: _____ Date: _____ Grade: _____

Instructor: _____ Course: _____ Section: _____

Necessary Lab Equipment
None required.

Objective
To determine your stress vulnerability rating and identify areas where you can reduce your vulnerability to stress.

Instructions
Carefully read each statement and circle the number that best describes your feelings or behaviour. Please be completely honest with your answers.

I. Stress Vulnerability Questionnaire

Item	Strongly Agree	Mildly Agree	Mildly Disagree	Strongly Disagree
1. I try to incorporate as much physical activity as possible in my daily schedule.	1	2	3	4
2. I exercise aerobically for 20 minutes or more at least three times per week.	1	2	3	4
3. I regularly sleep seven to eight hours per night.	1	2	3	4
4. I take my time eating at least one hot, balanced meal a day.	1	2	3	4
5. I drink fewer than two cups of coffee (or equivalent) per day.	1	2	3	4
6. I am at recommended body weight.	1	2	3	4
7. I enjoy good health.	1	2	3	4
8. I do not use tobacco in any form.	1	2	3	4
9. I limit my alcohol intake to no more than one drink per day.	1	2	3	4
10. I do not use hard drugs (chemical dependency).	1	2	3	4
11. There is someone I love, trust, and can rely on for help if I have a problem or need to make an essential decision.	1	2	3	4
12. There is love in my family.	1	2	3	4
13. I routinely give and receive affection.	1	2	3	4
14. I have close personal relationships with other people that provide me with a sense of emotional security.	1	2	3	4
15. There are people close by whom I can turn to for guidance in time of stress.	1	2	3	4
16. I can speak openly about feelings, emotions, and problems with people I trust.	1	2	3	4
17. Other people rely on me for help.	1	2	3	4
18. I am able to keep my feelings of anger and hostility under control.	1	2	3	4
19. I have a network of friends who enjoy the same social activities that I do.	1	2	3	4
20. I take time to do something fun at least once a week.	1	2	3	4
21. My religious beliefs provide guidance and strength in my life.	1	2	3	4
22. I often provide service to others.	1	2	3	4
23. I enjoy my job (or major or school).	1	2	3	4
24. I am a competent worker.	1	2	3	4
25. I get along well with co-workers (or students).	1	2	3	4
26. My income is sufficient for my needs.	1	2	3	4
27. I manage time adequately.	1	2	3	4

Item	Strongly Agree	Mildly Agree	Mildly Disagree	Strongly Disagree
28. I have learned to say "no" to additional commitments when I already am pressed for time.	1	2	3	4
29. I take daily quiet time for myself.	1	2	3	4
30. I practise stress management as needed.	1	2	3	4

Total Points: ____

Test Interpretation

Rating	Points
Excellent (great stress resistance)	0–30 points
Good (little vulnerability to stress)	31–40 points
Average (somewhat vulnerable to stress)	41–50 points
Fair (vulnerable to stress)	51–60 points
Poor (very vulnerable to stress)	≥61 points

This questionnaire helps you identify areas where improvements can be made to help you cope with stress more effectively. As you take this test, you will notice that most of the items describe situations and behaviours that are within your control. To make yourself less vulnerable to stress, improve the behaviours that make you more vulnerable to stress. Start by modifying behaviours that are easiest to change before undertaking the most difficult ones.

II. In the space provided below, list, in order of priority, behaviours that you would like to change to help you decrease your vulnerability to stress. Also, briefly outline how you intend to accomplish these changes.

Lab 10C

GOALS AND TIME MANAGEMENT SKILLS

Name: _____ **Date:** _____ **Grade:** _____

Instructor: _____ **Course:** _____ **Section:** _____

Necessary Lab Equipment

None required.

Objective

To help you develop time management skills.

Instructions

If you think you don't have enough hours during the day to get everything done, this lab is for you. Be sure to read the Time Management section and fill out all the forms provided with this lab.

I. Long- and Short-Term Goals

In the spaces provided below, list your goals as indicated. You may want to keep this form and review it in years to come.

1. List three goals you wish to accomplish in this life:

_____

_____

_____

2. List three goals you wish to see accomplished 10 years from now:

_____

_____

_____

3. List three goals you wish to accomplish this year:

_____

_____

_____

4. List three goals you wish to accomplish this month:

_____

_____

_____

5. List three goals you wish to accomplish this week:

_____

_____

_____

Signature: _____ **Date:** _____

II. Finding Time Killers

Keep a four- to seven-day log and record at half-hour intervals the activities you do (make additional copies of this form as needed). Record the activities as you go through your typical day, so you will remember them all. At the end of each day, decide when you wasted time. Using a highlighter, identify the time killers on this form and plan necessary changes for the next day.

6:00	
6:30	
7:00	
7:30	
8:00	
8:30	
9:00	
9:30	
10:00	
10:30	
11:00	
11:30	
12:00	
12:30	
1:00	
1:30	
2:00	
2:30	
3:00	
3:30	
4:00	
4:30	
5:00	
5:30	
6:00	
6:30	
7:00	
7:30	
8:00	
8:30	
9:00	
9:30	
10:00	
10:30	
11:00	
11:30	
12:00	

III. Daily and Weekly Goals and Priorities

Take 10 minutes each morning to write down the goals or tasks you wish to accomplish that day. Rank them as top, medium, low, or "trash" priorities. (Make as many copies of this form as needed.) At the end of the day, evaluate how well you accomplished your tasks for the day. Cross off the goals you accomplished and carry over to the next day those you did not get done.

Date: ___ / ___ / ___   Day of the Week: ___

Top-Priority Goals

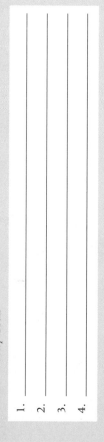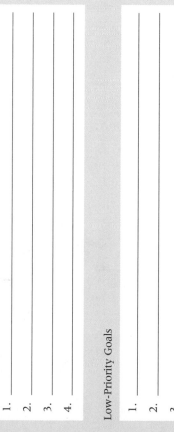

1. _____
2. _____
3. _____
4. _____

Medium-Priority Goals

1. _____
2. _____
3. _____
4. _____

Low-Priority Goals

1. _____
2. _____
3. _____
4. _____

Trash (do only after all other goals have been accomplished)

1. _____
2. _____
3. _____
4. _____

Take a few minutes each Sunday night to write down the goals or tasks you wish to accomplish that week. As with your daily goals, rank them as top, medium, low, or "trash" priorities. (Make as many copies of this form as needed.) At the end of the week, evaluate how well you accomplished your goals. Cross off the goals you accomplished and carry over to the next week those you did not get done.

Week: ___ / ___ / ___   to   ___ / ___ / ___

Top-Priority Goals

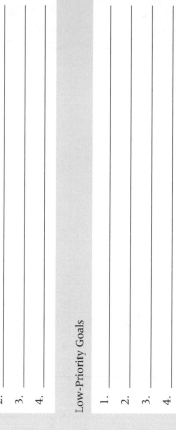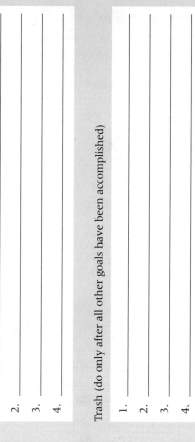

1. _____
2. _____
3. _____
4. _____

Medium-Priority Goals

1. _____
2. _____
3. _____
4. _____

Low-Priority Goals

1. _____
2. _____
3. _____
4. _____

Trash (do only after all other goals have been accomplished)

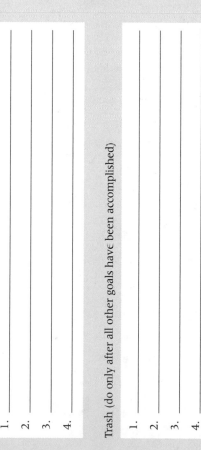

1. _____
2. _____
3. _____
4. _____

IV. Time Management Evaluation

On a weekly basis, go through the list of strategies below and provide a "yes" or "no" answer to each statement. If you are able to answer "yes" to most questions, congratulations, you are becoming a good time manager.

Strategy Date:															
1. I evaluate my time killers periodically.															
2. I have written down my long-range goals.															
3. I have written down my short-range goals.															
4. I use a daily planner.															
5. I conduct nightly audits.															
6. I conduct weekly audits.															
7. I delegate activities that others can do.															
8. I have learned to say "no" to additional tasks when I am already in "overload."															
9. I plan activities to avoid boredom.															
10. I plan ahead for distractions.															
11. I work on one task at a time, until it's done.															
12. I have removed distractions from my work.															
13. I set aside "overtimes."															
14. I set aside special time for myself daily.															
15. I reward myself for a job well done.															

Lab 10D
STRESS MANAGEMENT

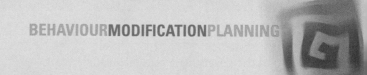

Name: _____   Date: _____   Grade: _____

Instructor: _____   Course: _____   Section: _____

Necessary Lab Equipment
None required.

Objective
To participate in a stress management session.

I. Stage of Change for Stress Management

Using Figure 2.4 (page 41) and Table 2.3 (page 41), identify your current stage of change for a stress management program:

_____

II. Stress Management

Instructions: The class should be divided into groups of about five students per group. Each group should select and go through a minimum of two of the following stress management techniques outlined in Chapter 10:

1. Progressive Muscle Relaxation
2. Breathing Techniques for Relaxation
3. Visual Imagery
4. Autogenic Training
5. Meditation
6. Yoga

A group leader is chosen who will lead the exercise according to the instructions provided for each relaxation technique in Chapter 10. Be sure this experience is conducted in a comfortable room that is as free of noise as possible. If trained personnel or a tape-recording for progressive muscle relaxation exercises is available. the entire class may participate in this experience at once. Institutions that have biofeedback equipment may use it in this laboratory as well. After completing this lab, answer the four questions given below.

1. Indicate the two relaxation techniques used in your lab:

    A. _____   B. _____

2. In your own words, relate your feelings as you were going through exercises A and B above:

    Exercise A: _____
    _____

    Exercise B: _____
    _____

3. Indicate how you felt mentally, emotionally, and physically after participating in this experience:

    _____
    _____

4. Are there situations in your daily life in which you think you would benefit from practising the selected stress-management exercises?

    _____
    _____

III. Self-Assessment Stress Evaluation

1. Do you currently perceive stress to be a problem in your life? ☐ Yes ☐ No

2. Do you experience any of the typical stress symptoms listed in the box on page 309? If so, which ones?

3. Indicate any specific events in your life that trigger a stress response.

4. Write specific objectives to either avoid or help you manage the various stress-inducing events listed above, including one or more stress-management techniques.

5. Do you have any behaviour patterns you would like to modify? List those you would like to change.

6. List specific techniques of change you will use to change undesirable behaviours (see Table 2.2, page 40).

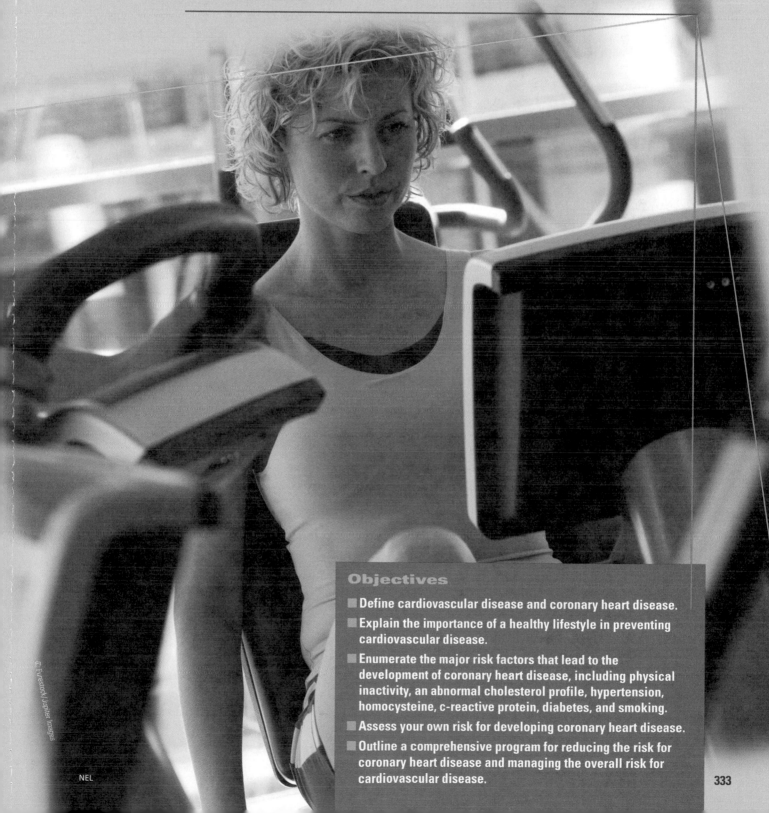

Chapter 11

Preventing Cardiovascular Disease

Objectives

- Define cardiovascular disease and coronary heart disease.
- Explain the importance of a healthy lifestyle in preventing cardiovascular disease.
- Enumerate the major risk factors that lead to the development of coronary heart disease, including physical inactivity, an abnormal cholesterol profile, hypertension, homocysteine, c-reactive protein, diabetes, and smoking.
- Assess your own risk for developing coronary heart disease.
- Outline a comprehensive program for reducing the risk for coronary heart disease and managing the overall risk for cardiovascular disease.

Cardiovascular disease is the leading cause of death in Canada and is responsible for about 37 percent of all deaths. About 1.2 million people in Canada suffer from some form of cardiovascular diseases, making them the most prevalent degenerative condition. Based on 2002 statistics, 34 percent of all female deaths and 32 percent of all male deaths were attributable to some form of cardiovascular disease (see Figure 11.1). According to the Canadian Heart and Stroke Foundation, Canadians experience between 40,000 and 50,000 heart attacks (myocardial infarction) per year and about half die from the attack. The attack and/or death is often sudden and unexpected with patients often having no previous symptoms of the disease. People often fail to recognize the early warning symptoms of a heart attack so deaths often occurred outside of the hospital.

Some examples of cardiovascular diseases are coronary heart disease, **peripheral vascular disease**, congenital heart disease, rheumatic heart disease, atherosclerosis, strokes, high blood pressure, and congestive heart failure. According to a recent study, the reduction in life expectancy from cardiovascular disease was 4.8 years.[1] This suggests that if all cardiovascular disease were eradicated, on average life expectancy would increase by almost five years.

In 2001, the economic burden related to the direct and indirect costs of cardiovascular disease was $6.8 billion and $11.6 billion, respectively. Every year, tens of thousands of Canadians have heart attacks either a first or subsequent attack, and many die as a result. One American study showed that half of heart attack deaths occur within one hour of onset of symptoms, before the person reaches the hospital (Canadian data are not available).

Although heart and blood vessel disease is a major problem throughout North America, the incidence has declined. In Canada, between 1970 and 1989, the mortality rate for males and females dropped by over 45 percent. This decrease was likely due to increased health education. More people are now aware of the risk factors for cardiovascular disease and are changing their lifestyle to lower their potential risk for these diseases. However, less than 5 percent of Canadian adults have no major risk factors for cardiovascular disease.

The heart and the coronary arteries are illustrated in Figure 11.2. The major form of cardiovascular disease is **coronary heart disease (CHD)**,

FIGURE 11.1 Mortality rates for cardiovascular diseases in Canada from 2000–2004

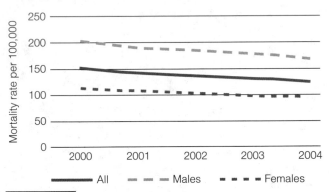

Source: Adapted from Statistics Canada publication *Mortality, Summary List of Causes*, 2004, Catalogue 84F0209XIE, p. 12, http://www.statcan.ca/english/freepub/84F0209XIE/84F0209XIE2004000.pdf

FIGURE 11.2 The heart and its blood vessels

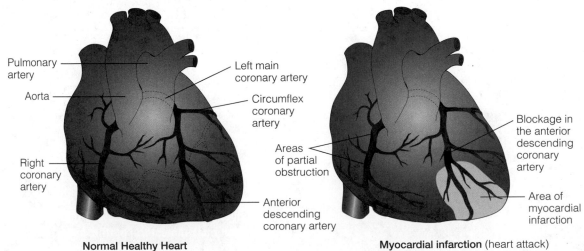

Normal Healthy Heart

Myocardial infarction (heart attack)
The result of acute reduction in blood flow through the anterior descending coronary artery.

in which the arteries that supply the heart muscle with oxygen and nutrients are narrowed by fatty deposits, such as cholesterol and triglycerides. Narrowing of the coronary arteries diminishes the blood supply to the heart muscle, which can precipitate a heart attack.

CHD is a major cause of death in Canada, accounting for more than 30 percent of all deaths and approximately half of all deaths related to cardiovascular diseases. Unfortunately, for people under age 65, a first heart attack often results in death. The risk of death is also greater in the least-educated segment of our population. Given that CHD is so common it should not be surprising that between 1990 and 1995, about 15,000 coronary bypass operations and about 20,000 **angioplasty** procedures were performed every year in Canada.

Coronary Heart Disease Risk Profile

Although genetic inheritance plays a role in CHD, the most important determinant is personal lifestyle. Several of the major risk factors for CHD are preventable and reversible. In this regard, CHD risk-factor analyses are administered to evaluate the impact of a person's lifestyle and genetic endowment as potential contributors to the development of coronary disease. The specific objectives of a CHD risk factor analysis are the following:

- To screen individuals who may be at high risk for the disease.
- To educate people regarding the leading risk factors for developing CHD.
- To implement programs aimed at reducing the risks.
- To use the analysis as a starting point from which to compare changes induced by the intervention program.

Leading Risk Factors for CHD

The leading **risk factors** contributing to CHD are listed in Table 11.1. A self-assessment of risk factors for CHD is given in Lab 11A. This analysis can be done by people who have little or no medical information about their cardiovascular health, as well as those who have had a thorough medical examination. The guidelines for zero risk are outlined for each factor, making this self-analysis a valuable tool for managing CHD risk factors.

The roles of HDL and LDL cholesterol in protecting against and causing heart disease are discussed later in this chapter.

To provide a meaningful score for CHD risk, a weighting system was developed to show the impact of each risk factor on developing the disease. This

TABLE 11.1 Weighing System for Coronary Heart Disease Risk Factors

Risk Factors	Maximal Risk Points
Abnormal cholesterol profile	12
Low HDL cholesterol	6
High LDL cholesterol	6
Inflammation	8
Physical inactivity	8
Smoking	8
Body mass index	8
Hypertension	8
Systolic blood pressure	4
Diastolic blood pressure	4
Personal history of heart disease	8
Abnormal stress electrocardiogram	8
Diabetes	6
High blood glucose	3
Known diabetes	3
Family history of heart disease	8
Elevated homocysteine	4
Age	4
Tension and stress	3
Abnormal resting electrocardiogram	3
Elevated triglycerides	2

system is based on current research and on the work done at leading preventive medical facilities in the United States. The most significant risk factors are given the heaviest numerical weight.

For example, a poor cholesterol profile seems to be the largest predictor for developing CHD. Up to 12 risk points are assigned to individuals with very high LDL cholesterol levels and very low HDL cholesterol levels. The least heavily weighted risk factor is triglycerides, with a maximum of only two risk points assigned to this factor. Each risk factor also is assigned a zero-risk level—the level at which it apparently does not increase the risk for disease at all.

Based on actual test results, a person receives a score anywhere from zero to the maximum number of points for each factor. When the risk points from all the risk factors are totalled, the final number is used to place an individual in one of five overall risk categories for potential development of CHD (see Lab 11A).

Cardiovascular diseases The array of conditions that affect the heart and the blood vessels.

Peripheral vascular disease Narrowing of the peripheral blood vessels, excluding the cerebral and coronary arteries.

Coronary heart disease (CHD) Condition in which the arteries that supply the heart muscle with oxygen and nutrients are narrowed by fatty deposits, such as cholesterol and triglycerides.

Angioplasty A procedure in which a balloon-tipped catheter is inserted, then inflated, to widen the inner lumen of one or more arteries.

Risk factors Lifestyle and genetic variables that may lead to disease.

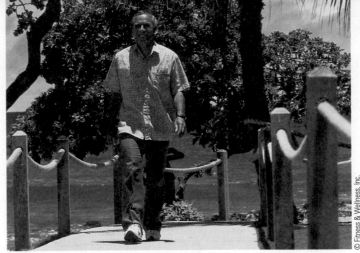

Regular physical activity helps to control most of the major risk factors that lead to heart disease.

BEHAVIOUR MODIFICATION PLANNING

SIGNS OF HEART ATTACK AND STROKE

Any or all of the following signs may occur during a heart attack or a stroke. If you experience any of these and they last longer than a few minutes, call 911 and seek medical attention immediately. Failure to do so may cause irreparable damage and even result in death.

Warning Signs of a Heart Attack

■ Chest pain, discomfort, pressure, or squeezing that lasts for several minutes. These feelings may go away and return later.
■ Pain that radiates to the shoulders, neck, or arms.
■ Chest discomfort with shortness of breath, lightheadedness, sweating, nausea, or fainting.

Warning Signs of Stroke

■ Sudden weakness or numbness of the face, arm, or leg— particularly on one side of the body.
■ Sudden severe headache.
■ Sudden confusion, dizziness, or difficulty in speech and understanding.
■ Sudden difficulty walking, loss of balance or coordination.
■ Sudden visual difficulty.

CRITICAL THINKING

What do you think about your own risk for diseases of the cardiovascular system? Is this something you need to concern yourself with at this point in your life? Why or why not?

The "Very Low" CHD risk category designates the group at lowest risk for developing heart disease based on age and gender. Low CHD suggests that, even though people in this category are taking good care of their cardiovascular health, they can improve it (unless all the risk points come from age and family history). "Moderate" CHD risk means that the person can definitely improve his or her lifestyle to lower the risk for disease, or medical treatment may be required. A score in the "High" or "Very High" CHD risk category points to a strong probability of developing heart disease within the next few years and calls for immediate implementation of a personal risk-reduction program, including professional medical, nutritional, and exercise intervention.

The leading risk factors for CHD are discussed next, along with the general recommendations for risk reduction.

Physical Inactivity

Physical inactivity is responsible for low levels of cardiorespiratory endurance (the ability of the heart, lungs, and blood vessels to deliver enough oxygen to the cells to meet the demands of prolonged physical activity). The level of cardiorespiratory endurance (or fitness) is given most commonly by the maximal amount of oxygen (in millilitres) that every kilogram of body weight is able to utilize per minute of physical activity (mL/kg/min). As maximal oxygen uptake increases, so does efficiency of the cardiorespiratory system.

Even though physical inactivity has not been assigned the most risk points (8 points for a poor level of fitness, versus 12 for a poor cholesterol profile—see Table 11.1), improving cardiorespiratory endurance through daily physical activity and aerobic exercise greatly reduces the overall risk for heart disease.

Although specific recommendations can be followed to improve each risk factor, daily physical activity and a regular aerobic exercise program help to control most of the major risk factors that lead to heart disease. Physical activity and aerobic exercise will

■ Increase cardiorespiratory endurance.
■ Decrease and control blood pressure.
■ Reduce body fat.
■ Lower blood lipids (cholesterol and triglycerides).
■ Improve HDL cholesterol.
■ Help control diabetes.
■ Decrease low-grade (hidden) inflammation in the body.
■ Increase and maintain good heart function, sometimes improving certain ECG abnormalities.
■ Motivate toward smoking cessation.
■ Alleviate tension and stress.
■ Counteract a personal history of heart disease.

Data from the research summarized in Figure 1.7, page 10, clearly show the tie between physical activity and mortality, regardless of age and other risk factors.[2] A higher level of physical fitness benefits even those who exhibit other risk factors, such as high blood pressure and serum cholesterol, cigarette smoking, and a family history of heart disease. In most cases, less-fit people in the study without these risk factors had higher death rates than highly fit people with these same risk factors.

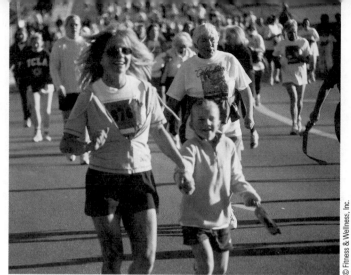
Lifetime participation in aerobic activity is one of the most important factors in preventing cardiovascular disease.

The findings show that the higher the level of cardiorespiratory fitness, the longer the life, but the largest drop in premature death is seen between the "Unfit" and the "Moderately Fit" groups. Even small improvements in cardiorespiratory endurance greatly decrease the risk for cardiovascular mortality. Most adults who engage in a moderate exercise program can attain these fitness levels easily. A 1 km walk in 30 to 40 minutes, five to seven days a week, is adequate to decrease risk.

Subsequent research published in the *New England Journal of Medicine* substantiated the importance of exercise in preventing CHD.[3] The benefits to previously inactive adults of starting a moderate-to-vigorous physical activity program were as important as quitting smoking, managing blood pressure, or controlling cholesterol. In relative risk for death from CHD, the increase in physical activity led to the same decrease as giving up cigarette smoking. Based on the overwhelming amount of scientific data in this area, evidence of the benefits of aerobic exercise in reducing heart disease is far too impressive to be ignored.

Even though aerobically fit individuals have a lower incidence of cardiovascular disease, regular physical activity and aerobic exercise by themselves do not guarantee a lifetime free of cardiovascular problems. Poor lifestyle habits—such as smoking; eating too many fatty, salty, or sweet foods; being overweight; and having high stress levels—increase cardiovascular risk and will not be eliminated completely through an active lifestyle.

Overall management of risk factors is the best guideline to lower the risk for cardiovascular disease. Still, aerobic exercise is one of the most important factors in preventing and reducing cardiovascular problems. The basic principles for cardiorespiratory exercise are given in Chapter 6.

As more research studies are conducted, the addition of strength training is increasingly recommended for good heart function. The American Heart Association recommends strength training even for individuals who have had a heart attack or have high blood pressure, as long as they do so under a physician's advice. Strength training helps control body weight and blood sugar and lowers cholesterol and blood pressure.

Abnormal Electrocardiograms

The **electrocardiogram (ECG** or **EKG)** is a valuable measure of the heart's function. The ECG provides a record of the electrical impulses that stimulate the heart to contract (see Figure 11.3 and 11.4). In reading an ECG, doctors interpret five general areas: heart rate, heart rhythm, axis of the heart, enlargement or hypertrophy of the heart, and myocardial infarction.

During a standard 12-lead ECG, 10 electrodes are placed on the person's chest. From these 10 electrodes, 12 tracings, or "leads," of the electrical

FIGURE 11.3 Normal electrocardiogram

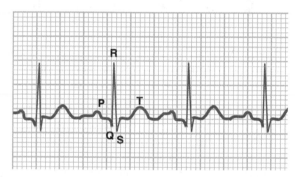

P wave = atrial depolarization
QRS complex = ventricular depolarization
T wave = ventricular repolarization

FIGURE 11.4 Abnormal electrocardiogram showing a depressed S-T segment

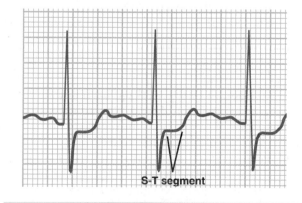

Electrocardiogram (ECG or EKG) A recording of the electrical activity of the heart.

impulses as they travel through the heart muscle, or **myocardium,** are studied from 12 different positions. By looking at ECG tracings, doctors can identify abnormalities in heart functioning (see Figure 11.4). Based on the findings, the ECG may be interpreted as normal, equivocal, or abnormal. An ECG will not always identify problems, so a normal tracing is not an absolute guarantee. Conversely, an abnormal tracing does not necessarily signal a serious condition.

ECGs are taken at rest, during the stress of exercise, and during recovery. A **stress electrocardiogram** is also known as a "graded exercise stress test" or a "maximal exercise tolerance test." Similar to a high-speed test on a car, a stress ECG reveals the tolerance of the heart to increased physical activity. It is a much better test than a resting ECG to discover CHD.

Stress ECGs also are used to assess cardiorespiratory fitness levels, to screen individuals for preventive and cardiac rehabilitation programs, to detect abnormal blood pressure response during exercise, and to establish actual or functional maximal heart rate for exercise prescription. The recovery ECG is another important diagnostic tool to monitor the return of the heart's activity to normal conditions.

Not every adult who wishes to start or continue an exercise program needs a stress ECG. This type of test, however, should be administered to the following:

1. Men over age 45 and women over age 55.
2. Anyone with total cholesterol level above 200 mg/dL or an HDL cholesterol below 35 mg/dL.
3. Hypertensive and diabetic patients.
4. Cigarette smokers.
5. Individuals with a family history of CHD, syncope, or sudden death before age 60.
6. People with an abnormal resting ECG.
7. All individuals with symptoms of chest discomfort, dysrhythmias (abnormal heartbeat), syncope (brief loss of consciousness), or chronotropic incompetence (heart rate that increases slowly during exercise and never reaches maximum).

At times, the stress ECG has been questioned as a reliable predictor of CHD. Nevertheless, it remains the most practical, inexpensive, non-invasive procedure available to diagnose latent (undiagnosed/unknown) CHD. The test is accurate in diagnosing CHD about 65 percent of the time. The sensitivity of the test increases along with the severity of the disease, and more accurate results are seen in people who are at high risk for cardiovascular disease, in particular men over age 45 and women over age 55.

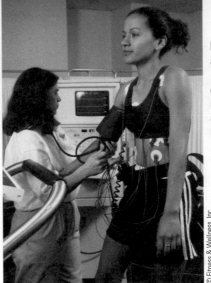

Exercise tolerance test with 12-lead electrocardiographic monitoring (an exercise stress-ECG).

Abnormal Cholesterol Profile

Cholesterol has received much attention because of its direct relationships to heart disease. **Blood lipids** (cholesterol and triglycerides) are carried in the bloodstream by molecules of protein known as **high-density lipoproteins (HDLs), low-density lipoproteins (LDLs), very low-density lipoproteins (VLDLs),** and **chylomicrons**. An increased risk for CHD has been established in people with high total cholesterol, high LDL cholesterol, and low HDL cholesterol.

An abnormal cholesterol profile contributes to **atherosclerosis**, the build-up of fatty tissue in the walls of the arteries (see Figures 11.5 and 11.6). As the plaque builds up, it blocks the blood vessels that supply the myocardium with oxygen and nutrients (the coronary arteries), and these obstructions

Myocardium Heart muscle.

Stress electrocardiogram An exercise test during which the workload is gradually increased until the individual reaches maximal fatigue, with blood pressure and 12-lead electrocardiographic monitoring throughout the test.

Cholesterol A waxy substance, technically a steroid alcohol, found only in animal fats and oil; used in making cell membranes, as a building block for some hormones, in the fatty sheath around nerve fibres, and in other necessary substances.

Blood lipids (fat) Cholesterol and triglycerides.

High-density lipoproteins (HDLs) Cholesterol-transporting molecules in the blood ("good" cholesterol) that help clear cholesterol from the blood.

Low-density lipoproteins (LDLs) Cholesterol-transporting molecules in the blood ("bad" cholesterol) that tend to increase blood cholesterol.

Very low-density lipoproteins (VLDLs) Triglyceride, cholesterol, and phospholipid-transporting molecules in the blood that tend to increase blood cholesterol.

Chylomicron Triglyceride-transporting molecule.

Atherosclerosis Fatty/cholesterol deposits in the walls of the arteries leading to formation of plaque.

FIGURE 11.5 The atherosclerotic process

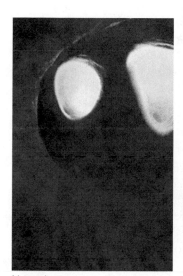

Early stage of atherosclerosis

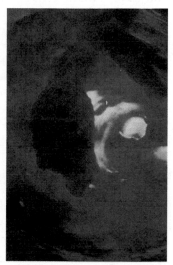

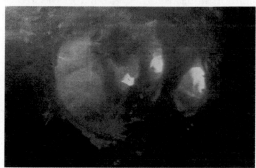

Normal artery

Progression of the atherosclerotic plaque

Advanced stage of atherosclerosis

FIGURE 11.6 Comparison of a normal healthy artery (A) and diseased arteries (B and C)

The Atherosclerotic Process

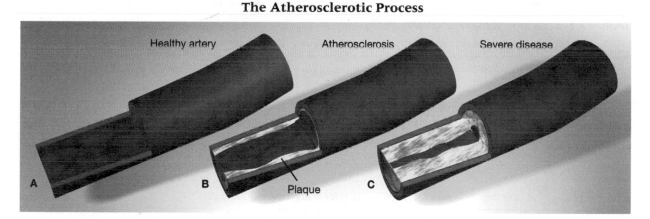

Healthy artery   Atherosclerosis   Severe disease

A   B   Plaque   C

can trigger a **myocardial infarction**, or heart attack.

Unfortunately, the heart disguises its problems quite well, and typical symptoms of heart disease, such as **angina pectoris**, do not start until the arteries are about 75 percent blocked. In many cases, the first symptom is sudden death.

It has been estimated that over 40 percent of all adult Canadians have unhealthy cholesterol levels. As important as it is, total cholesterol is not the best predictor for cardiovascular disease. Many heart attacks occur in people with only slightly elevated total cholesterol. More significant

is the way in which cholesterol is carried in the bloodstream.

Cholesterol is transported primarily in the form of high-density lipoprotein (HDL) cholesterol and low-density lipoprotein (LDL) cholesterol.

Myocardial infarction Heart attack; damage to or death of an area of the heart muscle as a result of an obstructed artery to that area.

Angina pectoris Chest pain associated with coronary heart disease.

Reverse cholesterol transport A process in which HDL molecules attract cholesterol and carry it to the liver, where it is changed to bile and eventually excreted in the stool.

In a process known as **reverse cholesterol transport**, HDLs, on the one hand, act as "scavengers," removing cholesterol from the body and preventing plaque from forming in the arteries. The strength of HDL is in the protein molecules found in its coating. When HDL comes in contact with cholesterol-filled cells, these protein molecules attach to the cells and take their cholesterol.

LDL-cholesterol, on the other hand, tends to release cholesterol, which then may penetrate the lining of the arteries and speed up the process of atherosclerosis. Table 11.2 will help you interpret your cholesterol levels. This information from the Canadian Heart and Stroke Foundation states that an optimal LDL reading is less than 3.0 mmol/L.

LDL-cholesterol particles are of two types: large or type A, and small or type B. Small particles are thought to pass through the inner lining of the coronary arteries more readily, thereby increasing the risk for a heart attack. Predominance of small particles can lead to a threefold to fivefold increase in the risk for CHD.[4] For individuals at risk for heart disease, LDL particle size should be included in the blood lipid analysis.

A genetic variation of LDL cholesterol, known as Lipoprotein-a or Lp(a), is also noteworthy because a high level of these particles promotes blood clots and earlier development of atherosclerosis. It is thought that certain substances in the arterial wall interact with Lp(a) and lead to premature formation of plaque. About 10 percent of the population has elevated levels of Lp(a). Only medications help decrease Lp(a), and drug options should be discussed with a physician.

The more HDL cholesterol (particularly the subcategory HDL_2), the better. HDL cholesterol, the "good cholesterol," offers some protection against heart disease. A low level of HDL cholesterol (less than 0.9 mmol/L) is one of the strongest predictors of CHD at all levels of total cholesterol. See Table 11.2 for recommended levels of HDL.[5]

For the most part, HDL cholesterol is determined genetically. Generally, women have higher levels than men. The female sex hormone estrogen tends to raise HDL, so premenopausal women have a much lower incidence of heart disease. HDL cholesterol also decreases with age.

Increasing HDL cholesterol improves the cholesterol profile and lessens the risk for CHD. Habitual aerobic exercise, weight loss, high-dose niacin, and quitting smoking help raise HDL cholesterol. Drug

TABLE 11.2 Interpreting Cholesterol Levels

	Normal	Secondary Action Plan: Change of Diet and Lifestyle Recommended	Action Plan: Change of Diet and Lifestyle Essential; Medication May Be Needed
18–29 Years of Age			
Total Cholesterol	Less than 4.7 mmol/L (180 mg/dL)	4.7–5.7 mmol/L (180–220 mg/dL)	Greater than 5.7 mmol/L (220 mg/dL)
LDL Cholesterol	Less than 3.0 mmol/L (115 mg/dL)	Greater than 3.0 mmol/L (115mg/dL)	—
HDL Cholesterol	Less than 0.9 mmol/L (35 mg/dL)	Less than 0.9 mmol/L (35 mg/dL)	—
Triglyceride	Less than 2.3 mmol/L (200 mg/dL)	Greater than 2.3 mmol/L (200 mg/dL)	—
30 Years of Age or Older			
Total Cholesterol	Less than 5.2 mmol/L (200 mg/dL)	5.2–6.2 mmol/L (200–240 mg/dL)	Greater than 6.2 mmol/L (240 mg/dL)
LDL Cholesterol	Less than 3.4 mmol/L (130 mg/dL)	Greater than 3.4 mmol/L (130 mg/dL)	—
HDL Cholesterol	Less than 0.9 mmol/L (35 mg/dL)	Less than 0.9 mmol/L (35 mg/dL)	—
Triglyceride	Less than 2.3 mmol/L (200 mg/dL)	Greater than 2.3 mmol/L (200 mg/dL)	—

(U.S. values shown in brackets)

Source: Heart and Stroke. Living With Cholesterol. Cholesterol and Healthy Living. Retrieved June 2008 at: http://www.heartandstroke.com/atf/cf/%7b99452D8B-E7F1-4BD6-A57D-B136CE6C95BF%7d/Living_with_Cholesterol_ENG.pdf (page 6). © Reproduced with the permission of the Heart and Stroke Foundation of Canada, 2008, www.heartandstroke.ca

therapy may also promote higher HDL cholesterol levels.

Improved HDL cholesterol is clearly related to a regular aerobic exercise program (preferably high intensity, or above 6 METs, for at least 20 minutes 3 times per week—see Chapter 6). Individual responses to aerobic exercise differ, but, generally, the more you exercise, the higher your HDL cholesterol level.

Even when more LDL cholesterol is present than the cells can use, cholesterol seems not to cause a problem until it is oxidized by free radicals (see discussion on Antioxidants, Chapter 3, page 73–74). After cholesterol is oxidized, white blood cells invade the arterial wall, take up the cholesterol, and clog the arteries.

The antioxidant effect of vitamins C and E may provide benefits. Data suggest that a single unstable free radical (an oxygen compound produced during metabolism—see Chapter 3) can damage LDL particles, accelerating the atherosclerotic process. Vitamin C may inactivate free radicals and slow the oxidation of LDL cholesterol. Vitamin E seems to protect LDL from oxidation, preventing heart disease, but studies suggest that it does not seem to be helpful in reversing damage once it has taken place.[6]

Although the average adult in Canada consumes between 200 and 400 mg of cholesterol daily, the body actually manufactures more than that. Saturated fats raise cholesterol levels more than anything else in the diet. Saturated fats produce approximately 1,000 mg of cholesterol per day. Because of individual differences, some people can have a higher-than-normal intake of saturated fats and still maintain normal levels. Others who have a lower intake can have abnormally high levels.

Saturated fats are found mostly in meats and dairy products and seldom in foods of plant origin (see Table 11.3). Poultry and fish contain less saturated fat than beef does, but should be eaten in moderation (about 85 to 170 g per day—see Chapter 3). Unsaturated fats are mainly of plant origin and cannot be converted to cholesterol. Two or three omega-3-rich fish meals per week also help lower LDL cholesterol and triglycerides.

Foods that contain trans fatty acids, hydrogenated fat, or partially hydrogenated vegetable oil should be avoided. Studies indicate that these foods elevate cholesterol as much as saturated fats do. Hydrogen is frequently added to monounsaturated and polyunsaturated fats to increase shelf life and to solidify them so they are more spreadable. Hydrogenation can change the position of hydrogen atoms along the carbon chain, transforming the fat into a trans fatty acid. Margarine and

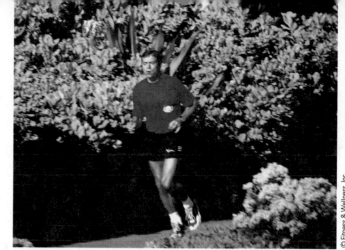

© Fitness & Wellness, Inc.

Habitual aerobic exercise helps increase HDL cholesterol ("good" cholesterol).

spreads, commercially produced crackers and cookies, dairy products, meats, and fast foods often contain trans fatty acids. The label "partially hydrogenated" and "trans fatty acids" indicates that the product carries a health risk just as high as that of saturated fat.

LDL cholesterol that is higher than ideal can be lowered through dietary changes, by losing body fat, by taking medication, and by participating in a regular aerobic exercise program. Based on research conducted at the Aerobics Research Institute in Dallas, Texas, the data showed a higher relative risk of mortality in unfit individuals with low cholesterol than fit people with high cholesterol.[7] The lowest mortality rate, of course, is seen in fit people with low total cholesterol levels.

With regard to dietary modifications, a diet lower in saturated fat and cholesterol and high in fibre is recommended. Saturated fat should be replaced with monounsaturated and polyunsaturated fats because the latter tend to decrease LDL cholesterol and increase HDL cholesterol (see the discussion of "Simple Fats" in Chapter 3). Exercise is important because dietary manipulation by itself is not as effective in lowering LDL cholesterol as a combination of diet plus aerobic exercise.

To lower LDL cholesterol significantly, total daily fibre intake must be in the range of 25 to 38 g per day (see "Fibre" in Chapter 3), total fat consumption can be in the range of 30 percent of total daily caloric intake, as long as most of the fat is unsaturated fat and the average cholesterol consumption is lower than 200 mg per day.

Among people in Canada, the average fibre intake is about 14 g per day. Fibre, in particular the soluble type, has been shown to lower cholesterol. Soluble fibre dissolves in water and forms a gel-like substance that encloses food particles. This property helps bind and excrete fats from the body. Soluble fibres also bind intestinal bile acids that could be recycled into additional cholesterol. Soluble fibres

TABLE 11.3 Cholesterol and Saturated Fat Content of Selected Foods

Food	Serving Size	Cholesterol (mg)	Sat. Fat (gr)
Avocado	1/8 med.	—	3.2
Bacon	2 slices	30	2.7
Beans (all types)	any	—	—
Beef—lean, fat trimmed off	85 g	75	6.0
Beef heart (cooked)	85 g	150	1.6
Beef liver (cooked)	85 g	255	1.3
Butter	5 mL	12	0.4
Caviar	28 g	85	—
Cheese			
Sliced processed	55 g	54	11.2
Cheddar	55 g	60	12.0
Cottage (1% fat)	250 mL	10	0.4
Cottage (4% fat)	250 mL	31	6.0
Cream	55 g	62	6.0
Muenster	55 g	54	10.8
Parmesan	55 g	38	9.3
Swiss	55 g	52	10.0
Chicken (no skin)	85 g	45	0.4
Chicken liver	85 g	472	1.1
Chicken thigh, wing	85 g	69	3.3
Egg (yolk)	1	250	1.8
Frankfurter	2	90	11.2
Fruits	any	—	—
Grains (all types)	any	—	—
Halibut, flounder	85 g	43	0.7
Ice cream	125 mL	27	4.4
Lamb	85 g	60	7.2
Lard	5 mL	5	1.9
Lobster	85 g	170	0.5
Margarine (all vegetable)	5 mL	—	0.7
Mayonnaise	15 mL	10	2.1
Milk			
Skim	250 mL	5	0.3
Low fat (2%)	250 mL	18	2.9
Whole	250 mL	34	5.1
Nuts	28 g	—	1.0
Oysters	85 g	42	—
Salmon	85 g	30	0.8
Scallops	85 g	29	—
Sherbet	125 mL	7	1.2
Shrimp	85 g	128	0.1
Trout	85 g	45	2.1
Tuna (canned—drained)	85 g	55	—
Turkey dark meat	85 g	60	0.6
Turkey light meat	85 g	50	0.4
Vegetables (except avocado)	any	—	—

BEHAVIOUR MODIFICATION PLANNING

BLOOD CHEMISTRY TEST GUIDELINES

People who have never had a blood chemistry test should do so to establish a baseline for future reference. The blood test should include total cholesterol, LDL cholesterol, HDL cholesterol, triglycerides, and blood glucose.

Following an initial normal baseline test no later than age 20, for a person who adheres to the recommended dietary and exercise guidelines, a blood analysis at least every 5 years prior to age 40 should suffice. Thereafter, a blood lipid test is recommended every year, in conjunction with a regular preventive medicine physical examination.

A single baseline test is not necessarily a valid measure. Cholesterol levels vary from month to month and sometimes even from day to day. If the initial test reveals cholesterol abnormalities, the test should be repeated within a few weeks to confirm the results.

are found primarily in oats, fruits, barley, legumes, and psyllium.

Psyllium, a grain that is added to some multi-grain breakfast cereals, also helps lower LDL cholesterol. As little as 3 daily grams of psyllium can lower LDL cholesterol by 20 percent. Commercially available fibre supplements that contain psyllium (such as Metamucil) can be used to increase soluble fibre intake. Forty-five millilitres daily will add about 10 g of soluble fibre to the diet.

The incidence of heart disease is very low in populations in which daily fibre intake exceeds 30 g per day. Further, a Harvard University Medical School study of 43,000 middle-aged men who were followed for more than 6 years showed that increasing fibre intake to 30 daily grams resulted in a 41 percent reduction in heart attacks.[8]

Research on the effects of a "typical" 30-percent-fat diet (including saturated fat) have shown that it has little or no effect in lowering cholesterol, and that CHD actually continues to progress in people who have the disease. Thus, some practitioners recommend a 10 percent or less fat-calorie diet combined with a regular aerobic exercise program while trying to lower cholesterol.

A daily 10 percent total-fat diet requires the person to limit fat intake to an absolute minimum. Some health care professionals contend that a diet like this is difficult to follow indefinitely. People with high cholesterol levels, however, may not have to follow that diet indefinitely but should adopt the 10-percent-fat diet while attempting to lower cholesterol. Thereafter, a 20- to 30-percent-fat diet may be adequate to maintain recommended cholesterol levels as long as most of the intake is from unsaturated fats (national data indicate that current fat consumption in Canada averages 38 percent of total calories).

A drawback of very low-fat diets (less than 25 percent fat) is that they tend to lower HDL cholesterol and increase triglycerides. If HDL cholesterol is already low, monounsaturated and polyunsaturated fats should be added to the diet. Examples of food items that are high in monounsaturated fats and polyunsaturated fats are olive, canola, corn, and soybean oils and nuts.

The 2001 American NCEP guidelines for people who are trying to decrease LDL cholesterol allow for a diet with up to 35 percent of calories from fat, including 10 percent from polyunsaturated fats and 20 percent from monounsaturated fats.[9] While attempting to lower LDL cholesterol, saturated fats should be kept to an absolute minimum. Carbohydrate intake can be in the range of 45 to 65 percent of total calories.

Soy protein is also recommended to lower total and LDL cholesterol. Soy protein increases the rate at which the liver removes LDL cholesterol from the blood, and it decreases LDL cholesterol production in the liver. Over time, a diet low in saturated fat and cholesterol that includes 25 g of soy protein a day will lower cholesterol by an additional 5 to 7 percent, compared to the same diet without the soy protein. This benefit is seen primarily in people with total cholesterol levels above 200 mg/dL. Some people have to consume up to 60 g a day to see an effect. Additional information on soy foods and their health benefits is given in Chapters 3 and 12.

Margarines and salad dressings that contain stanol ester, a plant-derived compound that interferes with cholesterol absorption in the intestine, are now also on the market. Over the course of several weeks, daily intake of about 3 g of margarine or 90 mL of salad dressing containing stanol ester lowers LDL cholesterol by 14 percent. Dietary guidelines to lower LDL cholesterol levels are provided in the accompanying box.

The best prescription for controlling blood lipids is the combination of a healthy diet, a sound aerobic exercise program, and weight control. If this does not work, a physician can recommend appropriate drug therapies based on a blood test to analyze the various subcategories of lipoproteins.

The American NCEP guidelines recommend that people consider drug therapy if, after six months on a low-cholesterol, low-saturated-fat diet, cholesterol remains unacceptably high. An unacceptable level is an LDL cholesterol above 190 mg/dL for individuals with fewer than two risk factors and no signs of heart disease. For individuals with more than two risk factors and with a history of heart disease, LDL cholesterol above 160 mg/dL is unacceptable.

ELEVATED TRIGLYCERIDES

Triglycerides, also known as free fatty acids, make up most of the fat in our diet and most of the fat

---

BEHAVIOUR MODIFICATION PLANNING

DIETARY GUIDELINES TO LOWER LDL CHOLESTEROL

- Consume between 25 and 38 g of fibre daily, including a minimum of 10 g of soluble fibre (good sources are oats, fruits, barley, legumes, and psyllium).
- Do not consume more than 200 mg of dietary cholesterol a day.
- Consume red meats (85 g per serving) fewer than three times per week and no organ meats (such as liver and kidneys).
- Do not eat commercially baked foods.
- Avoid foods that contain trans fatty acids, hydrogenated fat, or partially hydrogenated vegetable oil.
- Increase intake of omega-3 fatty acids (see Chapter 3) by eating two to three omega-3–rich fish meals per week.
- Consume 25 g of soy protein a day.
- Drink low-fat milk (1 percent or less fat, preferably) and use low-fat dairy products.
- Do not use coconut oil, palm oil, or cocoa butter.
- Limit egg consumption to fewer than three eggs per week (this is for people with high cholesterol only; others may consume eggs in moderation).
- Use margarines and salad dressings that contain stanol ester instead of butter and regular margarine.
- Bake, broil, grill, poach, or steam food instead of frying.
- Refrigerate cooked meat before adding to other dishes. Remove fat hardened in the refrigerator before mixing the meat with other foods.
- Avoid fatty sauces made with butter, cream, or cheese.
- Maintain recommended body weight.

---

that circulates in the blood. In combination with cholesterol, triglycerides speed up formation of plaque in the arteries. Triglycerides are carried in the bloodstream primarily by very low-density lipoproteins (VLDLs) and chylomicrons.

Although they are found in poultry skin, lunch meats, and shellfish, these fatty acids are manufactured mainly in the liver from refined sugars, starches, and alcohol. High intake of alcohol and sugars (honey and fruit juices included) significantly raises triglyceride levels. To lower triglycerides, avoid pastries, candies, soft drinks, fruit juices, white bread, pasta, and alcohol. In addition, cutting down on overall fat consumption, quitting smoking, reducing weight (if overweight), and doing aerobic exercise are helpful.

The desirable blood triglyceride level is less than 150 mg/dL (see Table 11.4). For people with cardiovascular problems, this level should be below 100 mg/dL. Levels above 1,000 mg/dL pose an immediate risk for

CRITICAL THINKING

Are you aware of your blood lipid profile? If not, what keeps you from getting a blood chemistry test? What are the benefits of having it done now as opposed to later in life?

Triglycerides Fats formed by glycerol and three fatty acids; also called free fatty acids.

TABLE 11.4 Triglycerides Guidelines

Amount	Rating
≤125 mg/dL	Desirable
126–499 mg/dL	Borderline high
≥500 mg/dL	High risk

potentially fatal sudden inflammation of the pancreas.

Some people consistently have slightly elevated triglyceride levels (above 140 mg/dL) and HDL cholesterol levels below 35 mg/dL. About 80 percent of these people have a genetic condition called LDL phenotype B. Although the blood lipids may not be notably high, these people are at higher risk for atherosclerosis and CHD.

CHOLESTEROL-LOWERING MEDICATIONS

Effective medications are available to treat elevated cholesterol and triglycerides. Most notable among them are the statins group (Lipitor, Mevacor, Pravachol, Lescol, and Zocor), which can lower cholesterol by up to 60 percent in 2 to 3 months. Statins slow down cholesterol production and increase the liver's ability to remove blood cholesterol. They also decrease triglycerides and produce a small increase in HDL levels.

In general, it is better to lower LDL cholesterol without medication, because drugs often cause undesirable side effects. Many people with heart disease, however, must take cholesterol-lowering medication, but it is best if medication is combined with lifestyle changes to augment the cholesterol-lowering effect. For example, when Zocor was taken alone over 3 months, LDL cholesterol decreased by 30 percent; but when a Mediterranean diet was adopted in combination with Zocor therapy, LDL cholesterol decreased by 41 percent.[10]

Other drugs effective in reducing LDL cholesterol are *bile acid sequestrans* that bind cholesterol found in bile acids. Cholesterol is subsequently excreted in the stools. These drugs are often used in combination with statin drugs.

High doses (1.5 to 3 g per day) of nicotinic acid or niacin (a B vitamin) also help lower LDL cholesterol, triglycerides, and increase HDL cholesterol. A fourth group of drugs, known as *fibrates*, is used primarily to lower triglycerides.

Elevated Homocysteine

Clinical data indicating that many heart attack and stroke victims have normal cholesterol levels has led researchers to look for other risk factors that may contribute to atherosclerosis. Although it is not a blood lipid, one of these factors is a high concentration of the amino acid **homocysteine** in the blood. It is thought to enhance plaque formation and subsequent blockage of the arteries.

The body uses homocysteine to help build proteins and carry out cellular metabolism. It is an intermediate amino acid in the interconversion of two other amino acids—methionine and cysteine. This interconversion requires the B vitamin folate (folic acid) and vitamins B_6 and B_{12}. Typically, homocysteine is metabolized rapidly, so it does not accumulate in the blood or damage the arteries.

A large number of people, however, have high blood levels of homocysteine. This might result from either a genetic inability to metabolize homocysteine or a deficiency in the vitamins required for its conversion.

Homocysteine is typically measured in micromoles per litre (µmol/L). Guidelines to interpret homocysteine levels are provided in Table 11.5. A 10-year follow-up study of people with high homocysteine levels showed that those individuals with a level above 14.25 µmol/L had almost twice the risk of stroke compared with individuals whose level was below 9.25 µmol/L.[11] Homocysteine accumulation is theorized to be toxic because it may

1. cause damage to the inner lining of the arteries (the initial step in the process of atherosclerosis),
2. stimulate the proliferation of cells that contribute to plaque formation, and
3. encourage clotting, which could completely obstruct an artery and lead to a heart attack or stroke.

Keeping homocysteine from accumulating in the blood seems to be as simple as eating the recommended daily servings of vegetables, fruits, grains, and some meat and legumes. Five servings of fruits and vegetables daily can provide sufficient levels of folate and vitamin B_6 to remove and clear homocysteine from the blood. Vitamin B_{12} is found

TABLE 11.5 Homocysteine Guidelines

Level	Rating
<9.0 µmol/L	Desirable
9–12 µmol/L	Mild elevation
13–15 µmol/L	Elevated
>15 µmol/L	Extreme elevation

Adapted from K. S. McCully, "What You Must Know Now About Homocysteine," *Bottom Line/Health* 18 (January 2004): 7–9.

primarily in animal flesh and animal products. Vitamin B_{12} deficiency is rarely a problem because 250 mL of milk or an egg provides the daily requirement. The body also recycles most of this vitamin; therefore, a deficiency takes years to develop. People who consume five servings of fruits and vegetables daily are unlikely to derive extra benefits from a vitamin-B-complex supplement.

Increasing evidence that folate can prevent heart attacks has led to the recommendation that people (especially women of childbearing age) consume 400 mcg per day—obtainable from five daily servings of fruits and vegetables. Unfortunately, estimates indicate that more than 80 percent of North Americans do not get 400 daily mcg of folate.

Inflammation

In addition to homocysteine, scientists are looking at inflammation as a major risk factor for heart attacks. Low-grade inflammation can occur in a variety of places throughout the body. For years it has been known that inflammation plays a role in CHD and that inflammation hidden deep in the body is a common trigger of heart attacks, even when cholesterol levels are normal or low and arterial plaque is minimal.

To evaluate ongoing inflammation in the body, physicians have turned to **C-reactive protein (CRP)**, a protein whose levels in the blood increase with inflammation. People with elevated CRP are more prone to cardiovascular events. The evidence shows that CRP blood levels elevate years before a first heart attack or stroke and that individuals with elevated CRP have twice the risk of a heart attack. The risk of a heart attack is even higher in people with both elevated CRP and cholesterol, resulting in an almost ninefold increase in risk (see Figure 11.7).

Because high CRP levels might be a better predictor of future heart attacks than high cholesterol alone, a new test known as high-sensitivity CRP (hs-CRP), which measures inflammation in the blood vessels is also available. The term "high-sensitivity" was derived from the test's capability to detect small amounts of CRP in the blood.

Hs-CRP test results provide a good measure of the probability of plaque rupture within the arterial wall. There are two main types of plaque: soft and hard. Soft plaque is the most likely to rupture. Ruptured plaque releases clots into the bloodstream that can lead to a heart attack or a stroke. Other evidence has linked high CRP levels to high blood pressure and colon cancer.

Excessive intake of alcohol and high-protein diets also increase CRP. Recent evidence further indicates that high-fat, fast-food meals increase CRP

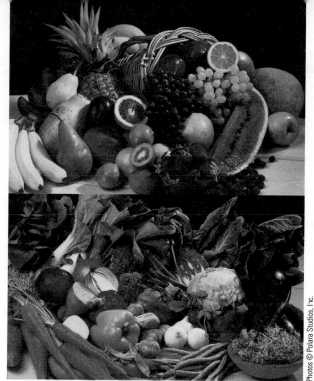

Five daily servings of fruits and vegetables can provide the necessary nutrients to keep homocysteine from causing heart disease or strokes.

FIGURE 11.7 Relationship between C-reactive protein and cholesterol and risk of cardiovascular disease

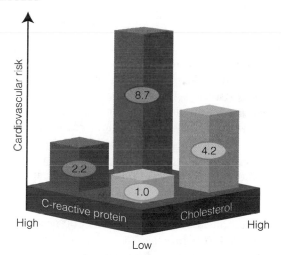

Source: Adapted from P. Libby, P. M. Ridker, and A. Maseri, "Inflammation and Atherosclerosis," *Circulation* 105 (2002): 1135–1143. Used with permission.

levels for several hours following the meals.[12] And cooking meat and poultry at high temperatures creates damaged proteins (AGEs or advanced glycosylation end products) that trigger inflammation.

Homocysteine An amino acid that, when allowed to accumulate in the blood, may lead to plaque formation and blockage of arteries.

C-reactive protein (CRP) A protein whose blood levels increase with inflammation, at times hidden deep in the body; elevation of this protein is an indicator of potential cardiovascular events.

TABLE 11.6 High-Sensitivity CRP Guidelines

Amount	Rating
<1 mg/L	Low risk
1–3 mg/L	Average risk
>3 mg/L	High risk

Source: T. A. Pearson, et. al. "Markers of Inflammation and Cardiovascular Disease." *Circulation* 107 (2003): 499–511. Used with permission.

TABLE 11.7 Blood Glucose Guidelines

Amount	Rating
≤126 mg/dL	Desirable
127–149 mg/dL	High
≥150 mg/dL	Very High

Obesity increases inflammation. With weight loss, CRP levels decrease proportional to the amount of fat lost.

An hs-CRP test is relatively inexpensive, and it is highly recommended for patients at risk for heart attack. Guidelines for hs-CRP levels are given in Table 11.6.

CRP levels decrease with statin drugs, which also lower cholesterol and reduce inflammation. Exercise, weight loss, proper nutrition, and aspirin are helpful in reducing hs-CRP. Omega-3 fatty acids (found in salmon, tuna, and mackerel fish) inhibit proteins that cause inflammation. Aspirin therapy also helps by controlling inflammation.

Diabetes

Diabetes mellitus is a condition in which blood glucose is unable to enter the cells because the pancreas totally stops producing **insulin**, or it does not produce enough to meet the body's needs, or the cells develop **insulin resistance**. The role of insulin is to "unlock" the cells and escort glucose into the cell.

It has been estimated that diabetes affects over 2 million people in Canada with about a third unaware that they have the condition. With more than 60,000 new cases diagnosed each year, it is not surprising that the cost of diabetes in Canada is estimated to be close to $9 billion annually. Diabetes and its complications account for 25,000 person years of life lost before age 75.

The incidence of cardiovascular disease and death in the diabetic population is quite high. Two of three diabetics will die from cardiovascular disease. People with chronically elevated blood glucose levels may have problems metabolizing fats, which can make them more susceptible to atherosclerosis, coronary heart disease, heart attacks, high blood pressure, and strokes. Diabetics also have lower HDL cholesterol and higher triglyceride levels.

Further, chronic high blood sugar can lead to nerve damage, vision loss, kidney damage, sexual dysfunction, and decreased immune function (making the individual more susceptible to infections). Diabetics are four times more likely to become blind and 20 times more likely to develop kidney failure.

Nerve damage in the lower extremities decreases the person's awareness of injury and infection, and a small, untreated sore can result in severe infection, gangrene, and even lead to an amputation.

An 8-hour fasting blood glucose level above 126 mg/dL on two separate tests confirms a diagnosis of diabetes (see Table 11.7). A level of 127 or higher should be brought to the attention of a physician.

TYPES OF DIABETES

Diabetes is of two types: **type 1**, or insulin-dependent diabetes mellitus (IDDM), and **type 2**, or non-insulin-dependent diabetes mellitus (NIDDM). Type 1 also has been called "juvenile diabetes," because it is found mainly in young people. With type 1, the pancreas produces little or no insulin. With type 2, the pancreas either does not produce sufficient insulin or produces adequate amounts but the cells become insulin-resistant, thereby keeping glucose from entering the cell. Type 2 accounts for 90 to 95 percent of all cases of diabetes.

Although diabetes has a genetic predisposition, 60 to 80 percent of type 2 diabetes is related closely to overeating, obesity, and lack of physical activity. Type 2 diabetes, once limited primarily to overweight adults, now accounts for almost half of the new cases diagnosed in children. In recent years, the prevalence of type 2 diabetes in youths has increased, particularly in those living in urban areas.

More than 80 percent of all type 2 diabetics are overweight or have a history of excessive weight. In most cases, this condition can be corrected through regular exercise, a special diet, and weight loss.

Aerobic exercise helps prevent type 2 diabetes. The protective effect is even greater in those with risk factors such as obesity, high blood pressure, and family propensity. The preventive effect is attributed to less body fat and to better sugar and fat metabolism resulting from the regular exercise program. At 3,500 Calories of energy expenditure per week through exercise, the risk is cut in half versus that of a sedentary lifestyle.

Both moderate-intensity and vigorous physical activity are associated with increased insulin sensitivity and decreased risk for diabetes. The key to increase and maintain proper insulin sensitivity, however, is regularity of the exercise program.

Failure to maintain habitual physical activity voids these benefits. Thus, a simple aerobic exercise program (walking, cycling, or swimming four or five times per week) often is prescribed because it increases the body's sensitivity to insulin. Exercise guidelines for diabetic patients are discussed in detail in Chapter 9.

A diet high in complex carbohydrates (unrefined whole grains) and water-soluble fibres (found in fruits, vegetables, oats, beans, and psyllium), low in saturated fat, and low in sugar is helpful in treating diabetes. Aggressive weight loss, especially if combined with exercise, often allows diabetic patients to normalize their blood sugar level without the use of medication.

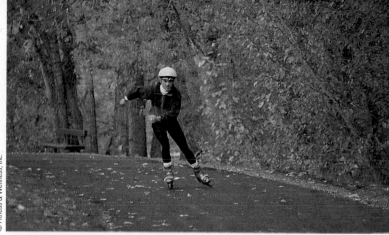

Habitual aerobic exercise increases insulin sensitivity and decreases the risk for diabetes.

GLYCEMIC INDEX

Although complex carbohydrates are recommended in the diet, diabetics need to pay careful attention to the glycemic index (explained in Chapter 5 and detailed in Table 5.1, page 126). Refined and starchy foods (small-particle carbohydrates, which are quickly digested) rank high in the glycemic index, whereas grains, fruits, and vegetables are low-glycemic foods.

Foods high in the glycemic index cause a rapid increase in blood sugar. A diet that includes many high-glycemic foods increases the risk for cardiovascular disease in people with high insulin resistance and **glucose intolerance**.[13] Combining a moderate amount of high-glycemic foods with low-glycemic foods or with some fat and protein, however, can bring down the average index.

A1c TEST

Individuals who have high blood glucose levels should consult a physician to decide on the best treatment. They also might obtain information about a new hemoglobin *A1c test* (also called Hb A1c) that measures the amount of glucose that has been in a person's blood over the last three months. Blood glucose can become attached to hemoglobin in the red blood cells. Once attached, it remains there for the life of the red blood cell, which is about three months. The higher the blood glucose, the higher is the concentration of glucose in the red blood cells. Results of this test are given in percentages.

The Hb A1c goal for diabetic patients is to keep it at less than 7 percent. At this level, or below, diabetics have a lower risk of developing diabetic-related problems of the eyes, kidneys, and nerves. Because the test tells a person how well blood glucose has been controlled over the last three months, a change in treatment is almost always recommended if the Hb A1c results are above 8 percent. All people with type 2 diabetes should have an Hb A1c test twice per year.

METABOLIC SYNDROME

As the cells resist the actions of insulin, the pancreas releases even more insulin in an attempt to keep blood glucose from rising. A chronic rise in insulin seems to trigger a series of abnormalities referred to as the **metabolic syndrome** or **syndrome X**. These abnormal conditions include abdominal obesity, elevated blood pressure, high blood glucose, low HDL cholesterol, high triglycerides, and an increased blood-clotting mechanism. All of these conditions increase the risk for CHD and other diabetic-related conditions (blindness, infection, nerve damage, and kidney failure). Approximately one in four Canadians is afflicted with this condition.

People with metabolic syndrome have an abnormal insulin response to carbohydrates, in particular high-glycemic foods. In contrast to some dietary guidelines, researchers on metabolic syndrome indicate that a low-fat, high-carbohydrate diet may not be the best for preventing CHD and

Diabetes mellitus A disease in which the body doesn't produce or utilize insulin properly.

Insulin A hormone secreted by the pancreas; essential for proper metabolism of blood glucose (sugar) and maintenance of blood glucose level.

Insulin resistance Inability of the cells to respond appropriately to insulin.

Type 1 diabetes Insulin-dependent diabetes mellitus (IDDM), a condition in which the pancreas produces little or no insulin; also known as juvenile diabetes.

Type 2 diabetes Non-insulin-dependent diabetes mellitus (NIDDM), a condition in which insulin is not processed properly; also known as adult-onset diabetes.

Glucose intolerance A condition characterized by slightly elevated blood glucose levels.

Syndrome X (metabolic syndrome) An array of metabolic abnormalities that contribute to the development of atherosclerosis triggered by insulin resistance. These conditions include low HDL-cholesterol, high triglycerides, high blood pressure, and an increased blood clotting mechanism.

TABLE 11.8 Blood Pressure Guidelines (expressed in mm Hg)

Rating	Systolic	Diastolic
Normal	≤120	≤80
Prehypertension	121–139	81–89
Hypertension	≥140	≥90

National Heart, Lung and Blood Institute, April 2008

FIGURE 11.8 Incidence of High Blood Pressure in Canada, 2005

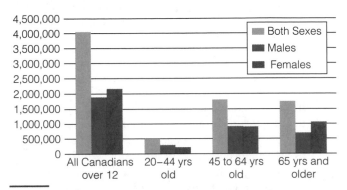

Adapted from Statistics Canada, Persons with high blood pressure, by age and sex, 2005, Statistics Canada Website, http://www40.statcan.ca/l01/cst01/health03.htm

could actually increase the risk for disease in people with high insulin resistance and glucose intolerance.[14] It might be best for these people to distribute daily caloric intake so that 45 percent of the calories are derived from carbohydrates (primarily low-glycemic), 40 percent from fat, and 15 percent from protein.[15] Of the 40 percent fat calories, most of the fat should come from mono- and polyunsaturated fats and less than 7 percent from saturated fat.

Metabolic syndrome patients also benefit from weight loss (if overweight), exercise, and smoking cessation.[16] Insulin resistance drops by about 40 percent in overweight people who lose 9 kg. Forty-five minutes of daily aerobic exercise enhances insulin efficiency by 25 percent. Quitting smoking also decreases insulin resistance.

Hypertension

Almost 100,000 km of blood vessels run through the human body. As the heart forces the blood through these vessels, the fluid is under pressure. **Blood pressure** is measured in millilitres of mercury (mm Hg), usually expressed in two numbers. **Systolic blood pressure** is the higher number, and **diastolic blood pressure** is the lower number. Ideal blood pressure is 120/80 or lower.

STANDARDS

Statistical evidence indicates that damage to the arteries starts at blood pressures above 120/80. The risk for cardiovascular disease doubles with each increment of 20/10, starting with a blood pressure of 115/75.[17] All blood pressures above 140/90 are considered to be **hypertension** (see Table 11.8). Blood pressures ranging from 120/80 to 139/89 are referred to as prehypertension.

Based on estimates released in 2005, approximately 1 in every 3 adults is hypertensive (Figure 11.8), up from 1 in 4 a decade earlier.[18]

Even though the threshold for hypertension has been set at 140/90, many experts believe that the lower the blood pressure, the better. Even if the pressure is around 90/50, as long as that person does not have any symptoms of **hypotension**, he or she need not be concerned. Typical symptoms of hypotension are dizziness, lightheadedness, and fainting.

Blood pressure also may fluctuate during a regular day. Many factors affect blood pressure, and one single reading may not be a true indicator of the real pressure. For example, physical activity and stress increase blood pressure, and rest and relaxation decrease it. Consequently, several measurements should be taken before diagnosing high pressure.

INCIDENCE AND PATHOLOGY

Based on data from the Public Health Agency of Canada (PHAC), over 5 million Canadians between the ages of 18 and 74 are hypertensive, and about 40 percent of them do not even know they have high blood pressure. This high rate of hypertension in Canada is likely related to the growing epidemic of obesity and the aging population. Unless appropriate, healthy, lifestyle

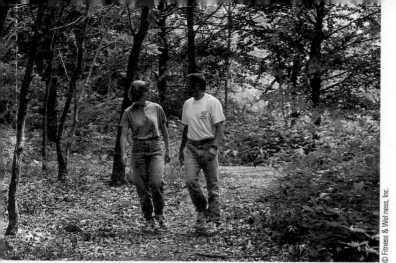
Regular physical activity is an important way to maintain healthy blood pressure.

strategies are implemented, people who do not have high blood pressure at age 55 have a 90 percent chance of developing it at some point in their lives.[19]

Hypertension has been referred to as "the silent killer." It does not hurt; it does not make you feel sick; and, unless you check it, years may go by before you even realize you have a problem. High blood pressure is a risk factor for CHD and also for congestive heart failure, strokes, kidney failure, and osteoporosis.

All inner walls of arteries are lined by a layer of smooth endothelial cells. Blood lipids cannot penetrate the healthy lining and start to build up on the walls unless the cells are damaged. High blood pressure is thought to be a leading contributor to destruction of this lining. As blood pressure rises, so does the risk for atherosclerosis. The higher the pressure, the greater is the damage to the arterial wall, making the vessels susceptible to fat deposits, especially if serum cholesterol is also high. Blockage of the coronary vessels decreases blood supply to the heart muscle and can lead to heart attacks. When brain arteries are involved, strokes may follow.

A clear example of the connection between high blood pressure and atherosclerosis can be seen by comparing blood vessels in the human body. Even when atherosclerosis is present throughout major arteries, fatty plaques rarely are seen in the pulmonary artery, which goes from the right part of the heart to the lungs. The pressure in this artery normally is below 40 mm Hg, and at such low pressure, significant deposits do not occur. This is one of the reasons people with low blood pressure have a lower incidence of cardiovascular disease.

Constantly elevated blood pressure also causes the heart to work much harder. At first the heart does well, but in time this continual strain produces an enlarged heart, followed by congestive heart

failure. Furthermore, high blood pressure damages blood vessels to the kidneys and eyes, which can result in kidney failure and loss of vision.

TREATMENT

Of all hypertension, 90 percent has no definite cause. Called "essential hypertension," it is treatable. Aerobic exercise, weight reduction, a low-salt/low-fat and high-potassium/high-calcium diet, lower alcohol and caffeine intake, smoking cessation, stress management, and antihypertensive medication all have been used effectively to treat essential hypertension.

The remaining 10 percent of hypertensive cases are caused by pathological conditions, such as narrowing of the kidney arteries, glomerulonephritis (a kidney disease), tumours of the adrenal glands, and narrowing of the aortic artery. With this type of hypertension, the pathological cause has to be treated before the blood pressure problem can be corrected.

Antihypertensive medicines often are the first choice of treatment, but they produce many side effects. These include lethargy, sleepiness, sexual difficulties, higher blood cholesterol and glucose levels, lower potassium levels, and elevated uric acid levels. A physician may end up treating these side effects as much as the hypertension itself. Because of the many side effects, about half of the patients stop taking the medication within the first year of treatment.

Another factor contributing to elevated blood pressure is too much sodium in the diet (salt, or sodium chloride, contains approximately 40 percent sodium). With a high sodium intake, the body retains more water, which increases the blood volume and, in turn, drives up the pressure. High intake of potassium seems to regulate water retention and lower the pressure slightly. According to the U.S. Institute of Medicine of the National Academy

CRITICAL THINKING

Do you know what your most recent blood pressure reading was, and did you know at the time what the numbers meant? How would you react if your doctor were to instruct you to take blood pressure medication?

Blood pressure A measure of the force exerted against the walls of the vessels by the blood flowing through them.

Systolic blood pressure Pressure exerted by blood against walls of arteries during forceful contraction (systole) of the heart; higher of the two numbers in blood pressure readings.

Diastolic blood pressure Pressure exerted by blood against walls of arteries during relaxation phase (diastole) of the heart; lower of the two numbers in blood pressure readings.

Hypertension Chronically elevated blood pressure.

Hypotension Low blood pressure.

PREVENTING CARDIOVASCULAR DISEASE

of Sciences, we need to consume at least 4,700 mg of potassium per day. Most Canadians get only half that amount.[20] Food items high in potassium include vegetables (especially leafy green), citrus fruit, dairy products, fish, beans, and nuts.

Although sodium is essential for normal body functions, the body can function with as little as 200 mg daily. Even under strenuous conditions of job and sports participation that incite heavy perspiration, the amount of sodium required is seldom more than 3,000 mg per day. Yet, sodium intake in the typical Canadian diet is at the high end—about 3,000 mg per day.

A 2004 U.S. government report now indicates that, to either prevent or postpone the onset of hypertension and to help some hypertensives control their blood pressure, people should consume even less sodium than previously recommended.[21] These new guidelines are provided in Table 11.9. The upper limit has been set at 2,300 mg per day. Among Americans and Canadians, about 95 percent of men and 75 percent of women exceed this limit.

Where does all the sodium come from? Part of the answer is given in Table 11.10. People do not realize the amount of sodium in various foods (the list in Table 11.10 does not include salt added at the table). Unfortunately, most of the sodium in our diets comes from prepared foods, in which the consumer does not have control over the ingredients.

When treating high blood pressure (unless it is extremely high), before recommending medication, many sports medicine physicians suggest a combination of aerobic exercise, weight loss, and less sodium in the diet. In most instances, this treatment brings blood pressure under control.

The relative risk for mortality ranked by blood pressure and fitness levels is similar to that of physical fitness and cholesterol. The data show that, in men and women alike, the relative risk of early mortality is lower in fit people with high systolic blood pressure (140 mm Hg or higher) than in unfit people with a healthy systolic blood pressure (120 mm Hg or lower).[22]

TABLE 11.10 Sodium and Potassium Levels of Selected Foods

Food	Serving Size	Sodium (mg)	Potassium (mg)
Asparagus	230 g	2	330
Avocado	1/2	4	680
Banana	1 med	1	440
Beans			
Kidney (canned)	115 g	436	330
Lima (cooked)	115 g	2	478
Pinto (cooked)	115 g	2	398
Refried (canned)	115 g	16	336
Bologna	85 g	1,107	133
Bouillon cube	1	960	4
Brussels sprouts (cooked)	115 g	16	247
Cantaloupe	1/4	17	341
Carrot (raw)	1	34	225
Cheese			
Sliced processed	55 g	614	93
Cheddar	55 g	342	56
Muenster	55 g	356	77
Parmesan	55 g	1,056	53
Swiss	55 g	148	64
Chicken (light meat)	170 g	108	700
Corn (natural)	115 g	3	136
Frankfurter	1	627	136
Haddock	170 g	300	594
Hamburger (reg)	1	500	321
Milk (whole)	250 mL	120	351
Milk (skim)	250 mL	126	406
Nuts			
Brazil	1 nut	1	120
Walnuts	230 g	1	327
Orange	1 med	1	263
Peach	1 med	2	308
Peas (canned)	115 g	200	82
Pizza (cheese—35 cm diam.)	1/8	456	85
Potato	1 med	6	763
Salami	85 g	1,047	170
Salmon (baked)	110 g	75	424
Salmon (canned)	170 g	198	756
Salt	5 mL	2,132	0
Soups			
Chicken Noodle	250 mL	979	55
Cream of Mushroom	250 mL	955	98
Vegetable Beef	250 mL	1,046	162
Soy sauce	5 mL	1,123	22
Spaghetti (tomato sauce and cheese)	170 g	648	276
Spinach (cooked, fresh)	230 g	126	838
Strawberries	230 g	1	244
Tomato (raw)	1 med	3	444
Tuna (drained)	85 g	38	255

The link between hypertension and obesity seems to be quite strong. Blood volume increases with excess body fat, and each additional 500 g of fat requires an estimated extra 1.6 km of blood vessels to feed this tissue. Furthermore, blood capillaries are constricted by the adipose tissues as these vessels run through them. As a result, the heart muscle must work harder to pump the blood through a longer, constricted network of blood vessels.

The role of regular physical activity in managing blood pressure is becoming more important each day. On the average, fit individuals have a lower blood pressure than unfit people do. Aerobic exercise of moderate intensity supplemented by strength training is recommended for individuals with high blood pressure.[23]

Comprehensive reviews on the effects of aerobic exercise on blood pressure found that, in general, an individual can expect exercise-induced reductions of approximately 4 to 5 mm Hg in resting systolic blood pressure and 3 to 4 mm Hg in resting diastolic blood pressure.[24] Although these reductions do not seem large, a decrease of about 5 mm Hg in resting diastolic blood pressure has been associated with a 40 percent decrease in the risk for stroke and a 15 percent reduction in the risk for coronary heart disease.[25] Even in the absence of any decrease in resting blood pressure, hypertensive individuals who exercise have a lower risk of all-cause mortality compared to hypertensive/ sedentary individuals. The research data also show that exercise, not weight loss, is the major contributor to the lower blood pressure of exercisers. If they discontinue aerobic exercise, they do not maintain these changes.

Another extensive review of research studies on the effects of at least four weeks of strength training on resting blood pressure yielded similar results.[26] Both systolic and diastolic blood pressures decreased by an average of 3 mm Hg. Participants in these studies, however, were primarily individuals with normal blood pressure. Of greater significance, the results showed that strength training did not cause an increase in resting blood pressure. More research remains to be done on hypertensive subjects.

The effects of long-term participation in exercise are apparently much more remarkable. An 18-year follow-up study on exercising and non-exercising subjects showed much lower blood pressures in the active group.[27] The exercise group had an average resting blood pressure of 120/78 compared to 150/90 for the non-exercise group (see Table 11.11).

Aerobic exercise programs for hypertensive patients should be of moderate intensity. Training at 40 to 60 percent intensity (12 to 13 on the RPE scale) seems to have the same effect in lowering blood pressure as training at 70 percent. High-intensity training

TABLE 11.11 Effects of Long-term (14–18 years) Aerobic Exercise on Resting Blood Pressure

	Initial	Final
Exercise Group		
Age	44.6	68.0
Blood Pressure	120/79	120/78
Non-exercise Group		
Age	51.6	69.7
Blood Pressure	135/85	150/90

Note: The aerobic exercise program consisted of an average four training sessions per week, each 66 minutes long, at about 76 percent of heart rate reserve.

Based on data from F. W. Kash, J. L. Boyer, S. P. Van Camp, L. S. Verity, and J. P. Wallace, "The Effect of Physical Activity on Aerobic Power in Older Men (A Longitudinal Study)," *The Physician and Sportsmedicine* 18, no. 4 (1990): 73–83.

(above 70 percent) in hypertensive patients may not lower the blood pressure as much as moderate-intensity exercise. Even so, a person may be better off being highly fit and having high blood pressure than being unfit and having low blood pressure. The death rates for unfit individuals with low systolic blood pressure are much higher than for highly fit people with high systolic blood pressure. Strength training for hypertensive individuals should be performed with a minimum of one set of 10 to 15 repetitions that elicit a "somewhat hard" RPE rating, using 8 to 10 exercises involving multi-joint exercises, two to three times per week.

Most important is a preventive approach. Keeping blood pressure under control is easier than trying to bring it down once it is high. Regardless of your blood pressure history, high or low, you should have it checked routinely. To keep your blood pressure as low as possible, exercise regularly, lose excess weight, eat less salt and sodium-containing foods, do not smoke, practise stress management, do not consume more than two alcoholic beverages a day if you are a man, or one if you are a woman, and consume more potassium-rich foods such as potatoes, bananas, orange juice, cantaloupe, tomatoes, and beans (see "Guidelines to Stop Hypertension"). The Dietary Approach to Stop Hypertension (DASH)—which emphasizes fruits, vegetables, grains, and dairy products—lowers systolic blood pressure by 11 points and diastolic pressure by 5.5 points.[28]

Those who are taking medication for hypertension should not stop unless the prescribing physician gives the go-ahead. If it is not treated properly, high blood pressure can kill. By combining medication with the other treatments, drug therapy eventually may be reduced or completely eliminated.

1. Increase daily physical activity, and participate in aerobic and strength-training programs.
2. Follow a diet lower in fat and refined sugars and high in complex carbohydrates and fibre.
3. Reduce total caloric intake moderately while getting the necessary nutrients to sustain normal body functions.

Additional recommendations for weight reduction and weight control are discussed in Chapter 5.

Excessive Body Fat

Body composition refers to the ratio of lean body weight to fat weight. If the body contains too much fat, the person is considered overweight or obese (see Table 4.10, page 107).

Although some experts recognize obesity as an independent risk factor for CHD, the risks attributed to obesity may actually be augmented by other risk factors that usually accompany excessive body fat. Risk factors such as high blood lipids, hypertension, and diabetes are typically seen in conjunction with obesity. All of these risk factors usually improve with increased physical activity.

Attaining recommended body composition helps to improve some of the CHD risk factors and also helps to reach a better state of health and wellness. People who have a weight problem and want to get down to recommended weight must implement the following:

Smoking

In Canada, there are more than 6.5 million smokers aged 12 years and over. In 2000, about 24 percent of females and about 28 percent of males smoked cigarettes daily or occasionally. Smoking is the single most significant and preventable cause of morbidity and mortality in Canada. Smoking has been linked to cardiovascular disease, cancer, bronchitis, emphysema, and peptic ulcers. In relation to coronary disease, smoking speeds up the process of atherosclerosis and carries a threefold increase in the risk of sudden death following a myocardial infarction.

According to estimates, about 20 percent of all deaths from cardiovascular diseases are attributable to smoking. Smoking prompts the release of nicotine and another 1,200 toxic compounds into the bloodstream. Similar to hypertension, many of these substances are destructive to the inner membrane that protects the walls of the arteries. Once the lining is damaged, cholesterol and triglycerides can be deposited readily in the arterial wall. As the plaque builds up, it obstructs blood flow through the arteries.

Furthermore, smoking encourages the formation of blood clots, which can completely block an artery already narrowed by atherosclerosis. In addition, carbon monoxide, a byproduct of cigarette smoke, decreases the blood's oxygen-carrying capacity. A combination of obstructed arteries, less oxygen, and nicotine in the heart muscle heightens the risk for a serious heart problem.

Smoking also increases heart rate, raises blood pressure, and irritates the heart, which can trigger fatal cardiac **arrhythmias**. Another harmful effect is a decrease in HDL cholesterol, the "good" type that helps control blood lipids. Smoking actually presents a much greater risk of death from heart disease than from lung disease.

Pipe and cigar smoking and chewing tobacco also increase the risk for heart disease. Even if the smoker inhales no smoke, he or she absorbs toxic substances through the membranes of the mouth, and these end up in the bloodstream. Individuals who use tobacco in any of these three forms also have a much greater risk for cancer of the oral cavity.

The risks for both cardiovascular disease and cancer start to decrease the moment a person quits smoking. One year after quitting, the risk of CHD decreases by half, and within 15 years, the relative risk of dying from cardiovascular disease and cancer approaches that of a lifetime non-smoker.

Tension and Stress

Tension and stress have become a part of life. Everyone has to deal daily with goals, deadlines, responsibilities, pressures. Almost everything in life (whether positive or negative) can be a source of stress. The stressor itself is not what creates the health hazard but, rather, the individual's response to it.

The human body responds to stress by producing more **catecholamines**, which prepare the body for quick physical action—often called "fight or flight." These hormones increase heart rate, blood pressure, and blood glucose levels, enabling the person to take action. If the person actually fights or flees, the higher levels of catecholamines are metabolized and the body can return to a normal state. If, however, a person is under constant stress and unable to take action (as in the death of a close relative or friend, loss of a job, trouble at work, or financial insecurity), the catecholamines remain elevated in the bloodstream.

People who are not able to relax place a constant low-level strain on the cardiovascular system that could manifest itself as heart disease. In addition, when a person is in a stressful situation, the coronary arteries that feed the heart muscle constrict, reducing the oxygen supply to the heart. If the blood vessels are largely blocked by atherosclerosis, arrhythmias or even a heart attack may follow.

Individuals who are under a lot of stress and do not cope well with it need to take measures to counteract the effects of stress in their lives. One way is to identify the sources of stress and learn how to cope with them. People need to take control of themselves, examine and act upon the things that are most important in their lives, and ignore less meaningful details.

Physical activity is one of the best ways to relieve stress. When a person takes part in physical activity, the body metabolizes excess catecholamines and is able to return to a normal state. Exercise also steps up muscular activity, which contributes to muscular relaxation after completing the physical activity.

Many executives in large cities are choosing the evening hours for their physical activity programs,

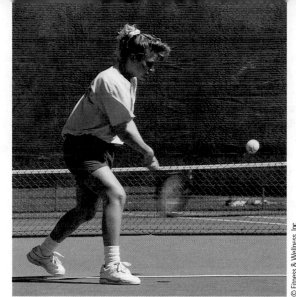

Physical activity is one of the best ways to relieve stress.

stopping after work at the health or fitness club. In doing this, they are able to "burn up" the excess tension accumulated during the day and enjoy the evening hours. This has proved to be one of the best stress-management techniques. More information on stress management techniques is presented in Chapter 10.

Personal and Family History

Individuals who have had cardiovascular problems are at higher risk than those who have never had a problem. People with this history should control the other risk factors as much as they can. Many of the risk factors are reversible, so this will greatly decrease the risk for future problems. The more time that passes after the cardiovascular problem occurred, the lower is the risk for recurrence.

A genetic predisposition toward heart disease has been demonstrated clearly. All other factors being equal, a person with blood relatives who now have or did have heart disease run a greater risk than someone with no such history. Premature CHD is defined as a heart attack before age 55 in a close male relative or before age 65 in a close female relative. The younger the age at which the relative incurred the cardiovascular incident, the greater is the risk for the disease.

Arrhythmias Irregular heart rhythms.

Catecholamines "Fight-or-flight" hormones, including epinephrine and norepinephrine.

PREVENTING CARDIOVASCULAR DISEASE

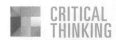

CRITICAL THINKING

Do you have any relatives with cardiovascular disease? If so, what steps are you taking to prevent a cardiovascular event in your life? Can you do anything to help others in your family do the same?

In some cases, there is no way of knowing whether the heart problem resulted from a person's genetic predisposition or simply poor lifestyle habits. A person may have been physically inactive, been overweight, smoked, and had bad dietary habits—all of which contributed to a heart attack. Regardless, blood relatives fall in the "family history" category. Because we have no reliable way to differentiate all the factors contributing to cardiovascular disease, a person with a family history should watch all other factors closely and maintain the lowest risk level possible. In addition, the person should have a blood chemistry analysis annually to make sure the body is handling blood lipids properly.

Age

Age is a risk factor because of the higher incidence of heart disease as people get older. This tendency may be induced partly by other factors stemming from changes in lifestyle as we get older—less physical activity, poorer nutrition, obesity, and so on. Young people should not think they are exempt from heart disease, though. The process begins early in life. Autopsies conducted on soldiers killed at age 22 and younger revealed that approximately 70 percent had early stages of atherosclerosis. Other studies found elevated blood cholesterol levels in children as young as 10 years old.

Although the aging process cannot be stopped, it certainly can be slowed. Physiological age versus chronological age is important in preventing disease. Some individuals in their 60s or older have the body of a 30-year-old. And 30-year-olds often are in such poor condition and health that they almost seem to have the body of 60-year-olds. The best ways to slow the natural aging process are to engage in risk-factor management and positive lifestyle habits.

Other Risk Factors for CHD

Additional evidence points to a few other factors that may be linked to coronary heart disease. One of these factors is gum disease. The oral bacteria that build up with dental plaque can enter the bloodstream and contribute to inflammation, formation of blood vessel plaque, blood clotting, and thus increase the risk for heart attack. Data on women who have periodontal disease indicate that these women also have higher blood levels of CRP and lower HDL cholesterol. Daily flossing, using a power brush, scraping the tongue, and irrigating the gums with water are all preventive measures that will help protect you from gum disease.

Another factor that has been linked to cardiovascular disease is loud snoring. People who snore heavily may suffer from sleep apnea, a sleep disorder in which the throat closes for a brief moment, causing breathing to stop. Individuals who snore heavily may triple their risk of a heart attack and quadruple the risk of a stroke.

Low birth weight, considered to be under 2.5 kg, also has been linked to heart disease, hypertension, and diabetes. Individuals with low birth weight should bring this information to the attention of their personal physician and regularly monitor the risk factors for CHD.

Aspirin therapy is also recommended to prevent heart disease. For individuals at moderate risk or higher, a daily aspirin dose of about 81 mg per day (the equivalent of a baby aspirin) can prevent or dissolve clots that cause heart attack or stroke. With daily use, the incidence of nonfatal heart attack is decreased by about a third.

Cardiovascular Risk Reduction

Using Lab 11A, you can chart a program to reduce your own cardiovascular risk. Most of the risk factors are reversible and preventable. Having a family history of heart disease and/or possessing some of the other risk factors because of neglect in lifestyle does not mean you are doomed. A healthier lifestyle—free of cardiovascular problems—is something over which you have extensive control. Be persistent! Willpower and commitment are required to develop patterns that eventually will turn into healthy habits and contribute to your total well-being and longevity.

ASSESS YOUR KNOWLEDGE

1. Coronary heart disease
   a. is the single leading cause of death in Canada.
   b. is the leading cause of sudden cardiac deaths.
   c. is a condition in which the arteries that supply the heart muscle with oxygen and nutrients are narrowed by fatty deposits.
   d. accounts for approximately 20 percent of all cardiovascular deaths.
   e. All of the above.

2. The incidence of cardiovascular disease in Canada has
   a. increased.
   b. decreased.
   c. remained constant.
   d. increased in some years and decreased in others.
   e. fluctuated according to medical technology.

3. Regular aerobic activity helps
   a. lower LDL cholesterol.
   b. lower HDL cholesterol.
   c. increase triglycerides.
   d. decrease insulin sensitivity.
   e. All of the above.

4. The risk of heart disease increases with
   a. high LDL cholesterol.
   b. low HDL cholesterol.
   c. high concentration of homocysteine.
   d. high levels of hs-CRP.
   e. All of the above factors.

5. An optimal level of LDL cholesterol is
   a. between 200 and 239 mg/dL.
   b. at about 200 mg/dL.
   c. between 150 and 200 mg/dL.
   d. between 100 and 150 mg/dL.
   e. below 100 mg/dL.

6. As a part of a CHD-prevention program, saturated fat intake should be kept below
   a. 35 percent.
   b. 30 percent.
   c. 22 percent.
   d. 15 percent.
   e. 7 percent.

7. Statin drugs
   a. increase the liver's ability to remove blood cholesterol.
   b. decrease LDL cholesterol.
   c. slow cholesterol production.
   d. help reduce inflammation.
   e. All of the above.

8. Type 1 diabetes is related closely to
   a. overeating.
   b. obesity.
   c. lack of physical activity.
   d. insulin resistance.
   e. All of the above factors.

9. Metabolic syndrome is related to
   a. low HDL cholesterol.
   b. high triglycerides.
   c. increased blood-clotting mechanism.
   d. an abnormal insulin response to carbohydrates.
   e. All of the above.

10. Comprehensive reviews on the effects of aerobic exercise on blood pressure found that, in general, an individual can expect exercise-induced reductions of approximately
    a. 3 to 5 mm Hg.
    b. 5 to 10 mm Hg.
    c. 10 to 15 mm Hg.
    d. over 15 mm Hg.
    e. There is no significant change in blood pressure with exercise.

Correct answers can be found at the back of the book.

MEDIA MENU

INTERNET CONNECTIONS

■ The Heart and Stroke Foundation of Canada. The mission of this national voluntary non-profit organization is to improve the health of Canadians by preventing and reducing disability and death from heart disease and stroke through research, health promotion, and advocacy. The website provides information about heart, stroke, and healthy living in Canada.

   www.heartandstroke.ca/

■ National Cholesterol Education Program. This comprehensive site features interactive sessions on planning a low-cholesterol diet and lots more. It provides you with information to prevent heart disease as well as information for people who already have heart disease. You can also hear radio messages from the Heart Beat Radio Network. This site is highly recommended.

   http://rover.nhlbi.nih.gov/chd

■ Check Your Healthy Heart IQ. This site is sponsored by the National Heart, Lung, and Blood Institute. Test your knowledge about heart disease and its risk factors (high blood pressure, high blood cholesterol, smoking, lack of exercise, and overweight) and learn ways to reduce your risk.

   http://www.nhlbi.nih.gov/health/public/heart/other/

Notes

1. D. G. Manuel, M. Leung, K. Nguyen, P. Tanuseputro, and H. Johansen, "Burden of Cardiovascular Disease in Canada," *Canadian Journal of Cardiology* 19 (2003): 997–1004.

2. S. N. Blair, H. W. Kohl III, R. S. Paffenbarger, Jr., D. G. Clark, K. H. Cooper, and L. W. Gibbons, "Physical Fitness and All-Cause Mortality: A Prospective Study of Healthy Men and Women," *Journal of the American Medical Association* 262 (1989): 2395–2401.

3. R. S. Paffenbarger, Jr., R. T. Hyde, A. L. Wing, I. Lee, D. L. Jung, and J. B. Kampert, "The Association of Changes in Physical-Activity Level and Other Lifestyle Characteristics with Mortality Among Men," *New England Journal of Medicine* 328 (1993): 538–545.

4. M. Mogadam, "5 Little-Known Ways to Lower Heart Attack Risk," *Bottom Line/Health* 18 (May 2004): 5–6.

5. Heart and Stroke Foundation, "Take Charge to Protect Your Heart." Retrieved January 30, 2008, from http://www.heartandstroke.com/site/c.ikIQLcMWJtE/b.3532103/apps/s/content.asp?ct=4763847.

6. "From Starring Role to Bit Part: Has the Curtain Come Down on Vitamin E?" *Environmental Nutrition* 25 no. 5 (May 2002): 1, 4.

7. Blair et al., "Physical Fitness and All-Cause Mortality."

8. E. B. Rimm, A. Ascherio, E. Giovannucci, D. Spiegelman, M. J. Stampfer, and W. C. Willett, "Vegetable, Fruit, and Cereal Fiber Intake and Risk of Coronary Heart Disease Among Men," *Journal of the American Medical Association* 275 (1996): 447–451.

9. National Cholesterol Education Program Expert Panel, "Summary of the Third Report of the National Cholesterol Education Program (NCEP) Expert Panel on Detection, Evaluation, and Treatment of High Blood Cholesterol in Adults (Adult Treatment Panel III)," *Journal of the American Medical Association* 285 (2001): 2486–2497.

10. A. Jula et al., "Effects of Diet and Simvastatin on Serum Lipids, Insulin, and Antioxidants in Hypercholesterolemic Men," *Journal of the American Medical Association* 287 (2002): 598–605.

11. "The Homocysteine–CVD Connection," *HealthNews* (October 25, 1999).

12. "Inflammation May Be Key Cause of Heart Disease and More: Diet's Role" *Environmental Nutrition* 27 no. 7 (July 2004): 1, 4.

13. S. Liu et al., "A Prospective Study of Dietary Glycemic Load, Carbohydrate Intake, and Risk of Coronary Heart Disease in the U.S.," *American Journal of Clinical Nutrition* 71 (2000): 1455–1461.

14. E. J. Mayer et al., "Intensity and Amount of Physical Activity in Relation to Insulin Sensitivity," *Journal of the American Medical Association* 279 (1998): 669–674.

15. G. M. Reaven, T. K. Strom, and B. Fox, *Syndrome X: Overcoming the Silent Killer That Can Give You a Heart Attack* (Englewood Cliffs, NJ: Simon & Schuster, 2000).

16. G. M. Reaven, "Syndrome X: The Little Known Cause of Many Heart Attacks," *Bottom Line/Health* 14 (June 2000).

17. A. V. Chobanian, et al., "The Seventh Report of the Joint National Committee on Prevention, Detection, Evaluation, and Treatment of High Blood Pressure," *Journal of the American Medical Association* 289 (2003): 2560–2571.

18. L. E. Fields, et al., "The Burden of Adult Hypertension in the United States 1999 to 2000: A Rising Tide," *Hypertension On Line First*, August 23, 2004.

19. Fields et al., "The Burden of Adult Hypertension in the United States 1999 to 2000."

20. "Water, Sodium, Potassium: The Verdict Is In," *University of California at Berkeley Wellness Letter* (Palm Coast, FL: The Editors, May 2004).

21. "Water, Sodium, Potassium."

22. Blair et al., "Physical Fitness and All-Cause Mortality."

23. L. S. Pescatello et al., "Exercise and Hypertension Position Stand," *Medicine and Science in Sports and Exercise* 36 (2004): 533–553.

24. G. Kelley, "Dynamic Resistance Exercise and Resting Blood Pressure in Adults: A Meta-analysis," *Journal of Applied Physiology* 82 (1997): 1559–1565.

    G. A. Kelley and Z. Tran, "Aerobic Exercise and Normotensive Adults: A Meta-analysis," *Medicine and Science in Sports and Exercise* 27 (1995): 1371–1377.

    G. Kelley and P. McClellan, "Antihypertensive Effects of Aerobic Exercise: A Brief Meta-analytic Review of Randomized Controlled Trials," *American Journal of Hypertension* 7 (1994): 115–119.

25. R. Collins et al., "Blood Pressure, Stroke, and Coronary Heart Disease; Part 2, Short-term Reductions in Blood Pressure: Overview of Randomized Drug Trials in Their Epidemiological Context," *Lancet* 335 (1990): 827–838.

26. G. A. Kelley and K. S. Kelley, "Progressive Resistance Exercise and Resting Blood Pressure: A Meta-Analysis of Randomized Controlled Trials," *Hypertension* 35 (2000): 838–843.

27. F. W. Kash, J. L. Boyer, S. P. Van Camp, L. S. Verity, and J. P. Wallace, "The Effect of Physical Activity on Aerobic Power in Older Men (A Longitudinal Study)," *Physician and Sportsmedicine* 18, no. 4 (1990): 73–83.

28. S. G. Sheps, "High Blood Pressure Can Often Be Controlled without Medication," *Bottom Line/Health*, November, 1999.

Suggested Readings

Cooper, K. H. "Control Your Cholesterol without Drugs." *Bottom Line/Health* 17 (August 2003): 3–4.

Goralski, K. B., and C. J. Sinal. "Type 2 Diabetes and Cardiovascular Disease: Getting to the Fat of the Matter." *Canadian Journal of Physiology and Pharmacology* 85 (2007): 113–132.

Heart and Stroke Foundation of Canada. "The Changing Face of Heart Disease and Stroke in Canada 2000." http://ww2.heartandstroke.ca/Page.asp?PageID=1613&ContentID=15935&ContentTypeID=1.

Kavanagh, T. *Take Heart*. Toronto: Key Porter Books, Ltd., 1998.

Kavanagh, T. "Exercise in Cardiac Rehabilitation." *British Journal of Sports Medicine* 34 (2000): 3.

National Cholesterol Education Program Expert Panel. "Summary of the Third Report of the National Cholesterol Education Program (NCEP) Expert Panel on Detection, Evaluation, and Treatment of High Blood Cholesterol in Adults (Adult Treatment Panel III)." *Journal of the American Medical Association* 285 (2001): 2486–2497.

Lab 11A

SELF-EVALUATION OF CARDIOVASCULAR RISK AND BEHAVIOUR MODIFICATION PROGRAM

Name: _____   Date: _____   Grade: _____

Instructor: _____   Course: _____   Section: _____

Necessary Lab Equipment

Basic lab equipment to repeat the body composition and blood pressure tests, and if possible, a blood chemistry analysis should be performed prior to this lab.

Objective

To assess your current risk for coronary heart disease (CHD) and develop a behaviour modification program.

I. Self-Assessment: Coronary Heart Disease Risk Factor Analysis

Instructions   The disease process for cardiovascular disease starts early in life, primarily as a result of poor lifestyle habits. Studies have shown beginning stages of atherosclerosis and elevated blood lipids in children as young as 10 years old. Consequently, the purpose of this lab is to establish a baseline CHD risk profile and to point out the "zero-risk" level for each coronary risk factor.

You may want to repeat the body composition and blood pressure tests to obtain current values for this lab experience. If time does not allow for reassessment of these parameters, use the results obtained in previous labs. In addition, if you have had a blood chemistry analysis performed recently that included total cholesterol, HDL cholesterol, triglycerides, and glucose levels, you may use the results for this lab.

		Score
1. Physical Activity	Do you participate in a regular aerobic exercise program (brisk walking, jogging, swimming, bicycling, aerobics, etc.) for more than 20 minutes:	
	Once a week or less 8	
	Two times per week 3	
	Three or more times per week 0	

2. Resting and Stress Electrocardiograms (ECG)	Add scores for both ECGs			
	ECG	Resting	Stress	
	Normal	(0)	(0) 0	
	Equivocal	(1)	(4) 1–5	
	Abnormal	(3)	(8) 3–11	

3. HDL Cholesterol	18–29 Years of Age	30 Years of Age and Older	
(If unknown, answer Question 6)	>0.9 mmol/L	>0.9 mmol/L 0	
	<0.9 mmol/L	<0.9 mmol/L 3	

4. LDL Cholesterol	18–29 Years of Age	30 Years of Age and Older	
(If unknown, answer Question 6)	<3.0 mmol/L	<3.4 mmol/L 0	
	>3.0 mmol/L	>3.4 mmol/L 3	

5. Triglycerides	18–29 Years of Age	30 Years of Age and Older	
(If unknown, answer Question 6)	<2.3 mmol/L	<2.3 mmol/L 0	
	>2.3 mmol/L	>2.3 mmol/L 1	

Subtotal Risk Score: _____

Self-Assessment: Coronary Heart Disease Risk Factor Analysis (continued)

Subtotal Risk Score (from previous page): ☐

6. Diet (Do not answer if Questions 3, 4, and 5 have been answered)	Does your regular diet include (high score if all apply): One or more daily servings of red meat; 7 or more eggs/week; daily butter, cheese, whole milk, sweets and alcohol	10–14
	Four to six servings of red meat/week; 4–6 eggs per week; 1% or 2% milk; some cheese, sweets, and alcohol	4–10
	Fish, poultry, red meat fewer than three times/week; fewer than 3 eggs/week; skim milk and skim milk products; moderate sweets and alcohol	0–3 ☐
7. Homocysteine	Does your daily diet include: 2 and 3 servings of fruits and vegetables respectively	0
	Less than 2 and 3 servings of fruits and vegetables respectively	4 ☐
8. Inflammation (as measured by High-Sensitivity C-Reactive Protein or hs-CRP)	<1 mg/L	0
	1–3 mg/L	2
	>3 mg/L	8 ☐
9. Diabetes/Glucose	≤120	0
	121–128	1
	129–136	1.5
	137–144	2
	145–149	2.5
	≥150	3
	Diabetics add another 3 points	3 ☐

10. Blood Pressure

Add scores for both readings (e.g., 144/88 score = 4)

Systolic	Diastolic	
≤120 ....(0)	≤80 ....(0)	0
121–130 ....(1)	81–90 ....(1)	1–2
131–140 ....(2)	91–98 ....(2)	2–4
141–150 ....(3)	99–106 ....(3)	3–6
≥151 ....(4)	≥107 ....(4)	4–8 ☐

11. Body Mass Index (BMI)

≤25.0	0
25.0–29.99	2
30.0–39.99	4
≥40.0	8 ☐

12. Smoking

Lifetime non-smoker	0
Ex-smoker more than 1 year	0
Ex-smoker less than 1 year	1
Smoke 1 cigarette/day or none	1
Nonsmoker, but live or work in smoking environment	2
Pipe or cigar smoker, or chew tobacco	3
Smoke 1–9 cigarettes/day	3
Smoke 10–19 cigarettes/day	4
Smoke 20–29 cigarettes/day	5
Smoke 30–39 cigarettes/day	6
Smoke 40 or more cigarettes/day	8 ☐

Subtotal Risk Score: ☐

Subtotal Risk Score (from previous page):

13. Tension and Stress	Are you:	
	Sometimes tense	0
	Often tense	1
	Nearly always tense	2
	Always tense	3

14. Personal History	Have you ever had a heart attack, stroke, coronary disease, or any known heart problem:	
	During the last year	8
	1–2 years ago	5
	2–5 years ago	3
	More than 5 years ago	2
	Never had heart disease	0

15. Family History	Have any of your blood relatives (parents, uncles, brothers, sisters, grandparents) had cardiovascular disease (heart attack, strokes, bypass surgery):	
	One or more before age 51	8
	One or more between 51 and 60	4
	One or more after age 60	2
	None had cardiovascular disease	0

16. Age	29 or younger	0
	30–39	1
	40–49	2
	50–59	3
	≥60	4

Total Risk Score:

How to Score

Risk Category	Total Risk Score
Very Low	5 or fewer points
Low	Between 6 and 15 points
Moderate	Between 16 and 25 points
High	Between 26 and 35 points
Very High....................................	36 or more points

II. Stage of Change for Cardiovascular Disease Prevention

Using Figure 2.4 (page 41) and Table 2.3 (page 41), identify your current stage of change for participation in a cardiovascular disease risk-reduction program:

III. In a few sentences, discuss your family and personal risk for cardiovascular disease:

IV. Discuss lifestyle changes that you have already implemented in this course, as well as additional changes that you can make to decrease your own risk of developing cardiovascular disease in the future.

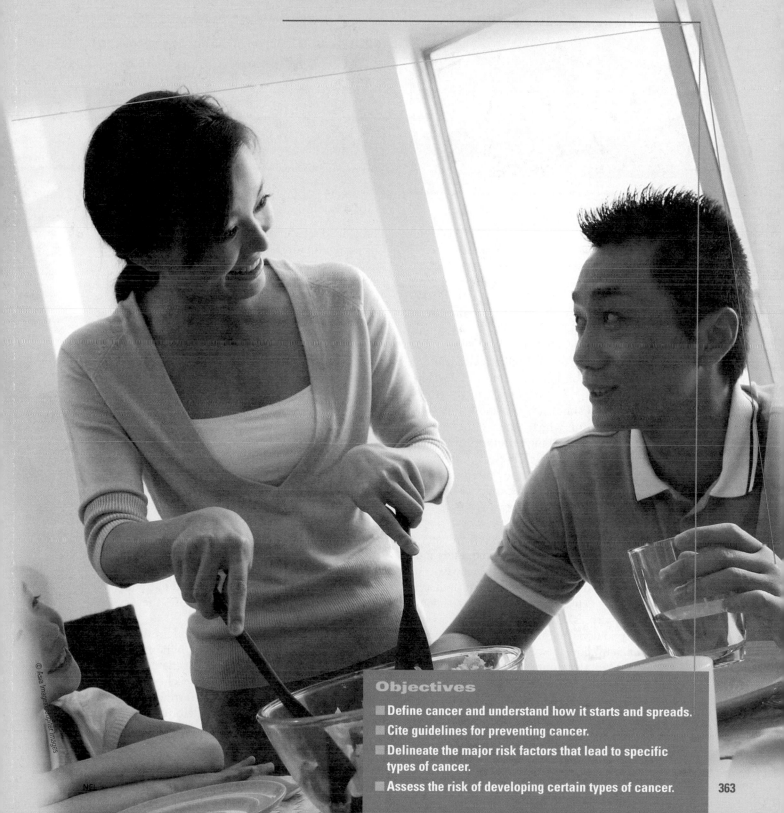

Chapter **12**

Cancer Prevention

Objectives

- Define cancer and understand how it starts and spreads.
- Cite guidelines for preventing cancer.
- Delineate the major risk factors that lead to specific types of cancer.
- Assess the risk of developing certain types of cancer.

363

FIGURE 12.1 Mutant (cancer) cells

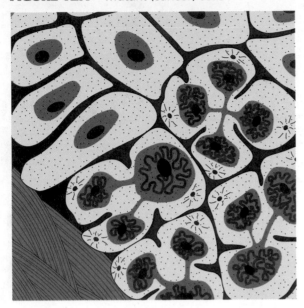

FIGURE 12.2 Erosion of chromosome telomeres in normal cells

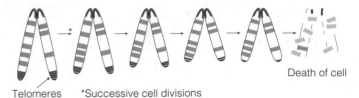

Telomeres   *Successive cell divisions

Death of cell

FIGURE 12.3 Action of the enzyme telomerase

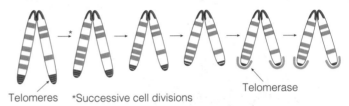

Telomeres   *Successive cell divisions   Telomerase

The human body has approximately 100 trillion cells. Under normal conditions, these cells reproduce themselves in an orderly way. Cell growth (cell reproduction) takes place to replace and repair old, worn-out tissue.

Cell growth is controlled by **deoxyribonucleic acid (DNA)** and **ribonucleic acid (RNA)**, found in the nucleus of each cell. When nuclei lose their ability to regulate and control cell growth, cell division is disrupted and mutant cells can develop (see Figure 12.1). Some of these cells might grow uncontrollably and abnormally, forming a mass of tissue called a tumour, which can be either **benign** or **malignant**. Benign tumours do not invade other tissues. Although they can interfere with normal bodily functions, they rarely cause death. A malignant tumour is a **cancer**. More than 100 types of cancer can develop in any tissue or organ of the human body.

The process of cancer actually begins with an alteration in DNA. Within DNA are **oncogenes** and tumour **suppressor genes**, which normally work together to repair and replace cells. Defects in these genes—caused by external factors such as radiation, chemicals, and viruses, as well as internal factors such as immune conditions, hormones, and genetic mutations—ultimately allow the cell to grow into a tumour.

A healthy cell can duplicate as many as 100 times in its lifetime. Normally, the DNA molecule is duplicated perfectly during cell division. In the few cases when the DNA molecule is not replicated exactly, specialized enzymes make repairs quickly. Occasionally, however, cells with defective DNA

keep dividing and ultimately form a small tumour. As more mutations occur, the altered cells continue to divide and can become malignant. A decade or more might pass between exposure to carcinogens or mutations and the time cancer is diagnosed.

The process of abnormal cell division is related indirectly to chromosome segments called **telomeres** (see Figure 12.2). Each time a cell divides, chromosomes lose some telomeres. After many cell divisions, chromosomes eventually run out of telomeres and the cell then invariably dies.

Scientists have discovered that human tumours make an enzyme known as **telomerase**. In cancer cells, telomerase keeps the chromosome from running out of telomeres entirely. The shortened strand of telomeres (see Figure 12.3) now allows cells to reproduce indefinitely, creating a malignant tumour.

Telomerase seems to have another function that is still under investigation: After many cell divisions, cancer cells grow old by nature, but telomerase keeps them from dying. If scientists can confirm that telomerase plays such a crucial role in the formation of tumours, research will be directed to finding a way to block the action of telomerase, thereby making cancerous cells die.

Cancer starts with the abnormal growth of one cell, which then can multiply into billions of cancerous cells. A critical turning point in the development of cancer occurs when a tumour reaches about one million cells. At this stage, it is referred to as **carcinoma in situ**. Such an undetected tumour may go for months or years without any significant growth. While it remains encapsulated, it does not pose a

FIGURE 12.4   How cancer starts and spreads

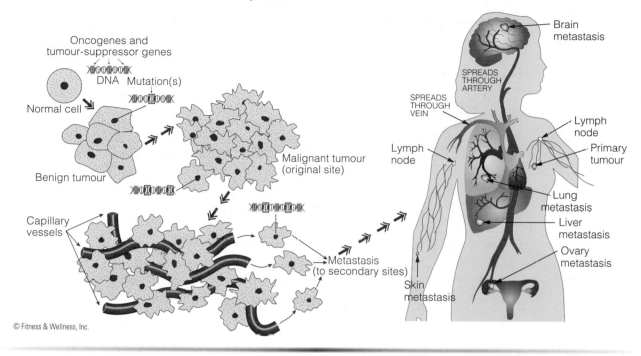

© Fitness & Wellness, Inc.

serious threat to human health. To grow, however, the tumour requires more oxygen and nutrients.

In time, a few of the cancer cells start producing chemicals that enhance **angiogenesis**, or capillary (blood vessel) formation into the tumour. Angiogenesis is the precursor of **metastasis**. Through the new blood vessels formed by angiogenesis, cancerous cells now can break away from a malignant tumour and migrate to other parts of the body, where they can cause new cancer (Figure 12.4).

Most adults have precancerous or cancerous cells in their bodies. By middle age, our bodies contain millions of precancerous cells. The immune system and the blood turbulence destroy most cancer cells, but only one abnormal cell lodging elsewhere is enough to start a new cancer. These cells grow and multiply uncontrollably, invading and destroying normal tissue. The rate at which cancer cells grow varies from one type to another. Some types grow fast, and others take years.

Once cancer cells metastasize, treatment becomes more difficult. Although therapy can kill most cancer cells, a few cells might become resistant to treatment. These cells then can grow into a new tumour that will not respond to the same treatment.

Incidence of Cancer

According to Statistics Canada, cancers were responsible for 29 percent of all deaths in Canada in 2001. Cancer is the second leading cause of adult deaths and, after unintentional injuries, the leading cause of death in children over one year. The major contributor to the increase in incidence of cancer during the last five decades is lung cancer. Tobacco use alone is responsible for 87 percent of lung cancer and accounts for 30 percent of all deaths from cancer. Death rates for most major cancer sites are declining, except for lung cancer in women (see Figure 12.5).

Deoxyribonucleic acid (DNA) Genetic substance of which genes are made; molecule that contains cell's genetic code.

Ribonucleic acid (RNA) Genetic material that guides the formation of cell proteins.

Benign Noncancerous.

Malignant Cancerous.

Cancer Group of diseases characterized by uncontrolled growth and spread of abnormal cells.

Oncogenes Genes that initiate cell division.

Suppressor genes Genes that deactivate the process of cell division.

Telomeres A strand of molecules at both ends of a chromosome.

Telomerase An enzyme that allows cells to reproduce indefinitely.

Carcinoma in situ Encapsulated malignant tumour that has not spread.

Angiogenesis Formation of blood vessels (capillaries).

Metastasis The movement of cells from one part of the body to another.

FIGURE 12.5 Breast, Prostate, and Lung Cancer Mortality (1984–2001) in Canada

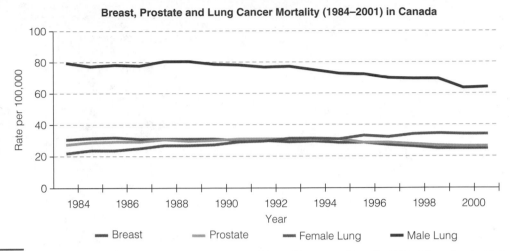

Source: Cancer Surveillance On-line: Cancer Mortality over Time, Public Health Agency of Canada, 2002. © Reproduced with the permission of the Minister of Public Works and Government Services Canada, 2008. Available from http://dsol-smed.hc-sc.gc.ca/dsol-smed/cancer/d_time_e.html

According to the best estimates, approximately two in five Canadian men and one in three Canadian women will develop cancer at some point in their lives. Also based on estimates, approximately 70,000 Canadians died from cancer and approximately 150,000 new cases were diagnosed in 2005. What this means is that one in 3.5 Canadian men and one in 4.3 Canadian women (approximately one in four of all Canadians) will die from some type of cancer.[1]

Statistical estimates of the incidence of cancer and deaths by sex and site for the year 2006 are given in Figure 12.6. These estimates exclude **non-melanoma skin cancer** and carcinoma in situ.

Like coronary heart disease, cancer is largely preventable. As much as 80 percent of all human cancer is related to lifestyle or environmental factors (including diet and obesity, tobacco use, sedentary lifestyle, excessive use of alcohol, and exposure to occupational hazards—see Figure 12.7). Most of these cancers could be prevented through positive lifestyle habits.

Research sponsored by the American Cancer Society and the National Cancer Institute showed that individuals who have a healthy lifestyle have some of the lowest cancer mortality rates ever reported in scientific studies. A group of about 10,000 members of the Church of Jesus Christ of Latter-Day Saints (commonly referred to as the Mormon church) in California was reported to have only about one-third (men) to one-half (women) the rate of cancer mortality of the general white population[2] (Figure 12.8). In this study, the investigators looked at three general health habits in the participants: lifetime abstinence from

smoking, regular physical activity, and sufficient sleep. In addition, healthy lifestyle guidelines (encouraged by the church since 1833) include abstaining from all forms of tobacco, alcohol, and drugs and adhering to a well-balanced diet based on grains, fruits, and vegetables, and moderate amounts of poultry and red meat. Lifestyle is definitely an important factor in the risk for cancer.

Equally important is that many people with a history of cancer are alive. Currently, 6 in 10 people diagnosed with cancer are expected to be alive 5 years after the initial diagnosis.[3] In the past when someone announced that they had cancer, there was silence as their prognosis was probably not good. Today, when someone announces they have cancer, the next question is always "What kind or type of cancer?" as many cancers, when detected early enough, are very treatable.

CRITICAL THINKING

Have you ever had, or do you now have, any family members with cancer? Can you identify lifestyle or environmental factors as possible contributors to the disease? If not, are you concerned about your genetic predisposition, and, if so, are you making lifestyle changes to decrease your risk?

Guidelines for Preventing Cancer

The biggest factor in fighting cancer today is health education. People need to be informed about the risk factors for cancer and the guidelines for early detection. The most effective way to protect against cancer is to change negative lifestyle habits and behaviours. Following are some guidelines for preventing cancer.

FIGURE 12.6 Deaths from various types of cancer in Canada

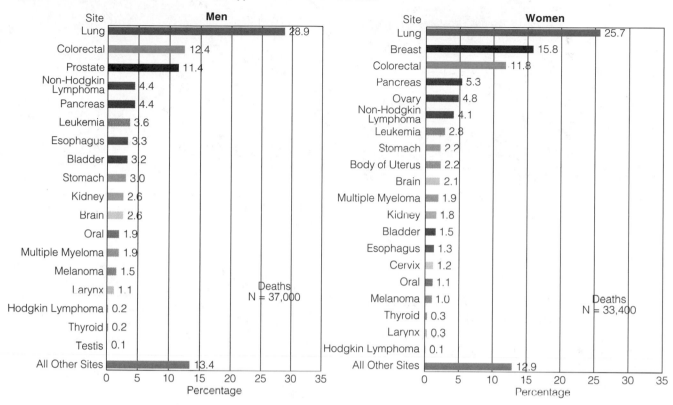

Canadian Cancer Society/National Cancer Institute of Canada: *Canadian Cancer Statistics 2006*, Toronto, Canada, 2006, pp.18–19
http://129.33.170.32/vgn/images/portal/cit_86751114/31/21/935505792cw_2006stats_en.pdf.pdf

FIGURE 12.7 Estimates of the relative role of the major cancer-causing factors

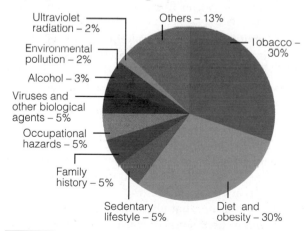

Source: Harvard Center for Cancer Prevention. *Causes of Human Cancer, Harvard Report on Cancer Prevention*, 1 (1996). Used with permission of the Harvard Center for Cancer Prevention.

FIGURE 12.8 Effects of a healthy lifestyle on cancer mortality rate

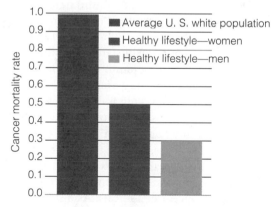

Note: Healthy lifestyle factors include proper nutrition, abstinence from cigarette smoking, regular sleep (7–8 hours per night), and regular physical activity.

Source: "Health Practices and Cancer Mortality Among Active California Mormons," *Journal of the National Cancer Institute* 81 (1989): 1807–1814, by permission of Oxford University Press.

Nonmelanoma skin cancer Cancer that spreads or grows at the original site but does not metastasize to other regions of the body.

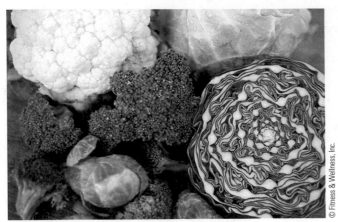

Cruciferous vegetables are recommended in a cancer-prevention diet.

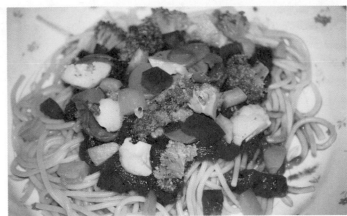

Nutrition guidelines for a cancer-prevention program include a diet low in fat and high in fibre, with ample amounts of fruits and vegetables.

Make Dietary Changes

Many cancers are related to nutrition. Therefore, a healthy diet is crucial to decrease the risk for cancer. The diet should be predominately vegetarian, high in fibre, and low in fat (particularly from animal sources). **Cruciferous vegetables**, tea, soy products, calcium, and omega-3 fats are encouraged. Protein intake should be kept within the recommended nutrient guidelines. If alcohol is used, it should be used in moderation. Obesity should be avoided.

Green and dark yellow vegetables, cruciferous vegetables (cauliflower, broccoli, cabbage, Brussels sprouts, and kohlrabi), and beans (legumes) seem to protect against cancer. Folate, found naturally in dark green leafy vegetables, dried beans, and orange juice, may reduce the risk for colon and cervical cancers. Brightly coloured fruits and vegetables also contain **carotenoids** and vitamin C. Lycopene, one of the many carotenoids (a phytochemical—see the following discussion), has been linked to lower risk of cancers of the prostate, colon, and cervix. Lycopene is especially abundant in cooked tomato products.

Researchers believe the antioxidant effect of vitamins and the mineral selenium help protect the body from oxygen free radicals. As discussed in Chapter 3 (under "Antioxidants," pages 73–74), during normal metabolism most of the oxygen in the human body is converted into stable forms of carbon dioxide and water. A small amount, however, ends up in an unstable form known as "oxygen free radicals," which are thought to attack and damage the cell membrane and DNA, leading to the formation of cancers. Antioxidants are thought to absorb free radicals before they can cause damage and also interrupt the sequence of reactions once damage has begun.

PHYTOCHEMICALS

A promising horizon in preventing cancer is the discovery of **phytochemicals**. These compounds, found in abundance in fruits and vegetables, apparently prevent cancer by blocking the formation of cancerous tumours and disrupting the process at almost every step of the way. Phytochemicals exert their protective action in the following ways:

- Removing **carcinogens** from cells before they cause damage.
- Activating enzymes that detoxify cancer-causing agents.
- Keeping carcinogens from locking onto cells.
- Preventing carcinogens from binding to DNA.
- Breaking up cancer-causing precursors to benign forms.
- Disrupting the chemical combination of cell molecules that can produce carcinogens.
- Keeping small tumours from accessing capillaries (small blood vessels) to get oxygen and nutrients.

Examples of phytochemicals and their effects are found in Table 12.1. Experts in this area recommend that to obtain the best possible protection, vegetables should be consumed several times during the day (instead of in one meal) to maintain phytochemicals at effective levels throughout the day. Research indicates that phytochemical blood levels drop within three hours of consuming the food containing phytochemicals.[4]

FIBRE

Although one recent study failed to show an association, many studies have linked low intake of fibre to increased risk for colon cancer. Fibre binds to bile acids in the intestine for excretion from the body in the stools. The interaction of bile acids with intestinal bacteria releases carcinogenic byproducts. The

TABLE 12.1 Selected Phytochemicals: Their Effects, and Sources

Phytochemical	Effect	Good Sources
Sulforaphane	Removes carcinogens from cells	Broccoli
PEITC	Keeps carcinogens from binding to DNA	Broccoli
Genistein	Prevents small tumours from accessing capillaries to get oxygen and nutrients	Soybeans
Flavonoids	Helps keep cancer-causing hormones from locking onto cells	Most fruits and vegetables
p-coumaric and chlorogenic acids	Disrupts the chemical combination of cell molecules that can produce carcinogens	Strawberries, green peppers, tomatoes, pineapple
Capsaicin	Keeps carcinogens from binding to DNA	Hot chili peppers

production of bile acid increases with higher fat content in the small intestine (created, of course, by higher fat content in the diet).

Daily consumption of 25 (women) to 38 (men) grams of fibre is recommended. Grains are high in fibre and contain vitamins and minerals—folate, selenium, and calcium—which seem to decrease the risk for colon cancer. Selenium protects against prostate cancer and, possibly, lung cancer. Calcium may protect against colon cancer by preventing the rapid growth of cells in the colon, especially in people with colon polyps.

TEA

Polyphenols (a phytochemical) are potent cancer-fighting antioxidants found in tea. Green, black, and red tea all seem to provide protection. Evidence also points to certain components in tea that can block the spread of cancers to other parts of the body.

Polyphenols are known to block the formation of **nitrosamines** and quell the activation of carcinogens. Green tea and black tea have similar amounts of polyphenols. Polyphenols are also thought to fight cancer by shutting off the formation of cancer cells, turning up the body's natural detoxification defences and thereby suppressing progression of the disease.

Green tea seems to be especially helpful in preventing gastrointestinal cancers, including those of the stomach, small intestines, pancreas, and colon. Consumption of green tea also has been linked to a lower incidence of lung, esophageal, and estrogen-related cancers, including most breast cancers.

Research on tea-drinking habits in China showed that people who regularly drank green tea had about half the risk for chronic gastritis and stomach cancer and the risk decreased further as the number of years of drinking green tea increased.[5]

In Japan, where people drink green tea regularly but smoke twice as much as people in the United States, the incidence of lung cancer is half that of the United States. The antioxidant effect of one of the polyphenols in green tea, epigallocatechin gallate, or EGCG, is at least 25 times more effective than vitamin E and 100 times more effective than vitamin C at protecting cells and the DNA from damage believed to cause cancer, heart disease, and other diseases associated with free radicals.[6] EGCG is also twice as strong as the red wine antioxidant resveratrol in helping prevent heart disease.

A cancer-prevention diet recommends drinking two or more cups of green tea daily. Herbal teas do not provide the same benefits as regular tea.

DIETARY FAT

High fat intake may promote cancer and excessive weight. Some experts actually recommend that total fat intake be limited to less than 20 percent of total daily calories.[7] Fat intake should consist of primarily monounsaturated and omega-3 fats (found in flaxseed and many types of fish), which seem to offer protection against colorectal, pancreatic, breast, oral, esophageal, and stomach cancers. Omega-3 fats block the synthesis of prostaglandins, bodily compounds that promote growth of tumours.

PROCESSED MEAT AND PROTEIN

Salt-cured, smoked, and nitrite-cured foods have been associated with cancers of the esophagus and stomach. Processed meats should be consumed sparingly and always with orange juice or other vitamin C-rich foods, as vitamin C seems to discourage the formation of nitrosamines. These potentially cancer-causing compounds are formed when nitrites

Cruciferous vegetables Plants that produce cross-shaped leaves (cauliflower, broccoli, cabbage, Brussels sprouts, and kohlrabi); they seem to have a protective effect against cancer.

Carotenoids Pigment substances in plants that are often precursors to vitamin A. More than 600 carotenoids are found in nature, about 50 of which are precursors to vitamin A, the most potent one being beta-carotene.

Phytochemicals Compounds found in fruits and vegetables that block formation of cancerous tumours and disrupt the progress of cancer.

Carcinogens Substances that contribute to the formation of cancers.

Nitrosamines Potentially cancer-causing compounds formed when nitrites and nitrates, which are used to prevent the growth of harmful bacteria in processed meats, combine with other chemicals in the stomach.

and nitrates, which are used to prevent the growth of harmful bacteria in processed meats, combine with other chemicals in the stomach.

Further, nutritional guidelines discourage the excessive intake of protein. The daily protein intake for some people is almost twice the amount the human body needs. Too much animal protein apparently decreases blood enzymes that prevent precancerous cells from developing into tumours. According to the U.S. National Cancer Institute, eating substantial amounts of red meat may increase the risk of colorectal, pancreatic, breast, prostate, and renal cancer.

Research also suggests that grilling protein (fat or lean) at high temperatures for a long time increases the formation of carcinogenic substances on the skin or surface of the meat. Microwaving the meat for a couple of minutes before barbecuing decreases the risk, as long as the fluid released by the meat is discarded. Most of the potential carcinogens collect in this solution. Removing the skin before serving and cooking at lower heat to "medium" rather than "well done" also seem to lower the risk.

SOY

Soy protein seems to decrease the formation of carcinogens during cooking of meats. Soy foods may help because soy contains chemicals that prevent cancer. Although further research is merited, isoflavones (phytochemicals) found in soy are structurally similar to estrogen and may prevent breast cancer, prostate, lung, and colon cancers. Isoflavones, frequently referred to as "phytoestrogens" or "plant estrogens," also block angiogenesis. Presently, it is not known if the health benefits of soy are derived from isoflavones by themselves or in combination with other nutrients found in soy.

One drawback of soy was found in animal studies in which animals with tumours were given very large amounts of soy. The estrogen-like activity of soy isoflavones actually led to the growth of estrogen-dependent tumours. Experts, therefore, caution women with breast cancer or a history of this disease to limit their soy intake because it could stimulate cancer cells by closely imitating the actions of estrogen. No specific recommendations are presently available as to the amount of daily soy protein intake for cancer prevention.

Based on the traditional diets of people (including children) in China and Japan who regularly consume soy foods, there doesn't appear to be an unsafe natural level of consumption. Soy protein powder supplementation, however, may elevate soy protein intake to an unnatural (and perhaps unsafe) level.

ALCOHOL

Alcohol should be consumed in moderation, because too much alcohol raises the risk for

BEHAVIOUR MODIFICATION PLANNING

TIPS FOR A HEALTHY CANCER-FIGHTING DIET

Increase intake of phytochemicals, fibre, cruciferous vegetables, and more antioxidants by

- Eating a predominantly vegetarian diet
- Eating more fruits and vegetables every day (six to eight servings per day maximize anticancer benefits)
- Increasing the consumption of broccoli, cauliflower, kale, turnips, cabbage, kohlrabi, Brussels sprouts, hot chili peppers, red and green peppers, carrots, sweet potatoes, winter squash, spinach, garlic, onions, strawberries, tomatoes, pineapple, and citrus fruits in your regular diet
- Eating vegetables raw or quickly cooked by steaming or stir-frying
- Substituting Tea, fruit, and vegetable juices for coffee and soda
- Eating whole-grain breads
- Including calcium in the diet (or from a supplement)
- Including soy products in the diet
- Using whole-wheat flour instead of refined white flour in baking
- Using brown (unpolished) rice instead of white (polished) rice

Decrease daily fat intake to 20 percent of total caloric intake by

- Limiting consumption of beef, poultry, or fish to no more than 85 to 170 g (about the size of a deck of cards) once or twice a week
- Trimming all visible fat from meat and removing skin from poultry prior to cooking
- Decreasing the amount of fat and oils used in cooking
- Substituting low-fat for high-fat dairy products
- Using salad dressings sparingly
- Using only half to three-quarters the amount of fat required in baking recipes
- Limiting fat intake to mostly monounsaturated (olive oil, canola oil, nuts, and seeds) and omega-3 fats (fish, flaxseed, and flaxseed oil)
- Eating fish once or twice a week
- Including flaxseed oil in the diet

developing certain cancers, especially when it is combined with tobacco smoking or smokeless tobacco. In combination, these substances significantly increase the risk for cancers of the mouth, larynx, throat, esophagus, and liver. In 1995, 3,443 alcohol-related deaths in Canada were attributed to cancers, cirrhosis, or other chronic conditions. The combined action of heavy alcohol and tobacco use can increase the odds of developing cancer of the oral cavity fifteenfold.

Maintaining recommended body weight is encouraged. Based on estimates, excess weight accounts for 14 percent of cancer deaths in men and 20 percent in women, respectively. Furthermore, obese men and women have an increased risk of

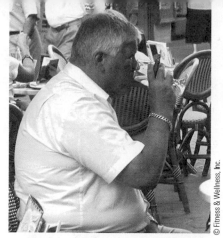

Heavy drinking and smoking greatly increase risk for oral cancer.

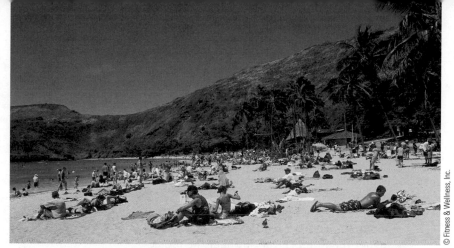

Tanning poses a risk for skin cancer from overexposure to ultraviolet rays. Tanned skin is the body's natural reaction to permanent and irreversible damage—a precursor to severe or fatal skin cancer.

more than 50 percent of dying from any form of cancer.[8] Obesity has been associated with cancers of the colon, rectum, breast, prostate, endometrium, and kidney.

Abstain from Tobacco

Cigarette smoking by itself is a major health hazard. Smoking was responsible for more than 45,000 unnecessary deaths in Canada in 2006. The World Health Organization estimates that smoking causes 5 million deaths worldwide annually. The average life expectancy for a chronic smoker is about 15 years shorter than for a non-smoker.[9]

The biggest carcinogenic exposure in the workplace is cigarette smoke. Of all cancers, at least 30 percent are tied to smoking, and 87 percent of lung cancers are linked to smoking. Use of smokeless tobacco also can lead to nicotine addiction and dependence as well as increased risk for mouth, larynx, throat, and esophageal cancers.

Avoid Excessive Exposure to Sun

Too much exposure to ultraviolet radiation (both UVB and UVA rays) is a major contributor to skin cancer. The most common sites of skin cancer are the areas exposed to the sun most often (face, neck, and back of the hands).

The three types of skin cancer are

1. Basal cell carcinoma
2. Squamous cell carcinoma
3. Malignant melanoma

In 2007, it was estimated that over 69,000 new cases of non-melanoma occurred in Canada.[10] Many of these cases were probably preventable by protecting the skin from the sun's rays. It was also estimated that **melanoma**, the most deadly type of

skin cancer, was responsible for over 900 deaths. Again, many of these deaths might have been prevented by either proper skin protection or early detection of the skin cancer.

Nothing is healthy about a "healthy tan." Tanning of the skin is the body's natural reaction to permanent and irreversible damage from too much exposure to the sun. Even small doses of sunlight add up to a greater risk for skin cancer and premature aging. The tan fades at the end of the summer season, but the underlying skin damage does not disappear. Ultraviolet rays are strongest when the sun is high in the sky. Therefore, you should avoid sun exposure between 10:00 A.M. and 4:00 P.M. Take the shadow test: If your shadow is shorter than you, the UV rays are at their strongest.

The stinging sunburn comes from **ultraviolet B (UVB) rays,** which also are thought to be the main cause of premature wrinkling and skin aging; roughened, leathery, and sagging skin; and skin cancer. Unfortunately, the damage may not become evident until up to 20 years later. By comparison, skin that has not been overexposed to the sun remains smooth and unblemished, and, over time, shows less evidence of aging.

Sun lamps and tanning parlours provide mainly ultraviolet A (UVA) rays. Once thought to be safe, they, too, are now known to be damaging and have been linked to melanoma. As little as 15 to 30 minutes of exposure to UVA can be as dangerous as a day spent in the sun. Similar to regular sun exposure, short-term exposure to recreational tanning at a salon causes DNA alterations that can lead to skin cancer.[11]

Melanoma The most virulent, rapidly spreading form of skin cancer.

Ultraviolet B (UVB) rays Portion of sunlight that causes sunburn and encourages skin cancers.

Sunscreen lotion should be applied about 30 minutes before lengthy exposure to the sun because the skin takes that long to absorb the protective ingredients. A **sun protection factor (SPF)** of at least 15 is recommended. SPF 15 means that the skin takes 15 times longer to burn than it would with no lotion. If you ordinarily get a mild sunburn after 20 minutes of noonday sun, an SPF 15 allows you to remain in the sun about 300 minutes before burning. The higher the number, the stronger the protection. When swimming or sweating, you should reapply waterproof sunscreens more often, because all sunscreens lose strength when they are diluted.

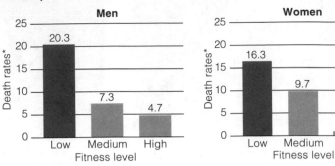

FIGURE 12.9 Association between physical fitness and cancer mortality

*Age-adjusted per 10,000 person-years at follow-up

Monitor Estrogen, Radiation Exposure, and Potential Occupational Hazards

Intake of estrogen has been linked to endometrial cancer in some studies, but other evidence contradicts those findings. As to exposure to radiation—although it increases the risk for cancer, the benefits of X-rays may outweigh the risk involved, and most medical facilities use the lowest dose possible to keep the risk to a minimum. Occupational hazards—such as asbestos fibres, nickel and uranium dusts, chromium compounds, vinyl chloride, and bischlormethyl ether—increase the risk for cancer. Cigarette smoking magnifies the risk from occupational hazards.

Engage in Physical Activity

An active lifestyle has been shown to have a protective effect against cancer. Although the mechanism is not clear, physical fitness and cancer mortality in men and women may have a graded and consistent inverse relationship (see Figure 12.9). A daily 30-minute, moderate-intensity exercise program lowers the risk for colon cancer and may lower the risk for cancers of the breast and reproductive system. Research has shown that regular exercise lowers the risk for breast cancer in women by 20 to 30 percent. In addition, growing evidence suggests that the body's autoimmune system may play a role in preventing cancer and that moderate exercise improves the autoimmune system.

Early Detection

Fortunately, many cancers can be controlled or cured through early detection. The real problem comes when cancerous cells spread, because they become

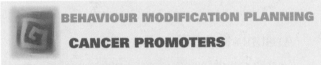

BEHAVIOUR MODIFICATION PLANNING

CANCER PROMOTERS

- Physical inactivity
- Being more than 4.5 kg overweight
- Frequent consumption of red meat
- A diet high in fat
- Charred/burned foods
- Frequent consumption of nitrate/nitrite-cured, salt-cured, or smoked foods
- Alcohol consumption
- Excessive sun exposure
- Estrogens
- Methyleugenol (flavouring agent in packaged foods)
- Radon
- Wood dust (high levels)

more difficult to destroy. Therefore, effective prevention, or at least early detection, is crucial. Herein lies the importance of periodic screening. Once a month, women should practise breast self-examination (BSE) (see Figure 12.12, page 377) and men, testicular self-examination (TSE) (see Figure 12.13, page 379). Men should pick a regular day each month (for example, the first day of each month) to practise TSE, and women should perform BSE two or three days after the menstrual period is over.

Other Factors

The contributions of many of the other much-publicized factors are not as significant as those just pointed out. Intentional food additives, sac-charin, processing agents, pesticides, and packaging materials currently used in developed countries seem to have minimal consequences. High levels of tension and stress and poor coping may affect the autoimmune system negatively and render the body less effective in dealing with the various cancers. In the workplace, the biggest carcinogenic exposure is cigarette smoke.

Genetics plays a role in susceptibility in about 10 percent of all cancers. Most of the effect is seen in the early childhood years. Some cancers are a combination of genetic and environmental liability; genetics may add to the environmental risk of certain types of cancers. "Environment," however, means more than pollution and smoke. It incorporates diet, lifestyle-related events, viruses, and physical agents such as X-rays and exposure to the sun.

Warning Signals of Cancer

Everyone should become familiar with the following seven warning signals for cancer and bring them to your physician's attention if any are present:

1. Change in bowel or bladder habits.
2. Sore that does not heal.
3. Unusual bleeding or discharge.
4. Thickening or lump in the breast or elsewhere.
5. Indigestion or difficulty in swallowing.
6. Obvious change in wart or mole.
7. Nagging cough or hoarseness.

The recommendations for early detection of cancer in asymptomatic people, outlined in Table 12.2, should be heeded in regular physical examinations as part of a cancer-prevention program. Although in most cases nothing serious will be found, any of the symptoms calls for a physician's attention as soon as possible. Scientific evidence and testing procedures for prevention and early detection of cancer do change. Studies continue to provide new information.

Treatment of cancer should always be left to specialized physicians and cancer clinics. Current treatment modalities include surgery, radiation, radioactive substances, chemotherapy, hormones, and immunotherapy.

In addition to becoming familiar with the warning signals of cancer, the Canadian Cancer Society also encourages lifestyle choices that will help prevent cancer and enable early detection of malignancy. In Lab 12A, you are encouraged to ask yourself how well you are doing with regard to a cancer-prevention program. The questions posed in this lab are based on information from the Canadian Cancer Society's Seven Steps to Health, presented in Table 12.3.

Assessing Your Risks

Explanations of the risk factors for a number of specific cancers are included in the following section, Common Sites of Cancer. These are the major risk factors for specific cancer sites and by no means represent the only ones that might be involved. As you read through this section, compare your personal status against the risk factors described. While there are certain risk factors that you cannot change such as your gender and age, there are other risk factors that you can control so that you reduce your risk of certain types of cancer. If you determine that many of the risk factors apply to you, you might want to discuss these risks with your family physician.

Common Sites of Cancer

Lung Cancer

RISK FACTORS

1. *Gender.* Men have a higher risk for developing lung cancer than women do, when type, amount, and duration of smoking are equal. Because more women are smoking cigarettes for a longer duration than previously, however, their incidence of lung and upper respiratory tract (mouth, tongue, and larynx) cancer is increasing. By type of cancer, lung cancer is now number one in mortality for women.
2. *Age.* The occurrence of lung and upper respiratory tract cancers increases with age.
3. *Smoking status.* Cigarette smokers have 20 times or even greater risk than non-smokers. The rates for ex-smokers who have not smoked for 10 years, however, approaches those for non-smokers.
4. *Type of smoking.* Pipe and cigar smokers are at higher risk for lung cancer than non-smokers. Cigarette smokers are at much higher risk than non-smokers or pipe and cigar smokers. All forms of tobacco, including chewing, markedly increase the user's risk of developing cancer of the mouth.
5. *Number of cigarettes smoked per day.* Males who smoke less than half a pack per day have lung cancer rates five times higher than nonsmokers. Males who smoke one to two packs per day have 15 times higher lung cancer rates than non-smokers. Males who smoke more than two packs per day are 20 times more likely than non-smokers to develop lung cancer.
6. *Type of cigarette.* Smokers of low-tar/nicotine cigarettes have slightly lower lung cancer rates.

Sun protection factor (SPF) Degree of protection offered by ingredients in sunscreen lotion; at least SPF 15 is recommended.

TABLE 12.2 Summary of Recommendations for Early Detection of Cancer in Asymptomatic People

Site	Recommendation
Breast	▪ Yearly mammograms are recommended starting at age 40. The age at which screening should be stopped should be individualized by considering the potential risks and benefits of screening in the context of overall health status and longevity.
	▪ Clinical breast exam should be part of a perodic health exam, about every three years for women in their 20s and 30s, and every year for women 40 and older.
	▪ Women should know how their breasts normally feel and report any breast change promptly to their health care providers. Breast self-exam is an option for women starting in their 20s.
	▪ Screening MRI is recommended in Canada for women with an approximate 20 to 25 percent or greater lifetime risk of breast cancer, including women with a strong family history of breast or ovarian cancer and women who were treated for Hodgkin disease.
Colon & Rectum	Beginning at age 50, men and women should follow one of the examination schedules below: ▪ A fecal occult blood test (FOBT) or fecal immunochemical test (FIT) every year ▪ A flexible sigmoidoscopy (FSIG) every five years ▪ Annual FOBT or FIT and flexible sigmoidoscopy every five years* ▪ A double-contrast barium enema every five years ▪ A colonoscopy every 10 years * Combined testing is preferred over either annual FOBT or FIT, or FSIG every five years, alone. People who are at moderate or high risk for colorectal cancer should talk with a doctor about a different testing schedule.
Prostate	The PSA test and the digital rectal exam should be offered annually, beginning at age 50, to men who have a life expectancy of at least 10 years. Men at high risk (and men with a strong family history of one or more first-degree relatives diagnosed with prostate cancer at an early age) should begin testing at age 45. For both men at average risk and high risk, information should be provided about what is known and what is uncertain about the benefits and limitations of early detection and treatment of prostate cancer so that they can make an informed decision about testing.
Uterus	**Cervix:** Screening should begin approximately three years after a woman begins having vaginal intercourse, but no later than 21 years of age. Screening should be done every year with regular Pap tests or every two years using liquid-based tests. At or after age 30, women who have had three normal test results in a row may get screened every two to three years. Alternatively, cervical cancer screening with HPV DNA testing and conventional or liquid-based cytology could be performed every three years. However, doctors may suggest a woman get screened more often if she has certain risk factors, such as HIV infection or a weak immune system. Women 70 years and older who have had three or more consecutive normal Pap tests in the last 10 years may choose to stop cervical cancer screening. Screening after total hysterectomy (with removal of the cervix) is not necessary unless the surgery was done as a treatment for cervical cancer.
	Endometrium: The American Cancer Society recommends that at the time of menopause all women should be informed about the risks and symptoms of endometrial cancer and strongly encouraged to report any unexpected bleeding or spotting to their physicians. Annual screening for endometrial cancer with endometrial biopsy beginning at age 35 should be offered to women with or at risk for hereditary nonpolyposis colon cancer (HNPCC).
Cancer-related Checkup	For individuals undergoing periodic health examinations, a cancer-related checkup should include health counselling and, depending on a person's age and gender, might include examinations for cancers of the thyroid, oral cavity, skin, lymph nodes, testes, and ovaries, as well as for some nonmalignant diseases.

American Cancer Society, *Cancer Facts & Figures 2008*, p. 68. Atlanta: American Cancer Society, Inc.

7. *Duration of smoking.* The frequency of lung and upper respiratory tract cancers increase with the length of time people have smoked.

8. *Type of industrial work.* Exposure to materials used in mining and asbestos industries and uranium and radioactive products have been demonstrated to be associated with lung cancer. Smokers who work in these industries have greatly increased risks. Exposure to arsenic, radon, radiation from occupational/medical/environmental sources, and air pollution increase the risk for lung cancer.

Colon/Rectum Cancer

RISK FACTORS

1. *Age.* Colon cancer occurs more frequently after 50 years of age.

2. *Family predisposition.* Colon cancer is more common in families that have a previous history of this disease.

3. *Personal history.* Polyps and bowel diseases are associated with colon cancer.

4. *Rectal bleeding.* Rectal bleeding may be a sign of colorectal cancer.

TABLE 12.3 Seven Steps to Health

Seven Steps to Health	Facts
1. Be a non-smoker and avoid second hand smoke.	Smoking causes about 30% of all cancer deaths in Canada. Lung cancer is the leading cause of cancer death for men and women in Canada. Smoking also increases your risk of developing cancers of the mouth, throat, larynx, cervix, pancreas, esophagus, colon, rectum, kidney and bladder. Non-smokers exposed to second-hand smoke are also at higher risk of getting cancer and other lung diseases. Health Canada estimates that more than 300 non-smokers die from lung cancer each year because of second hand smoke. If you are a smoker, quit. If you are a non-smoker, avoid second-hand smoke.
2. Eat 7–10 (19–50 years of age) servings of vegetables and fruit a day. Choose high fibre, lower fat foods. If you drink alcohol, limit your intake to 1–2 drinks a day	Research suggest as much as one third of all cancers may be related to what we eat and drink. Eat the recommended number of vegetables and fruit per day. Eat plenty of whole grain fibres and keep your dietary fat intake low. For a healthy diet, balance your daily meals with foods from the 4 food groups described in Canada's Food guide. If you drink alcohol, limit your consumption. Having one or more alcoholic drinks a day is associated with a slight increase in breast cancer risk. If you are pregnant or breast-feeding, avoid alcohol.
3. Be physically active on a regular basis: this will also help you maintain a healthy body weight.	Most people know that regular exercise is necessary to remain healthy. Studies strongly suggest that exercise reduces your risk of colon cancer. Also, the evidence of a link between physical activity and breast cancer is convincing.
4. Protect yourself and your family from the sun.	Be careful between the hours of 11 A.M. and 4 P.M. when the sun's rays are at their strongest or anytime of the day the UV Index™ is 3 or more. Check your skin regularly and report any changes to your doctor. Skin cancer is the most frequently diagnosed cancer in Canada.
5. Follow cancer screening guidelines	Even people with healthy lifestyles can develop cancer. One way to detect cancer early is to have regular screening tests. These tests can often find cancer when it is still at an early stage. The earlier the cancer is found, the more successful the treatment is likely to be. For women, discuss mammography, Pap tests, and clinical breast exams with a health professional. For men, discuss testicular exams and prostrate screening with a health professional. Both men and women should also discuss screening for colon and rectal cancers.
6. Visit your doctor or dentist if you notice any change in your normal state of health.	Know your body and report any changes to your doctor or dentist as soon as possible (for example, sores that do not heal, a cough which goes on for more than 4 weeks or a change in bowel habits). Health care professionals are trained to spot the early warning signs of cancer and other diseases.
7. Follow health and safety instructions at home and at work when using, storing, and disposing of hazardous materials.	Health Canada and Environment Canada have guidelines for handling cancer-causing substances. By following these guidelines, you can protect yourself against the risk posed by these materials. The guidelines are printed on the packaging and posted in workplaces.

Source: Based on information from the Canadian Cancer Society. Prevention. Seven Steps to Health. Retrieved May 19, 2008 at:
http://www.cancer.ca/ccs/internet/standard/0,3182,3172_12959__langId-en,00.html

A diet high in fat and low in fibre, inadequate consumption of fruits and vegetables, physical inactivity, a history of breast or endometrial cancer, and inflammatory bowel disease also increase the risk for colon or rectum cancer.

Skin Cancer

RISK FACTORS

1. *Sun exposure.* Excessive ultraviolet light is a culprit in skin cancer. Protect yourself with a sunscreen medication.

2. *Work environment.* Working in mines, around coal tar, or around radioactive materials can cause cancer of the skin.
3. *Complexion.* Individuals with light complexions need more protection than others.

The risk increases greatly with age, and family history also plays a role.

If any of these conditions apply to you, you need to protect your skin

CRITICAL THINKING

What significance does a "healthy tan" have in your social life? Are you a "sun worshiper" or are you concerned about skin damage, premature aging, and potential skin cancer in your future?

FIGURE 12.10 Warning signs of melanoma: ABCD rule

A. *Asymmetry:* One half of a mole or lesion doesn't look like the other half.

B. *Border:* A mole has an irregular, scalloped, or not clearly defined border.

C. *Colour:* The colour varies or is not uniform from one area of a mole or lesion to another, whether the colour is tan, brown, black, white, red, or blue.

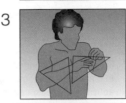

D. *Diameter:* The lesion is larger than 6 mm or larger than a pencil eraser.

¼"

Adapted from *FDA Consumer*, May 1991.

---

from the sun or any other toxic material. Changes in moles, warts, or skin sores are important and should be evaluated by your doctor (see Figure 12.10).

SKIN SELF-EXAM

One of the easiest and quickest self-exams is a brief survey to detect possible skin cancers (see Figure 12.11). A simple skin self-exam can reduce deaths from melanoma by as much as 63 percent.

- Make a drawing of yourself. Include a full frontal view, a full back view, and close-up views of your head (both sides), the soles of your feet, the tops of your feet, and the backs of your hands.
- After you get out of the bath or shower, examine yourself closely in a full-length mirror. On your sketch, make note of any moles, warts, or other skin marks you find anywhere on your body. Pay particular attention to areas that are exposed to the sun constantly, such as your face, the tops of your ears, and your hands.
- Briefly describe each mark on your sketch: its size, colour, texture, and so on.
- Repeat the exam about once a month. Watch for changes in the size, texture, or colour of moles, wart, or other skin mark. If you notice any difference, contact your physician. You also should contact a doctor if you have a sore that does not heal.

Breast Cancer

RISK FACTORS

1. *Age.* The risk for breast cancer increases significantly after 50 years of age.
2. *Race.* Breast cancer occurs more frequently in white women than any other group.

FIGURE 12.11 Self-exam for skin cancer

1 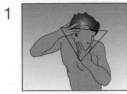 Examine your face, especially the nose, lips, mouth, and ears —front and back. Use one or both mirrors to get a clear view.

2 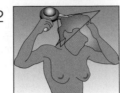 Thoroughly inspect your scalp, using a blow dryer and mirror to expose each section to view. Get a friend or family member to help, if you can.

3 Check your hands carefully: palms and backs, between the fingers, and under the fingernails. Continue up the wrists to examine both front and back of your forearms.

4 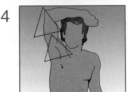 Standing in front of a full-length mirror, begin at the elbows and scan all sides of your upper arms. Don't forget the underarms.

5 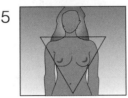 Next focus on the neck, chest, and torso. Women should lift breasts to view the underside.

6 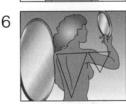 With your back to the full-length mirror, use the hand mirror to inspect the back of your neck, shoulders, upper back, and any part of the back of your upper arms you could not view in step 4.

7 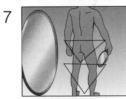 Still using both mirrors, scan your lower back, buttocks, and backs of both legs.

8 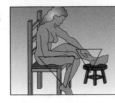 Sit down; prop each leg in turn on another stool or chair. Use the hand mirror to examine the genitals. Check front and sides of both legs, thigh to shin; ankles, tops of feet, between toes, and under toenails. Examine soles of feet and heels.

Reprinted with permission from *Family Practice Recertification* 14, no. 3 (March 1992).

3. *Family history.* The risk for breast cancer is higher in women with a family history of this type of cancer. The risk is even higher if more than one family member has developed breast cancer and is further enhanced by the closeness of the relationship of family member(s) (e.g., a mother or sister with breast cancer indicates a higher risk than a cousin with breast cancer).
4. *Personal history.* A previous history of breast or ovarian cancer indicates a greater risk.
5. *Maternity.* The risk is higher in women who never have had children and in women who bear children after 30 years of age.

Women should practise monthly breast self-examination (BSE—see Figure 12.12) and have their breasts examined by a doctor as part of a cancer-related check-up.

Clinical breast exams by a physician are recommended every 3 years for women between ages 20 and 40 and every year for women over age 40. The Canadian Cancer Society also recommends an annual **mammogram** for women over age 40. The latter is still an area of debate among health-care practitioners, and personal risk factors should be considered to determine the frequency of mammograms.

Other possible risk factors for breast cancer not listed in the questionnaire are a long menstrual

FIGURE 12.12   Breast self-examination

Looking
Stand in front of a mirror with your upper body unclothed. Look for changes in the shape and size of the breast, and for dimpling of the skin or "pulling in" of the nipples. Any changes in the breast may be made more noticeable by a change in position of the body or arms. Look for any of the above signs or for changes in shape from one breast to the other.

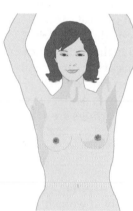
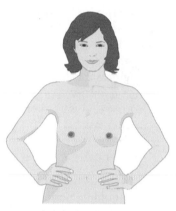

1. Stand with your arms down.

2. Raise your arms overhead.

3. Place your hands on your hips and tighten your chest and arm muscles by pressing firmly.

Feeling

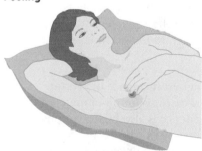
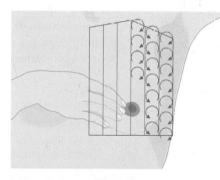
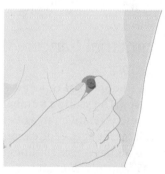

1. Lie flat on your back. Place a pillow or towel under one shoulder, and raise that arm over your head. With the opposite hand, you'll feel with the pads, not the fingertips, of the three middle fingers, for lumps or any change in the texture of the breast or skin.

2. The area you'll examine is from your collarbone to your bra line and from your breastbone to the centre of your armpit. Imagine the area divided into vertical strips. Using small circular motions (the size of a dime), move your fingers up and down the strips. Apply light, medium, and deep pressure to examine each spot. Repeat this same process for your other breast.

3. Gently squeeze the nipple of each breast between your thumb and index finger. Any discharge, clear or bloody, should be reported to your doctor immediately.

Source: From *An Invitation to Health,* 11th edition, by Hales. © 2005. Reprinted with permission of Wadsworth, a division of Thomson Learning, Inc.

Mammogram Low-dose X-rays of the breasts used as a screening technique for the early detection of breast cancer.

CANCER PREVENTION

history (onset of menstruation prior to age 13 and ending later in life), recent use of oral contraceptives or postmenopausal estrogens, drinking two or more alcoholic beverages per day, chronic cystic disease, and ionizing radiation. A diet high in fat has also been viewed as a predisposing factor, although more recent research has questioned its link to breast cancer.

Cervical Cancer (Women)

RISK FACTORS

1. *Age.* The highest occurrence is in the 40-and-over age group. The scoring numbers in the questionnaire represent the relative rates of cancer for different age groups—that is, a 45-year-old woman has a risk three times greater than a 20-year-old.
2. *Race.* Certain immigrant populations to North America have higher rates of cervical cancer.
3. *Number of pregnancies.* Women who have delivered several children have a higher occurrence.
4. *Viral infections.* Viral infections of the cervix and vagina are associated with cervical cancer.
5. *Age at first intercourse.* Women with earlier intercourse and with more sexual partners are at a higher risk.
6. *Bleeding.* Irregular vaginal bleeding may be a sign of uterine cancer.

Early detection through a Pap test during a pelvic exam should be performed annually in women who are or have been sexually active or who have reached the age of 18. Following three normal tests during three consecutive years, the Pap test may be done less frequently, at the discretion of the physician.

Endometrial Cancer (Women)

RISK FACTORS

1. *Age.* Endometrial cancer is seen in older age groups. The scoring numbers by the age groups represent relative rates of endometrial cancer at different ages—for example, a 50-year-old woman has a risk 12 times higher than that of a 35-year-old woman.
2. *Race.* White women have a higher occurrence.
3. *Births.* The fewer children the woman has delivered, the greater is the risk for endometrial cancer.
4. *Weight.* Women who are overweight are at greater risk.
5. *Diabetes.* Cancer of the endometrium is associated with diabetes.
6. *Estrogen use.* Cancer of the endometrium may be associated with prolonged and continuous intake of the estrogen hormone. This occurs in only a small number of women. Hormone replacement

therapy (progesterone plus estrogen) is thought to offset the increased risk related to estrogen use. You should consult your physician before starting or stopping any estrogen medication.
7. *Abnormal bleeding.* Women who do not have cyclic menstrual periods are at greater risk.
8. *Hypertension.* Cancer of the endometrium is associated with high blood pressure.

Additional risk factors that may be associated with endometrial cancer but are not included in the questionnaire are infertility, a prolonged history of failure to ovulate, and menopause occurring after age 55. Women over age 40 should have a yearly pelvic exam by a physician.

Other Cancer Sites

Following are other types of cancers whose risk factors have been outlined in *The Causes of Cancer*,[12] as well as in a series of pamphlets titled "Facts on Cancer." These types of cancer are presented, along with the risk factors associated with each type and preventive techniques to decrease the risk. No numeric weights for the risk factors have been assigned. As you read the information, however, rate yourself on a scale from 1 to 3 (1 for low risk, 2 for moderate risk, 3 for high risk) for each cancer site, and record your results in Lab 12B.

Prostate Cancer (Men)

The prostate gland is actually a cluster of smaller glands that encircles the top section of the urethra (urinary channel) at the point where it leaves the bladder. Although the function of the prostate is not entirely clear, the muscles of these small glands help squeeze prostatic secretions into the urethra.

RISK FACTORS

1. *Advancing age.* The highest incidence of prostate cancer (75 percent of cases) is found in men over age 65. The incidence is also higher among men of African heritage than whites, and more married men than single men develop this type of cancer.
2. *Family history.*
3. *Race.* African Americans have the highest rate in the world.
4. *Diet.* A diet high in fat.

PREVENTION AND WARNING SIGNALS
Prostate cancer is difficult to detect and control because the causes are not known. Death rates can be lowered through early detection and awareness of the warning signals. Detection is done by a digital rectal exam of the gland and a prostate-specific antigen

(PSA) blood test once a year after the age of 50. Possible warning signals include difficulties in urination (especially at night), painful urination, blood in the urine, and constant pain in the lower back or hip area.

Other factors that decrease the risk include increasing the consumption of selenium-rich foods (up to 200 mg per day), including consumption of tomato-rich foods and fatty fish in the diet two or three times per week, avoiding a high-fat (especially animal fat) diet, increasing daily consumption of produce and grains, taking a daily supplement of vitamin E (preferably mixed tocopherols), and maintaining recommended vitamin D intake (found in multivitamins, fortified milk, and manufactured by the body when exposed to sunlight).

Testicular Cancer (Men)

Testicular cancer accounts for only 1 percent of all male cancers, but it is the most common type of cancer seen in men between ages 25 and 35. The incidence is slightly higher in whites than in men of African heritage, and it is rarely seen in middle-aged and older men. The malignancy rate of testicular tumours is 96 percent, but if it is diagnosed early, this type of cancer is highly curable.

RISK FACTORS

1. *Undescended testicle* not corrected before age six.
2. *Atrophy of the testicle* following mumps or virus infection.
3. *Family history* of testicular cancer.
4. *Recurring injury* to the testicle.
5. *Abnormalities of the endocrine system* (e.g., high hormone levels of pituitary gonadotropin or androgens).
6. *Incomplete testicular development.*

PREVENTION AND WARNING SIGNALS

The incidence of testicular cancer is quite high in males born with an undescended testicle. Therefore, this condition should be corrected early in life. Parents of infant males should make sure that the child is checked by a physician to ensure that the testes have descended into the scrotum. Testicular self-examination (TSE) once a month following a warm bath or shower (when the scrotal skin is relaxed) is recommended. Guidelines for performing a TSE are given in Figure 12.13.

Some of the warning signs associated with testicular cancer are a small lump on the testicle, slight enlargement (usually painless) and change in consistency of the testis, sudden build-up of blood or fluid in the scrotum, pain in the groin and lower abdomen or discomfort accompanied by a sensation of dragging and heaviness, breast enlargement or tenderness, and enlarged lymph glands.

FIGURE 12.13 Testicular self-examination

How To Examine the Testicles

You can increase your chances of early detection of testicular cancer by regularly performing a testicular self examination (TSE). The following procedure is recommended:

- Perform the self-exam once a month. Select an easy day to remember such as the first day or first Sunday of the month.

- Learn how your testicle feels normally so that it will be easier to identify changes. A normal testicle should feel oval, smooth, and uniformly firm, like a hard-boiled egg.

- Perform TSE following a warm shower or bath, when the scrotum is relaxed.

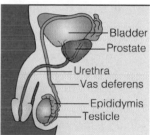

- Gently roll each testicle between your thumb and the first three fingers until you have felt the entire surface. Pay particular attention to any lumps, change in size or texture, pain, or a dragging or heavy sensation since your last self-exam. Do not confuse the epididymis at the rear of the testicle for an abnormality.

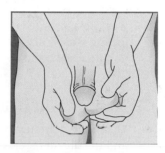

- Bring any changes to the attention of your physician. A change does not necessarily indicate a malignancy, but only a physician is able to determine that.

Early diagnosis of testicular cancer is essential, because this type of cancer spreads rapidly to other parts of the body. Because in most cases no early symptoms or pain is associated with testicular cancer, most people do not see a physician for months after discovering a lump or a slightly enlarged testis. Unfortunately, this delay allows almost 90 percent of testicular cancer to metastasize (spread) before a diagnosis is made.

Pancreatic Cancer

The pancreas is a thin gland that lies behind the stomach. This gland releases insulin and pancreatic juice. Insulin regulates blood sugar, and pancreatic juice contains enzymes that aid in digesting food.

POSSIBLE RISK FACTORS

1. *Increased incidence between ages 35 and 70*, but significantly higher around age 55.
2. *Cigarette smoking.*

3. *Chronic pancreatitis.*
4. *Cirrhosis.*
5. *Diabetes.*
6. *High-fat diet.*

Detection of pancreatic cancer is difficult because (a) no symptoms are apparent in the early stages, and (b) advanced disease symptoms are similar to those of other diseases. Only a biopsy can provide a definite diagnosis, but because it is primarily a "silent" disease, the need for a biopsy is apparent only when the disease is already in an advanced stage.

Warning signals that may be related to pancreatic cancer include pain in the abdomen or lower back, jaundice, loss of weight and appetite, nausea, weakness, agitated depression, loss of energy and feeling weary, dizziness, chills, muscles spasms, double vision, and coma.

Kidney and Bladder Cancer

The kidneys are the organs that filter the urine, and the bladder stores and empties the urine. Most of these two types of cancer are caused by environmental factors. Bladder cancer occurs most frequently between the ages of 50 and 70. Of all bladder cancers, 80 percent are seen in men, and the incidence among white males is twice that of men of African heritage.

POSSIBLE RISK FACTORS
1. *Heavy cigarette smoking.* Smoking is responsible for almost half of all deaths from bladder cancer in men and one-third of deaths from bladder cancer in women.
2. Congenital (inborn) abnormalities of either organ (these conditions are detected by a physician).
3. *Exposure to certain chemical compounds* such as aniline dyes, naphthalenes, or benzidines.
4. *History of schistosomiasis* (a parasitic bladder infection).
5. *Frequent urinary tract infections*, particularly after age 50.

PREVENTION AND WARNING SIGNALS
Avoiding cigarette smoking and occupational exposure to cancer-causing chemicals is important to decrease the risk. Bloody urine, especially in repeated occurrences, is always a warning sign and requires immediate evaluation. Bladder cancer is diagnosed through urine analysis and examination of the bladder with a cystoscope (a small tube that is inserted into the tract through the urethra).

Oral Cancer

Oral cancer includes the mouth, lips, tongue, salivary glands, pharynx, larynx, and floor of the mouth. Most of these cancers seem to be related to cigarette smoking and excessive consumption of alcohol.

RISK FACTORS
1. *Heavy use of tobacco* (cigarette, cigar, pipe, or smokeless) and/or alcohol drinking.
2. *Broken or ill-fitting dentures.*
3. *Broken tooth* that irritates the inside of the mouth.
4. *Excessive sun exposure* (lip cancer).

PREVENTION AND WARNING SIGNALS
Regular examinations and good dental hygiene help in prevention and early detection of oral cancer. Warning signals include a sore that doesn't heal or a white patch in the mouth, a lump, problems with chewing and swallowing, or a constant feeling of having "something" in the throat. A person with any of these conditions should be evaluated by a physician or a dentist. A tissue biopsy normally is conducted to diagnose the presence of cancer.

Esophageal and Stomach Cancer

The incidence of gastric cancer in Canada has declined in recent years. Cancer experts attribute this drastic decrease to changes in dietary habits and refrigeration. This type of cancer is more common in men, and the incidence is higher in men of African heritage than in white males.

RISK FACTORS
1. *A diet high in starch and low in fresh fruits and vegetables.*
2. *High consumption of salt-cured, smoked, and nitrate-cured foods.*
3. *Imbalance in stomach acid.*
4. *History of pernicious anemia.*
5. *Chronic gastritis or gastric polyps.*
6. *Family history* of these types of cancer.

PREVENTION AND WARNING SIGNALS
Prevention is accomplished primarily by increasing dietary intake of complex carbohydrates and fibre and decreasing the intake of salt-cured, smoked, and nitrate-cured foods. In addition, regular guaiac testing for occult blood (hemoccult test) is recommended. Warning signals for this type of cancer include indigestion for two weeks or longer, blood in the stools, vomiting, and rapid weight loss.

Ovarian Cancer (women)

The ovaries are part of the female reproductive system that produces and releases the egg and the hormone estrogen. Ovarian cancer develops more frequently after menopause, and the highest incidence is seen between ages 55 and 64.

RISK FACTORS

1. *Age.* Risk increases with age and peaks in the eighth decade of life.
2. *History of ovarian problems.*
3. *Extensive history* of menstrual irregularities.
4. *Family history* of breast or ovarian cancer.
5. *Personal history* of breast, bowel, or endometrial cancer.
6. *Nulliparity* (no pregnancies).
7. *Hereditary non-polyposis colon cancer.*

PREVENTION AND WARNING SIGNALS

In most cases, ovarian cancer has no signs or symptoms. Therefore, regular pelvic examinations to detect signs of enlargement or other abnormalities are highly recommended. Some warning signals may be an enlarged abdomen, abnormal vaginal bleeding, unexplained digestive disturbances in women over age 40, and "normal"-size (premenopause size) ovaries after menopause.

Thyroid Cancer

The thyroid gland, located in the lower portion of the front of the neck, helps regulate growth and metabolism. Thyroid cancer occurs almost twice as often in women as in men. The incidence also is higher in whites than people of African heritage.

RISK FACTORS

1. *Aging.*
2. *Radiation therapy* of the head and neck region received in childhood or adolescence.
3. *Family history* of thyroid cancer.

PREVENTION AND WARNING SIGNALS

Regular inspection for thyroid tumours is done by palpating the gland and surrounding areas during a physical examination. Thyroid cancer is slow-growing; therefore, it is highly treatable. Nevertheless, any unusual lumps in front of the neck should be reported promptly to a physician. Although thyroid cancer does not have many warning signals (besides a lump), these may include difficulty swallowing, choking, laboured breathing, and persistent hoarseness.

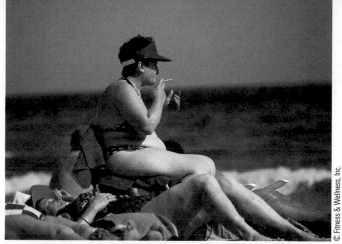

Cigarette smoking, obesity, and excessive sun exposure are major risk factors for cancer.

Liver Cancer

The incidence of liver cancer in Western countries is low. Men are more prone than women to liver cancer, and the disease is more common after age 60.

RISK FACTORS

1. *History of cirrhosis* of the liver.
2. *History of hepatitis B virus.*
3. *Exposure to vinyl chloride* (industrial gas used in plastics manufacturing) and aflatoxin (natural food contaminant).

PREVENTION AND WARNING SIGNALS

Prevention consists primarily of avoiding the risk factors and being aware of warning signals. Possible signs and symptoms are a lump or pain in the upper right abdomen (which may radiate into the back and the shoulder), fever, nausea, rapidly deteriorating health, jaundice, and tenderness of the liver.

Leukemia

Leukemia is a type of cancer that interferes with blood-forming tissues (bone marrow, lymph nodes, and spleen) by producing too many immature white blood cells. People who have leukemia cannot fight infection very well. The causes of leukemia are mostly unknown, although suspected risk factors have been identified.

POSSIBLE RISK FACTORS

1. *Inherited susceptibility,* but not transmitted directly from parent to child.
2. *Greater incidence in children with Down syndrome* (mongolism) and a few other genetic abnormalities.
3. *Excessive exposure to ionizing radiation.*
4. *Environmental exposure* to chemicals such as benzene.

PREVENTION AND WARNING SIGNALS

Detection is not easy because early symptoms can be associated with other serious ailments. When leukemia is suspected, the diagnosis is made through blood tests and a bone marrow biopsy.

Early warning signals include fatigue, pallor, weight loss, easy bruising, nosebleeds, paleness, loss of appetite, repeated infections, hemorrhages, night sweats, bone and joint pain, and fever. At a more advanced stage, fatigue increases, hemorrhages become more severe, pain and high fever continue, the gums swell, and various skin disorders occur.

Lymphoma

Lymphomas are cancers of the lymphatic system. The lymphatic system consists of lymph nodes found throughout the body and a network of vessels that link these nodes. The lymphatic system participates in the body's immune reaction to foreign cells, substances, and infectious agents.

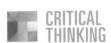

CRITICAL THINKING

You have learned about many of the risk factors for major cancer sites. How will this information affect your health choices in the future? Will it be valuable to you, or will you quickly forget all you have learned and remain in a Contemplation stage at the end of this course?

POSSIBLE RISK FACTORS

As with leukemia, the causes of lymphomas are unknown. People who have received organ transplants are at higher risk. Some researchers suspect that a form of herpes virus (called "Epstein–Barr virus") is active in the initial stages of lymphosarcomas. Risk of non-Hodgkin's lymphoma is higher in people who carry the human immunodeficiency virus (HIV) and human T-cell leukemia/lymphoma virus-I (HTLV-I) virus. Other researchers suggest that certain external factors may alter the immune system, making it more susceptible to the development and multiplication of cancer cells.

PREVENTION AND WARNING SIGNALS

Prevention of lymphoma is limited because little is known about its causes. Enlargement of a lymph node or a cluster of lymph nodes is the first sign of lymphoma. Other signs and symptoms are an enlarged spleen or liver, weakness, fever, back or abdominal pain, nausea/vomiting, unexplained weight loss, unexplained itching and sweating, and fever at night that lasts for a long time.

What Can You Do?

If you are at high risk for any form of cancer, you are advised to discuss this with your physician. An ounce of prevention is worth a pound of cure. Although cardiovascular disease is the number-one killer in the country, cancer is the number-one fear. Of all cancers, 60 to 80 percent is preventable, and about 50 percent is curable. Most cancers are lifestyle-related, so being aware of the risk factors and following the screening guidelines (Table 12.2, page 374) and basic recommendations for preventing cancer will greatly decrease your risk for developing cancer.

ASSESS YOUR KNOWLEDGE

1. Cancer can be defined as
   a. a process whereby some cells invade and destroy the immune system.
   b. an uncontrolled growth and spread of abnormal cells.
   c. the spread of benign tumours throughout the body.
   d. interference of normal body functions through blood-flow disruption caused by angiogenesis.
   e. All are correct choices.

2. Cancer treatment becomes more difficult when
   a. cancer cells metastasize.
   b. angiogenesis is disrupted.
   c. a tumour is encapsulated.
   d. cells are deficient in telomerase.
   e. cell division has stopped.

3. The leading cause of deaths from cancer in women is
   a. lung cancer.
   b. breast cancer.
   c. ovarian cancer.
   d. skin cancer.
   e. endometrial cancer.

4. Cancer
   a. is primarily a preventable disease.
   b. is often related to tobacco use.
   c. has been linked to dietary habits.
   d. risk increases with obesity.
   e. All are correct choices.

5. About 60 percent of cancers are related to
   a. genetics.
   b. environmental pollutants.
   c. viruses and other biological agents.
   d. ultraviolet radiation.
   e. diet, obesity, and tobacco use.

6. A cancer-prevention diet should include
   a. ample amounts of fruit and vegetables.
   b. cruciferous vegetables.
   c. phytochemicals.
   d. soy products.
   e. All of the above.

7. The biggest carcinogenic exposure in the workplace is
   a. asbestos fibres.
   b. cigarette smoke.
   c. biological agents.
   d. nitrosamines.
   e. pesticides.

8. Which of the following is *not* a warning signal for cancer?
   a. change in bowel or bladder habits
   b. nagging cough or hoarseness
   c. a sore that does not heal
   d. indigestion or difficulty in swallowing
   e. All of the above are warning signals for cancer.

9. The risk of breast cancer is higher in
   a. women under age 50.
   b. women with more than one family member with a history of breast cancer.
   c. minority groups than white women.
   d. women who had children prior to age 30.
   e. All of the above groups.

10. The risk for prostate cancer can be decreased by
    a. consuming selenium-rich foods.
    b. adding fatty fish to the diet.
    c. avoiding a high-fat diet.
    d. including tomato-rich foods in the diet.
    e. All of the above.

Correct answers can be found at the back of the book.

MEDIA MENU

INTERNET CONNECTIONS

■ Canadian Cancer Society. This comprehensive site features fact sheets and information on a variety of cancer types. The site explores treatment options. It features information for each province and territory network, and a search engine for local resources.

   http://www.cancer.ca

■ National Cancer Institute. This government site, from the National Institutes of Health, provides statistics, frequently asked questions, as well as information on research and support resources. It includes links to Web pages with information about specific cancers.

   http://www.nci.nih.gov

■ Susan G. Komen Breast Cancer Foundation. This site provides a wealth of breast cancer information including a video showing the correct way to perform a breast self exam, and the Komen NetQuiz, which allows you to test your breast cancer knowledge.

   http://www.komen.org/komen/index.htm

Notes

1. Canadian Cancer Society/National Cancer Institute of Canada: Canadian Cancer Statistics 2006.

2. J. E. Enstrom, "Health Practices and Cancer Mortality among Active California Mormons," *Journal of the National Cancer Institute* 81 (1989): 1807–1814.

3. American Cancer Society, *Cancer Facts & Figures—2004* (New York: ACS, 2004).

4. "Colorful Diet Helps Keep Cancer at Bay: Fruits and Vegetables Are Key," *Environmental Nutrition* 24, no. 6 (2001): 1, 6.

5. V. W. Setiawan et al., "Protective Effect of Green Tea on the Risks of Chronic Gastritis and Stomach Cancer," *International Journal of Cancer* 92 (2001): 600–604.

6. L. Mitscher and V. Dolby, *The Green Tea Book—China's Fountain of Youth* (New York: Avery Press, 1997).

7. J. H. Weisburger and G. M. Williams, "Causes of Cancer," *American Cancer Society Textbook of Clinical Oncology* (Atlanta: ACS, 1995): 10–39.

8. E. E. Calle, C. Rodriguez, K. Walker–Thurmond, and M. J. Thun, "Overweight, Obesity, and Mortality from Cancer in a Prospectively Studied Cohort of U.S. Adults," *New England Journal of Medicine* 348 (2003): 1625–1638.

9. American Cancer Society, *1995 Cancer Facts & Figures* (New York: ACS, 1995).

10. Canadian Cancer Society et al., "Canadian Cancer Statistics 2007," http://www.cancer.ca/vgn/images/portal/cit_86751114/36/15/1816216925cw_2007stats_en.pdf.

11. S. E. Whitmore, W. L. Morison, C. S. Potten, and C. Chadwick, "Tanning Salon Exposure and Molecular Alterations," *Journal of the American Academy of Dermatology* 44 (2001): 775–780.

12. Weisburger and Williams, "Causes of Cancer."

Suggested Readings

American Cancer Society. *Cancer Facts & Figures—2005*. New York: ACS, 2005.

American Cancer Society. "Causes of Cancer," *Textbook of Clinical Oncology*. Atlanta: ACS, 1995.

American Heart Association and American Cancer Society. *Living Well, Staying Well*. New York: Random House, 1999.

American Institute for Cancer Research. *Stopping Cancer Before It Starts*. New York: Griffin, 2000.

Canadian Cancer Society and National Cancer Institute of Canada. "Canadian Cancer Statistics 2007." http://www.cancer.ca/vgn/images/portal/cit_86751114/36/15/1816216925cw_2007stats_en.pdf.

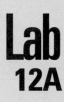

Lab 12A

CANCER PREVENTION—YOU CAN TAKE CONTROL

Name: _____   Date: _____

Instructor: _____   Course: _____   Section: _____

Necessary Lab Equipment
None required.

Objective
To encourage healthy lifestyle practises that will help decrease the risk for cancer.

I. Cancer Prevention: Are You Taking Control?

Today, scientists think most cancers may be related to lifestyle and environment—what you eat and drink, whether you smoke, and where you work and play. The good news, then, is that you can help reduce your own cancer risk by taking control of things in your daily life.

Ask yourself these questions and answer Yes or No   Yes   No

1. **Are you a non-smoker?** ☐ ☐

2. **Do you attempt to avoid second-hand smoke in work and play environments?** ☐ ☐

3. **If you are between 18 and 50 years of age, do you eat between 7 and 10 servings of vegetables and fruit a day?** ☐ ☐

4. **Do you choose high-fibre, low-fat foods?** ☐ ☐

5. **If you drink alcohol, do you limit your intake to 1 to 2 drinks per day?** ☐ ☐

6. **If you are pregnant or breast-feeding, do you abstain from alcohol?** ☐ ☐

7. **Are you physically active on a regular basis?** ☐ ☐

8. **If you are out in the sun do you protect yourself from the sun's rays, particularly between 11 A.M. and 4 P.M. when the sun's rays are at their strongest or when the UV Index is 3 or more?** ☐ ☐

9. **Do you check your skin regularly and report any changes to your doctor?** ☐ ☐

10. **Do you SLIP on clothing to cover your arms and legs?** ☐ ☐

11. **So you SLAP on a wide-brimmed hat?** ☐ ☐

12. **Do you SLOP on sunscreen (SPF 15 or higher)?** ☐ ☐

13. **Do you have regular cancer screening tests?** ☐ ☐

    Women—mammograms, Pap tests, clinical breast exams.

    Men—testicular exams and prostate screening. ☐ ☐

14. **Do you visit your doctor or dentist when you notice any changes in your normal state of health such as sores that do not heal, a cough that goes on for more than four weeks, or a change in bowel habits?** ☐ ☐

15. **Do you follow health and safety instructions at home and at work when you use, store, or dispose of hazardous materials such as household pesticides or any other chemicals?** ☐ ☐

If you answered "yes" to most of these questions, congratulations. You are taking control of simple lifestyle factors that will help you feel better and reduce your risk of cancer.

Lab 12B

CANCER RISK PROFILE

Name: _____ Date: _____ Grade: _____

Instructor: _____ Course: _____ Section: _____

Necessary Lab Equipment
None required.

Objective
To determine your stage of change for Cancer Prevention.

I. Stage of Change for Cancer Prevention

Identify your current stage of change for partcipation in a cancer-prevention program using information from Chapter 2.

_____

II. Personal Interpretation

In the space provided below, state your feelings about cancer and comment on any experiences that you may have had with cancer patients.

_____

_____

_____

_____

_____

_____

_____

_____

_____

III. Cancer Prevention

Discuss lifestyle habits that you should eliminate and habits that you might now adopt to reduce your own cancer risk. Also indicate how you can best implement and adhere to these changes.

_____

_____

_____

_____

_____

_____

_____

_____

_____

_____

_____

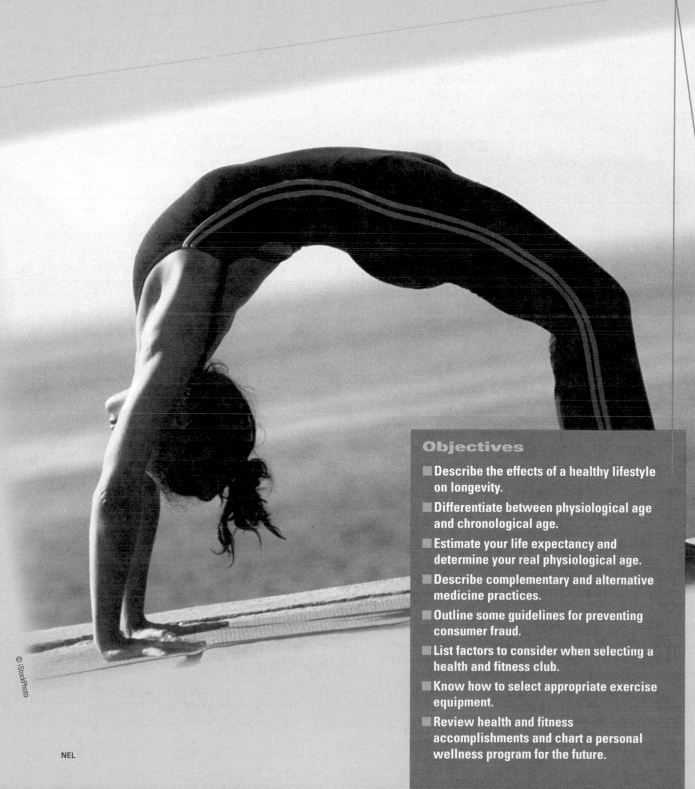

Chapter 13

Lifetime Fitness and Wellness

Objectives

- Describe the effects of a healthy lifestyle on longevity.
- Differentiate between physiological age and chronological age.
- Estimate your life expectancy and determine your real physiological age.
- Describe complementary and alternative medicine practices.
- Outline some guidelines for preventing consumer fraud.
- List factors to consider when selecting a health and fitness club.
- Know how to select appropriate exercise equipment.
- Review health and fitness accomplishments and chart a personal wellness program for the future.

© iStockPhoto

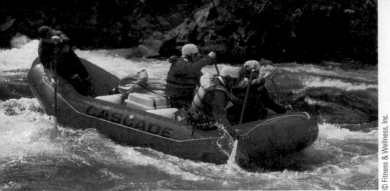

Good physical fitness provides freedom to enjoy many of life's recreational and leisure activities without limitations.

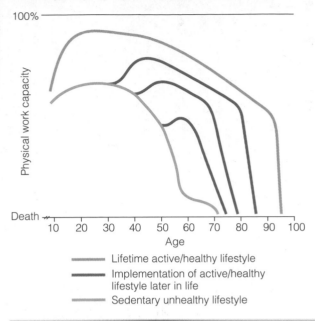

FIGURE 13.1 Relationships between physical work capacity, aging, and lifestyle habits

© Fitness & Wellness, Inc.

Physical work capacity

100%

Death

Age
10 20 30 40 50 60 70 80 90 100

——— Lifetime active/healthy lifestyle
——— Implementation of active/healthy lifestyle later in life
——— Sedentary unhealthy lifestyle

The three most important benefits to be derived from a lifetime fitness and wellness program are better health, a higher quality of life, and longevity. You have learned that physical fitness in itself does not always lower the risk for chronic diseases and ensure better health. Thus, implementation of healthy behaviours is the only way to attain your highest potential for well-being. The real challenge will come now that you are about to finish this course: maintaining your own lifetime commitment to fitness and wellness. Adhering to a program in a structured setting is a lot easier, but from now on, you will be on your own.

This chapter will help you evaluate how well you are adhering to health-promoting behaviours and the impact these behaviours may have on your **physiological age** and length of life. You will also learn how to chart a personal wellness program for the future.

Research data indicate that healthy (and unhealthy) lifestyle actions you take today will have an impact on your health and quality of life in middle and advanced age. In that most young people don't seem to worry much about health and longevity, you may want to take a closer look at the quality of life of your parents or other middle-aged and older friends and relatives you know. Though you may have a difficult time envisioning yourself at that age, their health status and **functional capacity** may help you determine how you would like to live when you reach your fourth, fifth, and subsequent decades of life.

Although previous research has documented declines in physiologic function and motor capacity as a result of aging, no hard evidence at present proves that large declines in physical work capacity are related primarily to aging alone. Lack of physical activity—a common phenomenon in our society as people age—is accompanied by decreases in physical work capacity that are greater by far than the effects of aging itself.

Data on individuals who have taken part in systematic physical activity throughout life indicate that these people maintain a higher level of functional capacity and do not experience the typical declines in later years. From a functional point of view, typical sedentary people in Canada or the United States are about 25 years older than their **chronological age** indicates. Thus, an active 60-year-old person can have a physical work capacity similar to that of a sedentary 35-year-old person.

Unhealthy behaviours precipitate premature aging. For sedentary people, any type of physical activity is seriously impaired by age 40 and productive life ends before age 60. Most of these people hope to live to be age 65 or 70 but often must cope with serious physical ailments. These people "stop living at age 60 but are buried at age 70" (see the theoretical model in Figure 13.1).

Scientists believe that a healthy lifestyle allows people to live a vibrant life—a physically, intellectually, emotionally, socially active, and functionally independent existence—to age 95. Such are the rewards of a wellness way of life. When death comes to active people, it usually is rather quick and not as a result of prolonged illness. In Figure 13.1, note the low, longer slope of the "unhealthy lifestyle" before death.

Life Expectancy and Physiological Age

Aging is a natural process, but some people seem to age better than others. Most likely, you know someone who looks much younger than his or her

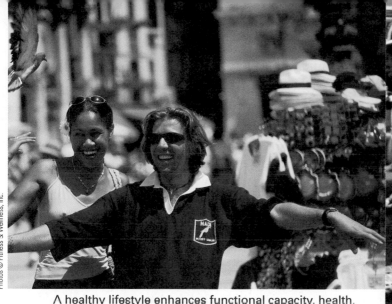

A healthy lifestyle enhances functional capacity, health, quality of life, and longevity.

chronological age indicates and, vice versa, someone who appears much older than their chronological age indicates. For example, you may have an instructor whom you would have guessed to be about 40, but in reality is 52 years old. Conversely, you may have a relative who looks 60 but who is actually 50 years old. Why the differences?

During the aging process, natural biological changes occur within the body. Although no one measurement can predict how long you will live, the rate at which the changes associated with aging take place depends on a combination of genetic and lifestyle factors. Your lifestyle habits will determine to a great extent how your genes will affect your aging process. Hundreds of research studies now point to critical lifestyle behaviours that will determine your statistical chances of dying at a younger age or living a longer life. Research also shows that lifestyle behaviours have a far greater impact on health and longevity than your genes alone.

CRITICAL THINKING

How long would you like to live, and are you concerned about how you will live the rest of your life?

Throughout this book, you have studied many of these factors. The question that you now need to ask yourself is: Are your lifestyle habits accelerating or decelerating the rate at which your body is aging? To help you determine how long and how well you may live the rest of your life, the Life Expectancy and Physiological Age Prediction Questionnaire, provided in Lab 13A, can help answer this question. By looking at 46 critical genetic and lifestyle factors, you will be able to estimate your **life expectancy** and your real physiological age. Of greater importance, most of these factors are under your own control and you can do something to make them work for you instead of against you.

As you fill out the questionnaire, you must be completely honest with yourself. Your life expectancy and physiological age prediction is based on your present lifestyle habits, should you continue those habits for life. Using the questionnaire, you will review factors that you can modify or implement in daily living and that may add years and health to your life. Please note that the questionnaire is not a precise scientific instrument but, rather, an estimated life expectancy analysis according to the impact of lifestyle factors on health and longevity. Also, the questionnaire is not intended as a substitute for advice and tests conducted by medical and health care practitioners.

Complementary and Alternative Health Care (CAHC)

Conventional Western medicine, also known as **allopathic medicine**, has seen major advances in care and treatment modalities during the last few decades. Conventional medicine is based on scientifically proven methods, wherein medical

Physiological age The biological and functional capacity of the body as it should be in relation to the person's maximal potential at any given age in the lifespan.

Functional capacity The ability to perform ordinary and unusual demands of daily living without limitations and excessive fatigue or injury.

Chronological age Calendar age.

Life expectancy How many years a person is expected to live.

Conventional Western medicine Traditional medical practice based on methods that are tested through rigorous scientific trials; also called **allopathic medicine**.

treatments are tested through rigorous scientific trials. In addition to a **primary care physician** (medical doctor), people seek advice from other practitioners of conventional medicine, including **osteopaths, dentists, oral surgeons, orthodontists, ophthalmologists, optometrists, physician assistants**, and **nurses**.

Notwithstanding modern technological and scientific advancements, some medical treatments either do not improve the patient's condition or create other ailments caused by the treatment itself.[1] Thus, many consumers are turning to **complementary and alternative medicine** or **CAM** or **complementary alternative health care** or **CAHC** (also called integrative health care) in search of answers to their health problems.

The reasons for seeking complementary and alternative treatments are diverse. Among the reasons commonly given by patients who seek unconventional treatments are lack of progress in curing illnesses and disease, frustration and dissatisfaction with physicians, lack of personal attention, testimonials about the effectiveness of alternative treatments, and rising health care costs. Some patients use it to either augment their regular medical care or to replace conventional practices.

According to Nadeem Esmail,[2] the author of a Fraser Institute report on complementary and alternative medicine in Canada, the majority of Canadians have used complementary and alternative health care services, with 74 percent of Canadians using at least one alternative therapy during their lifetime. Table 13.1 illustrates the percentage of Canadians using alternative therapies for wellness as a way of preventing future illness in 1997 and in 2006.

According to data collected by the American National Center for Complementary and Alternative Medicine (NCCAM) and the National Center for Health Statistics, 36 percent of American adults aged 18 and over used some form of CAM services in 2002.[3] People who use CAM tend to be more educated and believe that body, mind, and spirit all contribute to good health.

The NCCAM was established under the National Institutes of Health to examine methods of healing that previously were unexplored by science. CAM includes treatments and health care practices not widely taught in medical schools, not generally used in hospitals, and not usually reimbursed by U.S. medical insurance companies. CAM practices are grouped into four domains:[4]

1. **Mind-body medicine** used to enhance the mind's capacity in assisting the body to function. Mind-body techniques include cognitive-behaviour therapy (CBT), support groups, prayer, music, and dance.

2. **Biologically based practices** where herbs, foods, and vitamins are used to heal the body.
3. **Manipulative and body-based** practices, which include chiropractics and massage therapy.
4. **Energy medicine,** which includes biofield therapies such as Reiki therapy and therapeutic touch and bioelectromagnetic-based therapies, which involve the use of electromagnetic fields in unconventional ways.

Many alternative medicine practices have not gone through the same standard scrutiny as conventional medicine. Nonallopathic treatments are often based on theories that have not been scientifically proven. This does not imply that unconventional medicine practices are unhelpful. Many people have found relief from ailments or have been cured through unconventional treatments. More research studies are now being conducted using scientific trials similar to those in conventional medicine.

CAM includes a wide range of healing philosophies, approaches, and therapies. The practices most often associated with nonallopathic medicine are

TABLE 13.1 Use of Alternative Medicine or Therapies for Wellness in the Past 12 Months in Canada, by Therapy, 1997 and 2006

Practice	1997	2006
Yoga	86%	92%
Aromatherapy	66%	87%
Prayer/spiritual practice	83%	85%
Special diet programs	77%	83%
Lifestyle diet	87%	83%
Relaxation techniques	84%	81%
Naturopathy	69%	81%
Massage	66%	72%
High dose/mega vitamins	83%	71%
Herbal therapies	72%	70%
Self-help group	74%	67%
Chelation	100%	65%
Biofeedback	100%	64%
Energy healing	64%	63%
Osteopathy	100%	58%
Homeopathy	57%	58%
Imagery techniques	86%	56%
Spiritual or religious healing by others	59%	56%
Chiropractic care	46%	55%
Acupuncture	32%	48%
Hypnosis	78%	45%
Folk remedies	54%	43%

Base: Used therapy in past 12 months.

Esmail, Nadeem (2007). *Complementary and Alternative Medicine in Canada: Trends in Use and Public Attitudes, 1997–2006.* Fraser Institute. Public Policy Sources. Number 87/May 2007, Table 8, page 21. © The Fraser Institute, www.fraserinstitute.org. Retrieved May 2008 at: http://www.fraserinstitute.org/commerce.web/ publication_details.aspx?pubID=3213. Used with permission.

acupuncture, **chiropractics**, **herbal medicine**, **homeopathy**, **naturopathic medicine**, **ayurveda**, **magnetic therapy**, and **massage therapy**. Each of these practices offers a different approach to treatments, based on its beliefs about the body, some of which are hundreds or thousands of years old.

Many practitioners of these unconventional treatments believe that their modality aids the body in performing its own natural healing process. Inherent in these approaches, alternative treatments usually take longer than conventional allopathic medical care. Nonallopathic treatments are usually less harsh on the patient, and practitioners tend to avoid surgery and extensive use of medications.

Unconventional therapies are frequently called "holistic," implying that the practitioner looks at all the dimensions of wellness when evaluating a person's condition. Practitioners often persuade patients to adopt healthier lifestyle habits that will help them improve current conditions and also prevent other ailments from occurring. CAM further allows patients to better understand the treatments, and patients often are allowed to administer self-treatment.

Costs for CAM practices vary. Typically, patients pay directly for these services. According to Esmail[5] the average amount of money an individual Canadian paid to an alternative health care provider during the year before the Fraser Institute survey was conducted in 2006 was $173. This is an increase from $93 paid per user in 1997. These data suggest that overall, Canadians made more than $5.6 billion private payments to alternative health care providers. If payments for health books, herbs, vitamins, and special nutritional programs were included, the estimated total of private spending on alternative medicine in Canada could be calculated at approximately $7.84 billion in the last half of 2005 and the first half of 2006. If you are considering alternative medical therapies, some therapies may be reimbursable through your employer's health benefits plan.

CAM does have shortcomings, among them:

1. Many of the practitioners do not have the years of education given to conventional medical personnel and often know less about physiological responses that occur in the body.
2. Some practices are completely void of science; hence, the practitioner can rarely explain the specific physiologic benefits of the treatment used. Much of the knowledge is based on experiences with previous patients.
3. The practice of CAM is not regulated like that of conventional medicine. The training and certification of practitioners, malpractice liability, and evaluation of tests and methods used in treatments are not routinely standardized.

Many provinces do license practitioners in the areas of chiropractic services, acupuncture, naturopathy, homeopathy, herbal therapy, and massage therapy, but other therapies are unmonitored.

4. In Canada, we have just begun to monitor and regulate natural and herbal products. The word "natural" does not imply that the product is safe. Many products, including some herbs, can be toxic in large doses.

Primary care physician A medical practitioner who provides routine treatment of ailments; typically, the patient's first contact for health care.

Osteopath A medical practitioner with specialized training in musculoskeletal problems who uses diagnostic and therapeutic methods of conventional medicine in addition to manipulative measures.

Dentist Practitioner who specializes in diseases of the teeth, gums, and oral cavity.

Oral surgeon A dentist who specializes in surgical procedures of the oral–facial complex.

Orthodontist A dentist who specializes in the correction and prevention of teeth irregularities.

Ophthalmologist Medical specialist concerned with diseases of the eye and prescription of corrective lenses.

Optometrist Health care practitioner who specializes in the prescription and adaptation of lenses.

Physician assistant Health care practitioner trained to treat most standard cases of care.

Nurse Health care practitioner who assists in the diagnosis and treatment of health problems and provides many services to patients in a variety of settings.

Complementary and alternative medicine (CAM) or Complementary alternative health care (CAHC) A group of diverse medical and health care systems, practices, and products that are not presently considered to be part of conventional medicine; also called unconventional, nonallopathic, or integrative medicine.

Acupuncture Chinese medical system that requires body piercing with fine needles during therapy to relieve pain and treat ailments and diseases.

Chiropractics Health care system that believes that many diseases and ailments are related to misalignments of the vertebrae and emphasizes the manipulation of the spinal column.

Herbal medicine Unconventional system that uses herbs to treat ailments and disease.

Homeopathy System of treatment based on the use of minute quantities of remedies that in large amounts produce effects similar to the disease being treated.

Naturopathic medicine Unconventional system of medicine that relies exclusively on natural remedies to treat disease and ailments.

Ayurveda Hindu system of medicine based on herbs, diet, massage, meditation, and yoga to help the body boost its own natural healing.

Magnetic therapy Unconventional treatment that relies on magnetic energy to promote healing.

Massage therapy The rubbing or kneading of body parts to treat ailments.

5. A combination of high-dose vitamins and/or herbal supplements with prescription drugs can yield undesirable side effects. Therefore, individuals should always let their health care practitioners know which medications and alternative (including vitamin and mineral) supplements are being taken in combination.

Herbal medicine has been around for centuries. Through trial and error, by design, or by accident, people have found that certain plant substances have medicinal properties. Today, many of these plant substances have been replaced by products that are safer, more effective, and have fewer negative side effects. Although science has found the mechanisms whereby some herbs work, much research remains to be done.

Many herbs and herbal remedies are not safe for human use and continue to meet resistance from the scientific community. One of the main concerns is that active ingredients in drug therapy must be administered in accurate dosages. With herbal medicine, the potency cannot always be adequately controlled.

Also, some herbs produce undesirable side effects. For example, ephedra (ma huang), a previously popular weight loss and energy supplement, caused high blood pressure, rapid heart rate, tremors, seizures, headaches, insomnia, stroke, and even death. About 1,400 reports of adverse effects linked to herbal products containing ephedra, including 81 ephedra-related deaths, prompted its removal from the marketplace in the United States. St. John's wort, commonly taken as an antidepressant, can produce serious interactions with drugs used to treat heart disease. Ginkgo biloba impairs blood clotting; thus, it can cause bleeding in people who are already on regular blood-thinning medication or aspirin therapy. Other herbs, such as yohimbe, chaparral, comfrey, and jin bu juan have been linked to adverse events.

Increasingly, conventional health care providers will refer you to someone who is familiar with alternative treatments, but you have to be an informed consumer. Ask your primary care physician to obtain valid information regarding the safety and effectiveness of a given treatment. At times, the medical community will resist and reject unconventional therapies. If your physician is unable or unwilling to provide you with this information, other sources to search for this information include medical, college, or public libraries and popular bookstores. In any case, you need to educate yourself about the advantages and disadvantages of alternative treatments, risks, side effects, expected results, and length of therapy.

Information on complementary and alternative health therapies can be found on the Public Health

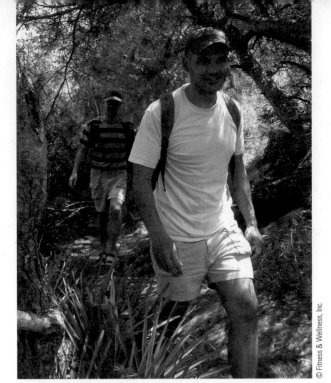

Frequent participation in recreational activities is important for health and wellness.

Agency of Canada Website at http://www.phac-aspc.gc.ca/chn-rcs/cah-acps-eng.php?rd= complement_eng. A document published by Health Canada titled the *Perspectives on Complementary and Alternative Health Care* also defines CAHC and provides some interesting information on the move toward an integrative health care approach in Canada. You can access this document at http://www.phac-aspc.gc.ca/publicat/pcahc-pacps/index.html.

The National Centre for Complementary and Alternative Medicine Health Information (NCCAM) housed within the National Institutes of Health (NIH) provides a comprehensive collection of information and research and can be accessed at http://nccam.nih.gov/

When you select a primary care physician or a nonallopathic practitioner, consult local and provincial medical boards, other health regulatory boards and agencies, and consumer affairs departments for information about a given practitioner's education, accreditation, and licence and about complaints that may have been filed against this health care provider. Many of the unconventional medical fields also have a national organization that provides guidelines for practitioners and health consumers. These organizations can guide you to the appropriate regulatory agencies in your province where you can obtain information regarding a specific practitioner.

You may also talk to other individuals who have undergone similar therapies and learn about the competence of the practitioner in question. Keep in mind, however, that patient testimonials do not adequately assess the safety and effectiveness of alternative treatments. Whenever possible, search for results of controlled scientific trials of the therapy in question and use this information in making your decision.

When undergoing any type of treatment or therapy, always disclose this information with all of your health care providers, whether conventional or unconventional. Adequate health care management requires that health care providers be informed of all concurrent therapies, so they will have a complete picture of the treatment plan. Lack of knowledge by one health care provider regarding treatments by another provider can interfere with the healing process or even worsen a given condition.

Many Canadians have benefited from CAM practices. You may also benefit from such services, but you need to make careful and educated decisions about the available options. By finding well-trained (and preferably licensed) practitioners, you increase your chances for recovery from ailments and disease.

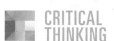

CRITICAL THINKING

Have you or someone you know ever used complementary or alternative medicine treatments? What experiences did you have with such treatment modalities, and would you use them in the future?

Quackery and Fraud

The rapid growth of the fitness and wellness industry during the last three decades has spurred the promotion of fraudulent products that deceive consumers into "miraculous," quick, and easy ways to achieve total well-being. **Quackery** and **fraud** are conscious promotions of unproven claims for profit.

Today's market is saturated with "special" foods, diets, supplements, pills, cures, equipment, books, and videos that promise quick, dramatic results. Advertisements for these products often are based on testimonials, unproven claims, secret research, half-truths, and quick-fix statements that the uneducated consumer wants to hear. In the meantime, the organization or enterprise making the claims stands to make a large profit from consumers' willingness to pay for astonishing and spectacular solutions to problems related to their unhealthy lifestyle.

Television, magazine, and newspaper advertisements are not necessarily reliable. For instance, one piece of equipment sold through television and newspaper advertisements promised to "bust the gut" through five minutes of daily exercise that appeared to target the abdominal muscle group. This piece of equipment consisted of a metal spring attached to the feet on one end and held in the hands on the other end. According to handling and shipping distributors, the equipment was "selling like hotcakes" and companies could barely keep up with consumer demands.

Three problems became apparent to the educated consumer: First, there is no such thing as spot reducing; therefore, the claims could not be true. Second, exercising five minutes daily burns hardly any calories and, therefore, has no effect on weight loss. Third, the intended abdominal (gut) muscles were not really involved; the exercise engaged mostly the gluteal and lower back muscles. This piece of equipment now can be found at garage sales for about a tenth of its original cost!

Although people in Western countries tend to be firm believers in the benefits of physical activity and positive lifestyle habits as a means to promote better health, most do not reap these benefits because they simply do not know how to put into practice a sound fitness and wellness program that will give them the results they want. Unfortunately, many uneducated wellness consumers are targets of deception by organizations making fraudulent claims for their products.

Deception is not limited to advertisements. Deceit is all around us—in newspaper and magazine articles, trade books, radio, and television. To make a profit, popular magazines occasionally exaggerate health claims or leave out pertinent information to avoid offending advertisers. Some publishers print books on diets or self-treatment approaches that have no scientific foundation. Consumers should even be cautious about news reports of the latest medical breakthroughs. Reporters have been known to overlook important information or give certain findings more credence than they deserve.

Precautions must also be taken when seeking health advice on the Internet. The Internet is full of both credible and dubious information. The following tips can help as you conduct a search on the Internet:

- Look for credentials of the person or organization sponsoring the site.
- Check when the site was last updated. Credible sites are updated often.
- Check the appearance of the information on the site. It should be presented in a professional manner. For instance, if every sentence ends with an exclamation mark, you have a good cause for suspicion.
- Be cautious if the site's sponsor is trying to sell a product. Be leery of opinions posted on the site. They could be biased, given that the company's main objective is to sell a product. Credible companies trying to sell a product on the Internet usually reference their sources of health information and provide additional links that support their product.
- Compare the content of a site to other credible sources. The content should be generally similar to that of other reputable sites or publications.

Quackery/fraud The conscious promotion of unproven claims for profit.

- Note the address and contact information for the company. A reliable company will list more than a post office box, an 800 number, and the company's email address. When only this information is provided, consumers may never be able to locate the company for questions, concerns, or refunds.
- Be on the alert for companies that claim to be innovators while criticizing competitors or the government for being close-minded or trying to keep them from doing business.
- Watch for advertisers that use valid medical terminology in an irrelevant context or use vague pseudomedical jargon to sell their products.

Not all people who promote fraudulent products, however, know they are doing so. Some may be convinced that the product they are promoting is effective. If you have questions or concerns about a health product, you may contact the Competition Bureau Canada (www.competitionbureau.gc.ca). The purpose of this organization is to provide the consumer with responsible, reliable, evidence-driven health information. The organization also monitors deceitful advertising, investigates complaints, and offers public information regarding fraudulent health claims.

Other consumer-protection organizations offer to follow up on complaints about quackery and fraud. The assurance of these organizations, however, should not give the consumer a false sense of security. The overwhelming number of complaints they receive each year makes it impossible for them to follow up on each case individually. The FDA's Center for Drug Evaluation Research in the United States, for example, has developed a priority system to determine which health fraud product it should regulate first. Products are rated on how great a risk they pose to the consumer. With this in mind, you can use the following list of U.S. organizations to make an educated decision before you spend your money. You can also report consumer fraud to these organizations:

- Food and Drug Administration (FDA). The FDA regulates safety and labelling of health products and cosmetics. You can search for the office closest to you in the federal government listings (blue pages) of the phone book.
- Better Business Bureau (BBB). The BBB can tell you whether other customers have lodged complaints about a product, a company, or a salesperson. You can find a listing for the local office in the business section of the phone book, or you can check the BBB Web site at http://www.betterbusinessbureau.com/.
- Consumer Product Safety Commission (CPS). This independent federal regulatory agency targets products that threaten the safety of American

RELIABLE SOURCES OF HEALTH, FITNESS, NUTRITION, AND WELLNESS INFORMATION

Health Canada is the federal department responsible for helping Canadians maintain and improve their health, while respecting individual choices and circumstances: http://www.hc-sc.gc.ca/ahc-asc/index_e.html.

The Canadian Council of Better Business Bureaus (CCBBB) governs 14 Better Business Bureaus across Canada. Its mission is to promote and foster the highest ethical relationship between businesses and the public through voluntary self-regulation, consumer and business education, and service excellence: http://www.ccbbb.ca/.

Consumer Product Safety is a branch of Health Canada that helps protect the Canadian public by researching, assessing, and collaborating in the management of the health risks and safety hazards associated with the many consumer products, including pest management products, that Canadians use every day: http://www.hc-sc.gc.ca/cps-spc/index_e.html.

Canada's Office of Consumer Affairs (OCA) is involved in supporting regulations for consumer protection and educates consumers in a range of areas: http://www.ic.gc.ca/epic/site/oca-bc.nsf/en/Home.

families. Unsafe products can be researched and reported on its Web site at http://www.cpsc.gov/.

Another way to get informed before making your purchase is to seek the advice of a reputable professional. Ask someone who understands the product but does not stand to profit from the transaction. As examples, a physical educator or an exercise physiologist can advise you regarding exercise equipment; a registered dietician can provide information on nutrition and weight-control programs; a physician can offer advice on nutritive supplements. Also, be alert to those who bill themselves as "experts." Look for qualifications, degrees, professional experience, certifications, and reputation.

Keep in mind that if it sounds too good to be true, it probably is. Fraudulent promotions often rely on testimonials or scare tactics and promise that their products will cure a long list of unrelated ailments; they use words like quick-fix, time-tested, new-found, miraculous, special, secret, all-natural, mail-order only, and money-back guarantee. Deceptive companies move often so customers have no way of contacting the company to request a reimbursement.

When claims are made, ask where the claims are published. Refereed scientific journals are the most reliable sources of information. When a researcher submits information for publication in a refereed journal, at least two qualified and reputable professionals in the field conduct blind reviews of the manuscript. A blind review means that the author does not know who will review the manuscript and the reviewers do not know who submitted the manuscript. Acceptance for publication is based on this input and relevant changes.

Deciding Your Fitness Future

Once you've decided to pursue a lifetime wellness program, you'll face several more decisions about exactly how to accomplish it. Following are some issues you'll encounter.

Health and Fitness Club Memberships

You may want to consider joining a health and fitness facility. Or, if you have mastered the contents of this book and your choice of fitness activity is one you can pursue on your own (walking, jogging, cycling), you may not need to join a health club. Barring injuries, you may continue your exercise program outside the walls of a health club for the rest of your life. You also can conduct strength training and stretching programs (see Chapters 7 and 8) in your own home.

To stay up-to-date on fitness and wellness developments, you probably should buy a reputable and updated fitness/wellness book every four to five years. You may subscribe to a credible health, fitness, nutrition, or wellness newsletter to stay current. You also can surf the World Wide Web, but be sure that the sites you are searching are from credible and reliable organizations.

If you are contemplating membership in a fitness facility, do all of the following:

■ Make sure that the facility complies with the standards established by the Canadian Society for Exercise Physiology (CSEP) or the American College of Sports Medicine (ACSM) for health and fitness facilities. These standards are given in Figure 13.2.

■ Examine all exercise options in your community: health clubs/spas, YMCAs, gyms, colleges, schools, community centres, seniors centres, and the like.

■ Check to see if the facility's atmosphere is pleasurable and nonthreatening to you. Will you feel comfortable with the instructors and other people who go there? Is it clean and well kept up? If the answer is no, this may not be the right place for you.

■ Analyze costs versus facilities, equipment, and programs. Take a look at your personal budget.

FIGURE 13.2 Standards for health and fitness facilities

1. A facility must have an appropriate emergency plan.
2. A facility must offer each adult member a preactivity screening that is relevant to the activities that will be performed by the member.
3. Each person who has supervisory responsibility must be professionally competent.
4. A facility must post appropriate signs in those areas of a facility that present potential increased risk.
5. A facility that offers services or programs to youths must provide appropriate supervision.
6. A facility must conform to all relevant laws, regulations, and published standards.
7. Accredited Fitness Appraisal Centres must follow CSEP (Canadian Society for Exercise Physiology) operation and safety guidelines and employ CSEP Certified Personal Trainers and Certified Exercise Physiologists.

Adapted from ACSM's *Health/Fitness Facility Standards and Guidelines*. (Champaign, IL: Human Kinetics, 1997) and CSEP Health and Fitness Program Certifications for Fitness Professionals, CSEP, Professional Certifications, www.csep.ca.

Will you really use the facility? Will you exercise there regularly? Many people obtain memberships and permit dues to be withdrawn automatically from a local bank account, yet seldom attend the fitness centre.

■ Find out what types of facilities are available: walking or running track; basketball, tennis, or racquetball courts; aerobic exercise room; strength training room; pool; locker rooms; saunas; hot tubs; handicapped access; and so on.

■ Check the aerobic and strength-training equipment available. Does the facility have treadmills, bicycle ergometers, stair climbers, cross-country skiing simulators, free weights, strength-training machines? Make sure the facilities and equipment meet your activity interests.

■ Consider the location. Is the facility close, or do you have to travel several kilometres to get there? Distance often discourages participation.

■ Check on times the facility is accessible. Is it open during your preferred exercise time (for example, early morning or late evening)?

■ Work out at the facility several times before becoming a member. Are people standing in line to use the equipment, or is it readily available during your exercise time?

■ Inquire about the instructors' qualifications. Do the fitness instructors have college degrees or professional certifications from organizations such as the Canadian Society for Exercise Physiology?

These organizations have rigorous standards to ensure professional preparation and quality of instruction.

- Consider the approach to fitness (including all health-related components of fitness). Is it well-rounded? Do the instructors spend time with members, or do members have to seek them out constantly for help and instruction?
- Ask about supplementary services. Does the facility provide or contract out for regular health and fitness assessments (cardiovascular endurance, body composition, blood pressure, blood chemistry analysis)? Does it offer wellness seminars (nutrition, weight control, stress management)? Do these have hidden costs?

Personal Trainers

In recent years, personal trainers have been in high demand by health and fitness participants. A **personal trainer** is a health and fitness professional who evaluates, motivates, educates, and trains clients to help them meet individualized healthy lifestyle goals. Rates typically start at $40 an hour and go up from there. Exercise sessions are usually conducted at a health and fitness facility or at the client's own home. Experience and the ability to design safe and effective programs based on the client's current fitness level, health status, and fitness goals are important. Personal trainers also recognize their limitations and refer clients to other health care professionals as necessary.

Currently, anyone who prescribes exercise can call himself or herself a personal trainer without proof of education, experience, or certification. Although good trainers should strive to maximize their own health and fitness, a good physique and previous athletic experience do not certify a person as a personal trainer. In 1981, a program was established by the Canadian Society for Exercise Physiology (CSEP) to address the needs and concerns of personnel working in the physical activity, fitness, and lifestyle appraisal industry in Canada. The CSEP Health and Fitness Program has the highest standards in the Canadian industry for fitness professionals and offers an introductory as well as an advanced level of certification.

Because of the high demand for personal trainers, more than 200 organizations now provide some type of certification to fitness specialists. This has led to great confusion by clients on how to evaluate the credentials of personal trainers. There is also a clear distinction between "certification" and a "certificate." Certification implies that the individual has met educational and professional standards of performance and competence. A certificate is typically awarded to individuals who attend a conference or workshop but are not required to meet any professional standards.

Presently, there is no licensing body that oversees personal trainers. Thus, it is easy to become a personal trainer. At a minimum, personal trainers should have an undergraduate degree and certification from a reputable organization such as the American College of Sports Medicine or the International Dance Exercise Association (IDEA). Undergraduate (and graduate) degrees should be conferred in a fitness-related area such as exercise science, exercise physiology, kinesiology, sports medicine, or physical education.

ACSM offers three certification levels: group exercise leader, health/fitness instructor, and health/fitness director. IDEA offers four levels: professional, advanced, elite, and master. For both ACSM and IDEA, each level of certification is progressively more difficult to obtain. A third organization, the National Strength and Conditioning Association (NSCA), also offers a personal trainer's certification program. When looking for a personal trainer, always inquire about the trainer's education and certification credentials.

As a final word of caution when seeking fitness advice from a health and fitness trainer via the Internet: Be aware that certain services cannot be provided over the Internet. An Internet trainer is not able to directly administer fitness tests, motivate, observe exercise limitations, or respond effectively in an emergency situation (spotting, administering first-aid or CPR), and thus, is not able to design the most safe and effective exercise program for you.

Purchasing Exercise Equipment

A final consideration addressed in this book is that of purchasing your own exercise equipment. The first question to ask yourself is whether you really need this piece of equipment. Most people buy on impulse because of television advertisements or because a salesperson has convinced them it is a great piece of equipment that will do wonders for their health and fitness. Ignore claims that an exercise device or machine can provide "easy/no-sweat" results in only a few minutes. Keep in mind that the benefits of exercise are obtained only if you do exercise. With some creativity, you can implement an excellent and comprehensive exercise program with little, if any, equipment (see Chapters 6, 7, 8, and 9).

Many people buy expensive equipment only to find that they really do not enjoy that mode of activity. They do not remain regular users. A few years ago, stationary bicycles (lower body only) and rowing ergometers were among the most popular pieces of equipment. Most of them now are seldom used and have become "fitness furniture" somewhere in the basement. Furthermore, be skeptical of testimonials and before-and-after pictures from "satisfied" customers. These results may not be typical, and they don't mean that you will like the equipment as well.

Exercise equipment does have its value for people who prefer to exercise indoors, especially during the winter months. It supports some people's motivation and adherence to exercise. The convenience of having equipment at home also allows for flexible scheduling. You can exercise before or after work or while you watch your favourite television show.

If you are going to purchase equipment, the best recommendation is to actually try it out several times before buying it. Ask yourself several questions: Did you enjoy the workout? Is the unit comfortable? Are you too short, tall, or heavy for it? Is it stable, sturdy, and strong? Do you have to assemble the machine? If so, how difficult is it to put together? How durable is it? Ask for references— people or clubs that have used the equipment extensively. Are they satisfied? Have they enjoyed using the equipment? Talk with professionals at colleges, sports medicine clinics, or health clubs.

Another consideration is to look at used units for signs of wear and tear. Quality is important. Cheaper brands may not be durable, so your investment would be wasted.

Finally, watch out for expensive gadgets. Monitors that provide exercise heart rate, work output, caloric expenditure, speed, grade, and distance may help motivate you, but they are expensive, need frequent repairs, and do not enhance the actual fitness benefits of the workout. Look at maintenance costs, and check for service personnel in your community.

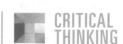

CRITICAL THINKING

Are there people around you whom you admire and would like to emulate for their wellness lifestyle? What behaviours do these people exhibit that would help you adopt a healthier lifestyle? What keeps you from emulating these behaviours, and how can you overcome these barriers?

Self-Evaluation and Behavioural Goals for the Future

The main objective of this book is to provide the information and experiences necessary to implement your personal fitness and wellness program. If you have implemented the programs in this book, including exercise, you should be convinced that a wellness lifestyle is the only way to attain a higher quality of life.

Most people who engage in a personal fitness and wellness program experience this new quality of life after only a few weeks of training and practising healthy lifestyle patterns. In some instances, however—especially for individuals who have led a poor lifestyle for a long time—a few months may be required to establish positive habits and feelings of well-being. In the end, though, everyone who applies the principles of fitness and wellness will reap the desired benefits.

Personal trainer A health/fitness professional who evaluates, motivates, educates, and trains clients to help them meet individualized, healthy, lifestyle goals.

Self-Evaluation

Throughout this course you have had an opportunity to assess various fitness and wellness components and write goals to improve your quality of life. You now should take the time to evaluate how well you have achieved your own goals. Ideally, if time allows and facilities and technicians are available, reassess the health-related components of physical fitness. If you are unable to reassess these components, determine subjectively how well you accomplished your objectives. You will find a self-evaluation form in part I of Lab 13B.

Behavioral Goals for the Future

If you have not yet achieved all your goals during this course, or if you need to reach beyond your current achievements, a final assignment should be conducted to help you chart the future. To complete this assignment, fill out the Wellness Compass in part II of Lab 13b. This compass provides a list of various wellness components, each illustrating a scale from 5 to 1; "5" indicates a low or poor rating and "1" indicates an excellent or "wellness" rating for that component. Using the Wellness Compass, rate yourself for each component according to the following instructions:

1. Colour in red a number from 5 to 1 to indicate where you stood on each component at the beginning of the semester. For example, if at the start of this course, you rated poor in cardio-respiratory endurance, colour the number 5 in red.
2. Colour in blue a second number from 5 to 1 to indicate where you stand on each component at the present time. If your level of cardiorespiratory endurance improved to average by the end of the semester, colour the number 3 in blue. If you were not able to work on a given component, simply colour in blue on top of the previous red.
3. Select one or two components you intend to work on during the next two months. Developing new behavioral patterns takes time, and trying to work on too many components at once most likely will lower your chances for success.

Start with components in which you think you will have a high chance for success. Next, colour in yellow the intended goal (number) to accomplish by the end of the two months. If your goal is to achieve a "good" level of cardiorespiratory endurance, colour the number 2 in yellow. When you achieve this level, you may later colour the number 1, also in yellow, to indicate your next goal.

After you have completed the previous exercise, write goals and objectives for the two components you intend to work on during the next two months

(use the form in part III of Lab 13B). As you write and work on these goals, review the SMART Goals section provided in Chapter 2, pages 42–43.

As a final assignment, to summarize your feelings about your past and present lifestyle, what you have learned in this course, and changes you were able to implement successfully, use part IV of Lab 13B for this evaluation. Keep this summary handy so you can review it in months and years to come.

The Fitness/Wellness Experience and a Challenge for the Future

Patty Neavill is a typical example of someone who often tried to change her life but was unable to do so because she did not know how to implement a sound exercise and weight control program. At age 24 and at 110 kg, she was discouraged with her weight, level of fitness, self-image, and quality of life in general. She had struggled with her weight most of her life. Like thousands of other people, she had made many unsuccessful attempts to lose weight.

Patty put her fears aside and decided to enroll in a fitness course. As part of the course requirement, a battery of fitness tests was administered at the beginning of the semester. Patty's cardiovascular fitness and strength ratings were poor, her flexibility classification was average, and her percent body fat was 41.

Following the initial fitness assessment, Patty met with her course instructor, who prescribed an exercise and nutrition program like the one in this book. Patty fully committed herself to carry out the prescription. She walked or jogged five times a week. She enrolled in a weight-training course that met twice a week. Her daily caloric intake was set in the range of 1,500 to 1,700 Calories.

Determined to increase her level of activity further, Patty signed up for recreational volleyball and basketball courses. Besides being fun, these classes provided four additional hours of activity per week.

She took care to meet the minimum required servings from the basic food groups each day, which contributed about 1,200 Calories to her diet. The remainder of the calories came primarily from complex carbohydrates.

At the end of the 16-week semester, Patty's cardiovascular fitness, strength, and flexibility ratings had all improved to the "good" category, she had lost 25 kg, and her percent body fat had decreased to 22.5!

Patty was tall. At 85 kg, most people would have thought she was too heavy. Her percent body fat, however, was lower than the average for university female physical education major students (about 23 percent body fat).

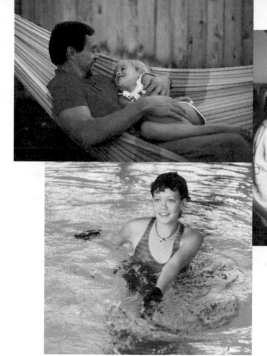
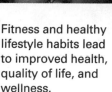
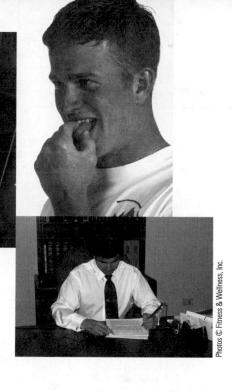

Fitness and healthy lifestyle habits lead to improved health, quality of life, and wellness.

A thank-you note from Patty to the course instructor at the end of the semester read:

Thank you for making me a new person. I truly appreciate the time you spent with me. Without your kindness and motivation, I would have never made it. It is great to be fit and trim. I've never had this feeling before, and I wish everyone could feel like this once in their life.

Thank you,
Your trim Patty!

Patty had never been taught the principles governing a sound weight-loss program. In Patty's case, not only did she need this knowledge, but, like most people who have not experienced the process of becoming physically fit, she needed to be in a structured exercise setting to truly feel the joy of fitness.

Even more significant, Patty maintained her aerobic and strength-training programs. A year after ending her calorie-restricted diet, her weight increased by 4.5 kg, but her body fat decreased from 22.5 to 21.2 percent. As you may recall from Chapter 5, this weight increase is related mostly to gains in lean tissue that she had lost during the weight-reduction phase.

In spite of only a slight drop in weight during the second year following the calorie-restricted diet, the two-year follow-up revealed a further decrease in body fat, to 19.5 percent. Patty understood the new quality of life reaped through a sound fitness program, and, at the same time, she finally learned how to apply the principles that regulate weight maintenance.

If you have read and successfully completed all the assignments set out in this book, including a regular exercise program, you should be convinced of the value of exercise and healthy lifestyle habits in achieving a new quality of life.

Perhaps this new quality of life was explained best by the late Dr. George Sheehan, when he wrote:[6]

For every runner who tours the world running marathons, there are thousands who run to hear the leaves and listen to the rain, and look to the day when it is all suddenly as easy as a bird in flight. For them, sport is not a test but a therapy, not a trial but a reward, not a question but an answer.

The real challenge will come now: a lifetime commitment to fitness and wellness. To make the commitment easier, enjoy yourself and have fun along the way. If you implement your program based on your interests and what you enjoy doing most, adhering to your new lifestyle will not be difficult.

Your activities over the last few weeks or months may have helped you develop "positive addictions" that will carry on throughout life. If you truly experience the feelings Dr. Sheehan expressed, there will be no looking back. If you don't get there, you won't know what it's like. Fitness and wellness is a process, and you need to put forth a constant and deliberate effort to achieve and maintain a higher quality of life. Improving the quality of your life, and most likely your longevity, is in your hands. Only you can take control of your lifestyle and thereby reap the benefits of wellness.

ASSESS YOUR KNOWLEDGE

1. From a functional point of view, typical sedentary people in Western countries are about _____ years older than their chronological age indicates.
   a. 2
   b. 8
   c. 15
   d. 20
   e. 25

2. Which one of the following factors has the greatest impact on health and longevity?
   a. genetics
   b. the environment
   c. lifestyle behaviours
   d. chronic diseases
   e. gender

3. Your real physiological age is determined by
   a. your birthdate.
   b. lifestyle habits.
   c. the amount of physical activity.
   d. your family's health history.
   e. your ability to obtain proper medical care.

4. Complementary and alternative medicine is
   a. also known as allopathic medicine.
   b. referred to as Western medicine.
   c. based on scientifically proven methods.
   d. a method of unconventional medicine.
   e. All are correct choices.

5. Complementary and alternative medicine health care practices and treatments are
   a. not widely taught in medical schools.
   b. endorsed by many physicians.
   c. not generally used in hospitals.
   d. not usually reimbursed by medical insurance companies.
   e. All of the above choices are correct.

6. In complementary and alternative medicine
   a. practitioners believe that their treatment modality aids the body as it performs its own natural healing process.
   b. treatments are usually shorter than with typical medical practices.
   c. practitioners rely extensively on the use of medications.
   d. patients are often discouraged from administering self-treatment.
   e. All of the above choices are correct.

7. When the word "natural" is used with a product
   a. it implies that the product is safe.
   b. it cannot be toxic, even when taken in large doses.
   c. it cannot yield undesirable side effects when combined with prescription drugs.
   d. there will be no negative side effects with its use.
   e. All of the above choices are incorrect.

8. To protect yourself from consumer fraud when buying a new product,
   a. get as much information as you can from the salesperson.
   b. obtain details about the product from another salesperson.
   c. ask someone who understands the product but does not stand to profit from the transaction.
   d. obtain all the research information from the manufacturer.
   e. All of these choices are correct.

9. Which of the following should you consider when looking to join a health and fitness centre?
   a. location
   b. instructor's certifications
   c. type and amount of equipment available
   d. verify that the facility complies with ACSM standards
   e. All choices are correct.

10. When purchasing exercise equipment, the most important factor is
    a. to try it out several times before buying it.
    b. a recommendation from an exercise specialist.
    c. cost-effectiveness.
    d. that it provides accurate exercise information.
    e. to find out how others like this piece of equipment.

Correct answers can be found at the back of the book.

MEDIA MENU

INTERNET CONNECTIONS

■ American College of Sports Medicine (ACSM). This site provides information on sport safety and research projects. This organization is committed to the practical application of sports medicine and exercise science to maintain and enhance physical fitness, health, and quality of life.

http://www.acsm.org

■ Canadian Society for Exercise Physiology. This voluntary organization is composed of professionals interested and involved in the scientific study of exercise physiology, exercise biochemistry, fitness, and health. Its mission is "to promote the generation, synthesis, transfer and application of knowledge and research related to exercise physiology (encompassing physical activity, fitness, health, nutrition, epidemiology, and human performance)".

http://www.csep.ca

■ Getting Started with an Exercise Program. This comprehensive site, from the Department of Kinesiology and Health of Georgia State University, features information on the benefits of exercise, how to choose a personal trainer, exercise safety and precautions, and lots more.

http://www.gsu.edu/~wwwfit/getstart.html

■ National Centre for Complementary and Alternative Medicine. This comprehensive site features information about a variety of complementary therapies geared for consumers, clinical practitioners, and investigators. The site also features a complementary medicine database, clinical trials information, and a list of resources.

http://nccam.nih.gov/

■ RealAge. This site features diet and exercise assessment tools, such as BMI calculator and exercise estimator, as well as RealAge assessment quizzes on a variety of health topics to help determine your risk of disease and what you can do to reduce this risk. The main feature is an interactive online personal assessment of a variety of lifestyle behaviours that also gives you options for growing younger.

http://www.realage.com

Notes

1. R. J. Donatelle and L. G. Davis, *Access to Health* (Boston: Allyn and Bacon, 2000).

2. N. Esmail, "Complementary and Alternative Medicine in Canada: Trends in Use and Public Attitudes, 1997–2006," Fraser Institute, *Public Policy Sources.* 87(May 2007): 3–53. Retrieved May 15, 2008, from http://www.fraserinstitute.org/commerce.web/publication_details.aspx?pubID=3213.

3. National Centre for Complementary and Alternative Medicine, "The Use of Complementary and Alternative Medicine in the United States," Retrieved May 15, 2008, from http://nccam.nih.gov/news/camsurvey_fs1.htm.

4. National Centre for Complementary and Alternative Medicine, "Cam Basics: What Is CAM?" Retrieved May 15, 2008, from http://nccam.nih.gov/health/whatiscam/.

5. Esmail, "Complementary and Alternative Medicine in Canada," pp. 4–5. Retrieved May 15, 2008, from http://www.fraserinstitute.org/commerce.web/publication_details.aspx?pubID=3213.

6. Human Relations Media, *Dynamics of Fitness: The Body in Action* (Pleasantville, NY, 1980).

Suggested Readings

Bloomer, R. "Successful Attributes of a Professional Fitness Trainer." *Fitness Management* 19 (1999): 40–45.

Buckman, R., and K. Sabbagh. *Magic or Medicine?: An Investigation of Healing and Healers.* Amherst, NY: Prometheus Books, 1995.

Janowiak, J. *Alternative Medicines: The Mindbody Prescription.* Belmont, CA: Wadsworth/Thomson, 2001.

Roizen, M. F. *Real Age: Are You As Young As You Can Be?* New York: Cliff Street Books, 1999.

Lab 13A

LIFE EXPECTANCY AND PHYSIOLOGICAL AGE PREDICTION QUESTIONNAIRE*

Name: _____   Date: _____   Grade: _____

Instructor: _____   Course: _____   Section: _____

Necessary Lab Equipment

None required.

Objective

To estimate the total number of years that you will live and your real physiological age based on your present lifestyle habits.

Instructions

Circle the points to the correct answer to each question. At the end of each page, obtain a net score for that page. Be completely honest with yourself. Your age prediction is based on your lifestyle habits, should you continue those habits for life. Using this questionnaire, you will learn about factors that you can modify or implement that can add years and health to your life. The scoring system is provided at the end of the questionnaire. Please note that the questionnaire is not a precise scientific instrument, but rather an estimated life expectancy analysis according to the impact of lifestyle factors on health and longevity. This questionnaire is not intended to substitute for advice and tests conducted by medical and health care practitioners.

I. Questionnaire

1. What is your current health status?
    - A. Excellent   + 2
    - B. Good   + 1
    - C. Average   0
    - D. Fair   − 1
    - E. Poor   − 2
    - F. Bad   − 3

2. How many days per week do you accumulate 30 minutes of moderate-intensity physical activity (50 to 60% of heart rate reserve—see Chapter 6)?
    - A. 6 to 7   + 3
    - B. 3 to 5   + 1
    - C. 1 to 2   0
    - D. Less than once per week   − 3

3. How often do you participate in a high-intensity cardio-respiratory exercise (over 60% of heart rate reserve) for at least 20 minutes?
    - A. 3 or more times per week   + 2
    - B. 2 times per week   + 1
    - C. Once a week   − 1
    - D. Less than once per week   − 2

4. How often do you perform strength-training exercises per week (a minimum of 8 exercises using 8 to 12 repetitions to near-fatigue on each exercise)?
    - A. 1–2 times   + 2
    - B. Less than once or less than 8 exercises with 8 to 12 reps per session   0
    - C. Do not strength train   − 1

5. How many times per week do you perform flexibility exercises (at least 15 minutes per stretching session)?
    - A. 3 or more   + 1
    - B. 1 to 3 times   +.5
    - C. Less than 1   0
    - D. Do not perform flexibility exercises   −.5

6. How many servings of fruits and vegetables do you eat on a daily basis?
    - A. 9 or more   + 3
    - B. 6 to 8   + 2
    - C. 5   + 1
    - D. 3 to 4   0
    - E. 2 or less   − 2

7. How many grams of fibre do you consume on an average day?
    - A. 25 or over   + 1
    - B. Between 13 and 24   0
    - C. 10 to 12 or don't know   − 1
    - D. Less than 10   − 2

8. As a percentage of total calories, what is your average fat intake on a daily basis?
    - A. 20% to 30%   + 1
    - B. 30%   0
    - C. 30% to 35% or don't know   − 1
    - D. Over 35%   − 2

9. As a percentage of total calories, what is your average saturated fat intake on a daily basis?
    - A. 5% or less   + 1
    - B. More than 5% but less than 10%   0
    - C. Don't know   − 1
    - D. Over 10%   − 2

10. How many servings of red meat (85 to 170 g) do you consume on a weekly basis?
    - A. 1 or less   + 1
    - B. 2 to 3   0
    - C. 4 to 7   − 1
    - D. More than 7   − 2

Page score: _____

11. How many servings of fish (85 to 170 g) do you consume on a weekly basis?
   A. 2 or more   + 1
   B. 1   0
   C. None   − 1

12. How many alcoholic drinks (a 350 mL bottle of beer, a 120 mL glass of wine, or a 45 mL shot of 80 proof liquor) do you consume per day?
   A. Men 2 or less, women 1 or less   + 1
   B. None   0
   C. Men 3–4, women 2–4   − 1
   D. 5 or more   − 3

13. How many international units of vitamin E do you get from supplements on a daily basis?
   A. 400   + 2
   B. Over 200 but less than 400   + 1
   C. Between 50 and 200   0
   D. None   − 1

14. How many milligrams of vitamin C do you get from food on a daily basis?
   A. Between 250 and 500   + 1
   B. Over 90 but less than 250   +.5
   C. Less than 90   − 1

15. How many micrograms of selenium do you get on a daily basis (preferably from food)?
   A. Between 100 and 200   + 1
   B. Between 50 and 99   +.5
   C. Less than 50   − 1

16. How many milligrams of calcium and how many international units of vitamin D do you get from food and supplements on an average day?
   A. Calcium = 1,200, Vitamin D = 400 or more   + 1
   B. Calcium = 1,200, Vitamin D = unknown   +.5
   C. Calcium = 800 to 1,200, Vitamin D = less than 400   0
   D. Calcium = less than 800, Vitamin D = less than 400   − 1

17. How many times per week do you eat breakfast?
   A. 7   + 1
   B. 5 to 6   +.5
   C. 3 to 5   0
   D. Less than 3   −.5

18. How many cigarettes do you smoke each day?
   A. Never smoked cigarettes or more than 15 years since giving up cigarettes   + 2
   B. None for 5 to 15 years   + 1
   C. None for 1 to 5 years   0
   D. None for 0 to 1 year   − 1
   E. Smoker, less than 1 pack per day   − 3
   F. Smoker, 1 pack per day   − 5
   G. Smoker, up to 2 packs per day   − 7
   H. Smoker, more than 2 packs per day   −10

19. Do you use tobacco products other than cigarettes?
   A. Never have   0
   B. Less than once per week   − 1
   C. Once per week   − 2
   D. 2 to 6 times per week   − 3
   E. More than 6 times per week   − 5

20. How often are you exposed to secondhand smoke or other environmental pollutants?
   A. Less than 1 hour per month   0
   B. Between 1 and 5 hours per month   − 1
   C. Between 5 and 29 hours per month   − 2
   D. Daily   − 3

21. Do you use addictive drugs, other than tobacco or alcohol?
   A. None   0
   B. 1   − 3
   C. 2 or more   − 5

22. What is the age of your parents (or how long did they live)?
   A. Both over 76   + 3
   B. Only one over 76   + 1
   C. Both are still alive and under 76   0
   D. Only one under 76   − 1
   E. Neither one lived past 76   − 3

23. What is your body composition category (see Table 4.13 in Chapter 4)?
   A. Excellent   + 2
   B. Good   + 1
   C. Average   0
   D. Overweight   − 1
   E. Significantly overweight   − 2

24. What is your blood pressure?
   A. 120/80 or less (both numbers)   + 2
   B. 120–140 or 80–90 (either number)   − 1
   C. Greater than 140/90 (either number)   − 3

25. What is your HDL cholesterol?
   A. Men greater than 45, women over 55   + 2
   B. Men 35 to 44, women 45 to 54   0
   C. Don't know   − 1
   D. Men less than 35, women below 45   − 2

26. What is your LDL cholesterol?
   A. Less than 130   + 2
   B. Don't know   − 1
   C. 130 to 159   − 1
   D. 160 or higher   − 2

27. Do you floss and brush your teeth regularly?
   A. Every day   +.5
   B. 3 to 6 days per week   0
   C. Less than 3 days per week   −.5

28. Are you a diabetic?
   A. No   0
   B. Yes, well-controlled   − 1
   C. Yes, poorly or not controlled   − 3

29. How often do you sunbathe (tan)?
   A. Not at all   + 1
   B. Between 1 and 3 times per year   −.5
   C. More than 3 times per year   − 1

30. How often do you wear a seat belt?
   A. All the time   + 1
   B. Most of the time   −.5
   C. Less than half the time   − 1

31. How fast do you drive?
   A. Always at or below the speed limit   0
   B. Up to 8 km/h over the speed limit   −.5
   C. Between 8 and 16 km/h over the speed limit   − 1
   D. More than 16 km/h over the speed limit   − 2

Page score:

32. Do you drink and drive?
    A. Never   0
    B. Yes (even if only once)   − 5

33. In terms of your sexual activity:
    A. I am not sexually active
       or I am in a monogamous
       sexual relationship   + 1
    B. I have more than one
       sexual partner but I always
       practise safer sex   − 1
    C. I have multiple sexual
       partners and I do not
       practise safer sex
       techniques   − 3

34. What is your marital status?
    A. Happily married   + 1
    B. Single and happy   0
    C. Single and unhappy   −.5
    D. Divorced   − 1
    E. Widowed with a belief
       in life hereafter   − 1
    F. Widowed   − 2
    G. Married and unhappy   − 2

35. On the average, how many
    hours of sleep do you get
    each night?
    A. 7 to 8   + 1
    B. 7   0
    C. 6 to 7   − 1
    D. Less than 6   − 2

36. Your stress rating according
    to the Life Experiences Survey
    (see Lab 10A) is:
    A. Excellent   + 1
    B. Good   0
    C. Average   −.5
    D. Fair   − 1
    E. Poor   − 2

37. Your Type A behaviour rating
    (see Lab 10A) is:
    A. Low   0
    B. Medium   − 1
    C. High   − 2

38. When under stress (distress),
    how often do you practise stress
    management techniques?
    A. Always   + 1
    B. Most of the time   +.5
    C. Not applicable (don't
       suffer from stress)   0
    D. Sometimes   − 1
    E. Never   − 2

39. Do you suffer from depression?
    A. Not at all   0
    B. Mild depression   − 1
    C. Severe depression   − 2

40. How often do you associate
    with people who have a
    positive attitude about life?
    A. Always   +.5
    B. Most of the time   0
    C. About half of the time   −.5
    D. Less than half the time   − 1

41. Do you have close family or
    personal relationships whom
    you can trust and rely on for
    help in times of need?
    A. Yes   + 1
    B. No   − 1

42. Do you feel loved and can
    you routinely give affection
    and love?
    A. Yes   + 1
    B. No   − 1

43. Do you have a good sense
    of humour?
    A. Yes   + 1
    B. No   − 1

44. How satisfied are you with
    your school work?
    A. Satisfied   +.5
    B. It's okay   0
    C. Not satisfied   −.5

45. How do you rate your
    present job satisfaction?
    A. Love it   + 1
    B. Like it   0
    C. It's okay   −.5
    D. Don't like it   − 1
    E. Hate it   − 2
    F. Not applicable   0

46. How do you rate yourself
    spiritually?
    A. Very spiritual   + 1
    B. Spiritual   0
    C. Somewhat spiritual   −.5
    D. Not spiritual at all   − 1

Page score:

Net score for all questions:

II. How To Score

To estimate the total number of years that you will live, (a) determine a net score by totalling the results from all 46 questions, (b) obtain an age change score by multiplying the net score by the age correction factor given below, and (c) add or subtract this number from your base life expectancy age (77 for men and 82 for women—the 2003 life expectancies in Canada). For example, if you are a 20-year-old male and the net score from the answers to all questions was −16, your estimated life expectancy would be 72.2 years (age change score = −16 × .3 = −4.8, life expectancy = 77 − 4.8 =72.2).

You can also determine your real physiological age by subtracting a positive age-change score or adding a negative age-change score to your current chronological (calendar) age. For instance, in the previous example, the real physiological age would be 24.8 years (20 + 4.8). If the age change score had been +4.8, the real physiological age would have been 16.2 years. Thus, a healthy lifestyle will always make your physiological age younger than your chronological age. Your real physiological age will have much greater significance in middle and older age, when it is not uncommon to see real-age reductions of 10 to 25 years in people who lead healthy lifestyles. Thus a 50-year-old person could easily have a real physiological age of 30.

Age Correction Factor (ACF)*

Age	ACF
≤30	.3
31–40	.4
41–50	.5
51–60	.6
61–70	.6
71–80	.5
81–90	.4
≥91	.3

Age Change Score (ACS) = [   ] (net score) × [   ] (ACF) = [   ]

Life expectancy

Men   = 77 ± [   ] (ACS) = [   ] years

Women = 82 ± [   ] (ACS) = [   ] years

Real physiological age**

Men   = [   ] (your age) ± [   ] (ACS) = [   ] years

Women = [   ] (your age) ± [   ] (ACS) = [   ] years

**Subtract a positive ACS from, or add a negative ACS to, your current age.

State your feelings about the experience of taking this questionnaire, analyze your results, and list lifestyle factors that you can work on that will positively affect your health and longevity.

Lab 13B

SELF-EVALUATION AND BEHAVIOURAL GOALS FOR THE FUTURE

Name: _____   Date: _____   Grade: _____

Instructor: _____   Course: _____   Section: _____

Necessary Lab Equipment

None required unless fitness tests are repeated.

Objective

To conduct a self-evaluation of the goals achieved in this course and to write behavioural goals for the future.

Lab Preparation

Review the section on SMART Goals in Chapter 2 (pages 42–43) prior to completing this lab. If time allows and technicians are available, repeat the assessments for the health-related components of fitness.

I. Fitness Evaluation

Conduct a self-evaluation of the fitness goals you accomplished in this course. Fill in the required information on the health-related fitness components below. If you were unable to repeat your fitness assessments, subjectively determine how well you reached your goals.

1. Did you accomplish your objective for:

   Cardiorespiratory Endurance (see Lab 6A)   ☐ Yes   ☐ No

   Pre-assessment VO_{2max}: _____ mL/kg/min   Fitness Classification: _____

   Post-assessment VO_{2max}: _____ mL/kg/min   Fitness Classification: _____

   Body Composition (see Labs 4A and 4B)   ☐ Yes   ☐ No

   Pre-assessment Percent Body Fat: _____   Body Composition Classification: _____

   Post-assessment Percent Body Fat: _____   Body Composition Classification: _____

   Muscular Strength and Endurance (see Lab 7A)   ☐ Yes   ☐ No

   Pre-assessment Percentile Total Points: _____   Fitness Classification: _____

   Post-assessment Percentile Total Points: _____   Fitness Classification: _____

   Muscular Flexibility (see Lab 8A)   ☐ Yes   ☐ No

   Pre-assessment Percentile Total Points: _____   Fitness Classification: _____

   Post-assessment Percentile Total Points: _____   Fitness Classification: _____

II. Wellness Evaluation

Using the Wellness Compass, rate yourself for each component and plan goals and objectives for the future according to the following instructions:

1. Colour in red a number from 5 to 1 to indicate where you stood on each component at the beginning of the semester (5 = poor rating, 1 = excellent or ideal rating).
2. Colour in blue a second number from 5 to 1 to indicate where you stand on each component at the present time.
3. Select one or two components that you intend to work on in the next two months. Start with components in which you think you will have a high chance for success. Colour in yellow the intended goal (number) to accomplish by the end of the two months. Once you achieve your objective, you later may colour another number, also in yellow, to indicate your next objective.

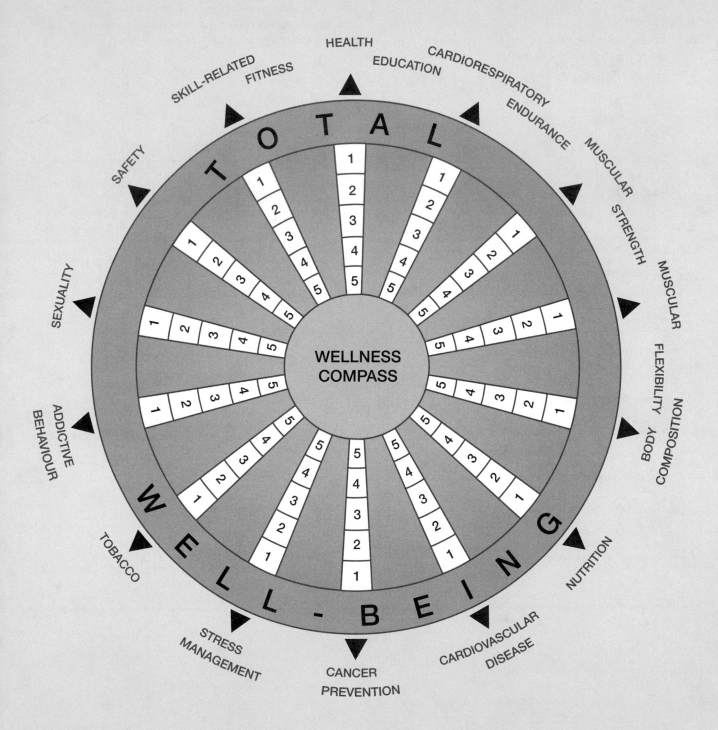

III. Wellness Lifestyle Self-Assessment

1. Explain the exercise program that you implemented in this course, indicate your feelings about the outcomes of this program, and evaluate how well you accomplished your fitness goals.

_____
_____
_____
_____
_____
_____
_____

2. List nutritional or dietary changes that you were able to implement this term and the effects of these changes on your body composition and personal wellness.

_____
_____
_____
_____
_____
_____
_____

3. List other lifestyle changes that you were able to make this term that may decrease your risk for disease. In a few sentences, explain how you feel about these changes and their impact on your overall well-being.

_____
_____
_____
_____
_____
_____
_____
_____
_____

IV. Behavioural Goals for the Future

Identify one or two goals you will work on during the next couple of months and write specific objectives that you will use to accomplish each goal (you may not need six objectives; write only as many as needed).

Goal:

Objectives:

1. _____
2. _____
3. _____
4. _____
5. _____
6. _____

Goal:

Objectives:

1. _____
2. _____
3. _____
4. _____
5. _____
6. _____

V. This Course and Your Future Lifestyle

Briefly evaluate this course and its impact on your quality of life. Indicate what you feel will be needed for you to continue to adhere to an active and healthy lifestyle.

_____
_____
_____
_____
_____
_____
_____
_____
_____

Nutrient Value of Some Common Foods

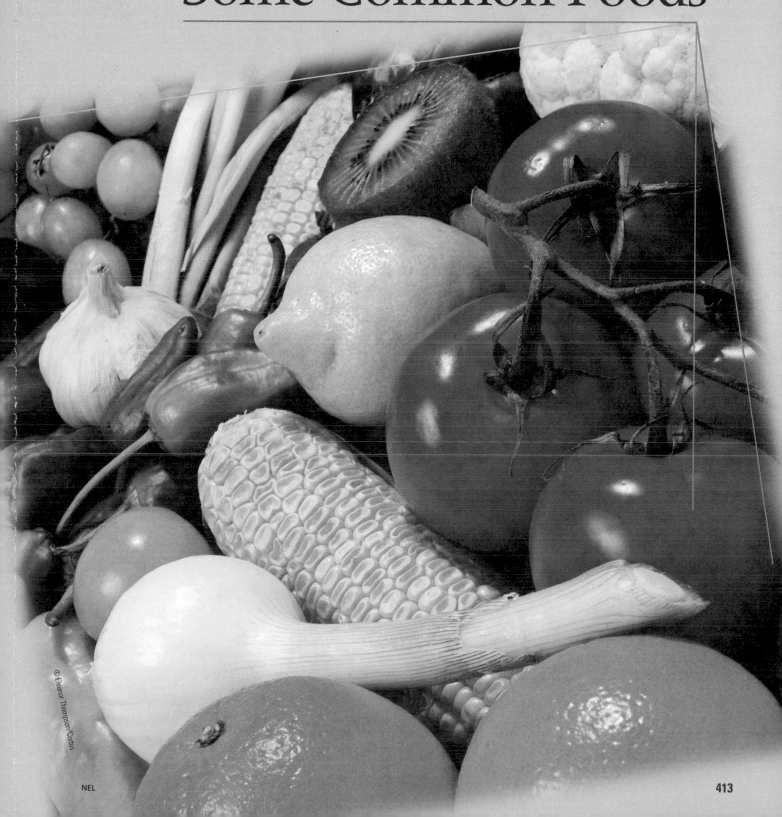

Breads, Cereals and Other Grain Products

Food Name	Measure	Weight g	Energy kcal	Energy kJ	Protein g	Carbohydrate g	Total Sugar g	Total Dietary Fibre g	Total Fat g	Saturated Fat g	Cholesterol mg	Calcium mg	Iron mg	Sodium mg	Potassium mg	Magnesium mg	Phosphorus mg	Thiamin mg	Riboflavin mg	Niacin NE	Folate DFE
Flours and Brans																					
Chickpea flour	125 mL	49	188	786	11	28	5	5.2	3	0.3	0	22	2.4	31	411	81	155	0.2	0.05	2.9	212
Cornmeal, dry	125 mL	73	267	1116	6	57	1	5.4	1	0.2	0	4	0.8	2	118	29	61	0.1	0.04	1.9	35
Oat bran, dry	125 mL	50	122	511	9	33	1	5.2	3	0.7	0	29	2.7	2	281	117	365	0.6	0.11	3.2	26
Oat flour	125 mL	53	200	838	7	35	1	5.3	4	0.7	0	27	2.2	2	199	78	226	0.3	0.08	1.8	15
Potato flour	125 mL	85	302	1262	6	70	3	0.1	tr	0.1	0	55	1.2	46	846	55	142	0.2	0.04	4.6	21
Rice flour	125 mL	83	305	1278	5	67	tr	2.0	1	0.3	0	8	0.3	0	63	29	82	0.1	0.02	3.2	3
Rye flour, light	125 mL	54	198	827	5	43	1	7.9	1	0.1	0	11	1.0	1	126	38	105	0.2	0.05	1.3	12
Soy flour	125 mL	53	174	729	25	20	11	9.2	1	0.1	0	127	4.9	11	1259	153	356	0.4	0.13	7.4	161
Wheat bran	15 mL	4	8	33	1	2	tr	1.6	tr	tr	0	3	0.4	tr	43	22	37	tr	0.02	0.7	3
Wheat flour, all purpose	125 mL	66	240	1005	7	50	tr	2.0	1	0.1	0	10	3.1	1	71	15	71	0.5	0.33	5.3	192
Wheat flour, bread	125 mL	72	261	1093	9	52	tr	1.7	1	0.2	0	11	3.2	1	72	18	70	0.6	0.37	7.1	208
Wheat flour, cake	125 mL	72	262	1096	6	56	tr	1.2	1	0.1	0	10	5.3	1	76	12	62	0.6	0.31	6.3	204
Wheat flour, whole grain	125 mL	63	215	899	9	46	tr	7.7	1	0.2	0	22	2.5	3	257	87	219	0.3	0.14	6.3	28
Wheat germ, toasted	15 mL	7	27	114	3	4	1	1.1	1	0.1	0	3	0.7	tr	68	23	82	0.1	0.06	0.9	25
Breads and Buns																					
Bagel, plain (10cm diam)	1	71	195	817	7	38	4	1.6	1	0.2	0	53	2.5	379	72	21	68	0.4	0.22	4.7	117
Bannock	1 medium	37	84	353	2	19	N/A	0.5	tr	0	1	84	0.7	N/A	N/A	N/A	60	0.1	0.06	1.4	N/A
Bread, French or Vienna	1 slice	35	96	401	3	18	tr	1.1	1	0.2	0	26	0.9	213	40	9	37	0.2	0.12	2.3	80
Bread, Italian	1 slice	35	95	397	3	18	tr	0.9	1	0.3	0	27	1.0	204	39	9	36	0.2	0.10	2.1	106
Bread, mixed-grain	1 slice	35	88	366	4	16	4	2.2	1	0.3	0	32	1.2	170	71	19	62	0.1	0.12	2.3	58
Bread, naan	1/2	63	192	803	7	36	2	1.4	2	0.8	3	78	2.3	208	115	16	89	0.3	0.33	5.6	115
Bread, oatmeal	1 slice	35	94	394	3	17	3	1.4	1	0.2	0	23	0.9	210	50	13	44	0.1	0.08	1.8	30
Bread, pita, white (17cm diam)	1	60	165	690	5	33	1	1.3	1	0.1	0	52	1.6	322	72	16	58	0.4	0.20	3.8	99
Bread, pita, whole wheat (17cm diam)	1	64	170	712	6	35	tr	4.7	2	0.3	0	10	2.0	340	109	44	115	0.2	0.05	3.4	22
Bread, pumpernickel	1 slice	35	88	366	3	17	1	2.3	1	0.2	0	24	1.0	235	73	19	62	0.1	0.11	1.6	47
Bread, raisin	1 slice	35	96	401	3	18	2	1.5	2	0.4	0	23	1.0	137	79	9	38	0.1	0.14	1.7	55
Bread, rye	1 slice	35	91	379	3	17	1	2.0	1	0.2	0	26	1.0	231	58	14	44	0.2	0.12	1.9	53

Canadian Nutrient File 2007. Nutrient Value of Some Common Foods. Health Canada, 2007. © Reproduced with the permission of the Minister of Public Works and Government Services Canada, 2008. Available online: http://www.hc-sc.gc.ca/fn-an/nutrition/fiche-nutri-data/index_e.html.

Breads, Cereals and Other Grain Products

Food Name	Measure	Weight g	Energy kcal	Energy kJ	Protein g	Carbohydrate g	Total Sugar g	Total Dietary Fibre g	Total Fat g	Saturated Fat g	Cholesterol mg	Calcium mg	Iron mg	Sodium mg	Potassium mg	Magnesium mg	Phosphorus mg	Thiamin mg	Riboflavin mg	Niacin NE	Folate DFE
Bread, white, Calorie-reduced	1 slice	35	72	303	3	16	2	3.4	1	0.2	0	33	1.1	159	27	8	42	0.1	0.10	1.9	48
Bread, white, commercial	1 slice	35	93	389	3	18	2	0.8	1	0.3	0	53	1.3	238	35	8	35	0.2	0.12	2.1	60
Bread, white, homemade with 2% milk	1 slice	35	100	417	3	17		0.7	2	0.4	1	20	1.0	126	51	7	40	0.1	0.13	1.8	44
Bread, whole wheat, commercial	1 slice	35	86	360	3	16	7	2.4	2	0.3	0	25	1.2	184	88	30	80	0.1	0.07	2.2	18
Bread, whole wheat, homemade with 2% milk	1 slice	35	97	407	3	18	1	2.1	2	0.3	0	12	1.1	121	110	28	65	0.1	0.08	2.1	27
English muffin, white, toasted	1	52	133	554	4	26	2	1.5	1	0.1	0	98	1.4	262	74	11	75	0.2	0.14	2.8	65
English muffin, whole wheat, toasted	1	52	126	528	5	25	1	2.6	2	0.2	0	100	1.6	216	105	22	65	0.2	0.15	2.8	41
Fry bread	1	37	122	511	2	18	1	1.0	5	1.7	3	21	1.5	122	28	7	46	0.2	0.08	2.2	73
Roll, crusty (kaiser)	1	57	167	698	6	30	1	1.3	2	0.3	0	54	1.9	310	62	15	57	0.3	0.19	3.5	86
Roll, dinner, white	1	28	85	356	2	14	2	0.9	2	0.5	tr	34	0.9	148	38	7	33	0.1	0.09	1.6	41
Roll, dinner, whole wheat	1	28	75	315	2	14	2	2.1	1	0.2	0	30	0.7	136	77	24	64	0.1	0.04	1.7	9
Roll, hamburger or hotdog, white	1	43	120	502	4	21	3	0.9	2	0.5	0	59	1.4	206	40	9	27	0.2	0.14	2.5	73
Roll, hamburger or hotdog, whole wheat	1	43	113	473	4	19	3	1.6	3	0.6	0	41	1.7	197	69	19	52	0.2	0.13	2.8	74

Other Bread Products

Food Name	Measure	Weight g	Energy kcal	Energy kJ	Protein g	Carbohydrate g	Total Sugar g	Total Dietary Fibre g	Total Fat g	Saturated Fat g	Cholesterol mg	Calcium mg	Iron mg	Sodium mg	Potassium mg	Magnesium mg	Phosphorus mg	Thiamin mg	Riboflavin mg	Niacin NE	Folate DFE
Bread stick, plain (19cm X 2cm)	1	10	41	172	1	7	tr	0.3	1	0.1	0	2	0.4	66	12	3	12	0.1	0.06	0.8	25
Bread stuffing, dry mix prepared	125 mL	106	188	786	3	23	2	3.1	9	1.8	0	34	1.2	574	78	13	44	0.1	0.11	2.3	56
Croutons, plain	60 mL	8	31	129	1	6	N/A	0.4	1	0.1	0	6	0.3	53	9	2	9	tr	0.02	0.6	16
Dumpling	1 dumpling	35	69	289	1	8	tr	0.3	4	1.0	1	23	0.4	138	23	3	22	0.1	0.06	0.8	19
Matzo, plain	1	28	112	468	3	24	tr	0.9	tr	0.1	0	4	0.9	1	32	7	25	0.1	0.08	1.7	5
Taco shell, baked (13cm diam)	1 shell	13	61	254	1	8	tr	1.0	3	0.4	0	21	0.3	48	23	14	32	tr	0.01	0.3	28
Tortilla, corn (15cm diam)	1	19	41	173	1	8	tr	1.2	1	0.1	0	15	0.2	9	35	14	60	tr	0.01	0.4	1
Tortilla, wheat (20cm diam)	1	49	159	666	2	27	N/A	1.6	3	0.9	0	19	1.6	234	64	13	61	0.3	0.14	2.6	98

Pancakes, Waffles and French Toast

Food Name	Measure	Weight g	Energy kcal	Energy kJ	Protein g	Carbohydrate g	Total Sugar g	Total Dietary Fibre g	Total Fat g	Saturated Fat g	Cholesterol mg	Calcium mg	Iron mg	Sodium mg	Potassium mg	Magnesium mg	Phosphorus mg	Thiamin mg	Riboflavin mg	Niacin NE	Folate DFE
French toast, frozen, ready to heat, heated	1 slice	59	126	526	4	19	N/A	0.6	4	0.9	48	63	1.3	292	79	10	82	0.2	0.22	2.5	42
French toast, homemade	1 slice	65	149	623	5	16	N/A	0.7	7	1.8	75	65	1.1	311	87	11	76	0.1	0.21	2.1	37
Pancake, buckwheat, prepared from mix (13cm diam)	1	40	73	305	3	10	2	1.1	3	0.6	20	89	0.7	191	80	27	143	0.1	0.09	1.2	9
Pancake, homemade with butter and syrup (13cm diam)	1	50	112	468	3	20	2	0.8	3	1.0	11	85	0.5	211	78	9	118	0.1	0.11	1.1	23
Pancake, plain, from complete mix (13cm diam)	1	40	64	266	1	11	N/A	0.4	2	0.2	3	36	0.4	180	50	6	96	0.1	0.06	0.8	15

Breads, Cereals and Other Grain Products

Food Name	Measure	Weight g	Energy kcal	Energy kJ	Protein g	Carbohydrate g	Total Sugar g	Total Dietary Fibre g	Total Fat g	Saturated Fat g	Cholesterol mg	Calcium mg	Iron mg	Sodium mg	Potassium mg	Magnesium mg	Phosphorus mg	Thiamin mg	Riboflavin mg	Niacin NE	Folate DFE
Pancake, plain, frozen, ready-to-heat (13cm diam), heated	1	41	94	393	2	18	4	0.7	1	0.3	4	25	1.4	209	30	6	153	0.2	0.19	2.1	27
Pancake, plain, homemade (13cm diam)	1	38	86	361	2	11	N/A	0.5	4	0.8	22	83	0.7	167	50	6	60	0.1	0.11	1.1	21
Potato pancake, homemade (8cm diam)	1	37	112	467	2	13	1	1.0	6	0.6	23	12	0.7	191	277	16	46	0.1	0.06	1.4	15
Waffle, homemade	1	37	103	432	2	14	2	0.5	4	0.7	33	44	0.9	146	58	7	53	0.1	0.15	1.7	37
Waffle, plain, frozen, ready-to-heat, heated	1	33	87	364	2	13	2	0.8	3	0.5	8	77	1.5	260	42	7	139	0.1	0.16	1.9	22

Rice, Pasta and Other Grains

Food Name	Measure	Weight g	Energy kcal	Energy kJ	Protein g	Carbohydrate g	Total Sugar g	Total Dietary Fibre g	Total Fat g	Saturated Fat g	Cholesterol mg	Calcium mg	Iron mg	Sodium mg	Potassium mg	Magnesium mg	Phosphorus mg	Thiamin mg	Riboflavin mg	Niacin NE	Folate DFE
Barley, pearled, cooked	125 mL	83	102	426	2	23	tr	2.0	tr	0.1	0	9	1.1	2	77	18	45	0.1	0.05	2.2	13
Bulgur, cooked	125 mL	96	80	334	3	18	tr	2.7	tr	tr	0	10	0.9	5	65	31	38	0.1	0.03	1.7	17
Couscous, cooked	125 mL	83	93	388	3	19	tr	0.7	tr	tr	0	7	0.3	4	48	7	18	0.1	0.02	1.5	12
Quinoa, cooked	125 mL	73	70	293	2	13	N/A	1.3	1	0.1	0	11	1.7	4	138	39	77	tr	0.07	1.0	9
Macaroni, cooked	250 mL	148	209	873	7	42	1	1.8	1	0.1	0	10	2.1	1	46	27	80	0.3	0.14	4.0	184
Noodles, Chinese, chow mein	60 mL	11	60	252	1	7	tr	0.4	4	0.5	0	2	0.5	50	14	6	18	0.1	0.05	0.9	16
Noodles, egg, cooked	250 mL	169	225	940	8	42	1	1.9	2	0.5	56	20	2.7	12	47	32	117	0.3	0.14	4.3	176
Pasta, fresh-refrigerated, cooked	250 mL	169	220	920	9	40	N/A	3.7	3	0.7	69	17	2.0	140	36	24	88	0.3	0.29	4.0	101
Pasta, fresh-refrigerated, spinach, cooked	250 mL	169	223	933	9	41	1	2.2	3	0.6	56	32	1.8	20	63	41	96	0.4	0.21	4.4	159
Ramen noodles, chicken flavour, dry	1 package	85	371	1554	9	54	1	2.0	13	6.0	N/A	23	3.3	1760	147	19	100	0.5	0.21	3.8	150
Rice noodles, cooked	250 mL	186	203	848	2	46	N/A	1.9	tr	tr	0	7	0.3	35	7	6	37	tr	0.01	0.5	6
Rice, brown, long-grain, cooked	125 mL	103	115	479	3	24	tr	1.5	1	0.2	0	10	0.4	5	44	44	86	0.1	0.03	2.1	4
Rice, white, long-grain, cooked	125 mL	83	109	454	2	24	tr	0.4	tr	0.1	0	8	0.2	1	29	10	36	tr	0.01	0.8	3
Rice, white, long-grain, instant, prepared	125 mL	87	85	357	2	19	0	0.5	tr	tr	0	7	0.2	3	3	4	12	tr	0.04	0.9	7
Rice, white, long-grain, parboiled, cooked	125 mL	92	105	441	2	23	tr	0.4	tr	0.1	0	18	0.2	3	34	11	39	tr	0.02	1.7	4
Rice, wild, cooked	125 mL	87	88	366	3	18	1	1.6	tr	tr	0	3	0.5	3	88	28	71	tr	0.08	1.8	23
Soba noodles, cooked	250 mL	120	119	499	6	26	N/A	N/A	tr	tr	0	5	0.6	72	42	11	30	0.1	0.03	2.1	8
Spaghetti, cooked	250 mL	148	209	873	7	42	1	2.5	1	0.1	0	10	2.1	1	46	27	80	0.3	0.14	4.0	184
Spaghetti, whole wheat, cooked	250 mL	148	183	768	8	39	1	4.8	1	0.1	0	22	1.6	4	65	44	132	0.2	0.07	2.7	7

Breakfast Cereals

Hot Cereal, cooked

Food Name	Measure	Weight g	Energy kcal	Energy kJ	Protein g	Carbohydrate g	Total Sugar g	Total Dietary Fibre g	Total Fat g	Saturated Fat g	Cholesterol mg	Calcium mg	Iron mg	Sodium mg	Potassium mg	Magnesium mg	Phosphorus mg	Thiamin mg	Riboflavin mg	Niacin NE	Folate DFE
Cream of wheat, regular	175 mL	186	46	195	2	9	tr	0.7	tr	0	0	2	1.6	tr	15	2	17	tr	0.01	0.4	N/A

Breads, Cereals and Other Grain Products

Food Name	Measure	Weight g	Energy kcal	Energy kJ	Protein g	Carbohydrate g	Total Sugar g	Total Dietary Fibre g	Total Fat g	Saturated Fat g	Cholesterol mg	Calcium mg	Iron mg	Sodium mg	Potassium mg	Magnesium mg	Phosphorus mg	Thiamin mg	Riboflavin mg	Niacin NE	Folate DFE
Oat bran, cooked	175 mL	179	73	306	3	12	tr	3.4	1	0.3	0	17	1.3	1	120	N/A	127	0.2	0.06	0.9	9
Oatmeal, instant, apple-cinnamon	1 packet	186	141	592	3	29	12	2.8	2	0.3	0	21	5.0	256	108	36	88	0.8	0.03	1.4	50
Oatmeal, instant, regular	1 packet	186	112	468	4	20	1	2.7	2	0.4	0	21	4.0	241	112	45	132	0.6	0.04	1.5	N/A
Oatmeal, large flakes/quick	175 mL	173	99	412	4	17	tr	2.6	2	0.3	0	13	1.0	1	98	N/A	111	0.2	0.04	0.9	8
Red River, Robin Hood™	175 mL	180	115	482	4	24	N/A	4.0	1	0.1	tr	15	1.3	27	N/A	18	63	0.1	0.02	1.4	19
Ready-to-eat																					
All Bran Buds with psyllium, Kellogg's™	75 mL	27	70	292	2	22	7	11.3	1	N/A	0	17	3.5	181	242	74	242	0.5	0.09	2.5	38
All Bran, Kellogg's™	125 mL	35	92	384	4	27	6	11.8	1	N/A	0	30	4.7	305	408	130	350	0.7	0.07	6.0	50
Almond Raisin Muslix, Kellogg's™	175 mL	44	173	722	4	34	13	3.0	3	N/A	0	24	5.9	140	191	30	86	0.9	0.07	2.1	N/A
Alpha-Bits, Post™	250 mL	34	139	580	2	30	14	1.1	1	0.2	0	3	4.5	126	21	24	74	0.7	0	2.0	41
Bran Flakes, Post™	250 mL	53	185	776	5	41	9	7.4	1	0.2	0	24	7.0	302	253	121	276	1.1	0.08	3.5	64
Cap'n Crunch, Quaker™	175 mL	27	108	452	1	23	10	0.7	1	1.1	0	0	3.6	213	30	11	22	0.5	0	1.3	32
Cheerios, Honey Nut, General Mills™	250 mL	35	134	561	3	28	12	2.1	1	N/A	0	128	4.7	252	99	38	115	0	0.06	1.6	41
Cheerios, regular, General Mills™	250 mL	24	95	396	3	18	1	2.2	2	N/A	0	44	3.2	219	78	32	105	tr	0.04	1.1	28
Cinnamon Toast Crunch, General Mills™	175 mL	28	123	514	1	22	9	1.0	3	N/A	0	103	3.8	193	41	12	93	0.8	0.01	1.3	33
Corn Bran, Quaker™	250 mL	38	124	520	3	30	8	6.1	2	0.8	0	0	5.0	349	91	N/A	42	0.8	0.02	1.7	45
Corn Flakes, Kellogg's™	250 mL	26	103	430	2	23	2	0.7	tr	0	0	1	3.5	190	28	2	12	0.5	0.71	1.6	32
Corn Pops, Kellogg's™	250 mL	33	130	544	1	30	12	0.4	tr	0	0	2	4.4	192	26	3	13	0.7	0.01	1.8	40
Fibre 1, General Mills™	125 mL	30	79	329	3	24	0	14.1	1	0.1	0	110	4.1	130	239	68	188	0.1	0.06	1.4	36
Froot Loops, Kellogg's™	250 mL	30	116	485	1	26	14	0.6	1	N/A	0	3	3.9	121	30	7	31	0.6	0.02	1.7	36
Frosted Flakes, Kellogg's™	250 mL	37	142	595	2	33	15	0.6	tr	0	0	1	4.9	196	28	2	9	0.7	0.67	2.1	45
Fruit & Fibre, Dates/Raisins/Walnuts, Post™	125 mL	29	93	389	3	22	7	4.3	3	N/A	0	16	3.9	134	145	55	126	0.6	0.05	1.9	35
Granola with Raisins, low fat, Kellogg's™	125 mL	59	226	944	5	46	17	3.5	3	N/A	0	24	7.8	147	173	47	135	1.2	0.14	3.7	71
Granola with Raisins, Rogers™	125 mL	59	245	1023	5	41	N/A	5.3	8	N/A	0	28	1.9	95	198	N/A	157	0.4	0.06	1.8	N/A
Grape-Nuts, Post™	125 mL	58	208	872	6	46	5	6.0	1	N/A	0	24	2.0	348	253	59	241	0.2	0.09	4.5	68
Harvest Crunch, regular, Quaker™	125 mL	47	218	911	5	31	12	3.3	9	6.7	1	51	1.1	45	226	N/A	N/A	0.1	0.07	1.5	14
Honeycomb, Post™	250 mL	23	92	384	1	21	8	0.2	tr	N/A	0	8	3.7	93	46	7	36	0.5	tr	1.4	28
Just Right, Kellogg's™	250 mL	45	172	720	4	38	10	2.2	1	N/A	0	11	6.0	250	105	28	93	0.9	0.10	2.9	55

Breads, Cereals and Other Grain Products

Food Name	Measure	Weight g	Energy kcal	Energy kJ	Protein g	Carbohydrate g	Total Sugar g	Total Dietary Fibre g	Total Fat g	Saturated Fat g	Cholesterol mg	Calcium mg	Iron mg	Sodium mg	Potassium mg	Magnesium mg	Phosphorus mg	Thiamin mg	Riboflavin mg	Niacin NE	Folate DFE
Life, Quaker™	175 mL	33	124	518	5	23	7	2.9	2	0.3	0	24	4.3	195	188	10	160	0.6	0.03	1.5	19
Lucky Charms, General Mills™	250 mL	34	132	550	2	28	15	1.7	1	N/A	0	124	4.6	227	64	28	87	0	0.02	1.6	40
Mini-Wheats with White Frosting, Kellogg's™	175 mL	35	121	505	3	29	3	3.6	1	N/A	0	14	4.7	4	135	31	102	0.7	0.02	2.3	42
Muesli, President's Choice™	75 mL	40	144	603	5	28	10	3.5	2	N/A	0	9	1.6	24	228	13	40	0.1	0.10	1.4	N/A
Nesquik, General Mills™	250 mL	30	120	502	1	27	14	0.6	1	N/A	0	33	4.1	192	49	8	44	0	0	1.4	36
Oatmeal Crisp Almond, General Mills™	125 mL	32	131	546	3	23	8	2.3	3	N/A	0	81	4.3	108	93	34	93	0.6	0.05	1.5	38
Oatmeal Crisp Maple Walnut, General Mills™	125 mL	32	133	557	3	25	9	2.3	3	0.3	0	81	4.3	142	101	29	81	0.6	0.05	1.5	38
Puffed Wheat, Quaker™	250 mL	13	45	188	2	9	tr	1.4	tr	0.1	0	9	0.5	0	60	18	40	0.1	0.01	1.0	1
Raisin Bran, Kellogg's™	250 mL	59	187	782	5	47	17	6.7	1	N/A	0	22	7.9	367	334	75	189	1.2	0.08	4.5	72
Reese's Puffs, General Mills™	175 mL	30	128	533	2	24	13	0.6	3	0.6	0	98	4.0	178	43	2	11	0	0	1.4	35
Rice Krispies, Kellogg's™	250 mL	29	110	458	2	24	3	0.3	tr	0	0	4	3.8	315	31	11	41	0.6	0.01	1.7	30
Shredded Wheat, Post™	1 biscuit	25	91	379	3	21	tr	3.5	1	0.1	0	9	1.5	1	92	31	83	0.1	0.06	2.3	11
Shreddies, Post™	175 mL	38	138	579	4	32	6	4.4	1	N/A	0	14	5.1	241	143	38	109	0.8	0.01	2.5	N/A
Special K, Kellogg's™	250 mL	24	94	392	4	18	2	0.3	tr	N/A	0	tr	3.2	226	34	13	49	0.5	0.03	1.9	29
Sugar Crisp, Post™	250 mL	26	103	432	1	24	14	0.8	1	N/A	0	3	0.3	33	1	11	44	0.5	tr	1.5	32
Trix, General Mills™	250 mL	30	117	491	1	27	13	1.0	3	N/A	0	98	4.0	195	16	2	22	0	0	1.4	35
Weetabix™	2 biscuits	35	130	543	4	29	2	4.4	1	0.1	0	14	1.1	126	141	58	144	0.7	N/A	2.6	13
Crackers																					
Cheese crackers, small	15	15	75	316	2	9	tr	0.4	4	1.4	2	23	0.7	149	22	5	33	0.1	0.06	1.0	36
Melba toast, plain	2	10	39	163	1	8	tr	0.6	tr	tr	0	9	0.4	83	20	6	20	tr	0.03	0.6	19
Milk crackers	2	24	109	457	2	17	4	0.5	4	0.6	3	41	0.9	142	27	5	73	0.1	0.10	1.5	34
Rusk toast	1	10	41	170	1	7	N/A	0.6	1	0.1	0	3	0.3	25	25	4	15	tr	0.04	0.7	10
Rye wafers, plain	2	20	67	279	2	16	tr	4.6	tr	tr	0	8	1.2	159	99	24	67	0.1	0.06	0.7	9
Saltine (oyster, soda, soup)	4	12	51	215	2	9	tr	0.4	1	0.2	0	8	0.7	129	18	3	12	tr	0.05	0.9	26
Saltine (oyster, soda, soup), unsalted top	4	12	52	218	1	9	0	0.4	1	0.4	0	14	0.6	92	15	3	13	0.1	0.06	0.9	23
Standard-type (snack-type) (Ritz™)	4	12	60	252	1	7	tr	0.2	3	0.5	0	14	0.4	102	16	3	27	tr	0.04	0.7	17
Standard-type, reduced sodium (Ritz™)	4	12	60	252	1	7	tr	0.2	3	0.5	0	14	0.4	45	43	3	27	tr	0.04	0.7	17
Wheat crackers	4	20	95	396	2	13	1	1.4	3	2.0	0	10	1.0	173	60	12	44	0.1	0.07	1.4	37

Food Name	Measure	Weight g	Energy kcal	Energy kJ	Protein g	Carbohydrate g	Total Sugar g	Total Dietary Fibre g	Total Fat g	Saturated Fat g	Cholesterol mg	Calcium mg	Iron mg	Sodium mg	Potassium mg	Magnesium mg	Phosphorus mg	Thiamin mg	Riboflavin mg	Niacin NE	Folate DFE
Breads, Cereals and Other Grain Products																					
Wheat crackers, low fat	4	18	79	330	2	12	2	0.9	2	1.2	tr	34	0.7	112	72	13	52	0.1	0.10	1.3	28
Whole wheat crackers	4	16	71	296	1	11	tr	1.7	3	0.5	0	8	0.5	105	48	16	47	tr	0.02	1.1	4
Baked Goods																					
Biscuits, Croissants, and Muffins																					
Biscuit, plain or buttermilk, fast food	1	51	186	776	3	25	2	0.7	8	1.3	1	25	1.7	537	114	9	219	0.2	0.15	2.4	58
Biscuit, plain or buttermilk, from mix, baked	1	30	97	404	2	14	3	0.4	4	1.0	2	54	0.6	273	55	7	136	0.1	0.11	1.4	31
Biscuit, plain or buttermilk, homemade	1	60	212	888	4	27	1	0.9	10	2.6	2	141	1.7	348	73	11	98	0.2	0.19	2.6	57
Biscuit, plain, refrigerated dough, baked	1	27	93	391	2	13	tr	0.4	4	1.0	0	5	0.7	325	42	4	104	0.1	0.06	1.2	37
Croissant, butter	1	57	231	968	5	26	6	1.5	12	6.6	38	21	1.2	424	67	9	60	0.2	0.14	2.2	74
Muffin, blueberry, from mix, prepared	1	54	149	623	3	24	N/A	N/A	5	1.2	32	14	0.6	216	41	6	93	0.1	0.17	1.9	61
Muffin, bran, from mix, prepared	1	55	159	666	4	27	N/A	N/A	5	1.4	32	18	1.5	271	84	33	189	0.1	0.13	2.9	38
Muffin, bran, homemade	1	57	199	833	4	32	13	3.7	8	0.9	23	82	2.3	242	363	80	129	0.1	0.16	3.0	37
Muffin, carrot, commercial	1	113	344	1439	7	49	17	1.9	14	1.6	34	100	2.2	396	208	18	117	0.3	0.31	4.1	90
Muffin, chocolate chip, commercial	1	113	366	1530	8	53	16	2.4	14	5.3	37	116	2.9	341	192	34	147	0.3	0.35	4.6	102
Muffin, fruit, commercial	1	113	313	1309	6	54	22	2.9	7	1.6	34	64	1.8	505	139	18	223	0.2	0.14	2.5	129
Muffin, fruit, homemade	1	57	162	679	4	23	N/A	0.9	6	1.2	21	108	1.3	251	70	9	83	0.2	0.16	2.0	42
Cookies, Granola Bars and Other Bars																					
Bars																					
Breakfast bar, Oatmeal to Go™	1	47	197	825	3	33	10	2.4	5	0.9	tr	17	4.2	202	102	N/A	N/A	0.7	N/A	1.7	N/A
Cereal bar, fruit filled (Nutri-Grain™)	1	37	135	566	2	26	14	1.2	3	0.5	tr	17	0.6	96	72	3	43	0.1	0.04	0.8	N/A
Granola bar, hard, chocolate chip	1	24	105	440	2	17	N/A	1.1	4	2.7	0	18	0.7	83	60	17	49	tr	0.02	0.7	3
Granola bar, hard, plain	1	25	118	493	3	16	N/A	1.3	5	0.6	0	15	0.7	74	84	24	69	0.1	0.03	1.1	6
Granola bar, soft, chocolate chip, graham and marshmallow	1	26	109	454	1	20	6	1.0	3	0.6	0	6	0.6	90	48	18	53	tr	0.04	0.5	3
Granola bar, soft, nuts and raisins	1	28	127	532	2	18	N/A	1.6	6	2.7	tr	24	0.6	71	110	25	67	0.1	0.05	1.2	8
Granola bar, soft, peanut butter, chocolate coated	1	37	188	788	4	20	N/A	1.0	12	6.3	4	40	0.5	71	125	25	84	tr	0.08	2.0	9
Granola bar, soft, plain	1	28	124	519	2	19	N/A	1.3	5	2.0	tr	29	0.7	78	91	21	64	0.1	0.05	0.6	7
Muffin bar (Hop&Go™, Sweet Mornings™)	1	50	178	746	2	30	18	0.6	6	1.0	20	7	0.8	175	64	7	26	0.1	0.10	1.4	33

Baked Goods

Food Name	Measure	Weight g	Energy kcal	Energy kJ	Protein g	Carbohydrate g	Total Sugar g	Total Dietary Fibre g	Total Fat g	Saturated Fat g	Cholesterol mg	Calcium mg	Iron mg	Sodium mg	Potassium mg	Magnesium mg	Phosphorus mg	Thiamin mg	Riboflavin mg	Niacin NE	Folate DFE
Cookies																					
Chocolate chip, commercial	2	20	98	409	1	13	7	0.6	5	1.5	N/A	7	0.7	59	30	10	23	tr	0.05	0.7	20
Chocolate chip, homemade	2	32	156	653	2	19	N/A	0.9	9	2.6	10	12	0.8	116	72	18	32	0.1	0.06	0.8	15
Chocolate chip, refrigerated dough, baked	2	24	118	494	1	16	N/A	0.4	5	1.9	6	7	0.6	56	48	6	18	tr	0.05	0.7	17
Chocolate coated marshmallow	2	30	129	541	1	21	14	0.6	4	2.2	tr	6	0.9	46	43	11	29	tr	0.06	0.4	11
Chocolate sandwich	2	20	93	390	1	14	8	0.6	4	1.8	0	4	2.1	97	37	10	18	tr	0.03	0.8	17
Coconut macaroons, homemade	2	48	194	811	2	35	34	0.9	6	5.4	0	3	0.4	119	75	10	21	tr	0.05	0.4	2
Fig	2	32	111	466	1	23	15	1.5	2	0.4	0	20	0.9	112	66	9	20	0.1	0.07	0.8	17
Ginger snaps	2	14	58	244	1	11	3	0.3	1	0.3	0	11	0.9	92	48	7	12	tr	0.04	0.6	20
Graham crackers, plain or honey	2	14	59	248	1	11	4	0.4	1	0.2	0	3	0.5	85	19	4	15	tr	0.04	0.8	9
Molasses	2	30	129	539	2	22	5	0.3	4	1.0	0	22	1.9	138	104	16	29	0.1	0.08	1.3	44
Oatmeal, with raisins, commercial	2	26	117	489	2	18	6	0.7	5	1.2	0	10	0.7	100	37	9	36	0.1	0.06	1.0	19
Oatmeal, without raisins, homemade	2	30	134	561	2	20	N/A	0.7	5	1.1	11	32	0.8	179	55	13	50	0.1	0.05	0.8	14
Peanut butter sandwich	2	28	134	560	2	18	10	0.5	6	1.4	0	15	0.7	103	54	14	53	0.1	0.07	1.6	26
Peanut butter, homemade	2	40	190	794	4	24	N/A	1.5	10	1.8	12	16	0.9	207	92	16	46	0.1	0.08	2.1	32
Shortbread, commercial, plain	2	16	80	336	1	10	2	0.3	4	1.0	3	6	0.4	73	16	3	17	0.1	0.05	0.8	18
Shortbread, homemade	2	33	185	773	2	19	7	0.5	12	7.3	31	6	0.7	130	20	4	20	0.1	0.08	1.3	32
Animal crackers (arrowroot, social tea)	2	10	45	187	1	7	1	0.2	1	0.3	0	4	0.3	39	10	2	11	tr	0.03	0.5	17
Sugar cookies, commercial	2	30	143	600	2	20	11	0.2	6	1.6	15	6	0.6	107	19	4	24	0.1	0.06	1.2	25
Sugar cookies, homemade	2	32	142	592	2	25	16	0.4	4	1.1	8	18	0.6	72	23	3	23	0.1	0.07	1.0	24
Vanilla wafers	2	12	57	237	1	9	N/A	0.2	2	0.6	8	3	0.3	37	13	1	8	tr	0.03	0.5	8
Cakes																					
Angelfood, commercial (25cm diam)	1/12	28	73	306	2	16	N/A	0.4	tr	tr	0	40	0.1	212	26	3	9	tr	0.14	0.6	16
Angelfood, from mix (25cm diam)	1/12	50	129	538	3	29	15	0.1	tr	tr	0	42	0.1	255	68	4	116	tr	0.10	0.7	14
Banana bread, homemade (11cm X 6cm X 1cm)	1 slice	60	196	818	3	33	N/A	0.7	6	1.3	26	13	0.8	181	80	8	35	0.1	0.12	1.4	29
Boston cream pie, commercial	1/6	92	232	970	2	39	33	1.3	8	2.2	34	21	0.3	132	36	6	45	0.4	0.25	0.7	17
Brownies, commercial (5cm X 5cm)	1 square	34	138	576	2	22	12	0.7	6	1.4	6	10	0.8	106	51	11	34	0	0.07	0.9	24
Brownies, homemade (5cm X 5cm)	1 square	36	168	702	2	18	N/A	0.8	10	2.6	26	21	0.7	123	63	19	48	0.1	0.07	0.8	14

Food Name	Measure	Weight g	Energy kcal	Energy kJ	Protein g	Carbohydrate g	Total Sugar g	Total Dietary Fibre g	Total Fat g	Saturated Fat g	Cholesterol mg	Calcium mg	Iron mg	Sodium mg	Potassium mg	Magnesium mg	Phosphorus mg	Thiamin mg	Riboflavin mg	Niacin NE	Folate DFE
Baked Goods																					
Carrot, homemade with cream cheese icing (2 layer, 23cm diam)	1/12	133	542	2266	5	70	52	1.5	28	3.8	73	49	1.6	201	131	10	70	0.2	0.22	2.7	57
Cheesecake, commercial (15 cm diam)	1/6	100	321	1342	6	26	N/A	0.4	23	9.9	55	51	0.6	207	90	11	93	tr	0.19	1.3	20
Cheesecake, from mix, no-bake type (20cm diam)	1/8	149	407	1702	3	53	N/A	2.8	19	9.9	43	255	0.7	564	313	28	347	0.2	0.39	2.4	57
Cheesecake, plain, homemade with cherry topping (20cm diam)	1/8	168	459	1920	11	55	45	0.8	23	8.8	75	65	1.6	496	146	12	124	tr	0.24	2.8	23
Chocolate, from mix, with icing (23cm diam)	1/12	109	362	1513	4	61	47	2.0	13	1.9	43	63	1.6	396	177	27	141	0.1	0.13	1.9	26
Chocolate, frozen, commercial, with chocolate icing (1 layer, 5cm X 20cm diam)	1/6	85	282	1180	3	48	37	2.0	10	1.0	33	49	1.0	309	138	21	110	N/A	N/A	1.0	20
Chocolate, homemade with icing (2 layer, 23cm diam)	1/12	109	408	1706	4	67	52	1.9	16	5.0	28	66	2.5	253	138	34	91	0.1	0.15	2.0	36
Coffee cake, cinnamon with crumb topping, commercial	1/10	57	237	991	4	26	N/A	1.1	13	3.3	18	31	1.1	199	70	12	61	0.1	0.13	1.7	46
Coffee cake, cinnamon with crumb topping, from mix (20cm X 15cm)	1/10	45	142	596	2	24	13	0.5	4	0.8	22	61	0.6	189	50	8	96	0.1	0.08	1.2	33
Fruitcake, commercial	1 piece	43	139	583	1	26	13	1.6	4	0.5	2	14	0.9	116	66	7	22	tr	0.04	0.6	14
Gingerbread, from mix (23cm X 23cm)	1/9	69	212	889	3	35	22	0.8	7	1.8	22	47	2.3	315	166	11	113	0.1	0.13	1.9	28
Pound cake, homemade (25cm X 13cm X 7.5cm)	1/10	91	391	1633	5	42	22	0.4	23	4.1	96	22	2.1	368	66	7	59	0.2	0.23	3.0	62
Shortcake, biscuit-type, homemade (4cm X 7.5cm diam)	1	75	234	978	5	34	8	1.0	8	2.4	28	106	1.7	459	96	12	100	0.2	0.24	3.1	72
Sponge, commercial, individual shell	1	25	72	302	1	15	9	0.1	1	0.2	26	18	0.7	61	25	3	34	0	0.07	0.8	18
Sponge, homemade (25cm diam)	1/12	63	187	782	5	36	N/A	0.2	3	0.8	107	26	1.0	144	89	6	63	0.1	0.19	1.7	33
White, from mix, with icing (2 layer, 23cm diam)	1/12	109	363	1518	3	66	51	0.9	10	1.6	N/A	41	0.9	342	76	15	138	0.1	0.12	1.9	47
White, homemade, with icing (2 layer, 23cm diam)	1/12	109	371	1553	3	70	56	0.3	9	2.5	1	50	1.3	205	55	5	41	0.1	0.14	1.9	33
White, frozen, commercial, with icing (1 layer, 5cm X 20cm diam)	1/6	85	283	1184	2	52	40	1.0	8	1.0	0	32	1.0	266	59	12	108	N/A	N/A	1.0	37
Yellow, from mix, with icing (2 layer, 23cm diam)	1/12	109	363	1519	4	64	47	0.9	11	2.0	46	60	1.1	338	74	15	137	0.1	0.14	2.0	57
Pies																					
Apple, commercial, 2 crust (23cm diam)	1/8	125	296	1239	2	43	20	2.0	14	4.7	0	14	0.6	333	81	9	30	tr	0.03	0.9	54
Apple, homemade, 2 crust (23cm diam)	1/8	155	411	1717	4	58	N/A	2.3	19	4.7	0	11	1.7	327	122	11	43	0.2	0.17	2.7	59
Banana cream, from mix, no-bake type (23cm diam)	1/8	92	231	966	3	29	N/A	0.6	12	6.4	27	67	0.4	267	104	11	154	0.1	0.13	1.4	28
Butter tart	1	54	243	1038	2	29	15	0.7	14	5.6	30	22	1.1	164	109	10	35	0.1	0.10	1.5	35
Cherry, commercial, 2 crust (23cm diam)	1/8	125	325	1359	3	50	18	1.0	14	3.2	0	15	2.0	308	101	10	36	0.2	0.16	2.5	50

Baked Goods

Food Name	Measure	Weight g	Energy kcal	Energy kJ	Protein g	Carbohydrate g	Total Sugar g	Total Dietary Fibre g	Total Fat g	Saturated Fat g	Cholesterol mg	Calcium mg	Iron mg	Sodium mg	Potassium mg	Magnesium mg	Phosphorus mg	Thiamin mg	Riboflavin mg	Niacin NE	Folate DFE
Chocolate cream, commercial (20cm diam)	1/6	113	344	1436	3	38	N/A	2.3	22	5.6	6	41	1.2	154	144	24	77	tr	0.12	1.4	19
Coconut cream, commercial (20cm diam)	1/6	64	191	797	1	24	23	0.8	11	4.5	0	19	0.5	163	42	13	54	tr	0.05	0.4	5
Fried pie, fruit (13cm X 10cm)	1	128	404	1692	4	55	27	3.3	21	3.1	0	28	1.6	479	83	13	55	0.2	0.14	2.7	36
Lemon meringue, commercial (20cm diam)	1/6	113	303	1267	2	53	27	1.4	10	2.0	51	63	0.7	165	101	17	119	0.1	0.24	1.1	40
Mincemeat pie, homemade, 2 crust (23cm diam)	1/8	165	477	1995	4	79	47	4.3	18	4.4	0	36	2.5	419	335	23	69	0.2	0.17	2.7	59
Pecan, commercial (20cm diam)	1/6	113	452	1890	5	65	32	4.0	21	4.0	36	19	1.2	479	84	20	87	0.1	0.14	1.5	61
Pumpkin, commercial (20cm diam)	1/6	109	229	957	4	30	15	2.9	10	1.9	22	65	1.5	307	168	16	77	0.2	0.22	1.9	35
Sugar pie, homemade, 1 crust	1/8	88	407	1703	3	31	18	0.5	31	17.3	84	61	1.1	81	139	13	59	0.1	0.15	1.6	34

Other Baked Goods

Food Name	Measure	Weight g	Energy kcal	Energy kJ	Protein g	Carbohydrate g	Total Sugar g	Total Dietary Fibre g	Total Fat g	Saturated Fat g	Cholesterol mg	Calcium mg	Iron mg	Sodium mg	Potassium mg	Magnesium mg	Phosphorus mg	Thiamin mg	Riboflavin mg	Niacin NE	Folate DFE
Apple crisp, homemade	125 mL	128	206	863	2	39	25	1.8	4	0.9	0	45	1.0	449	100	10	36	0.1	0.10	N/A	31
Bread pudding with raisins, homemade	125 mL	106	162	677	6	24	15	0.9	5	1.8	61	124	1.2	252	228	18	111	0.1	0.26	2.1	31
Danish pastry, cinnamon (11cm diam)	1	65	262	1095	5	29	13	0.8	15	3.7	14	46	1.3	241	81	12	70	0.2	0.17	2.8	60
Danish pastry, fruit (11cm diam)	1	71	263	1102	4	34	20	1.3	13	3.5	81	33	1.3	251	59	11	63	0.2	0.16	2.2	49
Date squares, homemade	1 square	61	226	944	3	37	N/A	2.3	8	4.7	20	21	2.0	241	154	23	61	0.2	0.08	1.7	31
Doughnut, cake-type, plain (8cm diam)	1	47	198	828	2	23	11	0.7	11	1.7	17	21	0.9	257	60	9	126	0.1	0.11	1.4	39
Doughnut, cake-type, plain, chocolate coated (9cm diam)	1	57	270	1130	3	27	13	1.1	18	4.6	35	20	1.4	245	112	23	115	0.1	0.06	1.4	39
Doughnut, yeast-leavened, honey bun, glazed (9cm x 6cm)	1	60	242	1011	4	27	14	0.7	14	3.5	4	26	1.2	205	65	13	56	0.2	0.13	2.5	41
Doughnut, yeast-leavened, jelly filled (9cm X 6cm)	1	85	289	1209	5	33	18	0.8	16	4.1	22	21	1.5	249	67	17	72	0.3	0.12	2.8	88
Eclairs, custard filled, chocolate glaze	1	100	262	1096	6	24	7	0.6	16	4.1	127	63	1.2	337	117	15	107	0.1	0.27	2.1	63
Rice Krispies Squares™, commercial	1 square	22	91	381	1	18	N/A	0.1	2	0.3	0	1	0.3	77	9	3	9	0.3	0.30	3.7	38
Toaster pastries (Pop-Tarts™), brown sugar & cinnamon	1	50	206	862	3	34	N/A	0.5	7	1.8	0	17	2.0	212	57	12	67	0.2	0.29	2.8	21
Toaster pastries (Pop-Tarts™), fruit, frosted	1	55	215	900	2	39	20	0.4	6	1.5	0	16	3.9	387	81	13	75	0.2	0.20	N/A	39

Vegetables and Vegetable Products

Vegetables

Food Name	Measure	Weight (g)	Energy (kcal)	Energy (kJ)	Protein (g)	Carbohydrate (g)	Total Sugar (g)	Total Dietary Fibre (g)	Total Fat (g)	Calcium (mg)	Iron (mg)	Sodium (mg)	Potassium (mg)	Magnesium (mg)	Phosphorus (mg)	Vitamin A (RAE)	Beta-carotene (mcg)	Lycopene (mcg)	Folate (DFE)	Vitamin C (mg)	Vitamin B12 (mcg)
Alfalfa sprouts, raw	60 mL	8	2	10	tr	tr	tr	0.2	tr	3	0.1	1	7	2	6	1	7	0	3	1	0
Artichoke hearts, canned in water	1 heart	27	13	56	1	3	tr	1.0	tr	12	0.3	74	95	16	23	2	28	0	14	3	0
Artichoke hearts, marinated in oil	1 heart	28	27	111	1	3	tr	1.0	2	12	0.3	79	93	16	23	2	28	0	13	3	0
Artichoke, boiled, drained	1 medium	120	60	251	4	13	1	4.7	tr	54	1.5	114	425	72	103	11	127	0	61	12	0
Asparagus, canned, drained	6 spears	108	21	85	2	3	1	1.5	1	17	2.0	310	186	11	46	44	532	26	104	20	0
Asparagus, fresh or frozen, boiled, drained	6 spears	90	18	75	2	3	tr	1.6	tr	18	0.7	8	178	11	46	41	489	24	128	14	0
Bean sprouts, stir-fried	125 mL	66	33	137	3	7	N/A	1.2	tr	9	1.2	6	143	22	52	1	12	N/A	46	10	0
Beans, lima, frozen, boiled, drained	125 mL	95	100	417	6	18	1	4.0	tr	27	1.9	28	391	53	107	8	95	0	15	6	0
Beans, snap (green, yellow, Italian), canned, drained	125 mL	71	14	60	1	3	1	1.5	tr	19	0.6	187	78	9	14	16	186	0	23	2	0
Beans, snap (green, yellow, Italian), fresh or frozen, boiled, drained	125 mL	71	22	94	1	5	1	1.9	tr	33	0.5	4	97	15	21	22	269	0	20	5	0
Beets, pickled, sliced, not drained	125 mL	120	78	326	1	20	N/A	2.2	tr	13	0.5	317	177	18	20	1	7	N/A	32	3	0
Beets, sliced, boiled, drained	125 mL	90	40	165	2	9	7	1.8	tr	14	0.7	69	274	21	34	2	19	0	72	3	0
Beets, sliced, canned, drained	125 mL	90	28	117	1	6	5	1.9	tr	13	1.6	174	133	15	15	1	13	0	27	6	0
Belgium endive, raw	1 endive	53	9	38	tr	2	N/A	1.6	tr	10	0.1	1	112	5	14	1	9	N/A	20	1	0
Bok Choy, Pak-Choi, shredded, boiled, drained	125 mL	90	11	45	1	2	1	0.9	tr	84	0.9	31	333	10	26	190	2289	0	37	23	0
Broccoli, chopped, boiled, drained	125 mL	82	29	120	2	6	1	2.0	tr	33	0.6	34	241	17	55	81	973	0	89	53	0
Broccoli, chopped, raw	125 mL	46	16	66	1	3	1	1.1	tr	22	0.3	15	147	10	31	15	178	0	29	41	0
Broccoli, frozen spears, boiled, drained	125 mL	97	27	114	3	5	1	2.3	tr	50	0.6	23	175	19	53	54	645	0	29	39	0
Brussels sprouts, fresh or frozen, boiled, drained	4 sprouts	84	33	137	3	6	2	3.2	tr	26	0.7	15	255	16	47	36	428	0	68	45	0
Cabbage, green, shredded, boiled, drained	125 mL	79	17	73	1	4	2	1.3	tr	25	0.1	6	77	6	12	6	59	0	16	16	0
Cabbage, green, shredded, raw	125 mL	37	9	37	1	2	1	0.7	tr	17	0.2	7	91	6	9	3	33	0	16	12	0
Cabbage, napa, shredded, boiled, drained	125 mL	58	7	29	1	1	N/A	N/A	tr	17	0.4	6	50	5	11	7	77	0	25	2	0
Cabbage, red, shredded, raw	125 mL	37	11	48	1	3	1	0.8	tr	17	0.3	10	90	6	11	21	248	7	7	21	0
Carrots, baby, raw	8	80	28	117	1	7	4	1.4	tr	26	0.7	62	190	8	22	552	5113	0	26	7	0
Carrots, fresh or frozen, boiled, drained	125 mL	77	28	116	1	6	3	1.9	tr	25	0.3	45	165	8	24	652	6333	1	10	2	0
Carrots, raw	1 medium	61	25	104	1	6	3	1.5	tr	20	0.2	42	195	7	21	367	3522	1	12	4	0

Food Name	Measure	Weight g	Energy kcal	Energy kJ	Protein g	Carbohydrate g	Total Sugar g	Total Dietary Fibre g	Total Fat g	Calcium mg	Iron mg	Sodium mg	Potassium mg	Magnesium mg	Phosphorus mg	Vitamin A RAE	Beta-carotene mcg	Lycopene mcg	Folate DFE	Vitamin C mg	Vitamin B12 mcg
Vegetables and Vegetable Products																					
Cauliflower, pieces, boiled, drained	125 mL	66	15	63	1	3	1	1.8	tr	10	0.2	10	93	6	21	1	5	0	29	29	0
Cauliflower, pieces, raw	125 mL	53	13	55	1	3	1	0.9	tr	12	0.2	16	160	8	23	1	4	0	30	25	0
Celery, raw	1 stalk	40	6	24	tr	1	tr	0.6	tr	16	0.1	32	104	4	10	9	108	0	14	1	0
Corn, sweet, canned, cream style	125 mL	135	97	407	2	25	4	1.8	1	4	0.5	385	181	23	69	5	41	0	61	6	0
Corn, sweet, canned, niblets	125 mL	111	88	366	3	22	4	2.3	1	6	0.5	302	206	26	71	4	37	0	54	6	0
Corn, sweet, on or off cob, fresh or frozen, boiled, drained	125 mL	87	82	343	3	19	3	2.0	1	2	0.5	8	209	26	79	7	50	0	35	4	0
Cucumber, peeled, raw	4 slices	28	3	14	tr	1	tr	0.2	tr	4	0.1	1	38	3	6	1	9	0	4	1	0
Edamame	125 mL	82	100	417	9	8	2	4.3	4	52	1.9	5	357	52	138	N/A	N/A	N/A	255	5	0
Eggplant, pieces, boiled, drained	125 mL	52	18	76	tr	5	2	1.3	tr	3	0.1	1	64	6	8	1	12	0	7	1	0
Fiddleheads, frozen, boiled	125 mL	98	33	139	4	6	N/A	0.9	tr	27	1.0	tr	244	26	78	171	1911	N/A	N/A	22	0
Fireweed leaves, raw	125 mL	12	13	52	1	2	N/A	1.3	tr	52	0.3	4	60	19	13	22	262	N/A	14	tr	0
Hearts of palm, canned	2	66	18	77	2	3	N/A	1.6	tr	38	2.1	281	117	25	43	0	0	N/A	26	5	0
Kale, chopped, boiled, drained	125 mL	69	19	80	1	4	1	1.4	tr	49	0.6	16	157	12	19	468	5613	0	9	28	0
Leeks, chopped, boiled, drained	125 mL	55	17	71	tr	4	N/A	0.5	tr	16	0.6	5	48	8	9	1	15	N/A	13	2	0
Lettuce, Boston, shredded	250 mL	58	8	31	1	1	1	0.6	tr	20	0.7	3	138	8	19	96	1155	0	42	2	0
Lettuce, iceberg, shredded	250 mL	58	8	34	1	2	1	0.7	tr	10	0.2	6	82	4	12	15	174	0	17	2	0
Lettuce, looseleaf, shredded	250 mL	59	9	37	1	2	tr	0.8	tr	21	0.5	17	115	8	17	219	2629	0	22	11	0
Lettuce, romaine, shredded	250 mL	59	10	42	1	2	2	1.2	tr	20	0.6	5	146	8	18	172	2062	0	80	14	0
Lettuce, spring mix (mesclun)	250 mL	58	12	50	1	2	tr	1.1	tr	43	0.7	21	202	19	23	124	1489	0	62	9	0
Mushrooms, pieces, canned, drained	125 mL	82	21	87	2	4	2	2.3	tr	9	0.7	350	106	12	54	0	0	0	10	1	0
Mushrooms, portobello, grilled	125 mL	85	30	124	4	4	0	1.9	1	3	0.5	9	443	13	128	0	0	0	16	0	0
Mushrooms, raw	3 medium	54	12	50	2	2	1	0.6	tr	2	0.3	2	170	5	46	0	0	0	9	1	0.02
Mushrooms, shiitake, sliced, stir-fried	125 mL	57	27	115	2	4	tr	2.1	tr	1	0.3	3	186	11	63	0	0	0	8	0	0
Mushrooms, white, sliced, stir-fried	125 mL	57	15	62	2	2	0	1.0	tr	2	0.1	7	226	6	60	0	0	0	11	0	0
Onions, green (scallion), raw	1 medium	15	5	20	tr	1	tr	0.4	tr	11	0.2	2	41	3	6	8	90	0	10	3	0
Onions, yellow, chopped, raw	60 mL	41	17	71	tr	4	2	0.6	tr	9	0.1	1	58	4	11	0	tr	0	8	3	0
Onions, yellow, chopped, sauteed	125 mL	46	61	254	tr	4	2	0.8	5	9	0.1	6	61	4	15	N/A	N/A	N/A	N/A	1	0

Vegetables and Vegetable Products

Food Name	Measure	Weight g	Energy kcal	Energy kJ	Protein g	Carbohydrate g	Total Sugar g	Total Dietary Fibre g	Total Fat g	Calcium mg	Iron mg	Sodium mg	Potassium mg	Magnesium mg	Phosphorus mg	Vitamin A RAE	Beta-carotene mcg	Lycopene mcg	Folate DFE	Vitamin C mg	Vitamin B12 mcg
Parsnip, sliced, boiled, drained	125 mL	82	59	245	1	14	4	2.7	tr	30	0.5	8	302	24	57	0	0	0	48	11	0
Peas, green, canned, drained	125 mL	90	62	260	4	11	4	4.0	tr	18	0.9	226	155	15	60	24	287	0	40	9	0
Peas, green, frozen, boiled, drained	125 mL	85	66	276	4	12	4	3.7	tr	20	1.3	61	93	19	65	89	1057	0	50	8	0
Peas, snowpeas, boiled, drained	125 mL	85	36	149	3	6	3	2.4	tr	36	1.7	3	203	22	46	44	505	0	25	40	0
Peas, snowpeas, raw	10	34	14	60	1	3	1	0.6	tr	15	0.7	1	68	8	18	18	214	0	14	20	0
Pepper, jalapeno, raw	1	14	4	18	tr	1	tr	0.4	tr	1	0.1	tr	30	3	4	6	64	0	7	6	0
Pepper, sweet, green, raw	1/2	82	16	69	1	4	2	1.2	tr	8	0.3	2	144	8	16	15	171	0	9	66	0
Pepper, sweet, green, sauteed	125 mL	74	95	396	1	3	2	1.3	9	6	0.2	13	100	6	11	8	101	0	1	132	0
Pepper, sweet, red, raw	1/2	60	15	65	1	4	2	0.8	tr	4	0.3	1	126	7	15	93	966	183	11	113	0
Pepper, sweet, red, sauteed	125 mL	74	99	413	1	5	3	1.3	9	5	0.4	16	144	9	17	98	1169	361	1	121	0
Pepper, sweet, yellow, raw	1/2	93	25	105	1	6	N/A	0.8	tr	10	0.4	2	197	-1	22	9	112	N/A	24	171	0
Pepper, sweet, yellow, sauteed	125 mL	74	36	149	1	5	3	0.6	2	9	0.3	175	153	9	18	30	86	0	19	132	tr
Potato, baked, flesh	1	156	145	607	3	34	3	3.4	tr	8	0.5	8	610	39	78	0	0	0	14	20	0
Potato, baked, flesh and skin	1	173	161	673	4	37	2	3.8	tr	26	1.9	17	926	48	121	2	10	0	48	17	0
Potato, boiled without skin	1	135	116	486	2	27	1	1.9	tr	11	0.4	7	443	27	54	0	3	0	12	10	0
Potato, boiled, flesh and skin	1	150	129	540	3	30	1	2.5	tr	13	1.3	7	572	34	67	0	0	0	15	18	0
Potato, canned, drained	4	140	84	351	2	19	N/A	1.3	tr	7	1.8	307	321	20	39	0	0	0	8	7	0
Potato, microwaved, flesh and skin	1	202	212	887	5	49	N/A	5.1	tr	22	2.5	16	903	55	212	0	0	0	24	31	0
Potato, microwaved, peeled after cooking	1	156	156	652	3	36	N/A	3.4	tr	8	0.6	11	641	39	170	0	0	0	19	24	0
Potatoes, French fried, frozen, home-prepared in oven	20 strips	48	96	403	2	15	tr	1.6	4	4	0.6	14	201	11	40	0	1	0	6	5	0
Potatoes, hashed brown, plain, frozen, heated	125 mL	82	180	752	3	23	1	1.8	9	12	1.2	28	359	14	59	0	0	0	6	5	0
Potatoes, mashed, dried, with 2% milk and margarine	125 mL	111	107	447	3	15	2	1.1	4	46	0.2	284	235	15	59	61	2	0	8	14	0.13
Potatoes, mashed, homemade with 2% milk and margarine	125 mL	111	116	487	2	19	N/A	2.2	4	29	0.3	327	321	20	51	19	N/A	0	9	7	0.06
Potatoes, scalloped, from mix with water, with 2% milk and margarine	125 mL	129	120	502	3	16	2	1.0	5	36	0.4	420	243	17	81	64	1	0	8	3	0.11
Potatoes, scalloped, homemade	125 mL	129	111	466	4	14	N/A	2.5	5	74	0.7	434	489	25	82	N/A	83	0	16	14	0
Pumpkin, canned	125 mL	129	44	184	1	10	4	3.8	tr	34	1.8	6	267	30	45	1007	8983	0	16	5	0
Radicchio, chopped	125 mL	21	5	20	tr	1	tr	0.2	tr	4	0.1	5	64	3	8	tr	3	0	13	2	0

Vegetables and Vegetable Products

Food Name	Measure	Weight g	Energy kcal	Energy kJ	Protein g	Carbohydrate g	Total Sugar g	Total Dietary Fibre g	Total Fat g	Calcium mg	Iron mg	Sodium mg	Potassium mg	Magnesium mg	Phosphorus mg	Vitamin A RAE	Beta-carotene mcg	Lycopene mcg	Folate DFE	Vitamin C mg	Vitamin B12 mcg
Radishes	3 medium	14	2	9	tr	tr	tr	0.2	tr	3	tr	5	5	31	1	3	0	1	0	3	2	0
Rutabaga (yellow turnip), diced, boiled, drained	125 mL	90	35	146	1	8	5	1.6	tr	43	0.5	18	293	21	50	13	1	0	13	17	0
Sauerkraut, canned, not drained	125 mL	75	14	59	1	3	1	1.9	tr	23	1.1	496	128	10	15	1	6	0	18	11	0
Seaweed, dulse, dried	60 mL	4	8	35	1	1	tr	0.1	tr	17	0.4	11	84	tr	14	62	740	N/A	35	9	0
Spinach, boiled, drained	125 mL	95	22	91	3	4	tr	2.3	tr	129	3.4	67	443	83	53	498	5980	0	139	9	0
Spinach, chopped, raw	250 mL	32	7	30	1	1	tr	0.7	tr	31	0.9	25	177	25	16	149	1783	0	61	9	0
Squash, acorn, cubed, baked	125 mL	108	61	253	1	16	N/A	2.1	tr	48	1.0	4	473	47	49	23	277	N/A	21	12	0
Squash, butternut, cubed, baked	125 mL	108	43	181	1	11	2	1.8	tr	44	0.6	4	308	31	29	413	4950	0	21	16	0
Squash, spaghetti, baked	125 mL	82	22	93	1	5	2	0.9	tr	17	0.3	15	96	9	11	5	48	0	7	3	0
Sweet potato, baked, peeled after cooking	1/2	57	51	214	1	12	5	1.9	tr	22	0.4	21	271	15	31	548	6560	0	3	11	0
Sweet potato, boiled without skin	1/2	76	57	240	1	13	4	1.9	tr	20	0.5	20	174	14	24	594	7130	0	5	10	0
Swiss chard, chopped, boiled, drained	125 mL	92	18	78	2	4	1	1.9	tr	54	2.1	165	508	80	31	283	3376	0	8	17	0
Tomatoes, canned, stewed	125 mL	135	35	147	1	8	6	1.4	tr	46	1.8	298	279	16	27	12	140	5436	7	11	0
Tomatoes, canned, whole	125 mL	127	22	90	1	5	3	1.0	tr	39	1.2	162	238	14	24	8	89	3423	10	18	0
Tomatoes, raw	1	123	22	92	1	5	3	1.5	tr	12	0.3	6	292	14	30	52	552	3165	18	16	0
Tomatoes, sun-dried	1 piece	2	5	22	tr	1	1	0.2	tr	2	0.2	42	69	4	7	1	10	815	1	1	0
Tomatoes, sun-dried, packed in oil, drained	1 piece	3	6	27	tr	1	N/A	0.2	tr	1	0.1	8	47	2	4	2	23	N/A	1	3	0
Turnip (white turnip), cubed, boiled, drained	125 mL	82	18	76	1	4	2	1.6	tr	27	0.1	13	146	7	21	0	0	0	7	10	0
Vegetables, Asian mix (broccoli, carrots, green beans, "mini corn", snow peas, sweet red pepper), frozen, boiled, drained	125 mL	74	29	122	2	6	2	1.8	tr	24	0.5	15	128	13	32	192	1878	tr	23	22	0
Vegetables, broccoli and cauliflower, frozen, boiled, drained	125 mL	95	22	93	2	4	1	2.4	tr	33	0.5	20	152	14	38	27	322	0	34	34	0
Vegetables, mixed (corn, lima beans, snap beans, peas, carrots), frozen, boiled, drained	125 mL	96	63	262	3	13	3	2.8	tr	24	0.8	34	163	21	49	206	2002	0	18	3	0
Vegetables, peas and carrots, canned, not drained	125 mL	135	51	214	3	11	N/A	2.7	tr	31	1.0	350	135	19	62	389	0	N/A	24	9	0
Zucchini, raw, slices	4	40	6	27	tr	1	2	0.4	tr	6	0.1	4	104	7	15	4	48	0	11	7	0
Zucchini, sliced, boiled, drained	125 mL	95	15	64	1	4	2	1.3	tr	12	0.3	3	241	21	38	53	637	0	16	4	0

Food Name	Measure	Weight g	Energy kcal	Energy kJ	Protein g	Carbohydrate g	Total Sugar g	Total Dietary Fibre g	Total Fat g	Calcium mg	Iron mg	Sodium mg	Potassium mg	Magnesium mg	Phosphorus mg	Vitamin A RAE	Beta-carotene mcg	Lycopene mcg	Folate DFE	Vitamin C mg	Vitamin B12 mcg
Vegetables and Vegetable Products																					
Vegetable Juices and Other Products																					
Carrot juice	125 mL	125	50	208	1	12	5	1.0	tr	30	0.6	36	364	17	52	966	11599	2	5	11	0
Coleslaw with dressing, homemade	125 mL	63	44	183	1	8	N/A	1.0	2	29	0.4	15	115	6	20	34	87	N/A	17	21	0
Potato salad, homemade	125 mL	132	205	858	4	14	3	1.4	15	28	0.7	579	276	17	66	57	183	0	22	17	0.20
Tomato clam cocktail	125 mL	128	61	257	1	14	4	0.5	tr	10	0.2	462	114	6	14	9	163	3807	10	6	0.04
Tomato juice	125 mL	128	22	91	2	5	5	0.9	tr	13	0.6	345	294	14	23	30	347	11602	26	10	0
Tomato juice, without added salt	125 mL	184	31	131	1	8	7	0.7	tr	18	0.8	18	421	20	33	42	N/A	16611	37	34	0
Tomato sauce for spaghetti, canned	125 mL	132	143	600	2	21	N/A	1.9	6	37	0.9	652	505	32	47	82	967	N/A	28	15	0
Tomato sauce, canned	125 mL	129	41	173	2	10	6	1.9	tr	17	1.3	678	428	21	34	22	271	19612	12	8	0
Vegetable juice cocktail	125 mL	128	24	101	1	6	2	0.7	tr	14	0.5	345	247	14	22	100	1061	12351	27	35	0
Vegetable juice cocktail, low sodium	125 mL	128	28	118	1	6	5	1.0	tr	14	0.5	89	247	14	22	66	1061	12350	27	35	0
Fruit and Fruit Juices																					
Fruit																					
Apple with skin (7cm diam)	1	138	72	300	tr	19	14	2.6	tr	8	0.2	1	148	7	15	4	37	0	4	6	0
Applesauce, unsweetened	125 mL	129	55	232	tr	15	13	1.5	tr	4	0.2	3	97	4	9	1	17	0	1	13	0
Apricots, dried	3	21	67	281	1	17	N/A	1.2	tr	13	1.3	3	389	13	33	133	0	0	1	2	0
Apricots, raw	3	105	50	211	1	12	10	2.1	tr	14	0.4	1	272	11	24	101	1149	0	9	11	0
Avocado	1/2	101	161	672	2	9	1	6.7	15	12	0.6	7	487	29	52	7	62	0	81	10	0
Banana	1	118	105	439	1	27	14	2.1	tr	6	0.3	1	422	32	26	4	31	0	24	10	0
Blackberries	125 mL	76	33	137	1	7	4	4.0	tr	22	0.5	1	123	15	17	8	97	0	19	16	0
Blueberries, frozen. unsweetened	125 mL	82	42	174	tr	10	7	2.6	1	7	0.1	1	44	4	9	2	23	0	6	2	0
Blueberries, raw	125 mL	77	44	182	1	11	8	2.0	tr	5	0.2	1	59	5	9	2	25	0	5	7	0
Cherries, sweet	10	68	43	179	1	11	9	1.4	tr	9	0.2	0	151	7	14	2	26	0	3	5	0
Clementine	1	74	35	146	tr	9	7	1.3	tr	22	0.1	1	131	7	16	N/A	N/A	N/A	18	36	0
Cranberries, dried, sweetened	60 mL	31	95	396	tr	25	20	1.8	tr	3	0.2	1	12	2	2	0	0	0	0	tr	0
Dates, dried	3	25	70	294	1	19	16	2.0	tr	10	0.3	tr	163	11	15	0	0	0	5	tr	0
Figs, dried	2	17	42	175	1	11	8	1.6	tr	27	0.3	2	114	11	11	tr	1	0	2	tr	0
Figs, raw	1	50	37	155	tr	10	8	1.5	tr	18	0.2	1	116	9	7	4	43	0	3	1	0

Fruit and Fruit Juices

Food Name	Measure	Weight g	Energy kcal	Energy kJ	Protein g	Carbohydrate g	Total Sugar g	Total Dietary Fibre g	Total Fat g	Calcium mg	Iron mg	Sodium mg	Potassium mg	Magnesium mg	Phosphorus mg	Vitamin A RAE	Beta-carotene mcg	Lycopene mcg	Folate DFE	Vitamin C mg	Vitamin B12 mcg
Fruit cocktail, canned, juice pack	125 mL	125	58	240	1	15	14	1.3	tr	10	0.3	5	119	9	18	19	193	0	4	3	0
Fruit cocktail, canned, light syrup pack	125 mL	128	73	304	1	19	18	1.3	tr	8	0.4	8	114	6	14	13	133	0	4	2	0
Fruit salad, tropical, canned, heavy syrup pack	125 mL	136	117	489	1	30	N/A	1.8	tr	18	0.7	3	178	18	10	8	102	N/A	12	24	0
Fruit salad, tropical, canned, juice pack	125 mL	131	70	272	1	18	16	1.1	tr	17	0.3	4	160	14	10	8	96	0	4	16	0
Grapefruit, pink or red	1/2	123	52	216	1	13	8	2.0	tr	27	0.1	0	166	11	22	71	844	1745	16	38	0
Grapefruit, white	1/2	118	39	163	1	10	9	2.1	tr	14	0.1	0	175	11	9	2	17	0	12	39	0
Grapes	20	100	69	289	1	18	15	1.2	tr	10	0.4	2	191	7	20	3	39	0	2	11	0
Groundcherries	10	49	26	108	1	5	N/A	N/A	tr	4	0.5	tr	75	N/A	19	17	210	N/A	3	5	0
Kiwifruit	1	76	46	194	1	11	7	2.3	tr	26	0.2	2	237	13	26	3	40	0	19	70	0
Lychees (litchis)	10	96	63	265	1	16	15	1.2	tr	5	0.3	1	164	10	30	0	0	0	13	69	0
Mango	1/2	104	67	282	1	18	15	1.9	tr	10	0.1	2	161	9	11	39	461	0	14	29	0
Melon, cantaloupe, cubes	125 mL	85	29	120	1	7	7	0.6	tr	8	0.2	14	226	10	13	143	1708	0	18	31	0
Melon, honeydew, cubes	125 mL	90	32	136	tr	8	7	0.7	tr	5	0.2	16	205	9	10	3	27	0	17	16	0
Melon, watermelon, cubes	125 mL	80	24	100	tr	6	5	0.3	tr	6	0.2	1	90	8	9	22	243	3639	2	7	0
Nectarine	1	136	60	250	1	14	11	2.3	tr	8	0.4	0	273	12	35	18	204	0	7	7	0
Orange	1	131	62	258	1	15	12	2.3	tr	52	0.1	0	237	13	18	8	93	0	39	70	0
Papaya, cubes	125 mL	74	29	121	tr	7	4	1.3	tr	18	0.1	2	190	7	4	17	204	0	28	46	0
Peach	1	98	38	160	1	9	8	1.9	tr	6	0.2	0	186	9	20	16	159	0	3	6	0
Peach, canned halves or slices, juice pack	125 mL	132	58	243	1	15	14	1.7	tr	8	0.4	5	169	9	22	25	250	0	4	5	0
Peach, canned halves or slices, light syrup pack	125 mL	133	72	300	1	19	18	1.7	tr	4	0.5	7	129	7	15	24	233	0	4	9	0
Peach, canned halves or slices, water pack	125 mL	129	31	129	1	8	6	1.7	tr	3	0.4	4	128	6	13	35	340	0	4	4	0
Pear with skin	1	166	96	403	1	26	16	5.0	tr	15	0.3	2	198	12	18	2	22	0	12	7	0
Pear, canned halves, juice pack	125 mL	131	66	274	tr	17	13	2.1	tr	12	0.4	5	126	9	16	0	4	0	1	2	0
Pear, canned halves, light syrup pack	125 mL	133	76	316	tr	20	16	2.1	tr	7	0.4	7	88	5	9	0	0	0	1	2	0
Pear, canned halves, water pack	125 mL	128	37	155	tr	10	8	2.0	tr	5	0.3	3	68	5	9	0	0	0	1	1	0
Pineapple, canned, juice pack	125 mL	132	79	330	1	21	19	1.2	tr	18	0.4	1	160	18	8	3	30	0	7	12	0
Pineapple, cubes	125 mL	82	42	174	tr	11	8	1.1	tr	11	0.2	1	88	10	7	2	28	0	16	46	0
Plantain, baked or boiled, sliced	125 mL	81	94	395	1	25	11	1.9	tr	2	0.5	4	378	26	23	37	300	0	21	9	0

Food Name	Measure		Weight g	Energy kcal	Energy kJ	Protein g	Carbohydrate g	Total Sugar g	Total Dietary Fibre g	Total Fat g	Calcium mg	Iron mg	Sodium mg	Potassium mg	Magnesium mg	Phosphorus mg	Vitamin A RAE	Beta-carotene mcg	Lycopene mcg	Folate DFE	Vitamin C mg	Vitamin B12 mcg
Fruit and Fruit Juices																						
Plum	1		66	30	127	tr	8	7	1.1	tr	4	0.1	0	104	5	11	11	125	0	3	6	0
Pomegranate (9.5cm diam)	1/2		77	53	220	1	13	13	0.5	tr	2	0.2	2	200	2	6	2	31	0	5	5	0
Prunes, dried	3		25	60	253	1	16	10	1.8	tr	11	0.2	1	184	10	17	10	99	0	1	tr	0
Prunes, dried, cooked, without added sugar	60 mL		63	67	281	1	18	16	3.6	tr	12	0.3	1	202	11	19	11	109	0	0	2	0
Raisins	60 mL		37	110	460	1	29	22	1.3	tr	18	0.7	4	275	12	37	0	0	0	2	1	0
Raspberries	125 mL		65	34	141	1	8	3	4.2	tr	16	0.4	1	98	14	19	1	8	0	14	17	0
Rhubarb, frozen, cooked, with added sugar	125 mL		127	147	615	tr	40	36	2.5	tr	184	0.3	1	122	15	10	5	56	0	6	4	0
Strawberries	7		84	27	113	tr	6	4	1.9	tr	13	0.4	1	129	11	20	2	6	0	20	49	0
Strawberries, frozen, unsweetened	125 mL		117	41	170	1	11	5	1.8	tr	19	0.9	2	173	13	15	2	32	0	20	48	0
Tangerine (mandarin)	1		84	45	186	1	11	9	1.5	tr	31	0.1	2	139	10	17	11	130	0	13	22	0
Tangerine (mandarin), canned, juice pack, drained	125 mL		100	38	159	1	9	8	1.2	tr	12	0.3	5	136	11	11	25	298	0	5	34	0
Fruit Juices																						
Apple juice, ready-to-drink, vitamin C added	125 mL		126	59	249	tr	15	14	0.1	tr	9	0.5	4	150	4	9	0	0	0	tr	52	0
Cranberry juice cocktail, ready-to-drink, vitamin C added	125 mL		134	76	318	0	19	16	0.1	tr	4	0.2	3	24	3	3	0	0	0	0	48	0
Cranberry juice, unsweetened, ready-to-drink	125 mL		134	61	257	tr	16	16	0.1	tr	11	0.3	3	103	8	17	3	36	0	1	12	0
Cranberry-apple juice-drink, ready-to-drink, low Calorie, vitamin C added	125 mL		127	24	100	tr	6	6	0.1	0	13	0.1	6	57	4	1	1	8	0	0	41	0
Grape juice, frozen, sweetened, diluted, vitamin C added	125 mL		132	67	281	tr	17	17	0.1	tr	5	0.1	3	28	5	5	0	7	0	1	20	0
Grape juice, ready-to-drink, vitamin C added	125 mL		132	81	337	1	20	20	0.1	tr	12	0.3	4	174	13	15	0	7	0	4	32	0
Grapefruit juice, ready-to-drink unsweetened or freshly squeezed	125 mL		130	50	210	1	12	12	0.4	tr	10	0.3	1	206	14	17	1	11	0	13	44	0
Grapefruit juice, ready-to-drink, sweetened	125 mL		132	61	254	1	15	15	0.1	tr	11	0.5	3	214	13	15	0	4	0	13	36	0
Lemon juice, canned or bottled	15 mL		15	3	14	tr	1	tr	0.1	tr	2	tr	3	16	1	1	tr	tr	0	2	4	0
Lime juice, canned or bottled	15 mL		16	3	14	tr	1	tr	0.1	tr	2	tr	2	12	1	2	tr	2	0	1	1	0
Nectar, apricot	125 mL		133	74	310	tr	19	18	0.8	tr	9	0.5	4	151	7	12	88	1042	0	1	44	0
Nectar, mango	125 mL		133	68	281	tr	17	17	0.4	tr	23	0.5	7	32	4	3	46	533	0	9	20	0
Orange and grapefruit juice, ready-to-drink	125 mL		130	56	235	1	13	13	0.1	tr	10	0.6	4	206	13	18	8	26	0	18	38	0
Orange juice, frozen, diluted	125 mL		132	59	247	1	14	11	0.3	tr	12	0.1	1	250	13	21	7	22	0	58	51	0
Orange juice, ready-to-drink	125 mL		132	58	242	1	13	N/A	0.3	tr	13	0.2	1	250	14	14	5	61	0	24	43	0

Fruit and Fruit Juices

Food Name	Measure	Weight (g)	Energy (kcal)	Energy (kJ)	Protein (g)	Carbohydrate (g)	Total Sugar (g)	Total Dietary Fibre (g)	Total Fat (g)	Calcium (mg)	Iron (mg)	Sodium (mg)	Potassium (mg)	Magnesium (mg)	Phosphorus (mg)	Vitamin A (RAE)	Beta-carotene (mcg)	Lycopene (mcg)	Folate (DFE)	Vitamin C (mg)	Vitamin B12 (mcg)
Orange juice, ready-to-drink, refrigerated, vitamin D and calcium added	125 mL	132	58	242	1	13	N/A	0.3	tr	185	0.2	1	250	14	14	5	N/A	0	N/A	43	0
Orange, strawberry and banana juice, ready-to-drink	125 mL	124	57	237	1	15	13	0.2	tr	14	0.3	5	124	12	15	1	21	0	21	31	0
Pineapple juice, ready-to-drink, vitamin C added	125 mL	132	74	309	tr	18	13	0.3	tr	22	0.3	1	177	17	11	0	4	0	30	32	0
Pomegranate juice, ready-to-drink	125 mL	128	72	300	0	20	17	0	0	0	0	5	215	N/A	N/A	0	N/A	N/A	N/A	0	0
Prune juice, ready-to-drink	125 mL	135	96	402	1	24	22	1.4	tr	16	1.6	5	373	19	34	0	3	0	0	6	0

Dairy Foods and Other Related Products

Milk and Substitutes

Food Name	Measure	Weight (g)	Energy (kcal)	Energy (kJ)	Protein (g)	Carbohydrate (g)	Total Sugar (g)	Total Fat (g)	Saturated Fat (g)	Cholesterol (mg)	Calcium (mg)	Iron (mg)	Sodium (mg)	Potassium (mg)	Magnesium (mg)	Phosphorus (mg)	Vitamin A (RAE)	Vitamin D (mcg)	Folate (DFE)	Vitamin B12 (mcg)	Riboflavin (mg)
Buttermilk	250 mL	259	104	432	9	12	12	2	1.4	10	300	0.1	272	391	28	230	18	0.2	13	0.57	0.40
Milk, chocolate, 1% M.F.	250 mL	264	166	695	9	28	26	3	1.6	8	304	0.6	161	449	34	272	153	2.6	13	0.90	0.44
Milk, chocolate, 2% M.F.	250 mL	264	190	795	8	27	26	5	3.3	18	301	0.6	158	446	34	269	145	2.6	13	0.90	0.43
Milk, skim	250 mL	259	88	368	9	13	13	tr	0.2	5	324	0.1	109	404	28	261	158	2.7	13	1.37	0.47
Milk, partly skimmed, 1% M.F.	250 mL	258	108	454	9	13	13	3	1.6	13	307	0.1	113	387	28	245	150	2.6	13	1.13	0.48
Milk, partly skimmed, 2% M.F.	250 mL	258	129	539	9	12	13	5	3.3	21	302	0.1	106	387	28	242	142	2.8	13	1.19	0.48
Milk, partly skimmed, 2% M.F., with added milk solids	250 mL	260	146	608	10	14	14	5	3.2	21	372	0.2	153	473	42	291	143	2.6	16	1.12	0.50
Milk, whole, 3.3% M.F.	250 mL	258	155	647	8	12	14	8	5.4	26	291	0.1	103	369	26	235	72	2.7	13	1.13	0.47
Rice beverage, flavoured and unflavoured, enriched	250 mL	259	127	531	tr	26	N/A	2	0.2	0	319	0.2	91	72	10	36	52	2.2	96	1.03	0.03
Soy beverage, chocolate, enriched	250 mL	257	162	673	6	26	20	4	0.6	0	323	1.2	136	367	38	131	180	2.6	29	1.80	0.67
Soy beverage, original and vanilla, enriched	250 mL	257	110	465	7	13	9	4	0.5	0	316	1.1	120	313	38	110	142	2.7	23	2.19	0.47
Soy beverage, unsweetened, enriched	250 mL	257	85	354	7	4	1	4	0.5	0	318	1.2	95	308	41	82	160	3.1	18	2.85	0.53

Processed Milk

Food Name	Measure	Weight (g)	Energy (kcal)	Energy (kJ)	Protein (g)	Carbohydrate (g)	Total Sugar (g)	Total Fat (g)	Saturated Fat (g)	Cholesterol (mg)	Calcium (mg)	Iron (mg)	Sodium (mg)	Potassium (mg)	Magnesium (mg)	Phosphorus (mg)	Vitamin A (RAE)	Vitamin D (mcg)	Folate (DFE)	Vitamin B12 (mcg)	Riboflavin (mg)
Milk, condensed, sweetened, canned (Eagle Brand™)	15 mL	19	62	260	2	11	11	2	1.1	7	55	tr	25	72	5	49	14	N/A	2	0.09	0.08
Milk, evaporated, partly skimmed, canned, diluted, 2% M.F.	250 mL	258	122	512	10	15	13	3	1.6	10	369	0.3	149	422	35	264	104	2.9	11	0.28	0.41

Dairy Foods and Other Related Products

Food Name	Measure	Weight g	Energy kcal	Energy kJ	Protein g	Carbohydrate g	Total Sugar g	Total Fat g	Saturated Fat g	Cholesterol mg	Calcium mg	Iron mg	Sodium mg	Potassium mg	Magnesium mg	Phosphorus mg	Vitamin A RAE	Vitamin D mcg	Folate DFE	Vitamin B12 mcg	Riboflavin mg
Milk, evaporated, partly skimmed, canned, undiluted, 2% M.F.	15 mL	16	15	62	1	2	2	tr	0.2	1	44	tr	18	51	4	32	12	0.3	1	0.03	0.05
Milk, evaporated, skim, canned, diluted, 0.2% M.F.	250 mL	259	105	438	10	15	15	tr	0.2	5	392	0.4	157	446	38	262	159	2.9	12	0.32	0.42
Milk, evaporated, skim, canned, undiluted, 0.2% M.F.	15 mL	16	13	53	1	2	2	tr	tr	1	47	tr	19	54	4	32	19	0.4	1	0.04	0.05
Milk, evaporated, whole, canned, diluted, 7.8% M.F.	250 mL	258	178	744	9	13	13	10	6.3	39	349	0.3	143	403	33	270	86	2.9	11	0.21	0.42
Milk, evaporated, whole, canned, undiluted, 7.8% M.F	15 mL	16	21	89	1	2	2	1	0.8	5	42	tr	17	48	4	32	10	0.3	1	0.03	0.05
Milk, reconstituted, from skim milk powder	250 mL	259	86	360	8	13	13	tr	0.1	4	301	0.1	137	410	30	237	170	2.6	12	0.96	0.42
Skim milk powder	5 mL	1	5	22	1	1	1	tr	tr	tr	18	tr	8	25	2	14	10	0.2	1	0.06	0.03

Milk Beverages

Food Name	Measure	Weight g	Energy kcal	Energy kJ	Protein g	Carbohydrate g	Total Sugar g	Total Fat g	Saturated Fat g	Cholesterol mg	Calcium mg	Iron mg	Sodium mg	Potassium mg	Magnesium mg	Phosphorus mg	Vitamin A RAE	Vitamin D mcg	Folate DFE	Vitamin B12 mcg	Riboflavin mg
Chocolate milk, chocolate flavour powder + 2% milk	250 mL	279	207	863	9	33	N/A	6	3.4	20	321	0.8	176	531	59	274	143	2.8	N/A	0.92	0.46
Chocolate milk, syrup + 2% milk	250 mL	298	238	998	10	38	N/A	5	3.3	21	319	1.0	158	489	60	298	146	2.8	15	0.95	0.45
Eggnog	250 mL	268	362	1516	10	36	23	20	11.9	158	349	0.5	145	443	51	293	121	1.1	3	1.21	0.51
Hot chocolate, aspartame sweetened, powder + water	250 mL	270	78	326	3	15	9	1	0	0	127	1.1	240	569	46	189	38	N/A	3	0.35	0.29
Hot chocolate, homemade with cocoa + 2% milk	250 mL	264	203	851	9	28	26	6	3.8	21	277	1.3	116	520	61	277	135	2.6	13	1.11	0.48
Hot chocolate, powder + 2% milk	250 mL	264	255	1068	10	41	37	6	3.8	20	318	0.5	272	595	55	327	126	2.5	11	1.52	0.62
Hot chocolate, powder + water	250 mL	291	160	669	2	34	30	2	0.9	3	64	0.5	206	285	35	125	0	N/A	0	0.52	0.23
Instant breakfast powder + 2% milk	250 mL	280	260	1087	16	36	12	5	3.1	24	555	3.9	286	811	61	459	444	2.6	12	2.21	1.41
Milk shake, chocolate	250 mL	249	296	1240	8	53	52	7	4.2	27	329	0.8	276	558	40	314	45	1.0	12	0.80	0.55
Milk shake, vanilla	250 mL	249	279	1166	10	44	44	8	4.7	30	364	0.2	237	456	30	286	62	0.5	17	1.30	0.49

Yogourts and Fermented Milk Products

Food Name	Measure	Weight g	Energy kcal	Energy kJ	Protein g	Carbohydrate g	Total Sugar g	Total Fat g	Saturated Fat g	Cholesterol mg	Calcium mg	Iron mg	Sodium mg	Potassium mg	Magnesium mg	Phosphorus mg	Vitamin A RAE	Vitamin D mcg	Folate DFE	Vitamin B12 mcg	Riboflavin mg
Drinkable yogourt	200 mL	207	145	607	5	24	24	3	2.1	12	191	0.2	81	257	23	157	N/A	0.2	25	0.58	0.23
Fresh cheese (Danimal™, Minigo™)	1	60	68	286	5	10	10	2	1.1	6	138	0.1	32	84	7	50	N/A	N/A	N/A	N/A	N/A
Kefir, plain	175 mL	165	104	433	6	7	6	6	3.8	25	187	0.1	70	250	19	148	58	0.2	23	0.33	0.30
Yogourt parfait with berries and granola	175 mL	188	233	973	7	40	3	5	2.7	14	208	2.2	119	337	36	201	23	0	40	0.59	0.31
Yogourt, plain, 1-2% M.F.	175 mL	181	114	477	10	13	13	3	1.8	11	332	0.1	127	424	31	261	25	N/A	20	1.01	0.39
Yogourt, plain, 2-4% M.F.	175 mL	181	129	538	9	12	8	5	3.3	17	292	0.1	111	412	28	246	31	N/A	21	1.03	0.42
Yogourt, plain, fat-free	175 mL	189	79	332	3	11	9	tr	0	6	253	0.1	113	368	26	215	N/A	1.8	N/A	0.89	0.32
Yogourt, vanilla or fruit, 1-2% M.F.	175 mL	185	183	767	7	30	25	4	2.3	17	227	0.1	98	335	20	167	N/A	N/A	N/A	0.31	0.15
Yogourt, vanilla or fruit, fat-free	175 mL	181	116	484	8	21	19	tr	tr	4	229	0.2	103	349	20	163	N/A	N/A	N/A	0.59	N/A

Food Name	Measure	Weight g	Energy kcal	Energy kJ	Protein g	Carbohydrate g	Total Sugar g	Total Fat g	Saturated Fat g	Cholesterol mg	Calcium mg	Iron mg	Sodium mg	Potassium mg	Magnesium mg	Phosphorus mg	Vitamin A RAE	Vitamin D mcg	Folate DFE	Vitamin B12 mcg	Riboflavin mg
Dairy Foods and Other Related Products																					
Yogourt, vanilla or fruit, fat-free with sugar substitute	175 mL	189	94	394	7	16	14	tr	0	6	205	0.2	92	311	22	179	N/A	1.4	N/A	0.72	0.27
Cheese																					
Blue	50 g	50	177	738	11	1	tr	14	9.3	38	264	0.2	698	128	12	194	99	0.2	18	0.61	0.19
Brick	50 g	50	186	776	12	1	tr	15	9.4	47	337	0.2	280	68	12	226	146	0.2	10	0.63	0.18
Brie	50 g	50	167	699	10	tr	tr	14	8.7	50	92	0.3	315	76	10	94	87	0.2	33	0.83	0.26
Camembert	50 g	50	150	628	10	tr	tr	12	7.6	36	194	0.2	421	94	10	174	121	0.2	31	0.65	0.24
Cheddar	50 g	50	202	843	12	1	tr	17	10.5	53	361	0.3	311	49	14	256	133	0.1	9	0.42	0.19
Cheddar, low fat (18% M.F.)	50 g	50	141	590	14	1	N/A	9	5.8	28	453	0.1	363	47	18	292	75	N/A	10	0.83	0.15
Cottage cheese (1% M.F.)	125 mL	119	86	359	15	3	3	1	0.8	5	73	0.2	500	103	6	160	13	N/A	14	0.75	0.20
Cream cheese, light	30 mL	30	70	294	3	2	tr	5	3.4	17	34	0.5	90	51	2	44	56	N/A	5	0.18	0.09
Cream cheese, regular	30 mL	29	103	430	2	1	tr	10	6.5	32	24	0.4	87	35	2	31	108	N/A	4	0.12	0.06
Edam	50 g	50	179	747	12	1	1	14	8.8	45	366	0.2	483	94	15	268	122	0.5	8	0.77	0.19
Feta	50 g	50	132	552	7	2	2	11	7.7	46	247	0.3	558	31	10	169	63	0.2	16	0.87	0.44
Goat cheese, soft	50 g	50	134	561	9	tr	tr	11	7.3	23	70	1.0	184	13	8	128	144	0.2	6	0.10	0.19
Gouda	50 g	50	178	745	13	1	1	14	9.0	58	350	0.1	410	61	15	273	83	0.2	11	0.78	0.17
Gruyere	50 g	50	207	864	15	tr	tr	16	9.5	55	506	0.1	168	41	18	303	136	0.2	5	0.80	0.14
Imitation cheese	50 g	50	120	500	8	6	4	7	4.4	18	281	0.2	673	121	15	356	57	0	4	0.20	0.22
Mozzarella (22.5% M.F.)	50 g	50	141	588	10	1	1	11	6.8	39	269	0.1	187	34	10	186	90	0.1	4	0.33	0.13
Mozzarella, partially skimmed (16.5% M.F.)	50 g	50	127	531	13	1	1	8	5.2	29	323	0.1	241	42	12	239	64	0.1	5	0.41	0.16
Parmesan, grated	15 mL	6	27	114	2	tr	tr	2	1.1	6	70	0.1	97	8	2	46	8	tr	1	0.14	0.03
Processed cheese food, thin slices	1	21	78	327	5	tr	tr	7	4.1	20	115	tr	310	35	6	107	53	tr	2	0.15	0.07
Processed cheese food, thin slices, light	1	21	50	209	4	2	2	3	1.8	11	110	tr	331	69	7	173	53	tr	4	0.23	0.10
Processed cheese spread (Cheez Whiz™)	30 mL	31	90	375	5	3	N/A	7	4.1	17	174	0.1	503	75	9	271	N/A	0.1	2	0.12	0.13
Processed cheese spread, light (Light Cheez Whiz™)	30 mL	31	69	287	6	4	3	3	2.2	13	178	tr	491	107	9	317	91	N/A	N/A	0.20	0.20
Ricotta cheese, partly skimmed milk	125 mL	131	181	756	15	7	tr	10	6.5	41	356	0.6	164	164	20	240	140	N/A	17	0.38	0.24
Romano, grated	15 mL	6	25	103	2	tr	tr	2	1.1	7	67	tr	76	5	3	48	6	tr	tr	0.07	0.02
Swiss (Emmental)	50 g	50	190	795	13	3	1	14	8.9	46	396	0.1	96	39	19	284	110	0.6	3	1.67	0.15
Swiss, processed, thin slices	1	21	70	291	5	tr	tr	5	3.3	18	161	0.1	285	45	6	159	41	0.2	1	0.26	0.06

Dairy Foods and Other Related Products

Food Name	Measure	Weight g	Energy kcal	Energy kJ	Protein g	Carbohydrate g	Total Sugar g	Total Fat g	Saturated Fat g	Cholesterol mg	Calcium mg	Iron mg	Sodium mg	Potassium mg	Magnesium mg	Phosphorus mg	Vitamin A RAE	Vitamin D mcg	Folate DFE	Vitamin B12 mcg	Riboflavin mg
Cream																					
Half and half, 10% M.F.	15 mL	15	18	76	tr	1	tr	2	1.0	5	16	tr	6	20	2	15	15	tr	2	0.05	0.02
Sour cream, 14% M.F.	15 mL	15	22	93	tr	1	tr	2	1.3	6	16	tr	6	19	1	14	17	0.1	2	0.04	0.02
Sour cream, light, 5% M.F.	15 mL	16	21	89	tr	1	tr	2	1.0	6	22	tr	11	33	2	11	14	N/A	2	0.07	0.02
Table cream (coffee cream), 18% M.F.	15 mL	15	28	118	tr	1	tr	3	1.7	9	15	tr	6	19	1	13	25	0.1	tr	0.04	0.02
Whipped, pressurized	60 mL	15	39	164	tr	2	1	3	2.1	12	15	tr	20	22	2	14	29	0.1	tr	0.04	0.01
Whipping cream, 35% M.F., not whipped	15 mL	15	49	207	tr	tr	tr	5	3.3	19	10	tr	5	12	1	9	62	0.1	1	0.03	0.02
Whipping cream, 35% M.F., sweetened, whipped	60 mL	30	100	419	1	3	2	10	6.2	36	19	tr	10	23	2	17	117	0.2	1	0.05	0.03
Imitation Cream Products																					
Coffee whitener, frozen liquid	15 mL	15	21	87	tr	2	2	2	0.3	0	1	tr	12	29	0	10	tr	0	0	0	0
Coffee whitener, powdered	5 mL	2	11	45	tr	1	1	1	0.6	0	tr	tr	4	16	tr	8	tr	0	0	0	tr
Coffee whitener, powdered, light	5 mL	2	9	36	tr	1	1	tr	0.1	0	tr	tr	5	18	0	3	tr	0	tr	0	0
Dessert topping, frozen	60 mL	19	60	253	tr	4	4	5	4.1	0	1	tr	5	3	tr	2	1	0	0	0	0
Dessert topping, frozen, low fat	60 mL	19	42	175	1	4	4	2	2.1	tr	14	tr	14	19	1	14	1	N/A	1	0.04	0.02
Dessert topping, powdered, prepared with 2% milk	60 mL	20	37	153	1	3	3	2	2.0	1	19	tr	12	31	2	18	9	0.2	1	0.07	0.03
Dessert topping, pressurized	60 mL	18	47	196	tr	3	3	4	3.4	0	1	tr	11	3	tr	3	1	0	0	0	0
Pudding																					
All flavours, instant, from mix, prepared with 2% milk	125 mL	139	149	623	4	27	23	3	1.6	9	141	0.2	391	206	18	307	65	1.3	6	0.54	0.23
Chocolate, ready-to-eat	1 unit	99	138	575	3	23	18	4	0.7	3	89	0.5	128	178	21	79	10	N/A	3	0	0.15
Chocolate, ready-to-eat, fat-free	1 unit	99	96	402	3	20	15	tr	0.2	1	72	0.8	168	139	19	75	47	N/A	4	0.22	0.15
Rice, homemade	125 mL	119	160	669	4	32	19	2	1.2	7	115	0.3	55	211	18	112	51	1.0	5	0.24	0.19
Rice, ready-to-eat	1 unit	99	161	675	2	22	N/A	7	1.2	1	51	0.3	84	59	8	67	25	0.1	3	0.21	0.07
Tapioca, ready-to-eat	1 unit	99	118	493	2	19	18	4	0.6	1	83	0.2	157	95	8	78	0	N/A	3	0.21	0.10
Tapioca, ready-to-eat, fat-free	1 unit	99	88	368	2	20	16	tr	0	1	50	0.3	210	52	5	40	32	N/A	2	0.15	0.10
Vanilla, ready-to-eat	1 unit	99	128	534	2	22	20	4	0.6	7	87	0.1	134	112	8	67	6	N/A	0	0.10	0.14
Vanilla, ready-to-eat, fat-free	1 unit	99	92	385	2	22	16	tr	tr	1	59	0.4	211	71	7	49	40	N/A	3	0.19	0.12

Eggs and Egg Dishes

Food Name	Measure	Weight (g)	Energy (kcal)	Energy (kJ)	Protein (g)	Carbohydrate (g)	Total Fat (g)	Saturated Fat (g)	Monounsaturated Fat (g)	Polyunsaturated Fat (g)	Cholesterol (mg)	Calcium (mg)	Iron (mg)	Sodium (mg)	Potassium (mg)	Phosphorus (mg)	Vitamin A (RAE)	Vitamin D (mcg)	Folate (DFE)	Vitamin B12 (mcg)	Vitamin E (mg)
Egg substitute, frozen (yolk replaced), cooked	2 eggs	111	226	947	14	4	17	2.9	4.6	8.8	2	89	2.4	291	258	88	60	1.9	14	0.35	2.2
Egg white, cooked	1 large	33	16	66	3	tr	0	0	0	0	0	3	tr	106	39	4	0	0	0	0.01	0
Egg yolk, cooked	1 large	17	59	249	3	1	6	1.7	2.3	0.8	202	22	0.7	34	17	64	106	0.8	30	0.88	1.4
Egg, fried	2 large	92	173	726	12	2	14	3.6	5.8	2.7	367	46	1.4	322	116	127	236	1.9	54	1.62	2.7
Egg, hard-boiled	1 large	50	78	324	6	1	5	1.6	2.0	0.7	216	25	0.6	62	63	86	85	0.7	22	0.56	0.5
Egg, poached	1 large	50	74	308	6	tr	5	1.5	1.9	0.7	215	27	0.9	147	67	95	70	0.4	24	0.64	0.5
Eggs benedict	2 eggs	310	572	2393	34	30	35	12.5	14.2	4.9	458	189	4.0	2015	456	453	265	2.1	113	1.96	1.7
Eggs, scrambled, made with 2 eggs	2 eggs	124	189	792	13	4	14	4.1	5.9	2.7	363	90	1.4	476	171	160	253	2.3	55	1.73	2.6
Omelet, cheese, made with 2 eggs	1 omelet	150	273	1142	18	5	20	8.0	7.8	2.8	376	238	1.6	890	241	356	304	2.3	56	1.99	2.7
Omelet, spanish, made with 2 eggs (mushrooms, onions, green peppers, tomatoes)	1 omelet	290	319	1336	15	13	24	5.7	10.4	6.3	353	111	1.8	607	514	211	403	4.3	72	1.70	3.7
Omelet, western, made with 2 eggs (green peppers, ham, onions)	1 omelet	158	237	993	17	5	17	5.1	7.3	2.9	346	86	1.5	720	258	202	231	2.2	53	1.72	2.5

Fish and Shellfish

Fish

Food Name	Measure	Weight (g)	Energy (kcal)	Energy (kJ)	Protein (g)	Carbohydrate (g)	Total Fat (g)	Saturated Fat (g)	Polyunsaturated Fat (g)	DHA (g)	EPA (g)	Cholesterol (mg)	Calcium (mg)	Iron (mg)	Sodium (mg)	Potassium (mg)	Phosphorus (mg)	Vitamin A (RAE)	Vitamin D (mcg)	Vitamin B12 (mcg)	Vitamin E (mg)
Anchovies, canned in oil, drained solids	2	8	17	70	2	0	1	0.2	0.2	0.10	0.06	7	19	0.4	293	44	20	20	0.1	0.07	0.3
Arctic char, cooked	75 g	75	119	496	20	0	4	0.7	0.9	0.30	0.38	N/A	23	0.4	38	N/A	188	68	2.8	N/A	N/A
Bass, mixed species, baked or broiled	75 g	75	110	458	18	0	4	0.8	1.0	0.34	0.23	65	77	1.4	68	342	192	26	N/A	1.73	N/A
Burbot (loche), raw	90 g	90	71	297	16	0	1	0.1	0.3	0.09	0.06	54	22	0.3	63	288	171	5	0.5	0.72	N/A
Catfish, channel, farmed, baked or broiled	75 g	75	114	477	14	0	6	1.3	1.0	0.10	0.04	48	7	0.6	60	241	184	11	N/A	2.10	1.0
Cisco (lake herring, tullibee), baked or broiled	75 g	75	98	408	17	0	3	N/A	N/A	N/A	N/A	N/A	38	0.5	38	312	188	0	N/A	N/A	N/A
Cisco (lake herring, tullibee), raw	90 g	90	88	369	17	0	2	1.1	1.2	0.46	0.11	45	10	0.4	50	319	137	27	N/A	0.90	N/A

Fish and Shellfish

Food Name	Measure	Weight g	Energy kcal	Energy kJ	Protein g	Carbohydrate g	Total Fat g	Saturated Fat g	Polyunsaturated Fat g	DHA g	EPA g	Cholesterol mg	Calcium mg	Iron mg	Sodium mg	Potassium mg	Phosphorus mg	Vitamin A RAE	Vitamin D mcg	Vitamin B12 mcg	Vitamin E mg
Cod, Atlantic, baked or broiled	75 g	75	79	329	17	0	1	0.1	0.2	0.12	tr	41	11	0.4	59	183	104	11	0.5	0.79	0.6
Cod, Atlantic, dried and salted, soaked in water	75 g	75	62	259	13	0	1	0.1	0.2	0.09	tr	32	35	0.5	1353	265	183	9	0.5	1.82	0.6
Gefiltefish	75 g	75	63	263	7	6	1	0.3	0.2	0.03	0.06	23	17	1.9	393	68	55	20	N/A	0.63	N/A
Grayling, baked or broiled	75 g	75	80	332	17	0	1	N/A	N/A	N/A	N/A	N/A	29	0.5	N/A	N/A	N/A	N/A	N/A	N/A	N/A
Haddock, baked or broiled	75 g	75	84	351	18	0	1	0.1	0.2	0.12	0.06	56	32	1.0	65	299	181	14	0.2	1.04	0.4
Halibut, Atlantic and Pacific, baked or broiled	75 g	75	105	439	20	0	2	0.3	0.7	0.28	0.07	31	45	0.8	52	432	214	41	3.6	1.03	2.2
Herring, Atlantic, kippered	75 g	75	163	680	18	0	9	2.1	2.2	0.88	0.73	62	63	1.1	689	335	244	30	1.6	14.03	1.2
Mackerel, Atlantic, baked or broiled	75 g	75	197	822	18	0	13	3.1	3.2	3.52	0.38	56	11	1.2	62	301	209	41	2.0	14.25	1.5
Ocean Perch, Atlantic, baked or broiled	75 g	75	91	380	18	0	2	0.2	0.4	0.20	0.08	41	103	0.9	72	263	208	11	N/A	0.86	1.2
Pickerel (Walleye), baked or broiled	75 g	75	89	374	18	0	1	0.2	0.4	0.22	0.08	83	106	1.3	49	374	202	18	3.5	1.73	0.2
Pike, northern, baked or broiled	75 g	75	71	298	16	0	1	0.2	0.2	0.08	0.08	38	33	0.3	23	323	180	1	2.4	1.73	0.2
Pollock, Atlantic, baked or broiled	75 g	75	89	370	19	0	1	0.1	0.5	0.34	0.07	68	58	0.4	83	342	212	9	1.4	2.76	0.2
Salmon, Atlantic, farmed, baked or broiled	75 g	75	155	646	17	0	9	1.9	3.3	1.09	0.52	47	11	0.3	46	288	189	11	5.1	2.10	1.2
Salmon, chum (keta), baked or broiled	75 g	75	116	483	19	0	4	0.8	0.9	0.38	0.22	71	11	0.5	48	413	272	26	14.0	2.60	1.1
Salmon, chum (keta), canned, drained solids with bone, salted	75 g	75	106	443	18	0	4	1.1	1.1	0.53	0.35	29	187	0.5	365	225	266	14	5.0	3.30	1.2
Salmon, chum (keta), canned, drained solids with bone, unsalted	75 g	75	106	443	18	0	4	1.1	1.1	0.53	0.35	29	187	0.5	56	225	266	14	4.2	3.30	1.2
Salmon, coho, farmed, baked or broiled	75 g	75	134	558	18	0	6	1.5	1.5	0.65	0.31	47	9	0.3	39	345	249	44	N/A	2.38	0.7
Salmon, eggs, raw	90 g	90	116	485	24	0	9	2.1	2.3	1.17	0.99	N/A	11	0.6	45	369	198	N/A	N/A	N/A	N/A
Salmon, king or chinook, smoked, canned	75 g	75	113	470	17	1	4	N/A	N/A	N/A	N/A	N/A	45	1.4	N/A	N/A	N/A	72	N/A	N/A	N/A
Salmon, pink, canned, drained with bones	75 g	75	102	427	17	0	4	0.6	1.1	0.52	0.27	62	208	0.7	299	233	274	17	N/A	3.71	1.0
Salmon, smoked	2 pieces	40	47	196	7	0	2	0.4	0.4	0.11	0.07	9	4	0.3	314	70	66	10	4.2	1.30	0.5
Salmon, smoked, lox	2 pieces	40	47	196	7	0	2	0.4	0.4	0.11	0.07	9	4	0.3	800	70	66	10	4.2	1.30	N/A
Salmon, sockeye, baked or broiled	75 g	75	162	677	20	0	8	1.4	1.8	0.53	0.40	65	5	0.4	50	281	207	47	17.0	4.35	2.3
Sardines, Atlantic, canned in oil, drained with bones	1 can	106	220	922	26	0	12	1.6	5.5	0.54	0.50	151	405	3.1	535	421	519	34	2.5	9.48	2.2
Sardines, Pacific, canned in tomato sauce, drained with bones	1 can	106	197	825	22	1	11	2.8	2.2	0.92	0.56	65	254	2.4	439	361	388	35	12.7	9.54	1.5
Smelt, breaded and fried	5	80	201	840	18	10	10	2.5	2.7	N/A	N/A	79	31	1.0	N/A	332	246	20	N/A	N/A	N/A
Snapper, mixed species, baked or broiled	75 g	75	96	401	20	0	1	0.3	0.4	0.20	0.04	35	30	0.2	43	392	151	26	2.2	2.63	0.5

Food Name	Measure	Weight (g)	Energy (kcal)	Energy (kJ)	Protein (g)	Carbohydrate (g)	Total Fat (g)	Saturated Fat (g)	Polyunsaturated Fat (g)	DHA (g)	EPA (g)	Cholesterol (mg)	Calcium (mg)	Iron (mg)	Sodium (mg)	Potassium (mg)	Phosphorus (mg)	Vitamin A (RAE)	Vitamin D (mcg)	Vitamin B12 (mcg)	Vitamin E (mg)
Fish and Shellfish																					
Sole (flatfish), baked or broiled	75 g	75	88	367	18	0	1	0.3	0.5	0.19	0.18	51	14	0.3	79	258	217	10	1.1	1.88	0.5
Trout, rainbow, farmed, baked or broiled	75 g	75	127	530	18	0	5	1.6	1.7	0.62	0.25	51	65	0.2	32	331	200	65	4.8	3.73	0
Tuna, light, canned in water, drained, salted	75 g	75	87	364	19	0	1	0.2	0.3	0.17	0.04	23	8	1.1	254	178	122	13	0.9	2.24	0.3
Tuna, light, canned with oil, drained, salted	75 g	75	149	621	22	0	6	1.2	2.2	0.08	0.02	14	10	1.0	266	155	233	17	0.7	1.65	0.7
Turbot, baked or broiled	75 g	75	92	383	15	0	3	N/A	N/A	N/A	N/A	47	17	0.3	144	229	124	9	N/A	1.91	N/A
Whitefish, lake, native, baked	75 g	75	100	417	17	0	3	0.9	2.1	0.90	0.30	58	12	0.3	33	294	168	8	11.3	0.72	N/A
Shellfish																					
Clams, mixed species, boiled or steamed	5 large	60	89	371	15	3	1	0.1	0.3	0.09	0.08	40	55	16.8	67	377	203	103	0.1	59.33	0.4
Clams, mixed species, canned, drained solids	125 mL	85	125	523	22	4	2	0.2	0.5	0.12	0.12	57	78	23.6	95	531	286	153	0.1	83.59	0.5
Crab, canned, drained	125 mL	71	71	295	15	0	1	0.2	0.3	0.12	0.14	63	72	0.6	238	267	185	1	N/A	0.33	1.3
Crab, snow, boiled or steamed	125 mL	62	72	300	15	0	1	0.1	0.3	0.09	0.21	44	21	1.8	431	125	80	32	N/A	6.47	N/A
Crayfish, mixed species, farmed, boiled or steamed	4 medium	60	52	218	11	0	1	0.1	0.2	0.02	0.07	82	31	0.7	58	143	145	9	N/A	1.86	N/A
Lobster, boiled or steamed	125 mL	77	75	314	16	1	tr	0.1	0.1	0.02	0.04	55	47	0.3	291	270	142	20	N/A	2.38	0.8
Mussels, boiled or steamed	15 small	75	129	539	18	6	3	0.6	0.9	0.38	0.21	42	25	5.0	277	201	214	68	0.2	18.00	0.8
Oysters, boiled or steamed	6 medium	42	58	241	6	3	2	0.6	0.8	0.25	0.23	44	38	5.0	177	118	85	23	3.4	14.71	0.7
Oysters, canned, solids and liquid	125 mL	131	90	379	9	5	3	0.8	1.0	0.30	0.28	72	59	8.8	147	300	182	118	N/A	25.06	1.1
Oysters, raw	6 medium	84	50	207	4	5	1	0.4	0.5	0.17	0.16	21	37	4.9	150	104	78	7	N/A	13.61	0.5
Scallops, cooked, steamed	6 medium	78	87	365	18	0	1	0.1	0.4	0.16	0.13	41	90	2.3	207	371	264	23	0	1.01	1.2
Shrimp, boiled or steamed	6 medium	30	30	124	6	0	tr	0.1	0.1	0.04	0.05	59	12	0.9	67	55	41	20	N/A	0.45	0.4
Fish Products																					
Calamari, breaded and fried	125 mL	79	156	651	14	9	7	1.7	1.6	0.27	0.11	197	45	1.0	303	216	194	17	0.1	1.02	1.0
Caviar, black or red	15 mL	16	41	171	4	1	3	0.7	1.2	0.62	0.44	95	45	1.9	243	29	58	91	0.5	3.25	1.1
Crab cake	1	60	93	389	12	tr	5	0.9	1.4	0.13	0.14	90	63	0.6	198	194	128	34	N/A	3.56	N/A
Crab, imitation, made from surimi	125 mL	67	68	284	8	7	1	0.2	0.4	0.24	0.16	13	9	0.3	560	60	188	13	1.2	1.07	0.1
Fish cake	1	120	240	1004	16	15	12	3.3	2.6	0.10	tr	63	30	0.8	290	526	201	28	1.5	0.73	0.7
Fish fillet, battered and fried	1	134	265	1108	22	9	15	3.6	3.4	0.14	0.08	71	42	1.0	133	508	266	23	0.8	1.02	1.0
Fish sticks, frozen, heated (10cm x 2.5cm x 1.3cm)	3 sticks	83	227	948	13	20	10	2.6	2.6	0.11	0.07	93	17	0.6	485	217	151	26	0.1	1.50	0.4
Shrimp, breaded and fried	6 medium	66	160	668	14	8	8	1.4	3.4	0.08	0.07	117	44	0.8	227	149	144	N/A	N/A	1.23	N/A
Tuna salad	125 mL	108	203	847	17	10	10	1.7	4.5	0.06	0.02	14	18	1.1	435	193	193	26	3.6	1.30	N/A

Meat and Poultry

Beef

Food Name	Measure	Weight (g)	Energy (kcal)	Energy (kJ)	Protein (g)	Carbohydrate (g)	Total Fat (g)	Saturated Fat (g)	Monounsaturated Fat (g)	Polyunsaturated Fat (g)	Cholesterol (mg)	Iron (mg)	Sodium (mg)	Potassium (mg)	Magnesium (mg)	Phosphorus (mg)	Vitamin A (RAE)	Vitamin D (mcg)	Vitamin B12 (mcg)	Folate (DFE)	Vitamin E (mg)
Blade roast, lean + fat, braised	75 g	75	200	834	26	0	10	4.0	5.0	0.4	71	2.5	46	202	18	142	0	0.5	2.38	4	0.1
Blade steak, lean + fat, braised	75 g	75	227	947	23	0	14	5.7	7.1	0.5	71	2.4	49	178	17	138	0	0.5	2.00	4	0.2
Composite, roast, lean + fat, cooked	75 g	75	181	756	24	0	8	3.5	4.2	0.4	61	2.3	40	230	19	155	0	0.5	1.89	4	0.1
Composite, steak, lean + fat, cooked	75 g	75	196	819	25	0	9	3.9	4.9	0.4	64	2.4	40	200	18	148	0	0.5	1.78	4	0.1
Cross rib roast, lean + fat, braised	75 g	75	197	825	27	0	9	3.6	4.5	0.5	70	2.6	52	242	21	164	0	0.5	1.89	5	0.6
Eye of round roast, lean + fat, roasted	75 g	75	148	618	24	0	5	2.1	2.5	0.2	50	1.5	40	243	19	152	0	0.5	1.44	5	0.2
Eye of round steak, lean + fat, braised	75 g	75	171	715	28	0	5	2.2	2.8	0.3	61	1.8	35	243	19	152	0	0.5	1.38	5	0.2
Flank steak, lean + fat, braised	75 g	75	184	769	25	0	8	3.6	4.1	0.3	54	2.2	45	243	19	152	0	0.5	2.15	5	0.3
Ground, extra lean, crumbled, pan-fried	75 g	75	167	696	23	0	8	3.2	3.3	0.3	59	2.1	65	311	22	180	0	0.3	2.06	5	N/A
Ground, lean, crumbled, pan-fried	75 g	75	194	809	22	0	11	4.5	5.1	0.3	59	2.1	70	293	21	174	0	0.5	2.16	0	N/A
Ground, medium, crumbled, pan-fried	75 g	75	214	894	22	0	13	5.6	6.0	0.4	61	2.0	68	303	21	173	0	0.6	1.88	6	N/A
Ground, regular, crumbled, pan-fried	75 g	75	243	1016	22	0	17	7.0	7.9	0.4	63	2.2	78	301	21	178	0	0.8	2.72	0	N/A
Inside (top) round roast, lean + fat, roasted	75 g	75	133	555	24	0	3	1.4	1.6	0.2	53	2.1	48	253	20	163	0	0.5	1.68	5	0.1
Inside (top) round steak, lean + fat, braised	75 g	75	175	731	30	0	5	2.1	2.6	0.3	68	2.4	38	204	20	157	0	0.5	1.43	5	0.4
Outside (bottom) round roast, lean + fat, roasted	75 g	75	158	659	25	0	5	2.1	2.8	0.3	58	2.9	42	243	19	152	0	0.5	1.67	5	0.2
Outside (bottom) round steak, lean + fat, braised	75 g	75	195	815	29	0	8	3.0	4.2	0.4	72	3.1	43	243	19	152	0	0.5	1.41	5	0.3
Rib eye steak, lean + fat, broiled	75 g	75	230	963	20	0	16	6.7	8.0	0.5	53	2.4	40	243	19	152	0	0.5	1.54	5	0.8
Rib steak, lean + fat, broiled	75 g	75	232	969	23	0	15	6.4	7.3	0.5	58	1.9	56	243	19	152	0	0.5	1.80	5	0.5
Rump roast, lean + fat, broiled	75 g	75	164	684	21	0	8	3.2	3.6	0.3	59	1.9	47	296	20	180	0	0.3	2.27	7	N/A
Short ribs, lean + fat, simmered	75 g	75	309	1292	17	0	26	11.2	11.8	1.0	57	1.4	29	146	10	86	0	1.7	1.97	4	N/A
Sirloin tip roast, lean + fat, roasted	75 g	75	156	653	25	0	5	2.2	2.8	0.3	58	2.7	44	243	19	152	0	0.5	1.85	5	0.1
Standing rib roast, lean + fat, roasted	75 g	75	237	992	21	0	16	6.9	8.0	0.5	55	1.7	53	243	19	152	0	0.5	1.73	5	0.5
Stewing beef, simmered	75 g	75	183	765	28	0	7	2.9	N/A	N/A	68	2.6	45	214	19	150	0	0.5	1.80	4	0.2
Strip loin (New York) steak, lean + fat, broiled	75 g	75	191	797	23	0	10	4.3	5.2	0.4	55	2.1	43	243	19	152	0	0.5	1.72	5	0.3
T-Bone (Porterhouse) steak, lean + fat, broiled	75 g	75	216	903	22	0	13	5.6	6.6	0.4	54	2.1	51	243	19	152	0	0.5	1.89	5	0.1
Tenderloin, steak, lean + fat, broiled	75 g	75	170	709	24	0	7	3.2	3.6	0.3	59	2.9	50	243	19	152	0	0.5	2.04	5	0.2
Top sirloin steak, lean + fat, broiled	75 g	75	146	611	21	0	6	2.6	3.1	0.3	52	2.0	43	257	20	160	0	0.5	2.33	5	0.2

Meat and Poultry

Food Name	Measure	Weight g	Energy kcal	Energy kJ	Protein g	Carbohydrate g	Total Fat g	Saturated Fat g	Monounsaturated Fat g	Polyunsaturated Fat g	Cholesterol mg	Iron mg	Sodium mg	Potassium mg	Magnesium mg	Phosphorus mg	Vitamin A RAE	Vitamin D mcg	Vitamin B12 mcg	Folate DFE	Vitamin E mg
Veal																					
Composite cuts, lean + fat, cooked	75 g	75	173	725	23	0	9	3.2	3.3	0.6	86	0.9	65	244	20	179	0	1.1	1.18	11	0.3
Cutlets, grain-fed, pan-fried	75 g	75	136	568	27	0	2	0.7	0.8	0.6	78	1.5	33	266	21	171	0	0.5	2.46	N/A	0.3
Cutlets, milk-fed, pan-fried	75 g	75	142	593	28	0	2	0.6	0.8	1.0	78	0.5	58	332	16	218	0	0.5	1.27	12	0.3
Ground, broiled	75 g	75	129	539	18	0	6	2.3	2.1	0.4	77	0.7	62	253	18	163	0	0.8	0.95	8	0.1
Leg, lean + fat, breaded, pan-fried	75 g	75	171	715	20	7	7	2.3	2.5	1.1	84	1.2	341	278	23	188	8	0.9	0.93	24	0.4
Leg, lean + fat, roasted	75 g	75	120	502	21	0	3	1.4	1.3	0.3	77	0.7	51	292	21	176	0	0.5	0.88	12	0.4
Loin, lean + fat, roasted	75 g	75	163	680	19	0	9	3.9	3.6	0.6	77	0.7	70	244	19	159	0	1.3	0.93	11	0.3
Shoulder, whole, lean + fat, roasted	75 g	75	142	593	23	0	5	2.2	1.8	0.3	65	0.7	56	266	17	140	0	0.7	2.50	N/A	0.4
Stewing meat, lean, braised	75 g	75	141	590	26	0	3	1.0	1.0	0.3	109	1.1	70	257	21	179	0	0.7	1.25	12	0.3
Pork																					
Back ribs, lean + fat, roasted	75 g	75	274	1145	21	0	20	7.9	8.9	2.6	85	0.9	100	251	18	147	2	0.8	0.83	2	N/A
Centre cut, loin, chop, lean + fat, broiled	75 g	75	180	753	22	0	10	3.6	4.4	0.7	62	0.6	44	269	19	174	2	0.4	0.55	5	0.1
Centre cut, loin, chop, lean + fat, pan-fried	75 g	75	208	869	22	0	12	4.5	5.3	1.4	69	0.7	60	319	22	194	2	0.5	0.55	5	0.2
Ground, lean, pan-fried	75 g	75	175	731	19	0	11	4.1	5.0	1.3	60	0.9	60	278	20	166	2	0.5	0.80	5	0.2
Ground, medium, pan-fried	75 g	75	224	938	18	0	16	6.0	7.3	2.2	66	0.8	68	275	19	164	2	0.5	0.86	5	0.2
Leg, butt end, lean + fat, roasted	75 g	75	189	791	22	0	11	3.9	4.8	1.0	72	0.8	47	281	20	204	2	0.4	0.54	2	0.2
Loin, rib end, lean + fat, broiled	75 g	75	197	825	22	0	12	4.3	5.2	0.9	62	0.6	47	301	20	178	2	0.4	0.55	2	0.3
Loin, rib end, lean + fat, pan-fried	75 g	75	199	831	20	0	13	4.8	5.6	1.4	55	0.5	38	323	19	177	2	0.5	0.53	2	0.2
Shoulder, butt, lean + fat, roasted	75 g	75	198	828	19	0	13	5.0	5.9	1.9	67	1.1	50	245	18	153	2	0.6	0.92	4	0.2
Shoulder, whole, lean + fat, roasted	75 g	75	219	916	17	0	16	5.9	7.1	1.5	68	1.0	51	247	14	159	2	0.5	0.60	4	0.1
Spareribs, lean + fat, braised	75 g	75	251	1048	20	0	18	7.0	7.8	2.5	74	1.1	49	118	14	107	2	0.6	0.68	3	N/A
Tenderloin, lean, roasted	75 g	75	108	452	21	0	2	0.8	0.9	0.4	52	1.0	44	302	23	184	2	0.1	0.41	5	0.2
Lamb																					
American, fresh, foreshank, lean + fat, cooked	75 g	75	182	762	21	0	10	4.2	4.3	0.7	80	1.6	54	193	17	125	0	0.2	1.71	13	0.1
American, fresh, ground, cooked	75 g	75	212	888	19	0	15	6.1	6.2	1.1	73	1.3	61	254	18	151	0	0.6	1.96	14	0.1
American, fresh, leg, whole, lean + fat, cooked	75 g	75	194	809	19	0	12	5.2	5.2	0.9	70	1.5	50	235	18	143	0	0.5	1.94	15	0.1
American, fresh, loin, lean + fat, cooked	75 g	75	232	969	17	0	18	7.7	7.3	1.4	71	1.6	48	185	17	135	0	0.5	1.66	14	0.1

Meat and Poultry

Food Name	Measure	Weight (g)	Energy (kcal)	Energy (kJ)	Protein (g)	Carbohydrate (g)	Total Fat (g)	Saturated Fat (g)	Monounsaturated Fat (g)	Polyunsaturated Fat (g)	Cholesterol (mg)	Iron (mg)	Sodium (mg)	Potassium (mg)	Magnesium (mg)	Phosphorus (mg)	Vitamin A (RAE)	Vitamin D (mcg)	Vitamin B12 (mcg)	Folate (DFE)	Vitamin E (mg)
American, fresh, rib, lean + fat, cooked	75 g	75	269	1126	16	0	22	9.6	9.4	1.6	73	1.2	55	203	15	125	0	0.5	1.67	11	0.1
American, fresh, shoulder, whole, lean+ fat, cooked	75 g	75	207	866	17	0	15	6.3	6.1	1.2	69	1.5	50	188	17	138	0	0.5	1.98	16	0.1
New Zealand, frozen, composite, lean + fat, cooked	75 g	75	203	847	19	0	13	6.6	5.2	0.7	80	1.6	35	121	14	158	0	0.5	2.03	1	0.1
New Zealand, frozen, foreshank, lean + fat, braised	75 g	75	194	809	20	0	12	5.9	4.6	0.5	77	1.6	35	89	11	131	0	0.3	1.83	1	0.1
New Zealand, frozen, leg, whole, lean + fat, roasted	75 g	75	176	734	19	0	10	5.1	4.1	0.5	76	1.6	33	128	15	166	0	0.5	1.96	1	0.1
New Zealand, frozen, loin, lean + fat, broiled	75 g	75	222	929	18	0	16	7.9	6.2	0.7	85	1.6	38	123	15	160	0	0.5	1.91	1	0.1
New Zealand, frozen, rib, lean + fat, roasted	75 g	75	238	995	15	0	19	9.6	7.4	0.9	74	1.3	33	96	11	130	0	0.4	1.74	1	0.1
New Zealand, frozen, shoulder, whole, lean + fat, braised	75 g	75	257	1073	22	0	18	8.6	7.0	0.9	92	1.6	39	113	14	150	0	0.4	2.60	1	0.2

Poultry and Game Birds

Food Name	Measure	Weight (g)	Energy (kcal)	Energy (kJ)	Protein (g)	Carbohydrate (g)	Total Fat (g)	Saturated Fat (g)	Monounsaturated Fat (g)	Polyunsaturated Fat (g)	Cholesterol (mg)	Iron (mg)	Sodium (mg)	Potassium (mg)	Magnesium (mg)	Phosphorus (mg)	Vitamin A (RAE)	Vitamin D (mcg)	Vitamin B12 (mcg)	Folate (DFE)	Vitamin E (mg)
Chicken, broiler, breast, meat and skin, roasted	75 g	75	142	593	19	0	7	1.8	2.6	1.4	63	0.4	45	241	20	N/A	20	0.2	0.24	3	0.2
Chicken, broiler, breast, meat, roasted	75 g	75	119	499	25	0	2	0.4	0.5	0.3	64	0.4	56	301	22	N/A	5	0.2	0.26	3	0.2
Chicken, broiler, drumstick, meat and skin, roasted	75 g	75	161	671	19	0	10	2.8	3.8	2.3	68	1.0	68	172	17	131	23	0.2	0.24	6	0.2
Chicken, broiler, drumstick, meat, roasted	75 g	75	127	530	19	0	5	1.4	1.7	1.3	70	1.0	71	185	18	N/A	14	0.2	0.26	7	0.2
Chicken, broiler, flesh and skin, roasted	75 g	75	179	749	20	0	10	2.8	4.0	2.2	66	0.9	62	167	17	137	35	0.2	0.23	4	0.2
Chicken, broiler, flesh, roasted	75 g	75	143	596	22	0	6	1.5	2.0	1.3	67	0.9	65	182	19	146	12	0.2	0.25	5	0.2
Chicken, broiler, thigh, meat and skin, roasted	75 g	75	187	781	15	0	14	3.8	5.4	3.0	70	1.0	63	167	17	131	36	0.2	0.22	5	0.2
Chicken, broiler, thigh, meat, roasted	75 g	75	127	530	19	0	5	1.5	2.0	1.2	71	1.0	66	179	18	N/A	15	0.1	0.23	6	0.2
Chicken, broiler, wing, meat and skin, roasted	75 g	75	218	910	20	0	15	4.1	5.7	3.1	63	1.0	62	138	14	113	35	0.5	0.22	2	0.2
Chicken, cornish game hens, flesh and skin, roasted	75 g	75	195	815	17	0	14	3.8	6.0	2.7	98	0.7	48	184	14	110	24	0.3	0.21	2	0.3
Chicken, ground, lean, cooked	75 g	75	153	640	16	0	9	N/A	N/A	N/A	59	1.2	51	212	12	N/A	9	0.2	N/A	N/A	N/A
Duck, domesticated, roasted	75 g	75	253	1057	14	0	21	7.3	9.7	2.7	63	2.0	44	153	23	117	47	4.1	0.23	5	0.5
Duck, wild, cooked	75 g	75	128	533	23	0	3	1.0	1.4	0.4	N/A	7.4	40	197	23	187	12	N/A	N/A	N/A	N/A
Goose, domesticated, flesh, roasted	75 g	75	179	746	22	0	10	3.4	3.3	1.2	72	2.2	57	291	19	232	9	0.1	0.37	9	N/A
Goose, wild (Canada goose), flesh, roasted	75 g	75	150	627	23	0	6	0.7	1.9	1.1	72	7.4	57	291	19	232	9	0.1	0.37	9	N/A
Ptarmigan, flesh, cooked	75 g	75	116	483	23	0	2	N/A	N/A	N/A	N/A	6.5	37	247	27	190	N/A	N/A	N/A	N/A	N/A
Spruce grouse, flesh, cooked	75 g	75	99	414	20	0	2	N/A	N/A	N/A	N/A	3.3	38	204	25	152	N/A	N/A	N/A	N/A	N/A
Turkey, dark meat and skin, roasted	75 g	75	162	677	17	0	9	2.0	2.6	1.4	82	1.7	60	207	17	148	0	0.5	0.28	7	N/A
Turkey, dark meat, roasted	75 g	75	139	581	19	0	6	1.6	2.0	1.0	82	1.7	62	220	17	154	0	0.2	0.29	8	N/A

Food Name	Measure	Weight g	Energy kcal	Energy kJ	Protein g	Carbohydrate g	Total Fat g	Saturated Fat g	Monounsaturated Fat g	Polyunsaturated Fat g	Cholesterol mg	Iron mg	Sodium mg	Potassium mg	Magnesium mg	Phosphorus mg	Vitamin A RAE	Vitamin D mcg	Vitamin B12 mcg	Folate DFE	Vitamin E mg
Meat and Poultry																					
Turkey, ground, cooked	75 g	75	176	737	21	0	10	2.5	3.7	2.4	77	1.4	80	203	18	147	0	0.8	0.25	5	0.3
Turkey, light meat and skin, roasted	75 g	75	143	599	21	0	4	0.9	1.2	0.6	58	1.1	50	215	20	157	0	0.2	0.27	5	N/A
Turkey, light meat, roasted	75 g	75	116	483	21	0	2	0.7	0.9	0.5	55	1.0	51	231	21	165	0	0.2	0.29	5	N/A
Game Meats and Other Meats																					
Bear, simmered	75 g	75	194	812	24	0	10	2.7	4.2	1.8	74	8.0	53	197	17	128	14	N/A	1.85	5	0.4
Beaver, roasted	75 g	75	95	398	20	0	1	1.6	1.4	1.0	88	3.6	68	255	17	135	N/A	N/A	6.23	8	0.3
Bison, roasted	75 g	75	107	449	21	0	2	0.7	0.7	0.2	62	2.6	43	271	20	157	0	N/A	2.15	6	0.3
Caribou (reindeer), roasted	75 g	75	122	512	24	0	2	1.9	1.4	0.9	82	4.2	35	268	23	168	4	0.2	4.98	4	0.3
Deer (venison), roasted	75 g	75	119	496	23	0	2	0.9	0.7	0.5	84	3.4	41	251	18	170	0	N/A	N/A	N/A	N/A
Emu, inside drum, broiled	75 g	75	117	489	24	0	2	0.5	0.6	0.3	68	5.5	89	234	25	230	2	N/A	1.80	8	0.2
Goat, roasted	75 g	75	107	449	20	0	2	0.7	1.0	0.2	56	2.8	65	304	0	151	0	N/A	0.89	4	0.3
Horsemeat, roasted	75 g	75	131	549	21	0	5	1.4	1.6	0.6	51	3.8	41	284	19	185	0	N/A	2.37	N/A	N/A
Moose, roasted	75 g	75	121	505	26	0	1	0.2	0.2	0.2	59	3.8	38	375	23	188	0	N/A	4.73	3	0.2
Narwhal skin (muktuk), raw	90 g	90	119	497	20	0	4	0.6	2.7	0.3	N/A	0.3	91	332	14	146	126	N/A	N/A	N/A	N/A
Ostrich, inside strip, cooked	75 g	75	123	515	22	0	3	1.3	1.3	0.6	73	3.6	55	275	20	190	0	N/A	4.83	12	0.2
Rabbit, composite cuts, roasted	75 g	75	148	618	22	0	6	1.8	1.6	1.2	62	1.7	35	287	16	197	0	0.1	6.23	8	N/A
Seal meat, boiled	75 g	75	129	539	26	0	2	0.8	1.6	0.3	133	17.6	33	212	20	139	11	N/A	N/A	N/A	N/A
Liver and Organ Meats																					
Heart, beef, simmered	75 g	75	124	518	21	tr	4	1.1	0.8	0.7	159	4.8	44	164	16	191	0	1.3	8.10	4	0.2
Kidney, beef, simmered	75 g	75	119	496	20	0	3	0.8	0.5	0.6	537	4.4	71	101	9	228	0	1.3	N/A	62	0.1
Liver, beef, pan-fried	75 g	75	131	549	20	4	4	1.1	0.5	0.4	286	4.6	58	263	17	364	5808	0.5	N/A	195	0.4
Liver, chicken, pan-fried	75 g	75	129	539	19	1	5	1.5	1.0	1.0	423	9.7	69	236	20	332	3972	N/A	N/A	420	0.6
Liver, veal, pan-fried	75 g	75	145	605	21	3	5	1.6	0.9	0.8	364	4.5	64	265	17	362	N/A	0.2	N/A	263	0.5
Thymus, veal, braised	75 g	75	94	392	17	0	2	0.7	0.7	0.2	263	0.9	44	326	18	470	0	N/A	2.14	15	0.1
Tongue, beef, canned or pickled	75 g	75	200	838	14	tr	15	7.5	6.8	0	71	1.6	55	148	11	137	0	N/A	N/A	4	0.3
Processed Meat Products																					
Back bacon, pork, grilled	2 slices	47	87	364	11	1	4	1.3	1.9	0.4	27	0.4	727	183	10	139	0	0.1	0.37	2	0.2
Bacon, pork, broiled, pan-fried or roasted	3 slices	24	130	543	9	tr	10	3.3	4.4	1.1	26	0.3	554	136	8	128	3	0.4	0.30	tr	tr

Meat and Poultry

Food Name	Measure	Weight g	Energy kcal	Energy kJ	Protein g	Carbohydrate g	Total Fat g	Saturated Fat g	Monounsaturated Fat g	Polyunsaturated Fat g	Cholesterol mg	Iron mg	Sodium mg	Potassium mg	Magnesium mg	Phosphorus mg	Vitamin A RAE	Vitamin D mcg	Vitamin B12 mcg	Folate DFE	Vitamin E mg
Bacon, pork, broiled, pan-fried or roasted, reduced sodium	3 slices	24	130	543	9	tr	10	3.3	4.4	1.1	26	0.3	247	136	8	128	3	0.1	0.30	tr	0.1
Bologna (baloney), beef and pork	2 slices	56	153	640	7	3	13	4.7	5.9	1.1	31	0.8	549	132	6	51	14	0.6	0.74	3	0.2
Bologna (baloney), beef and pork, light	2 slices	56	129	539	5	1	11	4.1	5.1	0.9	22	0.4	620	87	7	101	0	0.4	0.73	3	0.1
Bologna (baloney), chicken	2 slices	56	127	531	7	4	9	3.0	2.8	2.5	55	0.9	492	111	8	73	0	0.3	0.15	4	N/A
Chicken, canned, flaked	60 mL	52	89	372	9	tr	5	1.5	2.1	1.2	32	0.8	374	135	6	58	18	0.2	0.15	2	N/A
Corned beef, brisket, cooked	2 slices	56	101	422	11	1	6	2.0	2.9	0.2	55	1.0	653	112	7	70	0	0.2	0.91	3	0.1
Cottage roll, pork, lean and fat, roasted	2 slices	56	69	291	9	1	3	1.0	1.3	0.3	38	0.5	642	152	7	87	0	0.1	0.59	2	0.2
Creton	30 mL	34	198	808	5	tr	19	8.3	7.7	1.6	36	0.3	129	96	6	56	1	0.3	0.19	1	0.1
Deli meat, beef, thin sliced	4 slices	56	83	349	11	tr	4	1.6	1.7	0.2	39	1.2	791	240	11	94	0	0	1.44	6	0.1
Deli meat, chicken breast roll	2 slices	56	75	314	8	1	4	1.4	1.6	0.8	22	0.2	494	181	10	68	0	0.3	0.13	2	tr
Deli meat, chicken breast, low fat	2 slices	56	48	199	10	1	tr	0.1	0.1	tr	25	0.7	696	177	20	143	0	0	N/A	N/A	tr
Deli meat, ham, extra lean (5% fat)	2 slices	56	62	258	10	1	2	0.5	0.7	0.2	27	0.4	619	196	10	122	0	0.1	0.42	2	0.2
Deli meat, ham, regular (11% fat)	2 slices	56	91	382	9	2	5	1.6	2.4	0.4	32	0.6	730	161	12	86	0	0.1	0.24	4	tr
Deli meat, mock chicken, loaved	2 slices	56	147	616	7	2	12	7.4	N/A	1.7	33	N/A	536	129	N/A	N/A	0	0.4	N/A	N/A	0.1
Deli meat, turkey breast	2 slices	56	63	262	3	4	2	0.1	0.3	0.2	31	1.2	672	195	11	88	0	0	0.12	2	0.1
Ham, extra lean, canned	2 slices	56	62	260	9	tr	2	0.8	1.2	0.2	21	0.5	638	151	10	125	0	0.1	0.46	3	0.1
Ham, lean, canned	2 slices	56	81	337	10	0	4	1.4	2.0	0.4	21	0.5	715	187	9	116	0	0.2	0.45	3	0.1
Ham, flaked, canned	60 mL	35	48	199	6	tr	3	0.9	1.3	0.3	16	0.3	367	87	5	49	0	0.1	0.24	tr	0.1
Ham, lean and regular, roasted	75 g	75	124	518	15	tr	6	2.0	2.8	0.8	43	1.1	1039	272	14	186	0	0.2	0.51	2	0.2
Ham, lean, roasted	75 g	75	118	493	19	1	4	1.4	1.9	0.5	41	0.7	995	237	17	170	0	0.2	0.53	3	0.2
Kielbasa (Kolbassa), pork and beef	1 piece	56	124	517	5	2	9	3.1	4.1	1.0	38	1.7	520	155	9	83	0	0	0.90	3	0.1
Liver sausage (liverwurst), pork	30 mL	27	93	388	4	1	8	3.0	3.8	0.7	43	1.7	191	41	3	62	2248	0.2	3.64	8	0.1
Pastrami, beef	2 slices	56	74	309	10	1	3	1.3	1.8	0.1	52	1.1	694	121	10	84	0	0.2	0.99	4	N/A
Pate, liver, canned	30 mL	26	84	352	4	tr	7	2.5	3.3	0.8	67	1.4	184	36	3	53	261	0.2	0.84	16	N/A
Pepperoni, pork, beef	10 slices	55	252	1053	11	2	22	8.7	10.3	1.4	64	0.8	966	170	10	95	0	0	0.85	3	tr
Salami, beef and pork	2 slices	45	118	495	6	2	9	3.7	4.2	0.9	30	1.2	490	105	7	53	0	0.2	1.68	1	0.1
Salami, pork and beef, dry or hard	5 slices	50	185	774	12	1	15	5.1	7.2	1.4	40	0.8	900	194	9	71	0	0.4	0.95	1	0.1
Salami, pork and beef, reduced salt	2 slices	46	182	762	7	7	14	4.9	6.1	1.4	41	0.7	287	631	14	125	tr	0.4	0.81	4	0.1

Meat and Poultry

Food Name	Measure	Weight g	Energy kcal	Energy kJ	Protein g	Carbohydrate g	Total Fat g	Saturated Fat g	Monounsaturated Fat g	Polyunsaturated Fat g	Cholesterol mg	Iron mg	Sodium mg	Potassium mg	Magnesium mg	Phosphorus mg	Vitamin A RAE	Vitamin D mcg	Vitamin B12 mcg	Folate DFE	Vitamin E mg
Sausage, Bratwurst, pork, cooked	1	75	184	769	11	2	14	5.2	6.8	1.5	45	1.0	418	159	11	112	0	0.8	0.71	2	0
Sausage, Italian, pork, cooked	1	75	258	1079	14	3	20	7.2	9.0	2.5	43	1.1	905	228	14	128	8	0.8	0.98	4	0.2
Sausage, breakfast, pork and beef, cooked	1	13	51	215	2	tr	5	1.7	2.2	0.5	9	0.1	105	25	2	14	0	0.1	0.06	tr	tr
Sausage, breakfast, pork, cooked	1	13	35	145	2	tr	3	0.9	1.2	0.3	11	0.2	102	28	2	24	2	0.1	0.22	tr	0.1
Sausage, turkey, cooked	1	75	147	588	18	0	8	1.7	2.2	2.0	69	1.1	499	224	16	152	9	0.1	0.92	1	tr
Summer sausage, beef	2 slices	56	188	785	9	tr	17	6.7	7.3	0.7	42	1.4	696	152	8	62	0	0.5	3.08	1	N/A
Turkey, canned, flaked	60 mL	34	50	207	6	tr	3	0.8	0.9	0.7	23	0.6	229	92	7	55	0	0.2	0.10	2	N/A
Vienna sausage (cocktail), beef and pork, canned	3	48	110	462	5	1	9	3.4	4.6	0.6	42	0.4	465	48	3	24	0	0.4	0.49	2	0.1
Wiener (frankfurter), beef	1	38	104	436	5	2	8	3.3	4.0	0.5	23	0.6	343	54	5	60	0	0.3	0.65	2	0.1
Wiener (frankfurter), beef and pork	1	38	107	449	5	2	9	3.4	4.3	0.9	19	0.4	374	69	4	32	0	0.3	0.49	2	0.1
Wiener (frankfurter), beef and pork, light	1	38	58	242	4	2	4	1.4	1.8	0.4	17	0.5	471	56	4	53	0	0.1	0.49	2	tr
Wiener (frankfurter), chicken	1	38	93	390	4	2	7	2.1	3.2	1.5	38	0.8	514	32	4	40	14	0.2	0.09	2	0.1

Legumes, Nuts and Seeds

Meatless Products

Food Name	Measure	Weight g	Energy kcal	Energy kJ	Protein g	Carbohydrate g	Total Sugar g	Total Dietary Fibre g	Total Fat g	Saturated Fat g	Monounsaturated Fat g	Polyunsaturated Fat g	Calcium mg	Iron mg	Sodium mg	Potassium mg	Magnesium mg	Phosphorus mg	Folate DFE	Vitamin B12 mcg	Vitamin E mg
Meatless breaded chicken nuggets	2	72	168	705	15	6	0	3.1	9	0.8	2.3	3.3	30	2.8	288	216	9	176	40	3.68	1.4
Meatless ground beef	75 g	75	148	618	16	6	1	3.5	7	1.1	1.6	3.5	22	1.6	413	135	14	258	59	1.80	1.3
Soy patty	1	70	136	568	15	5	1	3.2	6	0.8	1.2	2.5	20	1.5	385	126	13	241	55	1.68	1.2
Tofu, regular, firm and extra firm	150 g	150	189	791	21	3	1	0	11	1.3	1.8	2.7	234	2.4	26	222	56	182	29	0	tr
Tofu, silken, soft	150 g	150	83	345	7	4	2	0.2	4	0.5	0.8	2.3	47	1.2	8	270	44	93	N/A	0	tr
Vegetable patty	1	90	138	576	18	7	N/A	5.7	4	1.0	2.1	0.3	102	3.9	411	432	70	225	22	0	N/A
Vegetarian luncheon meat	4 slices	56	106	442	10	2	1	0	6	0.7	1.2	2.5	23	1.0	398	112	13	248	56	2.24	1.7

Food Name	Measure	Weight (g)	Energy (kcal)	Energy (kJ)	Protein (g)	Carbohydrate (g)	Total Sugar (g)	Total Dietary Fibre (g)	Total Fat (g)	Saturated Fat (g)	Monounsaturated Fat (g)	Polyunsaturated Fat (g)	Calcium (mg)	Iron (mg)	Sodium (mg)	Potassium (mg)	Magnesium (mg)	Phosphorus (mg)	Folate (DFE)	Vitamin B12 (mcg)	Vitamin E (mg)
Legumes, Nuts and Seeds																					
Wiener, meatless	1	46	107	448	9	4	0	1.8	6	0.9	1.8	3.6	15	0.6	217	45	8	158	36	1.08	0.9
Beans, Peas and Lentils																					
Beans, baked, homemade	175 mL	187	283	1181	13	40	N/A	10.3	10	3.6	4.0	1.4	114	3.7	790	670	80	204	90	0	N/A
Beans, baked, plain or vegetarian, canned	175 mL	188	177	738	9	40	17	7.7	1	0.2	0.2	0.2	64	2.2	633	408	49	135	23	0	0.3
Beans, baked, with pork, canned	175 mL	187	198	829	10	37	N/A	10.4	3	1.1	1.3	0.4	99	3.2	775	578	64	202	67	0	N/A
Beans, black, canned, not drained	175 mL	178	162	676	11	29	N/A	12.2	1	0.1	tr	0.2	62	3.4	682	547	62	192	108	0	1.3
Beans, kidney, dark red, canned, not drained	175 mL	189	161	672	10	30	tr	12.1	1	0.1	0.1	0.4	45	2.4	646	487	53	178	97	0	1.1
Beans, navy, canned, not drained	175 mL	194	219	917	15	40	1	9.9	1	0.2	0.1	0.4	91	3.6	868	558	91	260	120	0	1.5
Beans, pinto, canned, not drained	175 mL	178	153	639	9	27	tr	8.2	1	0.3	0.3	0.5	76	2.6	522	431	48	163	107	0	1.1
Beans, refried, canned	175 mL	186	175	733	10	29	tr	9.9	2	0.9	1.0	0.3	65	3.1	557	498	62	160	21	0	N/A
Beans, white, canned, not drained	175 mL	194	227	948	14	43	N/A	9.3	1	0.1	tr	0.2	141	5.8	315	880	99	176	126	0	1.6
Black-eyed peas, canned, not drained	175 mL	178	137	572	8	24	N/A	5.9	1	0.3	0.1	0.4	36	1.7	531	305	50	124	91	0	0.5
Chickpeas (garbanzo beans), canned, not drained	175 mL	178	211	884	9	40	N/A	7.8	2	0.2	0.5	0.9	57	2.4	531	305	51	160	119	0	0.3
Falafel, homemade	1 ball	17	57	237	2	5	N/A	1.3	3	0.4	1.7	0.7	9	0.6	50	99	14	33	18	0	N/A
Hummus, commercial	60 mL	57	94	394	4	8	N/A	3.4	5	0.8	2.3	2.1	22	1.4	215	129	40	100	47	0	N/A
Lentils, boiled, salted	175 mL	146	170	710	13	29	3	6.2	1	0.1	0.1	0.3	28	4.9	349	540	53	264	265	0	N/A
Lentils, pink, boiled	175 mL	179	190	793	14	32	N/A	5.9	1	0.2	0.3	0.6	22	4.1	4	317	39	161	112	0	N/A
Peas, split, boiled	175 mL	145	171	715	12	31	4	4.2	1	0.1	0.1	0.2	20	1.9	3	525	52	144	94	0	N/A
Soybeans, boiled	175 mL	127	220	920	21	13	4	8.0	11	1.7	2.5	6.4	130	6.5	1	655	109	312	69	0	N/A
Peanuts																					
Peanut butter, chunk type, fat, sugar and salt added	30 mL	32	191	799	8	7	3	2.6	16	2.6	8.0	4.8	15	0.6	158	242	52	103	30	0	2.0
Peanut butter, natural	30 mL	31	184	770	7	7	1	2.5	16	2.2	7.8	4.9	17	0.7	2	207	55	113	46	0	2.2
Peanut butter, smooth type, fat, sugar and salt added	30 mL	32	191	798	8	6	3	1.8	16	3.3	7.7	4.5	14	0.6	149	210	50	116	24	0	2.9
Peanut butter, smooth type, light	30 mL	36	190	794	9	13	3	1.9	12	2.7	5.9	3.7	13	0.7	197	244	62	135	22	0	2.4
Peanuts, all types, shelled, oil-roasted, salted	60 mL	37	219	915	10	6	2	2.7	19	3.2	9.5	5.6	22	0.6	117	265	64	145	44	0	2.5
Peanuts, all types, shelled, roasted	60 mL	37	217	906	9	8	2	3.0	18	2.6	9.1	5.8	20	0.8	2	244	65	133	54	0	2.6
Nuts																					
Almonds, dried	60 mL	36	208	870	8	7	2	4.2	18	1.4	11.6	4.4	89	1.5	tr	262	99	171	10	0	9.3

Food Name	Measure	Weight (g)	Energy (kcal)	Energy (kJ)	Protein (g)	Carbohydrate (g)	Total Sugar (g)	Total Dietary Fibre (g)	Total Fat (g)	Saturated Fat (g)	Monounsaturated Fat (g)	Polyunsaturated Fat (g)	Calcium (mg)	Iron (mg)	Sodium (mg)	Potassium (mg)	Magnesium (mg)	Phosphorus (mg)	Folate (DFE)	Vitamin B12 (mcg)	Vitamin E (mg)
Legumes, Nuts and Seeds																					
Almonds, oil roasted	60 mL	40	242	1010	8	7	2	4.2	22	1.7	13.9	5.4	116	1.5	tr	278	109	186	11	0	10.3
Almonds, roasted, salted	60 mL	35	209	874	8	7	2	4.1	18	1.4	11.8	4.4	93	1.6	119	261	100	171	12	0	9.1
Brazil nuts, dried	60 mL	36	233	974	5	4	1	2.7	24	5.4	8.7	7.3	57	0.9	1	234	133	257	8	0	2.0
Cashews, roasted, salted	60 mL	35	199	834	5	11	2	1.0	16	3.2	9.5	2.7	16	2.1	222	196	90	170	24	0	0.3
Hazelnuts or filberts, dried	60 mL	34	215	899	5	6	1	3.3	21	1.5	15.6	2.7	39	1.6	0	233	56	99	39	0	5.2
Macadamia nuts, roasted, salted	60 mL	34	243	1017	3	4	1	2.7	26	4.1	20.1	0.5	24	0.9	90	123	40	67	3	0	0.2
Mixed nuts, oil roasted, salted	60 mL	36	222	929	6	8	2	3.2	20	3.1	11.4	4.8	39	1.2	151	209	85	167	30	0	2.6
Mixed nuts, roasted	60 mL	35	206	863	6	9	N/A	3.1	18	2.4	10.9	3.7	24	1.3	4	207	78	151	17	0	N/A
Mixed nuts, roasted, salted	60 mL	35	206	863	6	9	2	3.1	18	2.4	10.9	3.7	24	1.3	232	207	78	151	17	0	3.8
Pecans, dried	60 mL	25	173	726	2	3	1	2.4	18	1.6	10.2	5.4	18	0.6	0	103	30	70	6	0	0.4
Pine nuts, pignolia, dried	60 mL	34	230	963	5	4	1	1.3	23	1.7	6.4	11.7	5	1.9	1	204	86	197	12	0	3.2
Pistachios, shelled, roasted, salted	60 mL	31	177	741	7	8	2	3.2	14	1.7	7.6	4.3	34	1.3	126	325	37	151	16	0	0.6
Walnuts, dried	60 mL	25	166	694	4	3	1	1.7	17	1.6	2.3	12.0	25	0.7	1	112	40	88	25	0	0.2
Nut Butters																					
Almond butter	30 mL	32	205	858	5	7	N/A	1.2	19	1.8	12.4	4.0	88	1.2	4	246	98	170	21	0	N/A
Cashew butter	30 mL	32	190	796	6	9	N/A	0.6	16	3.2	9.4	2.7	14	1.6	5	177	84	148	22	0	0.5
Sesame butter, tahini	30 mL	30	181	757	5	6	tr	2.8	16	2.3	6.2	7.2	130	2.7	35	126	29	223	30	0	0.1
Seeds																					
Flaxseeds, whole and ground	15 mL	11	56	235	2	3	tr	3.0	4	0.4	0.8	3.2	36	0.5	3	89	39	53	30	0	tr
Pumpkin and squash seeds, kernels, dried	60 mL	35	189	792	9	6	tr	1.4	16	3.0	5.0	7.3	15	5.2	6	282	187	411	20	0	N/A
Sunflower seed kernels, roasted, salted	60 mL	32	189	790	6	8	1	2.9	16	1.7	3.1	10.7	23	1.2	133	276	42	375	77	0	8.5

Food Name	Measure	Weight (g)	Energy (kcal)	Energy (kJ)	Protein (g)	Carbohydrate (g)	Total Sugar (g)	Total Dietary Fibre (g)	Total Fat (g)	Saturated Fat (g)	Cholesterol (mg)	Calcium (mg)	Iron (mg)	Sodium (mg)	Potassium (mg)	Magnesium (mg)	Phosphorus (mg)	Vitamin A (RAE)	Folate (DFE)	Vitamin C (mg)	Vitamin B12 (mcg)
Fast Foods																					
Beverages																					
Milk shake, chocolate	250 mL	175	223	931	6	36	33	3.3	6	4.1	23	198	0.5	170	351	30	179	46	9	1	0.60
Milk shake, vanilla	250 mL	175	195	814	6	31	31	0.2	5	3.3	19	214	0.2	144	305	21	179	65	9	1	0.63
Side Dishes																					
French fries	20-25 fries	76	236	989	3	29	N/A	2.5	12	5.0	11	12	1.0	124	541	25	101	2	25	4	0.09
Garlic bread	2 slices	52	192	801	5	26	tr	1.5	8	1.3	0	40	1.3	384	65	14	56	74	97	tr	0.01
Onion rings, breaded and fried	8-9	83	276	1152	4	31	N/A	1.7	16	7.0	14	73	0.8	430	129	16	86	1	85	1	0.12
Zucchini, breaded and fried, sticks	4	36	60	250	1	3	1	0.3	5	0.5	5	18	0.2	44	81	6	36	8	9	3	0.05
Sandwiches																					
Breakfast bagel, with ham, egg and cheese	1	191	483	2019	27	52	7	0.4	18	7.8	243	185	4.1	1259	262	40	397	181	172	0	1.39
Breakfast biscuit with egg, cheese and bacon	1	144	477	1993	16	33	3	1.1	31	11.4	261	164	2.5	1260	230	20	459	N/A	64	2	1.05
Breakfast English muffin with egg, cheese and bacon	1	137	289	1208	17	27	3	1.5	13	4.7	234	151	2.4	729	199	23	270	177	86	2	0.67
Cheeseburger, double patty + condiments + vegetables	1	228	650	2718	30	53	N/A	1.8	35	12.8	93	169	4.7	921	390	36	349	N/A	131	3	2.07
Cheeseburger, single patty, plain	1	102	319	1335	15	32	6	1.3	15	6.5	50	141	2.4	500	164	21	196	0	N/A	0	0.97
Chicken sandwich, breaded chicken + condiments + vegetables	1	228	632	2640	29	42	N/A	2.2	39	12.4	78	258	3.6	1238	333	43	406	164	154	3	0.46
Chicken sandwich, grilled chicken + condiments + vegetables	1	169	335	1402	33	23	3	1.2	12	2.2	78	70	2.1	330	449	37	36	23	83	2	0.41
Donair / Gyro	1	195	310	1295	22	37	3	2.0	7	2.8	49	98	3.1	361	404	40	223	22	115	6	1.82
Fish sandwich with breaded fish	1	183	523	2189	21	48	N/A	2.4	29	8.1	68	185	3.5	939	353	37	311	N/A	134	3	1.08
Hamburger, double patty + condiments	1	215	576	2410	32	39	N/A	1.9	32	12.0	103	92	5.5	742	527	45	284	N/A	111	1	3.33
Hamburger, single patty, plain	1	90	275	1148	12	31	5	1.3	12	4.1	35	63	2.4	387	145	19	103	0	N/A	0	0.89
Submarine sandwich (6 inches), vegetarian	1	167	216	904	7	38	3	3.4	4	0.8	0	77	2.7	529	236	27	88	25	213	20	0
Submarine sandwich (6 inches), with cold cuts	1	228	456	1906	22	51	N/A	3.0	19	6.8	36	189	2.5	1651	394	68	287	71	109	12	1.09
Submarine sandwich (6 inches), with grilled/roasted chicken	1	229	417	1742	24	44	3	3.3	16	2.8	47	81	3.0	722	437	44	104	37	255	12	0.20
Submarine sandwich (6 inches), with tuna	1	256	534	2440	30	55	N/A	2.9	28	5.3	49	74	2.6	1293	335	79	220	46	135	4	1.61
Veggie burger, single patty + condiments + vegetables	1	157	359	1504	19	28	4	4.5	19	2.9	5	86	3.1	671	233	25	278	22	135	3	1.80
Wrap sandwich, chicken ranch	1	249	532	2227	32	44	3	3.5	25	6.7	77	134	3.3	847	544	50	235	50	146	12	0.47

APPENDIX NUTRIENT VALUE OF SOME COMMON FOODS

Food Name	Measure	Weight g	Energy kcal	Energy kJ	Protein g	Carbohydrate g	Total Sugar g	Total Dietary Fibre g	Total Fat g	Saturated Fat g	Cholesterol mg	Calcium mg	Iron mg	Sodium mg	Potassium mg	Magnesium mg	Phosphorus mg	Vitamin A RAE	Folate DFE	Vitamin C mg	Vitamin B12 mcg
Fast Foods																					
Chinese																					
Beef and broccoli stir fry	250 mL	229	266	1111	24	9	1	2.2	15	3.5	58	48	2.8	433	473	35	189	90	104	59	2.00
Chicken almond guy ding	250 mL	256	295	1232	22	18	3	2.6	15	1.6	42	58	1.7	510	591	61	123	14	27	7	0.29
Chicken chow mein	250 mL	232	200	837	21	10	7	2.2	9	1.6	51	38	1.7	982	423	35	191	17	50	8	0.26
Chicken fried rice	250 mL	209	343	1436	12	44	1	1.3	13	1.8	99	36	1.3	797	169	28	139	59	30	4	0.42
Egg roll	1	64	113	472	5	9	1	0.7	6	1.2	35	14	0.8	249	121	9	53	17	27	2	0.19
General Tao/Tso chicken	250 mL	258	806	3371	50	8	3	0.6	62	11.0	163	39	2.2	1285	476	47	340	38	13	11	0.56
Hot and sour soup	250 mL	258	167	697	17	5	1	0.5	8	2.8	36	45	1.8	1596	383	20	192	2	12	1	0.45
Sweet and sour chicken balls	3	75	199	831	9	17	7	0.5	10	2.7	46	24	1.0	390	90	13	23	18	19	1	0.17
Won ton soup	250 mL	255	191	798	15	15	1	1.0	7	2.4	53	37	1.8	810	339	23	159	74	55	2	0.49
Pizza																					
Pizza with cheese (medium - 12 inches)	1/6	84	210	880	9	25	2	1.5	8	3.4	14	171	2.0	515	180	19	161	32	70	4	0.13
Pizza with cheese and pepperoni (medium - 12 inches)	1/6	85	219	916	11	23	1	1.4	9	4.2	21	187	1.7	340	157	18	182	37	74	2	0.20
Pizza with cheese and vegetables (medium - 12 inches)	1/6	93	193	809	8	24	3	1.8	7	3.0	12	154	1.9	482	201	19	147	31	63	11	0.11
Pizza with cheese, meat and vegetables (medium - 12 inches)	1/6	105	250	1044	11	24	3	1.9	12	4.8	24	159	2.1	629	237	21	168	31	65	11	0.24
Other																					
Chicken, breaded and fried (pieces)	2 pieces	98	283	1184	22	9	0	0.3	17	4.6	85	20	1.3	286	181	20	151	0	N/A	0	0.27
Chicken, breaded and fried, boneless (nuggets)	6	96	285	1192	15	16	1	0.9	18	3.9	53	13	0.8	551	251	24	277	5	14	1	0.32
Chili con carne	250 mL	267	270	1128	26	23	N/A	4.9	9	3.6	142	72	5.5	1064	730	48	209	88	59	2	1.20
Corndog (Pogo™)	1	75	197	825	7	24	N/A	1.1	8	2.2	34	44	2.6	417	113	8	71	16	57	0	0.19
Hot-dog, plain	1	98	242	1012	10	18	N/A	0.9	15	5.1	44	24	2.3	670	143	13	97	tr	61	tr	0.51
Mixed Dishes																					
Mexican																					
Burrito with beans and cheese	1	93	189	790	8	27	N/A	3.8	6	3.4	14	107	1.1	583	248	40	90	49	52	1	0.45
Burrito with beef, cheese and chilli	1	152	316	1322	20	32	N/A	2.2	12	5.2	85	111	3.9	1046	333	35	158	99	99	2	1.03
Nachos with cheese	15-20 nachos	113	346	1446	9	36	N/A	4.1	19	7.8	18	272	1.3	816	172	55	276	N/A	N/A	1	0.82
Quesadilla with meat	1	184	627	2622	31	40	tr	2.5	38	17.3	95	442	3.9	1265	319	44	457	167	104	6	1.03

Food Name	Measure	Weight (g)	Energy (kcal)	Energy (kJ)	Protein (g)	Carbohydrate (g)	Total Sugar (g)	Total Dietary Fibre (g)	Total Fat (g)	Saturated Fat (g)	Cholesterol (mg)	Calcium (mg)	Iron (mg)	Sodium (mg)	Potassium (mg)	Magnesium (mg)	Phosphorus (mg)	Vitamin A (RAE)	Folate (DFE)	Vitamin C (mg)	Vitamin B12 (mcg)
Mixed Dishes																					
Taco salad	250 mL	129	193	807	12	13	2	2.0	11	4.1	35	92	1.3	452	275	29	138	40	18	4	0.58
Taco with beef, cheese, salsa + vegetables	1	78	168	704	9	12	N/A	N/A	9	5.2	26	101	1.1	366	216	32	93	N/A	45	1	0.48
Sandwiches																					
Club sandwich	1	246	558	2335	32	47	5	2.8	26	5.8	76	152	4.5	1152	480	47	347	43	163	6	0.48
Egg salad	1	157	479	2003	14	27	3	1.2	35	6.6	335	119	2.9	693	155	19	187	153	121	0	0.92
Hot chicken sandwich	1	284	388	1621	40	31	2	1.7	10	3.0	89	109	4.7	1344	519	43	327	0	96	0	0.54
Ham	1	121	260	1089	13	28	2	2.1	10	2.6	32	92	2.5	1132	229	25	139	49	93	3	0.24
Roast beef	1	139	346	1447	22	33	N/A	2.5	14	3.6	51	54	4.2	792	316	31	239	11	69	2	1.22
Salmon salad	1	162	340	1422	16	33	5	1.7	16	2.9	27	222	2.5	818	271	31	257	27	105	2	2.45
Tuna salad	1	162	371	1552	20	33	5	1.7	13	2.9	15	93	2.9	745	220	32	233	30	97	1	1.25
Salads																					
Caesar	250 mL	114	179	751	5	7	1	1.7	15	2.0	39	92	1.3	268	233	17	81	234	118	20	0.30
Caesar salad with chicken	500 mL	327	491	2055	41	12	3	3.7	31	4.3	137	147	2.9	718	890	61	146	504	249	42	0.76
Garden	250 mL	77	47	198	1	4	3	0.9	4	0.6	0	13	0.3	216	135	6	16	48	15	4	0
Greek	250 mL	111	139	580	4	4	2	1.1	13	3.9	19	121	0.6	315	130	12	85	43	20	11	0.36
Pasta salad with vegetables	250 mL	187	245	1001	5	33	5	2.2	14	1.6	0	27	1.8	1273	173	25	69	98	129	10	0
Pasta																					
Lasagna with meat (7.5cm x 9cm)	1 piece	232	364	1523	22	37	6	2.4	14	7.4	50	251	3.2	623	428	46	280	83	99	11	0.65
Lasagna, vegetarian (7.5cm x 9cm)	1 piece	256	355	1485	19	46	7	2.9	11	6.6	38	304	3.2	737	423	49	290	102	119	13	0.21
Macaroni and cheese (Kraft Dinner™)	250 mL	202	395	1653	11	49	6	2.0	17	4.1	9	158	2.2	784	162	36	194	165	191	tr	0.22
Macaroni casserole with beef and tomato soup	250 mL	263	319	1334	23	32	6	1.9	10	4.0	52	31	3.5	376	399	40	186	14	112	2	1.30
Spaghetti with cream sauce	250 mL	211	250	1047	9	47	4	1.9	2	0.9	5	81	2.2	111	140	34	140	33	192	tr	0.22
Spaghetti with meat sauce	250 mL	262	401	1678	19	50	9	4.9	14	4.5	56	101	4.7	1008	761	60	216	68	162	13	0.89
Other																					
Beef pot pie, commercial, individual	1 serving	227	638	2667	18	57	N/A	2.0	38	11.4	41	45	2.3	1203	293	N/A	109	279	88	0	N/A
Beef stew	250 mL	259	168	701	18	14	3	1.8	4	1.6	39	29	2.2	604	496	33	183	132	26	9	1.52
Butter chicken	250 mL	258	368	1538	28	13	3	1.5	23	9.9	116	125	2.4	740	669	54	307	147	15	11	0.44
Chicken fajita	1 fajita	223	350	1462	19	50	3	4.1	8	2.1	33	52	3.4	540	405	41	183	28	153	26	0.09

Mixed Dishes

Food Name	Measure	Weight (g)	Energy (kcal)	Energy (kJ)	Protein (g)	Carbohydrate (g)	Total Sugar (g)	Total Dietary Fibre (g)	Total Fat (g)	Saturated Fat (g)	Cholesterol (mg)	Calcium (mg)	Iron (mg)	Sodium (mg)	Potassium (mg)	Magnesium (mg)	Phosphorus (mg)	Vitamin A (RAE)	Folate (DFE)	Vitamin C (mg)	Vitamin B12 (mcg)
Chicken pot pie, commercial, individual	1 serving	227	494	2065	21	37	3	3.1	29	9.5	62	59	3.0	347	349	34	195	222	102	9	0.20
Pad Thai	250 mL	171	220	920	15	26	4	1.5	6	0.9	68	26	0.9	344	258	30	56	36	24	5	0.23
Poutine	250 mL	165	380	1587	13	25	1	1.9	26	9.9	40	282	1.4	755	387	26	261	97	16	7	0.38
Samosa, vegetarian	2	100	306	1280	5	32	1	2.1	18	5.6	8	33	1.8	795	178	17	70	36	68	3	0.06
Shepherd's pie	250 mL	257	389	1628	17	40	5	3.1	17	5.0	41	52	1.9	584	766	54	213	94	42	14	1.23
Stir fry with beef	250 mL	229	290	1213	22	20	11	2.2	14	2.3	46	45	2.7	888	534	37	211	30	43	69	1.77
Stir fry with chicken	250 mL	171	255	1067	18	8	2	1.5	17	4.0	63	27	1.3	552	387	25	165	109	16	22	0.19
Stir fry with tofu	250 mL	171	183	767	14	10	3	1.4	10	1.1	tr	142	1.8	493	326	36	141	72	22	20	0.02
Sushi with fish	4	104	164	684	5	35	7	0.8	tr	0.1	3	20	0.5	666	142	21	66	52	15	2	0.11
Sushi with vegetables, no fish	4	104	122	510	2	27	5	0.5	tr	0.1	0	13	0.2	100	60	13	38	16	7	2	tr
Sweet and sour meatballs	6	258	472	2322	26	33	19	0.7	26	10.6	95	76	3.3	931	409	37	243	33	34	1	2.60
Tourtiere, homemade (20cm diam)	1/6	113	307	1283	15	23	1	1.2	17	6.4	47	28	1.9	352	273	22	157	1	59	1	0.30

Soups

Ready-to-serve

Food Name	Measure	Weight (g)	Energy (kcal)	Energy (kJ)	Protein (g)	Carbohydrate (g)	Total Sugar (g)	Total Dietary Fibre (g)	Total Fat (g)	Saturated Fat (g)	Cholesterol (mg)	Calcium (mg)	Iron (mg)	Sodium (mg)	Potassium (mg)	Magnesium (mg)	Phosphorus (mg)	Vitamin A (RAE)	Folate (DFE)	Vitamin C (mg)	Vitamin B12 (mcg)
Beef or chicken, broth/bouillon	250 mL	254	18	74	3	tr	0	0	1	0.3	0	15	0.4	827	137	5	33	0	5	0	0.18
Beef, chunky	250 mL	254	180	753	12	21	2	1.5	5	2.7	15	33	2.5	915	355	5	127	137	15	7	0.66
Chicken noodle, chunky	250 mL	254	185	773	13	18	2	4.1	6	1.5	20	25	1.5	898	114	10	76	71	65	0	0.33
Chicken noodle, low fat, reduced salt	250 mL	257	105	444	9	13	1	2.1	2	1.0	13	21	0	501	N/A	N/A	N/A	N/A	N/A	0	N/A
Chicken vegetable, chunky	250 mL	254	175	733	13	20	N/A	0.9	5	1.5	18	28	1.5	1128	388	10	112	317	13	6	0.25
Clam chowder, Manhattan	250 mL	254	142	593	8	20	4	3.0	4	2.2	15	71	2.8	1057	406	20	89	178	10	13	8.37
Minestrone, chunky	250 mL	254	134	563	5	22	6	6.1	3	1.6	5	63	1.9	913	647	15	117	226	72	5	0
Split pea with ham, chunky	250 mL	254	195	817	12	28	5	4.1	4	1.7	8	36	2.3	1019	322	41	188	259	5	7	0.25
Vegetable, chunky	250 mL	254	129	540	4	20	4	1.3	4	0.6	0	58	1.7	1068	418	8	76	307	18	6	0

Condensed, prepared with water

Food Name	Measure	Weight (g)	Energy (kcal)	Energy (kJ)	Protein (g)	Carbohydrate (g)	Total Sugar (g)	Total Dietary Fibre (g)	Total Fat (g)	Saturated Fat (g)	Cholesterol (mg)	Calcium (mg)	Iron (mg)	Sodium (mg)	Potassium (mg)	Magnesium (mg)	Phosphorus (mg)	Vitamin A (RAE)	Folate (DFE)	Vitamin C (mg)	Vitamin B12 (mcg)
Beef noodle	250 mL	258	88	366	5	9	2	0.8	3	1.2	5	15	1.2	1005	106	5	49	8	31	tr	0.21
Chicken broth	250 mL	254	41	170	5	1	1	0	1	0.4	0	10	0.5	806	218	3	76	0	5	0	0.25
Chicken noodle	250 mL	255	79	331	4	10	N/A	0.8	3	0.7	8	18	0.8	1169	59	5	38	38	37	tr	0.15
Cream of mushroom	250 mL	258	137	572	2	10	2	0.5	9	2.6	3	49	0.5	931	106	5	52	15	5	1	0.05

Food Name	Measure	Weight g	Energy kcal	Energy kJ	Protein g	Carbohydrate g	Total Sugar g	Total Dietary Fibre g	Total Fat g	Saturated Fat g	Cholesterol mg	Calcium mg	Iron mg	Sodium mg	Potassium mg	Magnesium mg	Phosphorus mg	Vitamin A RAE	Folate DFE	Vitamin C mg	Vitamin B12 mcg
Soups																					
Tomato	250 mL	258	90	376	2	18	9	1.2	2	0.4	0	13	1.9	735	278	8	36	26	15	3	0
Tomato, reduced salt	250 mL	258	90	376	2	19	8	0.5	2	0.4	0	13	1.9	52	278	8	36	44	18	70	0
Vegetables with beef	250 mL	258	83	345	6	11	1	0.7	2	0.9	5	18	1.2	835	183	5	44	101	10	1	0.34
Vegetarian vegetable	250 mL	255	76	318	2	13	4	0.5	2	0.3	0	23	1.1	868	222	8	36	122	10	2	0
Condensed, prepared with 2% milk																					
Clam chowder, New England	250 mL	262	157	658	10	18	N/A	1.6	5	1.9	16	202	1.6	1051	320	26	168	71	10	4	10.85
Cream of chicken	250 mL	262	189	789	8	16	7	0.3	10	3.7	21	194	0.7	1108	293	21	162	86	N/A	1	0.58
Cream of mushroom	250 mL	262	202	844	6	16	N/A	0.5	13	4.2	10	191	0.6	983	288	24	168	86	10	2	0.52
Cream of mushroom, reduced salt	250 mL	262	134	558	6	17	9	0.8	5	2.4	14	168	0.7	562	691	21	189	74	21	tr	0.50
Cream of tomato	250 mL	262	155	647	6	24	16	1.3	5	1.9	10	173	1.9	802	480	26	160	69	22	4	0.47
Dehydrated, prepared with water																					
Chicken noodle	250 mL	254	58	243	2	9	1	0.3	1	0.3	10	5	0.5	581	33	8	30	3	28	0	0.05
Minestrone	250 mL	268	83	349	5	13	N/A	0.8	2	0.9	3	40	1.1	1084	360	8	64	16	51	1	0
Onion	250 mL	260	29	120	1	5	2	0.8	1	0.1	0	13	0.2	897	68	5	31	0	3	tr	0
Ramen noodles, chicken flavour, cooked	250 mL	258	162	678	3	20	N/A	6.2	8	3.5	0	N/A	1.2	792	N/A	N/A	N/A	72	N/A	0	N/A
Tomato vegetable	250 mL	255	56	234	2	10	2	0.5	1	0.4	0	8	0.6	1154	104	20	31	10	10	6	0
Homemade																					
Chicken noodle	250 mL	255	135	564	19	7	2	0.9	3	0.7	64	26	1.1	336	302	30	168	136	28	3	0.22
Cream of vegetable	250 mL	251	62	262	5	7	3	0.8	2	0.7	2	53	0.6	586	287	11	95	99	11	3	0.31
French onion	250 mL	255	204	852	10	28	3	1.9	6	2.9	13	159	1.5	904	204	25	157	30	69	2	0.58
Lentil	250 mL	262	193	805	12	27	3	5.1	5	0.4	0	41	3.3	654	365	41	171	45	69	6	0
Split pea with ham	250 mL	267	190	797	13	31	5	3.8	2	0.6	7	39	1.9	312	437	50	176	56	70	2	0.04
Vegetable	250 mL	252	49	204	3	8	2	1.4	1	0.2	0	34	0.7	692	336	16	58	93	20	11	0.14

Fats and Oils

Food Name	Measure	Weight (g)	Energy (kcal)	Energy (kJ)	Protein (g)	Carbohydrate (g)	Total Fat (g)	Saturated Fat (g)	Monounsaturated Fat (g)	Polyunsaturated Fat (g)	Trans Fat (g)	Cholesterol (mg)	Calcium (mg)	Iron (mg)	Sodium (mg)	Potassium (mg)	Magnesium (mg)	Phosphorus (mg)	Vitamin A (RAE)	Vitamin D (mcg)	Vitamin E (mg)
Butter and Margarine																					
Becel™, tub, calorie-reduced, canola and safflower oils (non-hydrogenated)	5 mL	5	17	70	tr	tr	2	0.3	0.8	0.6	tr	0	1	0	46	1	tr	1	48	0.6	0.2
Becel™, tub, canola and safflower oils (non-hydrogenated)	5 mL	5	34	144	tr	tr	4	0.5	1.7	1.2	tr	0	1	0	52	2	tr	1	48	0.6	0.2
Butter	5 mL	5	34	144	tr	tr	4	2.5	1.0	0.1	0.2	10	1	tr	28	1	tr	1	33	tr	0.1
Chefmaster™, tub, unspecified vegetable oils (hydrogenated)	5 mL	5	34	144	tr	tr	4	0.5	1.6	0.9	0.5	0	1	0	52	2	tr	1	48	0.6	0.2
Imperial™, stick, soy and canola oils (hydrogenated)	5 mL	5	34	141	tr	tr	4	0.5	2.5	0.4	1.5	0	tr	tr	31	1	tr	tr	48	0.6	0.3
Imperial™, tub, soya oil (non-hydrogenated)	5 mL	5	34	144	tr	tr	4	0.9	0.7	1.8	tr	0	1	0	52	2	tr	1	48	0.6	0.2
Lactantia™, tub, soya oil (hydrogenated)	5 mL	5	34	144	tr	tr	4	0.7	1.3	1.4	0.6	0	1	0	52	2	tr	1	48	0.6	0.2
Margarine, tub, composite	5 mL	5	34	144	tr	tr	4	0.6	1.7	1.3	tr	0	1	0	52	2	tr	1	48	0.6	0.2
Spread (20% butter / 80% margarine)	5 mL	5	34	141	tr	tr	4	1.0	2.2	0.4	1.0	2	1	tr	43	2	tr	1	47	N/A	0.4
Spread (50% butter / 50% margarine)	5 mL	5	33	137	tr	tr	4	1.5	1.8	0.2	0.7	5	1	tr	40	2	tr	1	16	0	0.2
Oils																					
Canola	15 mL	14	125	525	0	0	14	1.0	8.4	4.2	0.3	0	0	0	0	0	0	0	0	0	2.4
Corn	15 mL	14	122	510	0	0	14	1.8	3.8	7.5	0.1	0	0	0	0	0	0	0	0	0	2.0
Flaxseed	15 mL	14	122	511	0	0	14	1.4	2.5	9.9	tr	0	0	0	0	0	0	0	0	0	2.4
Grapeseed	15 mL	14	122	510	0	0	14	1.3	2.2	9.6	N/A	0	0	0	0	0	0	0	0	0	4.0
Olive	15 mL	14	121	506	0	0	14	1.8	10.1	1.4	tr	0	tr	0.1	tr	0	0	0	0	0	2.0
Peanut	15 mL	14	121	506	0	0	14	2.3	6.3	4.4	N/A	0	0	tr	0	0	0	0	0	0	2.2
Sesame	15 mL	14	122	510	0	0	14	2.0	5.5	5.7	N/A	0	0	0	0	0	0	0	0	0	0.2
Soybean	15 mL	14	122	510	0	0	14	2.0	3.2	8.0	0.2	0	0	tr	0	0	0	0	0	0	1.3
Sunflower	15 mL	14	122	510	0	0	14	1.4	2.7	9.1	0.1	0	0	0	0	0	0	0	0	0	5.7
Other																					
Bacon grease	15 mL	12	110	459	0	0	12	4.8	5.5	1.4	N/A	12	0	0	18	0	0	0	0	0	0.1
Lard	15 mL	13	117	489	0	0	13	5.2	5.9	1.5	0.2	12	0	0	0	0	0	0	0	0	0.1
Shortening	15 mL	13	115	481	0	0	13	3.2	5.4	3.7	N/A	0	tr	tr	1	0	0	0	0	0	0.1

Fats and Oils

Salad Dressings

Food Name	Measure	Weight (g)	Energy (kcal)	Energy (kJ)	Protein (g)	Carbohydrate (g)	Total Fat (g)	Saturated Fat (g)	Monounsaturated Fat (g)	Polyunsaturated Fat (g)	Trans Fat (g)	Cholesterol (mg)	Calcium (mg)	Iron (mg)	Sodium (mg)	Potassium (mg)	Magnesium (mg)	Phosphorus (mg)	Vitamin A (RAE)	Vitamin D (mcg)	Vitamin E (mg)
Blue cheese	15 mL	16	78	327	1	1	8	1.5	1.9	4.3	N/A	3	13	tr	170	6	0	11	10	N/A	0.9
Blue cheese, low Calorie	15 mL	16	15	64	1	tr	1	0.4	0.3	0.4	N/A	tr	14	0.1	186	1	1	13	N/A	N/A	tr
Creamy Caesar	15 mL	15	79	329	tr	tr	9	1.3	2.0	4.9	N/A	tr	4	tr	161	4	tr	3	tr	tr	0.8
Creamy Caesar, low Calorie	15 mL	15	17	70	tr	3	1	0.1	0.2	0.4	N/A	tr	4	tr	164	4	tr	3	tr	tr	0.1
Creamy dressing, fat-free	15 mL	16	21	90	tr	5	tr	tr	tr	tr	N/A	0	1	0.1	130	14	tr	0	tr	0	tr
French	15 mL	16	72	303	tr	2	7	0.9	1.3	3.3	N/A	0	4	0.1	133	11	1	3	4	0	0.8
French, low fat	15 mL	16	33	138	tr	4	2	0.3	0.5	1.2	N/A	0	2	0.1	165	13	0	2	2	0	0.5
Italian	15 mL	15	43	181	tr	2	4	0.7	0.9	1.9	N/A	0	1	0.1	246	7	tr	1	2	0	0.7
Italian, low Calorie	15 mL	15	11	48	tr	1	1	0.1	0.3	0.3	N/A	1	1	0.1	208	13	1	2	tr	0	tr
Mayonnaise	15 mL	14	100	419	tr	1	11	1.7	2.7	6.0	tr	5	3	0.1	79	5	tr	4	11	tr	0.7
Mayonnaise, light	15 mL	16	51	215	tr	1	5	0.8	1.3	2.8	tr	6	1	0.1	107	6	tr	6	3	N/A	0.5
Non creamy dressing, fat-free	15 mL	15	7	29	tr	1	tr	tr	tr	tr	N/A	tr	4	0.1	165	15	1	16	tr	0	0.1
Oil and vinegar	15 mL	16	73	305	0	tr	8	1.5	2.4	3.9	0	0	0	0	tr	1	0	0	0	0	0.8
Ranch	15 mL	15	71	297	tr	1	8	1.2	1.7	4.2	0	5	5	0.1	120	9	1	24	1	tr	0.7
Ranch, low fat	15 mL	16	35	149	tr	3	3	0.2	0.9	0.7	0.4	3	20	0.1	151	21	1	31	3	tr	0.3
Salad dressing, mayonnaise type	15 mL	15	53	243	tr	2	5	0.7	1.3	2.7	0.4	4	2	tr	106	1	tr	4	3	0.3	0.3
Salad dressing, mayonnaise type, fat-free	15 mL	16	14	57	tr	3	tr	0.1	0.3	tr	N/A	1	1	tr	128	8	tr	1	0	N/A	tr
Salad dressing, mayonnaise type, light	15 mL	15	44	184	0	2	4	0.2	2.2	1.1	N/A	0	tr	0	117	0	0	N/A	3	N/A	tr
Thousand Island	15 mL	16	59	245	tr	2	6	0.8	1.2	2.9	N/A	4	3	0.2	137	17	1	4	2	N/A	0.6
Thousand Island, low Calorie	15 mL	16	32	132	tr	3	2	0.1	1.0	0.4	N/A	tr	2	0.1	129	31	1	2	2	N/A	0.2

Sweets and Sugars

Sugar, Honey and Substitutes

Food Name	Measure	Weight g	Energy kcal	Energy kJ	Protein g	Carbohydrate g	Total Sugar g	Total Dietary Fibre g	Total Fat g	Saturated Fat g	Cholesterol mg	Calcium mg	Iron mg	Sodium mg	Potassium mg	Magnesium mg	Phosphorus mg	Vitamin A RAE	Vitamin C mg	Vitamin B12 mcg	Caffeine mg
Brown sugar	5 mL	5	18	73	0	5	4	0	0	0	0	4	0.1	2	16	1	1	0	0	0	0
Honey	5 mL	7	22	91	tr	6	6	tr	0	0	0	tr	tr	tr	4	tr	tr	0	tr	0	0
Icing sugar (powdered)	5 mL	3	10	41	0	2	2	0	tr	0	0	tr	tr	tr	0	0	tr	0	0	0	0
Sugar substitute, aspartame (Equal™)	1 packet	1	4	15	tr	1	1	0	0	0	0	0	0	tr	0	0	0	0	0	0	0
Sugar substitute, sucralose (Splenda™)	5 mL	1	2	7	0	tr	tr	0	0	0	0	0	0	0	0	0	0	0	0	0	0
White sugar (granulated)	5 mL	4	16	68	0	4	4	0	0	0	0	tr	0	0	0	0	0	0	0	0	0

Syrup and Molasses

Food Name	Measure	Weight g	Energy kcal	Energy kJ	Protein g	Carbohydrate g	Total Sugar g	Total Dietary Fibre g	Total Fat g	Saturated Fat g	Cholesterol mg	Calcium mg	Iron mg	Sodium mg	Potassium mg	Magnesium mg	Phosphorus mg	Vitamin A RAE	Vitamin C mg	Vitamin B12 mcg	Caffeine mg
Chocolate syrup, thin type	15 mL	20	110	461	1	26	20	1.0	tr	0.2	0	6	0.8	28	89	26	51	tr	tr	0	6
Corn syrup	15 mL	21	59	249	0	16	6	0	tr	0	0	4	0.1	32	9	2	2	0	0	0	0
Maple syrup	15 mL	20	55	230	0	14	12	0	tr	tr	0	22	0.2	2	46	4	tr	0	0	0	0
Molasses	15 mL	21	62	257	0	16	12	0	tr	tr	0	44	1.0	8	311	51	7	0	0	0	0
Pancake syrup	15 mL	20	47	195	0	12	7	0.1	0	0	0	1	tr	16	3	tr	2	0	0	0	0

Preserves

Food Name	Measure	Weight g	Energy kcal	Energy kJ	Protein g	Carbohydrate g	Total Sugar g	Total Dietary Fibre g	Total Fat g	Saturated Fat g	Cholesterol mg	Calcium mg	Iron mg	Sodium mg	Potassium mg	Magnesium mg	Phosphorus mg	Vitamin A RAE	Vitamin C mg	Vitamin B12 mcg	Caffeine mg
Double fruit jam type spread	15 mL	19	42	177	tr	10	9	0.5	tr	0	0	2	0.1	6	N/A	N/A	N/A	N/A	tr	N/A	N/A
Double fruit jam type spread, reduced sugar	15 mL	17	23	95	tr	7	5	0.4	tr	0	0	3	0.1	3	N/A	N/A	N/A	N/A	tr	N/A	N/A
Jams and preserves	15 mL	20	56	234	tr	14	10	0.2	tr	tr	0	4	0.1	6	16	1	4	tr	2	0	0
Jelly	15 mL	21	56	235	tr	15	11	0.2	0	0	0	1	tr	6	11	1	1	0	tr	0	0
Marmalade	15 mL	20	50	207	tr	13	12	0.1	0	0	0	8	tr	11	7	tr	1	1	1	0	0

Toppings and Spreads

Food Name	Measure	Weight g	Energy kcal	Energy kJ	Protein g	Carbohydrate g	Total Sugar g	Total Dietary Fibre g	Total Fat g	Saturated Fat g	Cholesterol mg	Calcium mg	Iron mg	Sodium mg	Potassium mg	Magnesium mg	Phosphorus mg	Vitamin A RAE	Vitamin C mg	Vitamin B12 mcg	Caffeine mg
Chocolate topping, fudge-type	30 mL	39	135	564	2	24	13	1.1	3	1.5	1	39	0.6	133	174	25	65	2	tr	0.11	3
Pie filling, cherry, canned	30 mL	25	29	121	tr	7	N/A	0.2	tr	tr	0	3	0.1	5	26	2	4	3	1	0	0
Spread, chocolate hazelnut (Nutella™)	30 mL	38	203	848	2	23	21	2.0	11	2.0	0	41	1.6	15	153	24	57	tr	0	0.11	3
Topping or spread, butterscotch	30 mL	42	105	438	1	27	N/A	0.4	tr	tr	tr	22	0.1	145	35	3	20	11	tr	0.04	0
Topping, strawberry	30 mL	43	110	458	tr	29	12	0.3	tr	tr	0	3	0.1	9	22	2	2	tr	6	0	0

Candies

Food Name	Measure	Weight g	Energy kcal	Energy kJ	Protein g	Carbohydrate g	Total Sugar g	Total Dietary Fibre g	Total Fat g	Saturated Fat g	Cholesterol mg	Calcium mg	Iron mg	Sodium mg	Potassium mg	Magnesium mg	Phosphorus mg	Vitamin A RAE	Vitamin C mg	Vitamin B12 mcg	Caffeine mg
Butterscotch	1 piece	5	21	87	tr	5	4	0	tr	0.1	tr	tr	tr	21	0	tr	tr	1	0	0	0
Candy, chocolate covered, sweetened with sorbitol	1 piece	5	29	120	1	2	1	0.2	2	1.1	1	15	0.1	5	30	5	17	3	tr	0.04	tr

APPENDIX NUTRIENT VALUE OF SOME COMMON FOODS

Food Name	Measure	Weight (g)	Energy (kcal)	Energy (kJ)	Protein (g)	Carbohydrate (g)	Total Sugar (g)	Total Dietary Fibre (g)	Total Fat (g)	Saturated Fat (g)	Cholesterol (mg)	Calcium (mg)	Iron (mg)	Sodium (mg)	Potassium (mg)	Magnesium (mg)	Phosphorus (mg)	Vitamin A (RAE)	Vitamin C (mg)	Vitamin B12 (mcg)	Caffeine (mg)
Sweets and Sugars																					
Caramel	4	40	154	646	2	31	26	0.5	3	2.7	3	56	0.1	99	86	7	46	tr	tr	0	0
Chewing gum	1 stick	3	7	31	0	2	2	0.1	tr	tr	0	0	0	tr	0	0	0	0	0	0	0
Chewing gum, sugarless	1 stick	2	5	22	0	2	0	tr	tr	tr	0	tr	0	tr	0	0	0	0	0	0	0
Fruit leather	1 roll	14	52	217	tr	12	7	0.5	tr	0.1	0	4	0.1	44	41	3	4	1	17	0	1
Fudge, chocolate, homemade	1 piece	17	70	292	tr	13	13	0.3	2	1.0	2	8	0.3	8	22	6	12	7	0	0.02	1
Fudge, vanilla, homemade	1 piece	22	84	353	tr	18	18	0	1	0.6	3	7	tr	11	10	1	6	10	0	0.02	0
Gumdrops	10 pieces	36	143	596	0	36	21	tr	0	0	0	1	0.1	16	2	tr	tr	0	0	0	0
Hard candy	1	6	24	99	0	6	4	0	tr	0	0	tr	tr	2	0	tr	tr	0	0	0	0
Hard candy, reduced sugar	1	3	11	47	0	3	3	0	0	0	0	tr	0.1	0	0	0	0	0	0	0	0
Jellybeans	10 beans	28	105	439	0	26	20	0.1	tr	0	0	1	tr	14	10	1	1	0	0	0	0
Licorice, strawberry (Twizzlers™)	3 strips	38	132	553	1	30	15	0	1	0	0	0	0.2	108	N/A	N/A	1	0	0	0	0
Marshmallows	1	7	23	96	tr	6	4	tr	tr	tr	0	tr	tr	6	1	tr	1	0	0	0	0
Sesame crunch (sesame snap)	4 pieces	35	181	757	4	18	11	2.8	12	1.6	0	229	1.5	58	113	88	148	0	tr	0	0
Skittles™	10 candies	11	43	181	tr	10	8	0	tr	0.1	0	0	tr	2	1	tr	tr	0	7	0	0
Toffee	1 piece	12	67	281	tr	8	8	0	4	2.5	12	4	tr	16	6	tr	4	38	tr	0.01	0
Chocolate Bars																					
Almonds, chocolate covered	10	32	180	752	4	15	12	1.4	12	4.8	4	64	0.8	16	N/A	N/A	N/A	0	0	N/A	N/A
Caramel coated cookies, chocolate covered (Twix™)	1 package	58	289	1210	3	38	28	0.6	14	5.2	3	52	0.5	112	110	19	63	13	tr	0.17	2
Caramel with nuts, chocolate covered (Turtles™)	2	28	132	550	3	17	12	1.2	6	1.3	0	22	0.5	7	125	23	46	12	tr	0	5
Caramel, chocolate covered (Rolo™, Caramilk™)	1 bar	52	246	1031	3	35	33	0.5	11	7.5	6	75	0.2	98	98	0	37	18	tr	0.14	2
Chocolate covered water (Kit Kat™, Coffee Crisp™)	1 bar	42	218	910	3	27	20	0.4	11	7.5	5	53	0.4	23	97	16	57	10	0	0.24	6
Chocolate malt-nougat and caramel, chocolate covered (Mars™)	1 bar	58	245	1026	3	42	35	1.0	9	4.5	8	75	0.4	139	140	20	84	10	1	0.19	5
Chocolate, candy coated (M&M'S™, Smarties™)	1 package	40	201	841	2	27	25	1.1	9	5.8	6	46	0.5	27	117	18	66	16	1	0.12	N/A
Chocolate, semisweet, bars or chips	60 mL	43	204	853	2	27	23	2.5	13	7.6	0	14	1.3	5	156	49	56	0	tr	0	26
Coconut candy, chocolate covered (Bounty™, Almond Joy™)	1 bar	49	235	981	2	29	24	2.5	13	8.6	2	31	0.6	70	124	N/A	55	N/A	tr	N/A	N/A
Fondant, chocolate covered (After Eight™)	2 pieces	16	59	246	tr	13	11	0.3	2	1.3	0	4	0.3	2	N/A	N/A	N/A	tr	0	N/A	N/A

Food Name

Food Name	Measure	Weight g	Energy kcal	Energy kJ	Protein g	Carbohydrate g	Total Sugar g	Total Dietary Fibre g	Total Fat g	Saturated Fat g	Cholesterol mg	Calcium mg	Iron mg	Sodium mg	Potassium mg	Magnesium mg	Phosphorus mg	Vitamin A RAE	Vitamin C mg	Vitamin B12 mcg	Caffeine mg
Sweets and Sugars																					
Fudge, caramel and nuts, chocolate covered (Oh Henry!™)	1 bar	63	289	1208	5	41	31	1.3	14	4.2	6	51	0.4	144	203	32	88	6	tr	0.13	3
Milk chocolate and crisped rice (Nestle Crunch™)	1 bar	40	209	873	2	26	22	1.0	11	6.1	5	68	0.2	53	138	23	81	8	tr	0.15	10
Milk chocolate, bars or chips	1 bar	50	268	1119	4	30	26	1.7	15	7.1	12	95	1.2	40	186	32	104	25	0	0.31	10
Peanut butter cups (Reese's™)	3 cups	51	263	1099	5	28	24	1.8	16	5.5	3	40	0.6	160	175	32	82	9	tr	0.29	9
Peanuts, chocolate covered	10	40	208	868	5	20	15	1.9	13	5.8	4	42	0.5	16	201	38	85	14	0	0.18	9
Raisins, chocolate covered (Glosette™)	10 pieces	10	39	163	tr	7	6	0.4	1	0.9	tr	9	0.2	4	51	5	14	2	tr	0.02	3
Toffee, chocolate covered (Skor™)	1 bar	39	209	872	1	24	23	0.5	13	7.3	21	51	0.2	124	60	4	24	60	tr	N/A	N/A
Frozen Desserts																					
Chocolate ice milk bar (Fudgesicle™)	1	51	65	271	3	14	10	0.9	tr	0.2	2	81	0.5	48	N/A	N/A	N/A	N/A	1	N/A	N/A
Frozen yogourt, chocolate	125 mL	91	116	484	3	20	20	1.2	3	2.1	12	91	0.4	57	213	23	81	36	6	0.06	3
Frozen yogourt, vanilla	125 mL	76	124	519	3	18	18	0	4	2.6	2	109	0.2	66	161	11	98	45	1	0.22	0
Fruit and juice bar	1	77	63	264	1	16	13	0.8	tr	0	0	4	0.1	3	41	3	5	1	7	0	0
Ice cream cone, vanilla, chocolate covered, with nuts	1	78	222	928	5	23	16	1.9	14	5.4	25	105	0.8	54	208	42	117	68	tr	0.23	4
Ice cream cone, vanilla, soft serve	1	150	266	1110	7	43	32	0.6	7	4.3	39	232	0.5	116	305	22	154	90	2	0.67	0
Ice cream sandwich	1	59	143	598	3	22	14	0.9	6	3.2	20	60	0.6	36	122	13	63	53	tr	0.18	1
Ice cream, chocolate	125 mL	70	151	630	3	20	18	0.8	8	4.7	24	76	0.6	53	174	20	75	82	tr	0.20	2
Ice cream, dairy free	125 mL	87	237	990	4	21	N/A	0.8	16	2.0	0	36	1.2	216	64	19	59	tr	tr	0	0
Ice cream, strawberry	125 mL	70	134	560	2	19	N/A	0.6	6	3.6	20	84	0.1	42	131	10	70	67	5	0.21	0
Ice cream, vanilla, low fat	125 mL	93	117	490	5	20	10	0	5	1.5	11	146	0.1	65	205	13	113	27	1	0.46	0
Ice cream, vanilla, low fat, aspartame sweetened	125 mL	69	106	445	3	15	4	0.5	5	2.8	19	93	0.1	66	135	6	52	1	1	0.36	0
Ice cream, vanilla, premium	125 mL	113	282	1177	4	25	23	0	18	11.7	104	132	0.4	69	178	12	119	206	0	0.44	0
Ice cream, vanilla, regular	125 mL	76	153	640	3	18	16	0.5	8	5.2	33	97	0.1	61	151	11	80	90	tr	0.30	0
Popsicles	1	75	54	226	0	14	10	0	0	0	0	0	0	9	3	1	0	0	0	0	0
Sherbet, orange	125 mL	78	113	471	1	24	19	2.6	2	0.9	9	42	0.1	36	75	6	31	8	5	0.09	0
Soft serve ice cream with Oreo™ cookies (Blizzard™, McFlurry™)	1 small	275	575	2404	13	89	68	1.9	20	10.5	63	386	4.7	368	564	52	279	148	3	1.12	5
Other Desserts																					
Chocolate mousse, homemade	125 mL	90	203	847	4	14	13	0.5	14	8.2	126	86	0.5	34	129	18	105	126	tr	0.42	6

Sweets and Sugars

Food Name	Measure	Weight (g)	Energy (kcal)	Energy (kJ)	Protein (g)	Carbohydrate (g)	Total Sugar (g)	Total Dietary Fibre (g)	Total Fat (g)	Saturated Fat (g)	Cholesterol (mg)	Calcium (mg)	Iron (mg)	Sodium (mg)	Potassium (mg)	Magnesium (mg)	Phosphorus (mg)	Vitamin A (RAE)	Vitamin C (mg)	Vitamin B12 (mcg)	Caffeine (mg)
Gelatin dessert, calorie-reduced, prepared (Jello™)	125 mL	124	25	104	1	5	0	0	0	0	0	4	tr	59	1	1	84	0	0	0	0
Gelatin dessert, prepared (Jello™)	125 mL	143	83	369	2	20	19	0	0	0	0	4	tr	107	1	1	31	0	0	0	0

Snacks

Food Name	Measure	Weight (g)	Energy (kcal)	Energy (kJ)	Protein (g)	Carbohydrate (g)	Total Sugar (g)	Total Dietary Fibre (g)	Total Fat (g)	Saturated Fat (g)	Cholesterol (mg)	Calcium (mg)	Iron (mg)	Sodium (mg)	Potassium (mg)	Magnesium (mg)	Phosphorus (mg)	Vitamin A (RAE)	Folate (DFE)	Vitamin C (mg)	Vitamin B12 (mcg)
Popcorn																					
Air-popped	250 mL	8	32	135	1	7	tr	1.3	tr	tr	0	1	0.2	tr	25	11	25	1	2	0	0
Caramel-coated	250 mL	37	160	670	1	29	20	1.9	5	1.3	2	16	0.6	77	41	13	31	1	2	0	tr
Microwave, low fat and reduced salt	250 mL	8	34	144	1	6	tr	1.1	1	0.1	0	1	0.2	39	19	12	21	tr	1	0	0
Oil-popped, regular and microwaved	250 mL	12	58	243	1	7	tr	1.2	3	0.6	0	1	0.3	103	26	13	29	1	2	tr	0
Chips																					
Corn-based puffs or twists, cheese (Cheesies™)	250 mL	37	205	857	3	20	1	0.4	13	2.4	1	21	0.9	388	61	7	40	2	2	tr	0.05
Potato chips made from dried potatoes, plain (Pringles™)	17 chips	28	156	654	2	14	1	1.0	11	2.6	0	7	0.4	184	282	16	44	0	2	2	0
Potato chips, baked, plain	1 small bag	43	202	843	2	31	2	2.1	8	1.1	0	54	0.3	394	310	18	118	0	0	0	0
Potato chips, flavoured	1 small bag	43	217	883	3	23	N/A	1.9	14	3.5	0	22	0.8	323	542	32	80	5	36	15	0
Potato chips, plain	1 small bag	43	230	964	3	21	tr	1.6	15	1.8	0	9	0.7	229	571	30	65	0	20	25	0
Tortilla chips, nacho flavoured (Doritos™)	1 small bag	50	249	1042	4	31	2	2.7	13	2.5	2	74	0.7	354	108	41	122	12	7	1	0
Tortilla chips, plain	26 small	47	234	980	3	29	tr	3.0	12	2.3	0	72	0.7	247	92	41	96	2	5	0	0
Other Snacks																					
Banana chips	10 chips	14	73	304	tr	8	5	1.1	5	4.1	0	3	0.2	1	75	11	8	1	2	1	0
Beef jerky (22cm long)	1 stick	20	81	340	7	2	2	0.4	5	2.1	10	4	1.1	438	118	10	81	0	27	0	0.20
Beer nuts	10 nuts	34	186	779	8	10	5	2.2	14	2.0	0	26	0.6	2	203	54	152	0	37	tr	0
Bits and bites snack bites (Bits & Bites™)	125 mL	31	132	554	4	21	3	1.9	4	1.0	1	18	2.6	263	92	24	71	2	37	tr	0.03

Snacks

Food Name	Measure	Weight (g)	Energy (kcal)	Energy (kJ)	Protein (g)	Carbohydrate (g)	Total Sugar (g)	Total Dietary Fibre (g)	Total Fat (g)	Saturated Fat (g)	Cholesterol (mg)	Calcium (mg)	Iron (mg)	Sodium (mg)	Potassium (mg)	Magnesium (mg)	Phosphorus (mg)	Vitamin A (RAE)	Folate (DFE)	Vitamin C (mg)	Vitamin B12 (mcg)
Fruit leather bar (Fruit to Go™)	1 bar	14	49	206	tr	11	N/A	0.5	1	0.6	0	4	0.1	11	19	3	8	1	1	1	0
Pretzels, hard, plain, salted	10 sticks	5	19	80	tr	4	tr	0.2	tr	tr	0	2	0.2	86	7	2	6	0	12	0	0
Pretzels, hard, plain, unsalted	10 sticks	5	19	80	tr	4	tr	0.2	tr	tr	0	2	0.2	15	7	2	6	0	12	0	0
Rice cakes, plain	1	9	35	146	1	7	tr	0.4	tr	0.1	0	1	0.1	29	26	12	32	0	2	0	0
Sesame sticks, salted	60 mL	14	75	316	2	6	tr	0.4	5	0.9	0	24	0.1	208	25	6	19	0	3	0	0
Soybeans, roasted, salted	60 mL	44	205	859	15	15	2	7.7	11	1.6	0	60	1.7	71	641	63	158	4	92	1	0
Trail mix, regular	60 mL	38	176	735	5	17	N/A	2.5	11	2.1	0	30	1.2	87	261	60	131	tr	27	1	0
Trail mix, tropical	60 mL	36	144	604	2	23	N/A	2.4	6	3.0	0	20	0.9	4	252	34	66	1	15	3	0

Beverages

Coffee, Tea and Substitutes

Food Name	Measure	Weight (g)	Energy (kcal)	Energy (kJ)	Protein (g)	Carbohydrate (g)	Total Sugar (g)	Total Dietary Fibre (g)	Total Fat (g)	Saturated Fat (g)	Cholesterol (mg)	Calcium (mg)	Iron (mg)	Sodium (mg)	Potassium (mg)	Magnesium (mg)	Phosphorus (mg)	Vitamin A (RAE)	Vitamin C (mg)	Alcohol (g)	Caffeine (mg)
Chai, latte	250 mL	242	149	624	5	26	26	0	3	2.0	13	186	0.1	67	263	19	150	88	tr	0	13
Coffee, brewed	250 mL	250	3	10	tr	0	0	0	tr	tr	0	5	tr	5	123	8	8	0	0	0	100
Coffee, brewed, decaffeinated	250 mL	251	3	10	tr	0	0	0	0	0	0	5	0.1	5	135	13	3	0	0	0	3
Coffee, instant, regular, powder + water	250 mL	253	5	20	tr	1	0	0	tr	tr	0	10	0.1	5	76	8	8	0	0	0	66
Coffee, latte	250 mL	256	101	420	5	7	9	0	6	3.5	16	188	0.2	79	340	89	156	46	tr	0	193
Coffee, substitute, powder + water	250 mL	254	13	53	tr	3	tr	0.8	tr	tr	0	8	0.2	8	79	10	18	0	0	0	0
Iced cappuccino - original - with cream (Tim Hortons™)	250 mL	N/A	211	886	2	28	28	0	9	5.0	38	80	0.3	42	N/A	N/A	N/A	N/A	0	N/A	N/A
Iced cappuccino - with 2% milk (Tim Hortons™)	250 mL	N/A	127	533	3	27	27	0	1	1.0	4	70	0.3	30	N/A	N/A	N/A	N/A	0	N/A	N/A
Iced coffee, Frappuccino (Starbucks™)	250 mL	N/A	127	533	3	26	22	0	2	1.0	7	110	0	120	N/A	N/A	N/A	N/A	0	N/A	60
Iced tea, lemon flavor, ready-to-drink	250 mL	254	91	383	0	23	23	0	0	tr	0	N/A	N/A	53	N/A	N/A	N/A	N/A	N/A	0	N/A
Iced tea, lemon flavour, powder + water	250 mL	274	93	389	tr	23	23	0	tr	tr	0	5	0.1	8	52	5	3	0	tr	0	30

Beverages

Food Name	Measure	Weight (g)	Energy (kcal)	Energy (kJ)	Protein (g)	Carbohydrate (g)	Total Sugar (g)	Total Dietary Fibre (g)	Total Fat (g)	Saturated Fat (g)	Cholesterol (mg)	Calcium (mg)	Iron (mg)	Sodium (mg)	Potassium (mg)	Magnesium (mg)	Phosphorus (mg)	Vitamin A (RAE)	Vitamin C (mg)	Alcohol (g)	Caffeine (mg)
Beverages																					
Tea, brewed	250 mL	250	3	10	0	1	0	0	tr	tr	0	0	0.1	8	93	8	3	0	0	0	50
Tea, brewed, herbal	250 mL	250	3	10	0	1	0	0	tr	tr	0	5	0.2	3	23	3	0	0	0	0	0
Carbonated Drinks																					
Club soda	250 mL	250	0	0	0	0	0	0	0	0	0	13	tr	53	5	3	0	0	0	0	0
Cola	250 mL	262	110	461	tr	28	24	0	0	0	0	8	0.1	10	3	3	34	0	0	0	26
Cola, aspartame sweetened	250 mL	250	3	10	tr	tr	0	0	0	0	0	8	0.1	13	15	3	28	0	0	0	35
Cola, decaffeinated	250 mL	262	107	448	0	28	28	0	0	0	0	5	0.1	10	8	3	29	0	0	0	0
Ginger ale	250 mL	258	88	366	0	23	22	0	0	0	0	8	0.5	18	3	3	0	0	0	0	0
Lemon-lime soda	250 mL	260	104	433	0	27	23	0	0	0	0	5	0.2	29	3	3	0	0	0	0	0
Non cola soda, aspartame sweetened	250 mL	250	0	0	0	tr	0	0	0	0	0	10	0.1	40	5	3	0	0	0	0	0
Orange soda	250 mL	262	126	527	0	32	N/A	0	0	0	0	13	0.2	31	5	3	3	0	0	0	0
Tonic water	250 mL	258	124	520	0	32	32	0	0	0	0	4	tr	15	5	3	3	0	0	0	0
Fruit Flavoured Drinks																					
Citrus juice drink, frozen, diluted (Five Alive™)	250 mL	262	131	548	tr	32	30	0.3	tr	0	0	13	1.8	5	128	10	10	N/A	38	0	0
Fruit flavour drink, low Calorie, powder + water (Crystal Light™)	250 mL	254	3	14	0	1	0	0	tr	0	0	6	tr	6	3	3	2	tr	0	0	0
Fruit punch flavour drink, powder (Kool-Aid™) + water	250 mL	276	102	427	0	26	N/A	0	tr	tr	0	44	0.1	39	3	3	55	0	0	0	0
Fruit punch flavour drink, vitamin C added, powder + water	250 mL	277	102	429	0	26	N/A	0	tr	tr	0	44	0.1	39	3	3	55	0	100	0	0
Fruit punch juice drink, ready-to-drink (Sunny D™)	250 mL	262	123	516	0	33	31	0	0	0	0	3	0.1	26	31	N/A	3	0	3	0	0
Lemonade, pink or white, frozen, diluted	250 mL	262	105	440	tr	27	13	0.2	tr	0	0	8	0.4	6	39	5	5	0	10	0	0
Mixed vegetable and fruit juice drink, ready-to-drink (V8 Splash™)	250 mL	257	113	472	tr	29	5	0.3	tr	0	0	10	0.2	41	62	5	8	N/A	81	0	0
Orange drink, vitamin C added (Hi-C™), ready-to-drink	250 mL	262	134	558	0	34	29	0	0	tr	0	16	0.7	42	47	5	3	N/A	94	0	0
Orange drink, vitamin C added (Tang™, Quench™, Rise'n Shine™), powder + water	250 mL	286	135	564	0	34	34	0	0	0	0	140	0.1	11	69	3	63	N/A	88	0	0
Other Beverages																					
Sports drink, fruit flavour, low Calorie, ready-to-drink (Gatorade™, Powerade™)	250 mL	261	29	120	0	8	0	0	0	0	0	0	0.1	91	26	3	23	0	16	0	0
Sports drink, fruit flavour, ready-to-drink (Gatorade™, Powerade™)	250 mL	258	67	281	0	16	14	0	tr	0	0	3	0.5	101	36	3	23	0	1	N/A	N/A

Food Name — Beverages

Food Name	Measure	Weight (g)	Energy (kcal)	Energy (kJ)	Protein (g)	Carbohydrate (g)	Total Sugar (g)	Total Dietary Fibre (g)	Total Fat (g)	Saturated Fat (g)	Cholesterol (mg)	Calcium (mg)	Iron (mg)	Sodium (mg)	Potassium (mg)	Magnesium (mg)	Phosphorus (mg)	Vitamin A (RAE)	Vitamin C (mg)	Alcohol (g)	Caffeine (mg)
Beverages																					
Water, mineral (Perrier™)	250 mL	250	0	0	0	0	0	0	0	0	0	35	0	3	0	0	0	0	0	0	0
Water, municipal	250 mL	250	0	0	0	0	0	0	0	0	0	5	0	5	0	3	0	0	0	0	0
Alcoholic																					
Beer, de-alcoholized, (Labbat .5™)	1 can	350	210	878	1	47	28	0	tr	0.1	0	24	0.2	45	28	24	56	0	2	1	0
Beer, high alcohol (7% alcohol by volume)	1 bottle	342	183	766	1	10	N/A	0.7	0	0	0	17	0.1	17	86	21	41	0	0	20	0
Beer, light (4% alcohol by volume)	1 bottle	340	99	412	1	5	tr	0	0	0	0	14	0.1	14	71	17	41	0	0	11	0
Beer, regular (5% alcohol by volume)	1 bottle	342	140	586	1	10	0	0	0	0	0	14	0.1	14	92	21	48	0	0	14	0
Cocktail, daiquiri	125 mL	128	237	993	tr	9	7	0.1	tr	tr	0	4	0.1	6	27	3	6	0	2	29	0
Cocktail, margarita	125 mL	131	246	1031	tr	6	4	0.1	tr	tr	0	4	0.1	527	23	2	7	tr	2	33	0
Liqueur, coffee and cream	45 mL	53	172	719	1	11	10	0	8	5.1	31	8	0.1	48	17	1	26	91	tr	7	4
Sangria	125 mL	123	87	365	tr	12	10	0.1	tr	tr	0	9	0.2	13	80	8	10	1	6	6	0
Spirits (gin, rum, vodka, whisky)	50 mL	47	109	456	0	0	0	0	0	0	0	0	tr	1	1	0	2	0	0	16	0
Vodka cooler	1 bottle	390	220	799	tr	33	12	0.3	1	tr	0	20	0.9	12	211	23	19	tr	11	13	0
Wine, dessert, sweet	125 mL	127	203	848	tr	17	10	0	0	0	0	10	0.3	11	117	11	11	0	0	19	0
Wine, table, red	125 mL	125	90	375	tr	2	1	0	0	0	0	10	0.5	6	140	16	17	0	0	12	0
Wine, table, white	125 mL	125	85	354	tr	1	1	0	0	0	0	11	0.4	6	100	12	17	0	11	12	0

Food Name — Miscellaneous

Food Name	Measure	Weight (g)	Energy (kcal)	Energy (kJ)	Protein (g)	Carbohydrate (g)	Total Sugar (g)	Total Fat (g)	Saturated Fat (g)	Monounsaturated Fat (g)	Polyunsaturated Fat (g)	Cholesterol (mg)	Calcium (mg)	Iron (mg)	Sodium (mg)	Potassium (mg)	Magnesium (mg)	Phosphorus (mg)	Vitamin A (RAE)	Lycopene (mcg)	Folate (DFE)
Miscellaneous																					
Condiments																					
Bacon bits, simulated meat	15 mL	7	34	141	2	2	0	2	0.3	0.4	1.0	0	7	0.1	126	10	7	15	0	0	9
Ketchup	15 mL	15	15	64	tr	4	3	tr	tr	tr	tr	0	3	0.1	169	57	3	5	7	2586	2
Mustard	15 mL	16	11	44	1	1	tr	1	tr	0.4	0.2	0	9	0.2	180	22	8	17	1	0	1

APPENDIX NUTRIENT VALUE OF SOME COMMON FOODS

Food Name	Measure	Weight (g)	Energy (kcal)	Energy (kJ)	Protein (g)	Carbohydrate (g)	Total Sugar (g)	Total Fat (g)	Saturated Fat (g)	Monounsaturated Fat (g)	Polyunsaturated Fat (g)	Cholesterol (mg)	Calcium (mg)	Iron (mg)	Sodium (mg)	Potassium (mg)	Magnesium (mg)	Phosphorus (mg)	Vitamin A (RAE)	Lycopene (mcg)	Folate (DFE)
Miscellaneous																					
Olives, pickled, canned or bottled	4	16	23	97	tr	1	tr	2	0.3	1.8	0.2	0	8	0.1	249	7	2	1	3	0	tr
Olives, ripe, canned, jumbo	2	16	13	54	tr	1	0	1	0.1	0.8	0.1	0	15	0.5	144	1	1	tr	3	0	0
Pickle relish, sweet	15 mL	15	20	83	tr	5	2	tr	tr	tr	tr	0	tr	0.1	123	4	1	2	1	0	tr
Pickles, cucumber, dill	1 medium pickle	65	12	49	tr	3	1	tr	tr	tr	0.1	0	6	0.3	833	75	7	14	6	0	1
Pickles, cucumber, sweet, slices	4	28	33	137	tr	8	5	tr	tr	tr	tr	0	1	0.2	263	9	1	3	3	0	1
Salsa	15 mL	17	5	19	tr	1	1	tr	tr	tr	tr	0	5	0.1	100	50	3	5	3	1758	1
Dips																					
Cream cheese dip	30 mL	30	108	451	2	1	tr	11	5.8	3.0	1.6	28	23	0.3	176	39	2	28	92	0	4
Onion dip	30 mL	31	50	211	1	3	tr	4	2.5	1.2	0.2	11	34	0.1	206	60	4	31	33	0	3
Spinach dip	30 mL	30	74	309	1	2	tr	7	1.6	1.9	3.3	6	26	0.3	84	57	8	17	75	tr	15
Gravies and Sauces																					
Gravy, beef, canned	60 mL	59	31	131	2	3	tr	1	0.7	0.6	tr	2	4	0.4	331	48	1	18	1	0	1
Gravy, beef, dehydrated, prepared with water	60 mL	65	20	85	1	3	0	tr	0.2	0.2	tr	tr	9	0.1	271	15	2	11	tr	0	2
Gravy, chicken, canned	60 mL	60	43	199	1	3	tr	3	0.9	1.5	0.9	1	12	0.3	348	66	1	18	1	0	1
Gravy, chicken, dehydrated, prepared with water	60 mL	66	22	93	1	4	0	1	0.2	0.3	0.1	1	10	0.1	244	24	3	15	2	0	8
Gravy, turkey, canned	60 mL	61	31	130	2	3	tr	1	0.4	0.6	0.3	1	2	0.4	353	67	1	18	0	0	3
Gravy, unspecified, dehydrated, prepared with water	60 mL	66	22	91	tr	4	0	tr	0.2	0.2	0.1	tr	11	0.1	362	16	3	13	0	0	3
Sauce, barbecue	15 mL	16	12	50	tr	2	4	tr	tr	0.1	0.1	0	3	0.1	129	28	3	3	tr	68	1
Sauce, cheese, dehydrated, prepared with 2% milk	60 mL	71	81	337	5	7	6	4	2.1	1.3	0.4	11	163	0.1	445	158	12	127	45	0	4
Sauce, cranberry, canned, sweetened	60 mL	70	105	443	tr	27	27	tr	tr	tr	tr	0	3	0.2	20	18	2	4	1	0	1
Sauce, nacho cheese, ready-to-serve	60 mL	64	121	505	5	3	0	10	4.3	3.1	2.1	20	120	0.2	499	20	6	107	66	N/A	3
Sauce, soy	15 mL	18	7	30	tr	1	tr	tr	0	0	0	0	1	0.3	1038	28	1	17	0	N/A	2
Sauce, steak (HP™, A1™)	15 mL	15	9	39	tr	2	N/A	tr	0.1	tr	tr	0	4	0.2	218	60	2	6	7	N/A	1
Sauce, sweet and sour	15 mL	17	20	85	tr	4	3	tr	0	0.1	0.2	0	3	0.1	59	11	1	2	1	N/A	tr
Sauce, teriyaki	15 mL	18	15	64	1	3	2	0	0	0	0	0	5	0.3	700	41	11	28	0	0	4
Sauce, white, medium, homemade with 2% milk	60 mL	61	89	374	2	6	3	6	1.7	2.7	1.7	4	72	0.2	215	95	9	60	55	0	6

glossary

A

Action stage Stage of change in the transtheoretical model in which people are actively changing a negative behaviour or adopting a new, healthy behaviour.

Activities of daily living Everyday behaviours that people normally do to function in life (cross the street, carry groceries, lift objects, do laundry, sweep floors).

Acupuncture Chinese medical system that requires body piercing with fine needles during therapy to relieve pain and treat ailments and diseases.

Adenosine triphosphate (ATP) A high-energy chemical compound that the body uses for immediate energy.

Adequate Intakes (AI) The recommended amount of a nutrient intake when sufficient evidence is not available to calculate the EAR and subsequent RDA.

Adipose tissue Fat cells in the body.

Aerobic Exercise that requires oxygen to produce the necessary energy (ATP) to carry out the activity.

Agility Ability to change body position and direction quickly and efficiently.

Air displacement Technique to assess body composition by calculating the body volume from the air displaced by an individual sitting inside a small chamber.

Allopathic medicine See Conventional Western medicine.

Altruism True concern for the welfare of others.

Amenorrhea Cessation of regular menstrual flow.

Amino acids Chemical compounds that contain nitrogen, carbon, hydrogen, and oxygen; the basic building blocks the body uses to build different types of protein.

Anabolic steroids Synthetic versions of the male sex hormone testosterone, which promotes muscle development and hypertrophy.

Anaerobic Exercise that does not require oxygen to produce the necessary energy (ATP) to carry out the activity.

Angina pectoris Chest pain associated with coronary heart disease.

Angiogenesis Formation of blood vessels (capillaries).

Angioplasty A procedure in which a balloon-tipped catheter is inserted, then inflated, to widen the inner lumen of one or more arteries.

Anorexia nervosa An eating disorder characterized by self-im<None>posed starvation to lose and maintain very low body weight.

Anthropometric measurement techniques Measurement of body girths at different sites.

Anticoagulant Any substance that inhibits blood clotting.

Antioxidants Compounds such as vitamins C and E, beta-carotene, and selenium that prevent oxygen from combining with other substances in the body to form harmful compounds.

Aquaphobic Having a fear of water.

Arrhythmias Irregular heart rhythms.

Arterial-venous oxygen difference (a-$\overline{v}O_2$diff) The amount of oxygen removed from the blood as determined by the difference in oxygen content between arterial and venous blood.

Atherosclerosis Fatty/cholesterol deposits in the walls of the arteries leading to formation of plaque.

Atrophy Decrease in the size of a cell.

Autogenic training A stress management technique using a form of self-suggestion, wherein an individual is able to place himself or herself in an autohypnotic state by repeating and concentrating on feelings of heaviness and warmth in the extremities.

Ayurveda Hindu system of medicine based on herbs, diet, massage, meditation, and yoga to help the body boost its own natural healing.

B

Balance Ability to maintain the body in proper equilibrium.

Ballistic (dynamic) stretching Exercises done with jerky, rapid, bouncy movements, or slow, short, and sustained movements.

Basal metabolic rate (BMR) The lowest level of oxygen consumption necessary to sustain life.

Behaviour modification The process of permanently changing negative behaviours to positive behaviours that will lead to better health and well-being.

Benign Noncancerous.

Binge-eating disorder An eating disorder characterized by uncontrollable episodes of eating excessive amounts of food within a relatively short time.

Bioelectrical impedance Technique to assess body composition by running a weak electrical current through the body.

Biofeedback A stress-management technique in which a person learns to influence physiological responses that are not typically under voluntary control or responses that typically are regulated but for which regulation has broken down as a result of injury, trauma, or illness.

Blood lipids (fat) Cholesterol and triglycerides.

Blood pressure A measure of the force exerted against the walls of the vessels by the blood flowing through them.

Bod Pod Commercial name of the equipment used for the assessment of body composition through the air displacement technique.

Body composition The fat and nonfat components of the human body; important in assessing recommended body weight.

Body mass index (BMI) A technique to determine thinness and excessive fatness that incorporates height and weight to estimate critical fat values at which the risk for disease increases.

Bradycardia Slower heart rate than normal.

Breathing exercise A stress management technique wherein the individual concentrates on "breathing away" the tension and inhaling fresh air to the entire body.

Bulimia nervosa An eating disorder characterized by a pattern of binge eating and purging in an attempt to lose weight and maintain low body weight.

C

Calorie The amount of heat necessary to raise the temperature of 1 gram of water 1 degree Centigrade; used to measure the energy value of food and cost (energy expenditure) of physical activity.

Cancer Group of diseases characterized by uncontrolled growth and spread of abnormal cells.

Capillaries Smallest blood vessels carrying oxygenated blood to the tissues in the body.

Carbohydrate loading Increasing intake of carbohydrates during heavy aerobic training or prior to aerobic endurance events that last longer than 90 minutes.

Carbohydrates A classification of dietary nutrient containing carbon, hydrogen, and oxygen; the major source of energy for the human body.

Carcinogens Substances that contribute to the formation of cancers.

Carcinoma in situ Encapsulated malignant tumor that has not spread.

Cardiac output Amount of blood pumped by the heart in one minute.

Cardiorespiratory endurance The ability of the lungs, heart, and blood vessels to deliver adequate amounts of oxygen to the cells to meet the demands of prolonged physical activity.

Cardiorespiratory training zone The recommended training intensity range, in terms of exercise heart rate, to obtain adequate cardiorespiratory endurance development.

Cardiovascular diseases The array of conditions that affect the heart and the blood vessels.

Carotenoids Pigment substances in plants that are often precursors to vitamin A. More than 600 carotenoids are found in nature, about 50 of which are precursors to vitamin A, the most potent one being beta-carotene.

Catecholamines "Fight-or-flight" hormones, including epinephrine and norepinephrine.

Cellulite Term frequently used in reference to fat deposits that "bulge out"; these deposits are nothing but enlarged fat cells from excessive accumulation of body fat.

Chiropractics Health care system that believes that many diseases and ailments are related to misalignments of the vertebrae and emphasizes the manipulation of the spinal column.

Cholesterol A waxy substance, technically a steroid alcohol, found only in animal fats and oil; used in making cell membranes, as a building block for some hormones, in the fatty sheath around nerve fibres, and in other necessary substances.

Chronic diseases Illnesses that develop and last a long time.

Chronic Lower Respiratory Disease (CLRD) A general term that includes chronic obstructive pulmonary disease, emphysema, and chronic bronchitis (all diseases of the respiratory system).

Chronological age Calendar age.

Chylomicron Triglyceride-transporting molecules.

Circuit training Alternating exercises by performing them in a sequence of three to six or more.

Circumference measurements Technique to assess body composition by measuring circumferences at specific body sites.

Complementary and alternative medicine (CAM) A group of diverse medical and health care systems, practices, and products that are not presently considered to be part of conventional medicine; also called unconventional, nonallopathic, or integrative medicine.

Complex carbohydrates Carbohydrates formed by three or more simple sugar molecules linked together; also referred to as polysaccharides.

Concentric Shortening of a muscle during muscle contraction.

Contemplation stage Stage of change in the transtheoretical model in which people are considering changing behaviour within the next 6 months.

Contraindicated exercises Exercises that are not recommended because they may cause injury to a person.

Controlled ballistic stretching Exercises done with slow, short, and sustained movements.

Conventional Western medicine Traditional medical practice based on methods that are tested through rigorous scientific trials; also called allopathic medicine.

Cool-down Tapering off an exercise session slowly.

Coordination The integration of the nervous and the muscular systems to produce correct, graceful, and harmonious body movements.

Core strength training A training program designed to strengthen the abdominal, hip, and spinal muscles (the core of the body).

Coronary heart disease (CHD) Condition in which the arteries that supply the heart muscle with oxygen and nutrients are narrowed by fatty deposits, such as cholesterol and triglycerides.

C-reactive protein (CRP) A protein whose blood levels increase with inflammation, at times hidden deep in the body; elevation of this protein is an indicator of potential cardiovascular events.

Creatine An organic compound derived from meat, fish, and amino acids that combines with inorganic phosphate to form creatine phosphate.

Creatine phosphate (CP) A high-energy compound that the cells use to resynthesize ATP during all-out activities of very short duration.

Cruciferous vegetables Plants that produce cross-shaped leaves (cauliflower, broccoli, cabbage, Brussels sprouts, and kohlrabi); they seem to have a protective effect against cancer.

D

Daily Values (DVs) Reference values for nutrients and food components used in food labels.

Dentist Practitioner who specializes in diseases of the teeth, gums, and oral cavity.

Deoxyribonucleic acid (DNA) Genetic substance of which genes are made; molecule that contains cell's genetic code.

Diabetes mellitus A disease in which the body doesn't produce or utilize insulin properly.

Diastolic blood pressure Pressure exerted by the blood against the walls of the arteries during the relaxation phase (diastole) of the heart; lower of the two numbers in blood pressure readings.

Dietary fibre A complex carbohydrate in plant foods that is not digested but is essential to the digestion process.

Dietary Reference Intakes (DRIs) A general term that describes four types of nutrient standards that establish adequate amounts and maximum safe nutrient intakes in the diet. These standards are Estimated Average Requirements (EAR), Recommended Dietary Allowances (RDA), Adequate Intakes (AI), and Tolerable Upper Intake Levels (UL).

Disaccharides Simple carbohydrates formed by two monosaccharide units linked together, one of which is glucose. The major disaccharides are sucrose, lactose, and maltose.

Distress Negative stress: Unpleasant or harmful stress under which health and performance begin to deteriorate.

Dual energy X-ray absorptiometry (DEXA) Method to assess body composition that uses very low-dose beams of X-ray energy to measure total body fat mass, fat distribution pattern, and bone density.

Dynamic training Strength-training method referring to a muscle contraction with movement.

Dysmenorrhea Painful menstruation.

E

Eccentric Lengthening of a muscle during muscle contraction.

Ecosystem A community of organisms interacting with each other in an environment.

Elastic elongation Temporary lengthening of soft tissue.

Electrocardiogram (ECG or EKG) A recording of the electrical activity of the heart.

Emotional wellness The ability to understand one's own feelings, accept limitations, and achieve emotional stability.

Endorphins Morphine-like substances released from the pituitary gland (in the brain) during prolonged aerobic exercise; thought to induce feelings of euphoria and natural well-being.

Energy-balancing equation A principle holding that as long as caloric input equals caloric output, the person will not gain or lose weight. If caloric intake exceeds output, the person gains weight; when output exceeds input, the person loses weight.

Environmental wellness The capability to live in a clean and safe environment that is not detrimental to health.

Enzymes Catalysts that facilitate chemical reactions in the body.

Essential fat Minimal amount of body fat needed for normal physiological functions; constitutes about 3 percent of total weight in men and 12 percent in women.

Estimated Average Requirements (EAR) The amount of a nutrient that meets the dietary needs in half the people.

Estimated Energy Requirement (EER) The average dietary energy (caloric) intake that is predicted to maintain energy balance in a healthy adult of defined age, gender, weight, height, and level of physical activity, consistent with good health.

Estrogen Female sex hormone essential for bone formation and conservation of bone density.

Eustress Positive stress: Health and performance continue to improve, even as stress increases.

Exercise A type of physical activity that requires planned, structured, and repetitive bodily movement with the intent of improving or maintaining one or more components of physical fitness.

Exercise intolerance Inability to function during exercise because of excessive fatigue or extreme feelings of discomfort.

F

Fast-twitch fibres Muscle fibres with greater anaerobic potential and fast speed of contraction.

Fats A classification of nutrients containing carbon, hydrogen, some oxygen, and sometimes other chemical elements.

Ferritin Iron stored in the body.

Fight or flight Physiological response of the body to stress that prepares the individual to take action by stimulating the body's vital defense systems.

Fixed resistance Type of exercise in which a constant resistance is moved through a joint's full range of motion.

Flexibility Refers to the achievable range of motion at a joint or group of joints without causing injury.

Folate One of the B vitamins.

Fortified foods Foods that have added nutrients that either were not present or were present in insignificant amounts with the intent of preventing nutrient deficiencies.

Fraud/quackery The conscious promotion of unproven claims for profit.

Free weights Barbells and dumbbells.

Frequency How many times per week a person engages in an exercise session.

Functional capacity The ability to perform ordinary and unusual demands of daily living without limitations and excessive fatigue or injury.

Functional foods Foods or food ingredients containing physiologically active substances that provide specific health benefits beyond those supplied by basic nutrition.

Functional independence Ability to carry out activities of daily living without assistance from other individuals.

G

General adaptation syndrome (GAS) A theoretical model that explains the body's adaptation to sustained stress which includes three stages: Alarm reaction, resistance, and exhaustion/recovery.

Genetically modified foods (GM foods)
Foods whose basic genetic material (DNA) is manipulated by inserting genes with desirable traits from one plant, animal, or microorganism into another one either to introduce new traits or to enhance existing ones.

Glucose intolerance A condition characterized by slightly elevated blood glucose levels.

Glycemic index An index that is used to rate the plasma glucose response of carbohydrate-containing foods with the response produced by the same amount of carbohydrate from a standard source, usually glucose or white bread.

Glycogen Form in which glucose is stored in the body.

Goals The ultimate aims toward which effort is directed.

H

Hatha yoga A form of yoga that incorporates specific sequences of static-stretching postures to help induce the relaxation response.

Health A state of complete well-being, and not just the absence of disease or infirmity.

Health fitness standards The lowest fitness requirements for maintaining good health, decreasing the risk for chronic diseases, and lowering the incidence of muscular-skeletal injuries; also referred to as criterion-referenced standards.

Health-related fitness Fitness programs that are prescribed to improve the individual's overall health; components are cardiorespiratory endurance, muscular strength and endurance, muscular flexibility, and body composition.

Healthy Life Expectancy (HLE) Number of years a person is expected to live in good health; this number is obtained by subtracting ill-health years from overall life expectancy.

Heart rate reserve (HRR) The difference between the maximal heart rate and the resting heart rate.

Heat cramps Muscle spasms caused by heat-induced changes in electrolyte balance in muscle cells.

Heat exhaustion Heat-related fatigue.

Heat stroke Emergency situation resulting from the body being subjected to high atmospheric temperatures.

Hemoglobin Protein–iron compound in red blood cells that transports oxygen in the blood.

Herbal medicine Unconventional system that uses herbs to treat ailments and disease.

High-density lipoproteins (HDLs) Cholesterol-transporting molecules in the blood ("good" cholesterol) that help clear cholesterol from the blood.

Homeopathy System of treatment based on the use of minute quantities of remedies that in large amounts produce effects similar to the disease being treated.

Homeostasis A natural state of equilibrium; the body attempts to maintain this equilibrium by constantly reacting to external forces that attempt to disrupt this fine balance.

Homocysteine An amino acid that, when allowed to accumulate in the blood, may lead to plaque formation and blockage of arteries.

Hydrostatic weighing Underwater technique to assess body composition; considered the most accurate of the body composition assessment techniques.

Hypertension Chronically elevated blood pressure.

Hypertrophy An increase in the size of the cell, as in muscle hypertrophy.

Hypokinetic diseases "Hypo" denotes "lack of"; therefore, lack of physical activity.

Hypotension Low blood pressure.

Hypothermia A breakdown in the body's ability to generate heat; a drop in body temperature below 35° C.

I

Imagery Mental visualization of relaxing images and scenes to induce body relaxation in times of stress or as an aid in the treatment of certain medical conditions such as cancer, hypertension, asthma, chronic pain, and obesity.

Insulin A hormone secreted by the pancreas; essential for proper metabolism of blood glucose (sugar) and maintenance of blood glucose level.

Insulin resistance Inability of the cells to respond appropriately to insulin.

Intensity In cardiorespiratory exercise, how hard a person has to exercise to improve or maintain fitness.

Intensity (for flexibility exercises) Degree of stretch when doing flexibility exercises.

International unit (IU) Measure of nutrients in foods.

Interval training A training program where high intensity speed intervals are followed by short recovery intervals.

Isokinetic training Strength-training method in which the speed of the muscle contraction is kept constant because the equipment (machine) provides an accommodating resistance to match the user's force (maximal) through the range of motion.

Isometric training Strength-training method referring to a muscle contraction that produces little or no movement, such as pushing or pulling against an immovable object.

L

Lactic acid End product of anaerobic glycolysis (metabolism).

Lactovegetarians Vegetarians who eat foods from the milk group.

Lean body mass Body weight without body fat.

Life expectancy Number of years a person is expected to live based on the person's birth year.

Life Experiences Survey A questionnaire used to assess sources of stress in life.

Lipoproteins Lipids covered by proteins, they transport fats in the blood; types are LDL, HDL, and VLDL.

Locus of control A concept examining the extent to which a person believes he or she can influence the external environment.

Low-density lipoproteins (LDLs) Cholesterol-transporting molecules in the blood ("bad" cholesterol) that tend to increase blood cholesterol.

M

Magnetic therapy Unconventional (CAM) treatment that relies on magnetic energy to promote healing.

Maintenance stage Stage of change in the transtheoretical model in which people maintain behavioural change for up to 5 years.

Malignant Cancerous.

Mammogram Low-dose X-rays of the breasts used as a screening technique for the early detection of breast cancer.

Massage therapy The rubbing or kneading of body parts to treat ailments.

Maximal heart rate (MHR) Highest heart rate for a person, related primarily to age.

Maximal oxygen uptake (VO$_2$max) Maximum amount of oxygen the body is able to utilize per minute of physical activity, commonly expressed in mL/kg/min; the best indicator of cardiorespiratory or aerobic fitness.

Meditation A stress management technique used to gain control over one's attention by clearing the mind and blocking out the stressor(s) responsible for the increased tension.

Mediterranean diet Typical diet of people around the Mediterranean region that focuses on olive oil, red wine, grains, legumes, vegetables, and fruits, with limited amounts of meat, fish, milk, and cheese.

Megadoses For most vitamins, 10 times the RDA or more; for vitamins A and D, 5 and 2 times the RDA, respectively.

Melanoma The most virulent, rapidly spreading form of skin cancer.

Mental wellness A state in which one's mind is engaged in lively interaction with the surrounding world; also called intellectual wellness.

MET Represents the rate of resting energy expenditure at rest; MET is the equivalent of 3.5 mL/kg/min.

Metabolic fitness Denotes improvements in the metabolic profile through a moderate-intensity exercise program in spite of little or no improvement in physical fitness standards.

Metabolic profile A measurement to assess risk for diabetes and cardiovascular disease through plasma insulin, glucose, lipid, and lipoprotein levels.

Metabolic syndrome *See* Syndrome X.

Metabolism All energy and material transformations that occur within living cells; necessary to sustain life.

Metastasis The movement of cells from one part of the body to another.

METs Short for metabolic equivalents, an alternative method of prescribing exercise intensity in multiples of the resting metabolic rate.

Minerals Inorganic nutrients essential for normal body functions; found in the body and in food.

Mitochondria Structures within the cells where energy transformations take place.

Mode Form or type of exercise.

Moderate physical activity Activity that uses 150 calories of energy per day, or 1,000 calories per week.

Monosaccharides The simplest carbohydrates (sugars), formed by five- or six-carbon skeletons. The three most common monosaccharides are glucose, fructose, and galactose.

Morbidity A condition related to, or caused by, illness or disease.

Motivation The desire and will to do something.

Motor neurons Nerves connecting the central nervous system to the muscle.

Motor unit The combination of a motor neuron and the muscle fibres that neuron innervates.

Muscular endurance The ability of a muscle to exert submaximal force repeatedly over time.

Muscular strength The ability of a muscle to exert maximum force against resistance (for example, 1 repetition maximum [or 1 RM] of the bench press exercise).

Myocardial infarction Heart attack; damage to or death of an area of the heart muscle as a result of an obstructed artery to that area.

Myocardium Heart muscle.

N

Naturopathic medicine Unconventional system of medicine that relies exclusively on natural remedies to treat disease and ailments.

Negative resistance The lowering or eccentric phase of a repetition during a strength training exercise.

Neustress Neutral stress; stress that is neither harmful nor helpful.

Nitrosamines Potentially cancer-causing compounds formed when nitrites and nitrates, which are used to prevent the growth of harmful bacteria in processed meats, combine with other chemicals in the stomach.

Nonallopathic medicine See complementary and alternative medicine.

Nonmelanoma skin cancer Cancer that spreads or grows at the original site but does not metastasize to other regions of the body.

Nonresponders Individuals who exhibit small or no improvements in fitness as compared to others who undergo the same training program.

Nurse Health care practitioner who assists in the diagnosis and treatment of health problems and provides many services to patients in a variety of settings.

Nutrient density A measure of the amount of nutrients and calories in various foods.

Nutrients Substances found in food that provide energy, regulate metabolism, and help with growth and repair of body tissues.

Nutrition Science that studies the relationship of foods to optimal health and performance.

O

Obesity An excessive accumulation of body fat, usually at least 30 percent above recommended body weight; body mass index (BMI) 30 or higher.

Objectives Steps required to reach a goal.

Occupational wellness The ability to perform one's job skillfully and effectively under conditions that provide personal and team satisfaction and adequately reward each individual.

Oligomenorrhea Irregular menstrual cycles.

Omega-3 fatty acids Polyunsaturated fatty acids found primarily in cold-water seafood, flaxseed, and flaxseed oil; thought to lower blood cholesterol and triglycerides.

Omega-6 fatty acids Polyunsaturated fatty acids found primarily in corn and sunflower oils and most oils in processed foods.

Oncogenes Genes that initiate cell division.

One repetition maximum (1 RM) The maximum amount of resistance an individual is able to lift in a single effort.

Ophthalmologist Medical specialist concerned with diseases of the eye and prescription of corrective lenses.

Optometrist Health care practitioner who specializes in the prescription and adaptation of lenses.

Oral surgeon A dentist who specializes in surgical procedures of the oral–facial complex.

Orthodontist A dentist who specializes in the correction and prevention of teeth irregularities.

Osteopath A medical practitioner with specialized training in musculoskeletal problems who uses diagnostic and therapeutic methods of conventional medicine in addition to manipulative measures.

Osteoporosis Softening, deterioration, or loss of bone mineral density that leads to disability, bone fractures, and even death from medical complications.

Other wellness Aspects of wellness that do not fall within the other six dimensions; for some people, other wellness may include spirituality.

Overload principle Training concept that the demands placed on a system (cardiorespiratory or muscular) must be increased systematically and progressively over time to cause physiological adaptation (development or improvement).

Overtraining An emotional, behavioural, and physical condition marked by increased fatigue, decreased performance, persistent muscle soreness, mood disturbances, and feelings of "staleness" or "burnout" as a result of excessive physical training.

Overweight An excess amount of weight against a given standard, such as height or recommended percent body fat; body mass index (BMI) greater than 25 but less than 30.

Ovolactovegetarians Vegetarians who include eggs and milk products in their diet.

Ovovegetarians Vegetarians who allow eggs in their diet.

Oxygen free radicals Substances formed during metabolism that attack and damage proteins and lipids, in particular the cell membrane and DNA, leading to diseases such as heart disease, cancer, and emphysema.

Oxygen uptake (VO_2) The amount of oxygen used by the human body.

P

Percent body fat Proportional amount of fat in the body based on the person's total weight; includes both essential fat and storage fat; also termed fat mass.

Periodization A training approach that divides the season into three cycles (macrocycles, mesocycles, and microcycles) using a systematic variation in intensity and volume of training to enhance fitness and performance.

Peripheral vascular disease Narrowing of the peripheral blood vessels, excluding the cerebral and coronary arteries.

Peristalsis Involuntary muscle contractions of intestinal walls that facilitate excretion of wastes.

Personal trainer A health/fitness professional who evaluates, motivates, educates, and trains clients to help them meet individualized, healthy, lifestyle goals.

Physical activity Bodily movement produced by skeletal muscles; requires expenditure of energy and produces progressive health benefits.

Physical fitness The ability to meet the ordinary as well as the unusual demands of daily life safely and effectively without being overly fatigued and still have energy left for leisure and recreational activities.

Physical fitness standards A fitness level that allows a person to sustain moderate-to-vigorous physical activity without undue fatigue and the ability to closely maintain this level throughout life.

Physical wellness Good physical fitness and confidence in one's personal ability to take care of health problems.

Physician assistant Health care practitioner trained to treat most standard cases of care.

Physiological age The biological and functional capacity of the body as it should be in relation to the person's maximal potential at any given age in the lifespan.

Phytochemicals Chemical compounds thought to prevent and fight cancer; found in large quantities in fruits and vegetables.

Pilates A training program that uses exercises designed to help strengthen the body's core by developing pelvic stability and abdominal control; exercises are coupled with focused breathing patterns.

Plastic elongation Permanent lengthening of soft tissue.

Plyometric exercise Explosive jump training, incorporating speed and strength training to enhance explosiveness.

Positive resistance The lifting, pushing, or concentric phase of a repetition during a strength-training exercise.

Power The ability to produce maximum force in the shortest time.

Prayer Sincere and humble communication with a higher power.

Precontemplation stage Stage of change in the transtheoretical model in which people are unwilling to change behaviour.

Preparation stage Stage of change in the transtheoretical model in which people are getting ready to make a change within the next month.

Primary care physician A medical practitioner who provides routine treatment of ailments; typically, the patient's first contact for health care.

Principle of individuality Training concept that states that genetics plays a major role in individual responses to exercise training and these differences must be considered when designing exercise programs for different people.

Processes of change Actions that help you achieve change in behaviour.

Progressive muscle relaxation A stress management technique that involves progressive contraction and relaxation of muscle groups throughout the body.

Progressive resistance training A gradual increase of resistance over a period of time.

Proprioceptive neuromuscular facilitation (PNF) Mode of stretching that uses reflexes and neuromuscular principles to relax the muscles that are being stretched.

Proteins A classification of nutrients consisting of complex organic compounds containing nitrogen and formed by combinations of amino acids; the main substances used in the body to build and repair tissues.

Pro-vitamin A compound that can be converted into a vitamin.

Q

Quackery/fraud The conscious promotion of unproven claims for profit.

R

Range of motion Entire arc of movement of a given joint.

Rate of perceived exertion (RPE) A perception scale to monitor or interpret the intensity of aerobic exercise.

Reaction time The time required to initiate a response to a given stimulus.

Recommended body weight Body weight at which there seems to be no harm to human health; healthy weight.

Recommended Dietary Allowances (RDA) The daily amount of a nutrient (statistically determined from the EARs) considered adequate to meet the known nutrient needs of almost 98 percent of all healthy people.

Recovery time Amount of time the body takes to return to resting levels after exercise.

Registered dietician (RD) A person with a college degree in dietetics who meets all certification and continuing education requirements of the American Dietetic Association or Dieticians of Canada.

Relapse (v.) To slip or fall back into unhealthy behaviour(s); or (n.) failure to maintain healthy behaviours.

Repetitions Number of times a given resistance is performed.

Resistance Amount of weight that is lifted.

Responders Individuals who exhibit improvements in fitness as a result of exercise training.

Resting heart rate (RHR) Heart rate after a person has been sitting quietly for 15–20 minutes.

Resting metabolic rate (RMR) The energy requirement to maintain the body's vital processes in the resting state.

Resting metabolism Amount of energy (expressed in millilitres of oxygen per minute or total calories per day) an individual requires during resting conditions to sustain proper body function.

Reverse cholesterol transport A process in which HDL molecules attract cholesterol and carry it to the liver, where it is changed to bile and eventually excreted in the stool.

Ribonucleic acid (RNA) Genetic material that guides the formation of cell proteins.

RICE An acronym used to describe the standard treatment procedure for acute sports injuries: Rest, Ice (cold application), Compression, and Elevation.

Risk factors Lifestyle and genetic variables that may lead to disease.

S

Sarcopenia Age-related loss of lean body mass, strength, and function.

Sedentary A lifestyle characterized by relative inactivity and a lot of sitting.

Sedentary Death Syndrome (SeDS) A term used to describe deaths that are attributed to a lack of regular physical activity.

Semivegetarians Vegetarians who include milk products, eggs, and fish and poultry in the diet.

Set A fixed number of repetitions; one set of bench presses might be 10 repetitions.

Setpoint Weight control theory that the body has an established weight and strongly attempts to maintain that weight.

Shin splints Injury to the lower leg characterized by pain and irritation in the shin region of the leg.

Side stitch A sharp pain in the side of the abdomen.

Simple carbohydrates Formed by simple or double sugar units with little nutritive value; divided into monosaccharides and disaccharides.

Skill-related fitness Fitness components important for success in activities and athletic events requiring high skill levels; encompasses agility, balance, coordination, power, reaction time, and speed.

Skinfold thickness Technique to assess body composition by measuring a double thickness of skin at specific body sites.

Slow-sustained stretching Exercises in which the muscles are lengthened gradually through a joint's complete range of motion.

Slow-twitch fibres Muscle fibres with greater aerobic potential and slow speed of contraction.

SMART An acronym used in reference to *S*pecific, *M*easurable, *A*ttainable, *R*ealistic, and *T*ime-specific goals.

Social wellness The ability to relate well to others, both within and outside the family unit.

Specific adaptation to imposed demand (SAID) training Training principle stating that, for improvements to occur in a specific activity, the exercises performed during a strength-training program should resemble as closely as possible the movement patterns encountered in that particular activity.

Specificity of training Principle that training must be done with the specific muscle the person is attempting to improve.

Speed The ability to propel the body or a part of the body rapidly from one point to another.

Sphygmomanometer Inflatable bladder contained within a cuff and a mercury gravity manometer (or aneroid manometer) from which the pressure is read.

Spot reducing Fallacious theory that exercising a specific body part will result in significant fat reduction in that area.

Sterols Derived fats, of which cholesterol is the best-known example.

Storage fat Body fat in excess of essential fat; stored in adipose tissue.

Strength training A program designed to improve muscular strength and/or endurance through a series of resistance (weight) training exercises that overload the muscular system and cause physiological development.

Stress The mental, emotional, and physiological response of the body to any situation that is new, threatening, frightening, or exciting.

Stress electrocardiogram An exercise test during which the workload is gradually increased until the individual reaches maximal fatigue, with blood pressure and 12-lead electrocardiographic monitoring throughout the test.

Stressor Stress-causing event.

Stretching Moving the joints beyond the accustomed range of motion.

Stroke volume Amount of blood pumped by the heart in one beat.

Structured interview Assessment tool used to determine behavioural patterns that define Type A and B personalities.

Subluxation Partial dislocation of a joint.

Substrates Substances acted upon by an enzyme (examples: carbohydrates, fats).

Sun protection factor (SPF) Degree of protection offered by ingredients in sunscreen lotion; at least SPF 15 is recommended.

Supplements Tablets, pills, capsules, liquids, or powders that contain vitamins, minerals, amino acids, herbs, or fibre that are taken to increase the intake of these nutrients.

Suppressor genes Genes that deactivate the process of cell division.

Syndrome X (metabolic syndrome) An array of metabolic abnormalities that contribute to the development of atherosclerosis triggered by insulin resistance. These conditions include low HDL-cholesterol, high triglycerides, high blood pressure, and an increased blood clotting mechanism.

Synergy A reaction in which the result is greater than the sum of its two parts.

Systolic blood pressure Pressure exerted by blood against walls of arteries during forceful contraction (systole) of the heart; higher of the two numbers in blood pressure readings.

T

Techniques of change Methods or procedures used during each process of change.

Telomerase An enzyme that allows cells to reproduce indefinitely.

Telomeres A strand of molecules at both ends of a chromosome.

Termination/adoption stage Stage of change in the transtheoretical model in which people have eliminated an undesirable behaviour or maintained a positive behaviour for more than 5 years.

Thermogenic response Amount of energy required to digest food.

Transfatty acid Solidified fat formed by adding hydrogen to monounsaturated and polyunsaturated fats to increase shelf life.

Triglycerides Fats formed by glycerol and three fatty acids; also called free fatty acids.

Type 1 diabetes Insulin-dependent diabetes mellitus (IDDM), a condition in which the pancreas produces little or no insulin; also known as juvenile diabetes.

Type 2 diabetes Non-insulin-dependent diabetes mellitus (NIDDM), a condition in which insulin is not processed properly; also known as adult-onset diabetes.

Type A Behaviour pattern characteristic of a hard-driving, overambitious, aggressive, at times hostile, and overly competitive person.

Type B Behaviour pattern characteristic of a calm, casual, relaxed, and easy-going individual.

Type C Behaviour pattern of individuals who are just as highly stressed as the Type A but do not seem to be at higher risk for disease than the Type B.

U

Ultraviolet B (UVB) rays Portion of sunlight that causes sunburn and encourages skin cancers.

Unconventional medicine See complementary and alternative medicine.

Underweight Extremely low body weight.

Upper Intake Level (UL) The highest level of nutrient intake that appears safe for most healthy people, beyond which exists an increased risk of adverse effects.

V

Variable resistance Training using special machines equipped with mechanical devices that provide differing amounts of resistance through the range of motion.

Vegans Vegetarians who eat no animal products at all.

Vegetarians Individuals whose diet is of vegetable or plant origin.

Very low-calorie diet A diet that only allows an energy intake (consumption) of 800 or less calories per day.

Very low-density lipoproteins (VLDLs) Triglyceride, cholesterol, and phospholipid-transporting molecules in the blood that tend to increase blood cholesterol.

Vigorous activity Any exercise that requires a MET level equal to or greater than 6 METs (21 mL/kg/min); 1 MET is the energy expenditure at rest, 3.5 mL/kg/min, whereas METs are defined as multiples of the resting metabolic rate (examples of activities that require a 6-MET level are aerobics, walking uphill at 5.6 km/h, cycling at 16 to 19.3 km/h, playing doubles in tennis, and vigorous strength training).

Vigorous exercise Cardiorespiratory exercise that requires an intensity level above 60 percent of maximal capacity.

Vitamins Organic nutrients essential for normal metabolism, growth, and development of the body.

Volume (in strength training) The sum of all the repetitions performed multiplied by the resistances used during a strength-training session.

Volume (of training) The total amount of training performed in a given work period (day, week, month, or season).

W

Waist-to-hip ratio (WHR) A measurement to assess potential risk for disease based on distribution of body fat.

Warm-up Starting a workout slowly.

Water The most important classification of essential body nutrients, involved in almost every vital body process.

Weight-regulating mechanism (WRM) A feature of the hypothalamus of the brain that controls how much the body should weigh.

Wellness The constant and deliberate effort to stay healthy and achieve the highest potential for well-being. It encompasses seven dimensions—physical, emotional, mental, social, environmental, occupational, and spiritual—and integrates them all into a quality life.

Workload Load (or intensity) placed on the body during physical activity.

Y

Yoga A school of thought in the Hindu religion that seeks to help the individual attain a higher level of spirituality and peace of mind.

Yo-yo dieting Constantly losing and gaining weight.

answer key

1	2	3	4	5	6	7	8	9	10	11	12	13
1. a	1. a	1. b	1. e	1. b	1. a	1. c	1. b	1. d	1. a	1. e	1. b	1. e
2. e	2. a	2. e	2. b	2. c	2. d	2. d	2. e	2. a	2. c	2. b	2. a	2. c
3. c	3. e	3. c	3. d	3. e	3. c	3. a	3. a	3. b	3. c	3. a	3. a	3. b
4. e	4. d	4. d	4. a	4. a	4. c	4. b	4. a	4. e	4. e	4. e	4. e	4. d
5. b	5. c	5. d	5. b	5. b	5. c	5. d	5. b	5. d	5. e	5. e	5. e	5. e
6. c	6. d	6. a	6. e	6. e	6. e	6. a	6. e	6. b	6. e	6. e	6. e	6. a
7. a	7. a	7. a	7. b	7. a	7. c	7. c	7. c	7. a	7. a	7. e	7. b	7. e
8. d	8. b	8. c	8. b	8. c	8. d	8. c	8. b	8. e	8. a	8. e	8. e	8. c
9. c	9. e	9. a	9. e	9. d	9. c	9. e	9. e	9. a	9. b	9. e	9. b	9. e
10. b	10. e	10. e	10. e	10. c	10. c	10. e	10. d	10. e	10. c	10. a	10. e	10. a

index

Note: *Italicized pages refer to illustrations and tables.*

multivitamins, 76
    health benefits of, 76
muscle building and nutrition, 81
muscle cramps, 282
muscle fibres, 137, 205
    types of, 206
muscle hypertrophy, 198
muscle soreness and stiffness, 281
muscular endurance, 200–202, *204*
muscular endurance test, 202–205
muscular flexibility, *11*, 291
Muscular Flexibility Assessment, 261–262 (Lab 8A)
muscular flexibility programs, 247–248
muscular hypertrophy, 210
muscular strength
    assessment of, 200–202
    definition of, 201
muscular strength and endurance, *11*, 288
Muscular Strength and Endurance Assessment, 235
        (Lab 7A)
muscular strength and endurance periodization
        program, 291
muscular strength and endurance scoring, 206
muscular strength and endurance test, 204–205
muscular system, *218*
myocardial infarction, 337–339

NAS, 62
NAS guidelines, 2002, 60, 61
National Academy of Sciences (NAS), 62
National Cancer Institute, 366
National Centre for Complementary and Alternative
        Medicine Health Information (NCCAM),
        The, 394
National Center for Health Statistics, 392
National Institute of Medicine, 177
National Strength and Conditioning Association
        (NSCA), 397
National Weight Control Registry, 141
natural breathing, complete, 314
naturopathic medicine
Nautilus machine, 209
Neavill, Patty, 400–401
negative resistance, 208
negative resistance excercises, 209
neural stimulation, 208
neustress, 305
New England Journal of Medicine, 127, 336
nitrosamines, 369
nonessential amino acids, 58
"non-insulin-dependent" diabetes, risk factors for, 108
nonmelanoma skin cancer, 366, 367
nonresponders, 163
normal heart rate, 164
nurse, 393
nutrient analysis, 64–66
nutrient density, 53
nutrient supplementation, 72–77
    for women, 72–73
nutrient value of foods, 409–456
nutrients, 52, 53–55
    Adequate Intakes (AI), *64*

carbohydrates, 53–56
Dietary Reference Intakes (DRIs), *64*
fuel nutrients, 53
in human body, *61*
Recommended Dietary Allowance (RDA), *64*
Tolerable Upper Intake Levels (UL) (for) adults, *64*
for women, 82–85
nutrition, 52
Nutrition Facts table, 65
Nutrition Facts table (Canadian), 67
nutritional recommendation (Canada), 52
nutritional standards, 62–64
nuts, 70

obesity, 94, *122*, *123*
    definition of, 123
    statistics on, 122
obesity and gender, statistics on, 122
obesity health care, cost of, 5, 122
obesity levels, 122
obesity rates, *111*
objectives, definition of, 43
occupational wellness, 8
    definition of, 9
Okinawan diet (Japan), 71
oligomenorrhea, 84, 85
omega-3 fats, 368
omega-3 fatty acids, 57
omega-6 fatty acids, 57
oncogenes, 364, 365
1 RM, 201
one repetition maximum (1 RM), 201
ophthalmologist, 393
optometrist, 393
oral cancer, 380
oral surgeon, 393
orthodontist, 393
osteopath, 393
osteoporosis, 82–84, *83*
    exercise in prevention of, 84
ovarian cancer, 380–381
overload principle, 206–207
overtraining, prevention of, 212, 213, 286, 287
    signs of, 286
overweight, 94, 95
overweight vs. obesity, 122–124
ovolactovegetarians, 69
ovovegetarians, 69
oxygen free radicals, 73
oxygen uptake (VO$_2$), 161, 164

pancreatic cancer, 379
pedometer, *180*
peer support, 39
Pelvic Clock exercise, 260
Pelvic Tilt, 225
Pelvic Tilt exercise, 260
periodization, 212, 213, 286–287
periodization program for strength, *287*
peripheral vascular disease, 334, 335
peristalsis, definition of, 55
personal trainers, 398–399

Calories Spent During Various Activities

To calculate the exercise calories you expend per hour, find your exercise in the left column and your weight in the right column. In the place where these parameters intersect is the figure indicating the calories burned per hour. For example, if you aerobic dance for 1 hour and weigh 50 kg, you will expend 250 calories.

WEIGHT (IN KILOGRAMS):	50	60	70	80	90
Exercise	CALORIES	EXPENDED	PER	HOUR	
Aerobic dancing	250	301	350	395	450
Basketball	415	497	581	660	750
Bowling	180	217	252	285	325
Calisthenics (vigorous)	225	270	313	360	410
Cross-country skiing					
moderately hilly	595	714	833	945	1080
indoor machine (17.5 km/hr)	330	397	463	525	600
Cycling					
outdoor (9 km/hr)	195	232	268	305	350
outdoor (15 km/hr)	300	360	422	475	545
outdoor racing (30.5 km/hr)	505	609	710	805	920
Schwinn Aerodyne	510	614	715	810	925
stationary (moderate tension)	330	397	463	525	600
Golf					
with cart (90-120 minutes)	145	175	206	230	265
no cart (90-120 minutes)	185	222	262	295	340
Hiking 6.5 km/hr, 9 kg pack	355	429	504	570	650
Ice skating	275	315	360	390	425
Racquetball	550	661	772	875	1000
Roller skating/blading	275	318	360	390	425
Rope skipping (100 skips/minute)	560	677	787	895	1020
Rowing (sculling or machine)	620	746	869	990	1130
Running (jogging)					
3.5 minutes/km (16 km/hr)	755	910	1060	1200	1375
4 minutes/km (13.5 km/hr)	685	825	962	1090	1245
5 minutes/km (12 km/hr)	625	751	875	990	1135
5.5 minutes/km (10.5 km/hr)	580	698	813	920	1050
6 minutes/km (9.5 km/hr)	535	640	751	850	970
7 minutes/km (8.5 km/hr)	470	560	658	745	850
7.5 minutes/km (8 km/hr)	375	450	525	600	680
Snow skiing—downhill	300	360	422	480	545
Softball	225	270	314	360	410
Stair climbing (moderate)	515	635	772	850	960
Step aerobics (120 steps/minute)	550	661	772	875	1000
Swimming					
28 minutes/km	385	460	540	610	700
37 minutes/km	300	355	417	475	540
Tennis					
doubles	225	270	314	360	410
singles	325	392	458	520	600
Treadmill					
7.5 minutes/km	375	450	525	600	680
8 minutes/km	330	397	463	525	600
Volleyball					
competitive	435	524	612	700	800
recreational	165	196	232	260	300
Walking/race walking					
7.5 minutes/km (8 km/hr)	435	524	612	700	800
Walking/jogging combination					
8.5 minutes/km (4.5 km/hr)	330	394	463	525	600
Walking					
9.5 minutes/km (6.5 km/hr) 10.5	300	366	427	480	550
minutes/km (5.5 km/hr)	250	302	355	400	450
12.5 minutes/km (5 km/hr)	225	270	319	360	410
18.5 minutes/km (3 km/hr)	145	175	206	230	265
Weight training/lifting (light)	270	328	381	430	500

Source: G. Kostas, MPH, RD, The Balancing Act Nutrition and Weight Guide, Dallas, TX, 1993.